Handbook of Dermatology

Handbook of Dermatology

Editor: Nicolas Webb

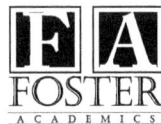

FA
FOSTER
ACADEMICS

www.fosteracademics.com

www.fosteracademics.com

F A
FOSTER
ACADEMICS

Cataloging-in-Publication Data

Handbook of dermatology / edited by Nicolas Webb.
    p. cm.
Includes bibliographical references and index.
ISBN 978-1-63242-623-9
1. Dermatology. 2. Skin--Diseases. I. Webb, Nicolas.
RL72 .H36 2019
616.5--dc23

Foster Academics,
118-35 Queens Blvd., Suite 400,
Forest Hills, NY 11375, USA

ISBN 978-1-63242-623-9 (Hardback)

Contents

Preface   IX

Chapter 1

Budget impact analysis of ustekinumab in the management of moderate to severe psoriasis in Greece   1
Georgia Avgerinou, Ioannis Bassukas, Georgios Chaidemenos, Andreas Katsampas, Marita Kosmadaki, Hara Kousoulakou, Athanasios Petridis, Brad Schenkel, Dimitrios Sotiriadis, Theofanis Spiliopoulos, Panagiotis Stavropoulos, Evgenia Toumpi and Loukas Xaplanteris

Chapter 2

Innate lymphoid cells and the skin   10
Maryam Salimi and Graham Ogg

Chapter 3

Longitudinal, mixed method study to look at the experiences and knowledge of non melanoma skin cancer from diagnosis to one year   18
Fiona Bath-Hextall, Claire Jenkinson, Arun Kumar, Jo Leonardi-Bee, William Perkins, Karen Cox and Cris Glazebrook

Chapter 4

miR-125b induces cellular senescence in malignant melanoma   28
Anne Marie Nyholm, Catharina M Lerche, Valentina Manfé, Edyta Biskup, Peter Johansen, Niels Morling, Birthe Mørk Thomsen, Martin Glud and Robert Gniadecki

Chapter 5

Survey and online discussion groups to develop a patient-rated outcome measure on acceptability of treatment response in vitiligo   39
Selina K Tour, Kim S Thomas, Dawn-Marie Walker, Paul Leighton, Adrian SW Yong and Jonathan M Batchelor

Chapter 6

What determines patient preferences for treating low risk basal cell carcinoma when comparing surgery vs imiquimod? A discrete choice experiment survey from the SINS trial   51
Michela Tinelli, Mara Ozolins, Fiona Bath-Hextall and Hywel C Williams

Chapter 7

Effects of tofacitinib on lymphocyte sub-populations, CMV and EBV viral load in patients with plaque psoriasis   62
Fernando Valenzuela, Kim A Papp, David Pariser, Stephen K Tyring, Robert Wolk, Marjorie Buonanno, Jeff Wang, Huaming Tan and Hernan Valdez

Chapter 8

HLA class II alleles may influence susceptibility to adult dermatomyositis and polymyositis in a Han Chinese population   73
Xiang Gao, Lei Han, Lan Yuan, Yongchen Yang, Guimei Gou, Hengjuan Sun, Ling Lu and Liming Bao

Chapter 9

Subjective stress reactivity in psoriasis – a cross sectional study of associated psychological traits   80
Charlotta Remröd, Karin Sjöström and Åke Svensson

Chapter 10

Prevalence, incidence and predictive factors for hand eczema in young adults   88
Arne Johannisson, Ann Pontén and Åke Svensson

Chapter 11

High glycemic load diet, milk and ice cream consumption are related to acne vulgaris in Malaysian young adults   99
Noor Hasnani Ismail, Zahara Abdul Manaf and Noor Zalmy Azizan

Chapter 12

Topical treatment with fresh human milk versus emollient on atopic eczema spots in young children: a small, randomized, split body, controlled, blinded pilot study   107
Teresa Løvold Berents, Jørgen Rønnevig, Elisabeth Søyland, Peter Gaustad, Gro Nylander and Beate Fossum Løland

Chapter 13

Comparison of publication trends in dermatology among Japan, South Korea and Mainland China   114
Huibin Man, Shujun Xin, Weiping Bi, Chengzhi Lv, Theodora M Mauro, Peter M Elias and Mao-Qiang Man

Chapter 14

Single application of 4% dimeticone liquid gel versus two applications of 1% permethrin crème rinse for treatment of head louse infestation   120
Ian F Burgess, Elizabeth R Brunton and Nazma A Burgess

Chapter 15

Association of variation in the LAMA3 gene, encoding the alpha-chain of laminin 5, with atopic dermatitis in a German case   127
Susanne Stemmler, Qumar Parwez, Elisabeth Petrasch-Parwez, Joerg T Epplen and Sabine Hoffjan

Chapter 16

Treatment and referral patterns for psoriasis in United Kingdom primary care   133
Javaria Mona Khalid, Gary Globe, Kathleen M Fox, Dina Chau, Andrew Maguire and Chio-Fang Chiou

Chapter 17

Topical application of RTA 408 lotion activates Nrf2 in human skin and is welltolerated by healthy human volunteers   140
Scott A. Reisman, Angela R. Goldsberry, Chun-Yue I. Lee, Megan L. O'Grady, Joel W. Proksch, Keith W. Ward and Colin J. Meyer

Chapter 18

Prevalence of head lice infestation and pediculicidal effect of permethrine shampoo in primary school girls in a low-income area in southeast of Iran   151
Moussa Soleimani-Ahmadi, Seyed Aghil Jaberhashemi, Mehdi Zare and Alireza Sanei-Dehkordi

Chapter 19

Enzymatic debridement for the treatment of severely burned upper extremities – early single center experiences   157
Tomke Cordts, Johannes Horter, Julian Vogelpohl, Thomas Kremer, Ulrich Kneser and Jochen-Frederick Hernekamp

Chapter 20

Risk factors of keloids in Syrians   164
Abeer Shaheen, Jamal Khaddam and Fadi Kesh

Chapter 21

Skin cancer knowledge and attitudes in the region of Fez, Morocco   175
Awatef kelati, Hanane Baybay, Mariam Atassi, Samira Elfakir, Salim Gallouj, Mariame Meziane and Fatima Zahra Mernissi

Chapter 22

Magnitude and associated factors of Atopic dermatitis among children in Ayder referral hospital, Mekelle, Ethiopia   182
Abraham Getachew Kelbore, Workalemahu Alemu, Ashenafi Shumye and Sefonias Getachew

Chapter 23

Expert Consensus on The Management of Dermatophytosis in India (ECTODERM India)   192
Murlidhar Rajagopalan, Arun Inamadar, Asit Mittal, Autar K. Miskeen, C. R. Srinivas, Kabir Sardana, Kiran Godse, Krina Patel, Madhu Rengasamy, Shivaprakash Rudramurthy and Sunil Dogra

Chapter 24

Treatment of plaque psoriasis with an ointment formulation of the Janus kinase inhibitor, tofacitinib: a Phase 2b randomized clinical trial   203
Kim A. Papp, Robert Bissonnette, Melinda Gooderham, Steven R. Feldman, Lars Iversen, Jennifer Soung, Zoe Draelos, Carla Mamolo, Vivek Purohit, Cunshan Wang and William C. Ports

Chapter 25

**Persistence rates and medical costs of biological therapies for psoriasis
treatment in Japan: a real-world data study using a claims database**   215
Rosarin Sruamsiri, Kosuke Iwasaki, Wentao Tang and Jörg Mahlich

Chapter 26

**A multicenter, randomized, open-label pilot trial assessing the efficacy and safety of
etanercept 50 mg twice weekly followed by etanercept 25 mg twice weekly,
the combination of etanercept 25 mg twice weekly and acitretin, and acitretin
alone in patients with moderate to severe psoriasis**   226
*Joo-Heung Lee, Jai-Il Youn, Tae-Yoon Kim, Jee-Ho Choi, Chul-Jong Park, Yong-Beom Choe,
Hae-Jun Song, Nack-In Kim, Kwang-Joong Kim, Jeung-Hoon Lee and Hyun-Jeong Yoo*

Chapter 27

Features of human scabies in resourcelimited settings: the Cameroon case   235
*Emmanuel Armand Kouotou, Jobert Richie N Nansseu, Isidore Sieleunou, Defo Defo,
Anne-Cécile Zoung-Kanyi Bissek and Elie Claude Ndjitoyap Ndam*

Chapter 28

**Cost and effectiveness of prescribing emollient therapy for atopic eczema in UK
primary care in children and adults: a large retrospective analysis of the Clinical
Practice Research Datalink**   241
*George Moncrieff, Annie Lied-Lied, Gill Nelson, Chantal E Holy, Rachel Weinstein,
David Wei and Simon Rowe*

Chapter 29

**Randomized placebo control study of insulin sensitizers (Metformin and Pioglitazone)
in psoriasis patients with metabolic syndrome (Topical Treatment Cohort)**   252
Surjit Singh and Anil Bhansali

Chapter 30

**Adherence to drug treatments and adjuvant barrier repair therapies are key
factors for clinical improvement in mild to moderate acne: the ACTUO
observational prospective multicenter cohort trial in 643 patients**   263
*Raúl de Lucas, Gerardo Moreno-Arias, Montserrat Perez-López, Ángel Vera-Casaño,
Sonia Aladren and Massimo Milani*

Chapter 31

Variation of mutant allele frequency in NRAS Q61 mutated melanomas   269
*Zofia Hélias-Rodzewicz, Elisa Funck-Brentano, Nathalie Terrones, Alain Beauchet,
Ute Zimmermann, Cristi Marin, Philippe Saiag and Jean-François Emile*

Permissions

Contributors

Index

Preface

I am honored to present to you this unique book which encompasses the most up-to-date data in the field. I was extremely pleased to get this opportunity of editing the work of experts from across the globe. I have also written papers in this field and researched the various aspects revolving around the progress of the discipline. I have tried to unify my knowledge along with that of stalwarts from every corner of the world, to produce a text which not only benefits the readers but also facilitates the growth of the field.

Diseases of the skin, hair and nails are clinically treated under the domain of dermatology. Dermatologic drugs can be categorized under antifungals, antipruritics, antiseptics and disinfectants, antipsoriatics, antibiotics and chemotherapeutics, hair loss medications, etc. Some dermatologic procedures are dermabrasion, facial rejuvenation, hydradermabrasion, ultraviolet light therapy, tattoo removal, etc. Most of these procedures fall under the domains of dermatologic surgery and cryotherapy. Dermatologic surgery includes cryosurgery, electrosurgery, photorejuvenation, electrodesiccation and curettage, etc. Cryotherapy refers to the use of low temperatures in medical therapy to destroy diseased or abnormal tissue, for the treatment of tissue lesions. Extreme cold is also used in cryosurgery for the treatment of warts, skin tags, moles and solar keratoses. This book is a valuable compilation of topics, ranging from the basic to the most recent advancements in the field of dermatology. It presents this complex subject in the most comprehensible and easy to understand language. For someone with an interest and eye for detail, this book covers the most significant aspects of dermatology.

Finally, I would like to thank all the contributing authors for their valuable time and contributions. This book would not have been possible without their efforts. I would also like to thank my friends and family for their constant support.

Editor

Budget impact analysis of ustekinumab in the management of moderate to severe psoriasis in Greece

Georgia Avgerinou[3†], Ioannis Bassukas[1†], Georgios Chaidemenos[2†], Andreas Katsampas[3†], Marita Kosmadaki[3†], Hara Kousoulakou[8*], Athanasios Petridis[1†], Brad Schenkel[9], Dimitrios Sotiriadis[4†], Theofanis Spiliopoulos[5†], Panagiotis Stavropoulos[3†], Evgenia Toumpi[6†] and Loukas Xaplanteris[7]

Abstract

Background: The purpose of this study was to estimate the annual and per-patient budget impact of the treatment of moderate to severe psoriasis in Greece before and after the introduction of ustekinumab.

Methods: A budget impact model was constructed from a national health system perspective to depict the clinical and economic aspects of psoriasis treatment over 5 years. The model included drug acquisition, monitoring, and administration costs for both the induction and maintenance years for patients in a treatment mix with etanercept, adalimumab, infliximab, with or without ustekinumab. It also considered the resource utilization for non-responders. Greek treatment patterns and resource utilization data were derived from 110 interviews with dermatologists conducted in February 2009 and evaluated by an expert panel of 18 key opinion leaders. Officially published sources were used to derive the unit costs. Costs of adverse events and indirect costs were excluded from the analysis. Treatment response was defined as the probability of achieving a PASI 50, PASI 75, or PASI 90 response, based on published clinical trial data.

Results: The inclusion of ustekinumab in the biological treatment mix for moderate to severe psoriasis is predicted to lead to total per-patient savings of €443 and €900 in years 1 and 5 of its introduction, respectively. The cost savings were attributed to reduced administration costs, reduced hospitalizations for non-responders, and improved efficacy. These results were mainly driven by the low number of administrations required with ustekinumab over a 5 year treatment period (22 for ustekinumab, compared with 272 for etanercept, 131 for adalimumab, and 36 for infliximab).

Conclusions: The inclusion of ustekinumab in the treatment of moderate to severe psoriasis in Greece is anticipated to have short- and long-term health and economic benefits, both on an annual and per-patient basis.

Background

Psoriasis is a chronic, currently incurable, inflammatory skin disease. It is characterized by relapses and remissions, and is affected by several genetic and environmental factors [1]. Estimates of the worldwide prevalence of psoriasis range from 0.5% to 4.6% [2], with males and females being equally affected [1]. In Greece, the relative prevalence of psoriasis is 2.8% based on an 8-year prevalence study in an outpatient setting of a general state hospital dermatological teaching clinic [3]. Ethnic variations have been identified and Caucasians are more likely to suffer from the disease. The median age of onset is 28 years [2].

The most common type of psoriasis, occurring in more than 80% of cases, is plaque psoriasis or psoriasis vulgaris, characterized by well-demarcated erythematous scaly plaques [4]. Thirty-five percent of those with plaque psoriasis suffer from moderate to severe disease [5], which is usually defined as psoriasis affecting at least 10% of body surface area or a Psoriasis Area and Severity Index (PASI) score of 10 or more [1].

The chronic and incurable nature of plaque psoriasis indicates that it has a major social and economic impact

* Correspondence: hkousoulakou@prmaconsulting.com
[†]Equal contributors
[8]PRMA Consulting Ltd, Hampshire, UK
Full list of author information is available at the end of the article

on the community [6]. The psychological impact of psoriasis can be profound. The extent to which psoriasis affects a person's health-related quality of life (HRQoL) is similar to that of other chronic diseases, such as arthritis, chronic lung disease, and type 2 diabetes [7]. Those with more severe psoriasis experience similar levels of anxiety to patients with conditions such as breast cancer, osteoporosis, or metastatic prostate cancer [8,9]. In a US study of 265 adults with psoriasis, 32% screened positive for depression and there was a graded relationship between depressive symptoms and HRQoL impairment ($P < 0.001$). More than 16% of those with high depression scores were treated with antidepressant medication. Both dissatisfaction with psoriasis treatment and illness-related stress were highly associated with depression [10]. Many people with psoriasis report moderate to severe feelings of stigmatization, anxiety, anger, and depression [11]. Increasing severity of psoriasis is closely correlated with suicidal ideation [12,13].

The annual, per-patient direct cost of psoriasis has been reported to be more than $14,600 in the US [14], £3,800 in the UK [15], and more than €5,000 in Italy [16]. The economic burden of psoriasis has not yet been evaluated in Greece.

One of the goals of psoriasis therapy is to reduce or clear plaques and induce remission [17]. The ideal therapy is an efficacious, long-lasting agent that is devoid of acute or long-term adverse effects, with minimal monitoring requirements and a dosing regimen that facilitates adherence [17]. These characteristics may help to reduce treatment costs while maintaining improvements in patients' HRQoL [18,19].

Currently available systemic treatments for moderate to severe psoriasis include conventional drug therapies (cyclosporine, methotrexate, retinoids, and phototherapy) and biologics. The former have demonstrated varying degrees of efficacy, and long-term use can lead to serious side-effects [17]. In addition, systemic therapies lack durable efficacy (the symptoms of psoriasis recur shortly after withdrawal of conventional therapies) and have inconvenient administration schedules (e.g., daily dosing, multiple weekly exposures) [17].

On the other hand, the available biologic agents (infliximab, etanercept, adalimumab, and ustekinumab) provide specific, targeted regulation of the cells in the immune system and pathophysiologically designed intervention in the immunological disease cascade of psoriasis. They thus offer a treatment choice for patients who have moderate to severe disease where "conventional" systemic treatments have failed, are contraindicated, or not tolerated [20].

The primary safety concern with biologic agents is immunosuppression. Biologic agents are associated with increased risk of infection, serious infection and possibly malignancies [21]. The safety of biologic agents compared with conventional therapies for the treatment of psoriasis has not yet been precisely defined [22].

Ustekinumab is the most recent biologic agent to come to market. It was approved in Europe in January 2009 and has been shown to be well tolerated, to improve moderate to severe psoriasis, and to have a favorable administration and monitoring schedule (one subcutaneous injection every 12 weeks during the maintenance period) [23,24]. Moreover, in the Phase 3 randomized clinical trials, the PASI 75 results achieved with ustekinumab were sustained through at least 52 weeks [25,26].

The objective of this study was to estimate the annual and per-patient budget impact of the introduction of ustekinumab as a treatment alternative for patients with moderate to severe psoriasis in Greece, and to test the hypothesis that a treatment with improved risk–benefit and administration profiles compared with existing treatments can lead to cost savings.

Methods

An economic model that estimated the annual and per-patient budget impact of ustekinumab was built in Excel 2007. The budget impact model estimated the impact of introducing ustekinumab into the treatment mix of biologic agents available for the treatment of moderate to severe plaque psoriasis in Greece, by comparing the costs incurred by the national health system before and after the introduction of ustekinumab.

All available biologic agents for the treatment of moderate to severe psoriasis in Greece, namely ustekinumab, etanercept, infliximab, and adalimumab, were included in the model as treatment options. Efalizumab was excluded from the analysis as its European marketing authorization was suspended in February 2009.

Model structure

The economic analysis was performed from a national health system perspective. The model time frame was 5 years (base year 2009), during which the prevalence of psoriasis was assumed to be constant. The treatment response to biologic therapies was measured in terms of the probability of achieving a PASI 75 response, and the annual costs and resource utilization of both responders and non-responders to biologic treatment were considered in the model.

Model inputs

Clinical data

Data on the clinical efficacy of biologic agents were taken from the meta-analysis conducted by Reich and colleagues [27]. This systematic literature review included all randomized controlled trials (until October 2008) that evaluated the efficacy of approved biologics for the treatment of moderate to severe psoriasis. A total of 20 studies enrolling 10,108 patients with psoriasis were included in the meta-analysis, including three Phase 3 trials of ustekinumab (PHOENIX 1, PHOENIX 2, and ACCEPT trials [25,26,28]). The estimated mean PASI 75 response rates per product are presented in Table 1.

Resource utilization data

Data on medical resource use were collected through face-to-face interviews with dermatologists, the results of which were validated by an expert panel of 18 dermatologists.

The interviews were undertaken during January–March 2009 and included two stages. The first stage involved 5 minutes of computer-assisted telephone interviews (CATI), which aimed to identify dermatologists who were eligible for the second stage of the survey. CATI participants were randomly selected through a database including contact details for all registered members of the Hellenic Society of Dermatology and Venereology, which is publicly available on the official website of the society (http://www.edae.gr/). Randomization was based on market research techniques and resulted in a total of 200 dermatologists, who were both office and hospital based, and were from Athens, Thessaloniki (Salonica), and other urban centers.

Following CATI, a sample of 110 dermatologists was selected for the second stage of the primary research, based on specific quotas, the most important of which were the number of patients with psoriasis treated by each physician and the number of psoriasis patients for the treatment of whom the physician was personally responsible. The reason behind that was to include in the survey experienced dermatologists, actively involved in the treatment of psoriasis. The second stage included 30-minute face-to-face interviews with the 110 dermatologists, the characteristics of whom are presented in Table 2.

A 40-item questionnaire (both quantitative and qualitative) was developed with the aim of exploring: a) epidemiologic data (number of patients with plaque psoriasis, percentage of patients with moderate to severe disease); b) treatment pathways (percentage of patients receiving pharmaceutical treatment, percentage receiving monotherapy versus combined treatment, percentage receiving biologic agents versus conventional systemic therapy); and c) resource utilization of both responders and non-responders (frequency and setting of administration, number of annual outpatient visits to physicians' offices and hospitals, duration of hospitalizations) (see Additional file 1: Primary research questionnaire). Non-responders were defined as patients who did not achieve a PASI 75 response.

The interviews were based on a retrospective analysis on the use of biologic agents and on a hypothetical projection regarding the use of ustekinumab. In particular, the dermatologists were asked to consider their workload over the last month and provide information on moderate to severe psoriasis epidemiology and resource utilization based on their own experiences. The aim was to gather information on usual practice as opposed to best practice, as the former is more informative for determining the actual costs of treatment.

All data collected in the interviews were validated by an expert panel of 18 key opinion leaders in dermatology, who were selected on the basis of being either distinguished academics or managers of psoriasis treatment centers. The experts included in the panel represented all major geographic regions of Greece. No Ethics Committee approval was requested for the primary research component of the study, as the conduct of interviews with physicians and Experts' Panel are not subject to any approval according to the Greek legislation.

The questionnaire used during the expert panel procedure was the same as that used in the interviews. The findings from the original interviews were projected on a screen and the expert panel was asked to either confirm or reject them using a tele-voting system. If more than 60% of the experts disagreed with the findings of the fieldwork, they were invited to answer the same question based on their experience. The average of the experts' answers was then included in the model. The experts' opinions were also used to inform the model on the market shares of the biologic agents, with and without ustekinumab.

Table 1 Mean percentage of patients achieving PASI 75 response with psoriasis biologic treatments

Agent	Mean (%)	95% CI
Adalimumab	58	49–68
Etanercept	52	45–59
Infliximab	80	70–87
Ustekinumab	69	62–75

[a]The relevant dosing scheme for each product is presented in Table 3.
CI, confidence interval; PASI, Psoriasis Area and Severity Index.
Source: Reich et al., 2012.

Table 2 Distribution of the 110 interviewed dermatologists by place of work and area

Place of work	Number of dermatologists	%
Office based	70	64
Hospital based	40	36
Area		
Athens	70	64
Thessaloniki	20	18
Other urban centers	20	18

Table 3 Dosing scheme per product used in the analysis

Agent	Dosing scheme
Adalimumab	80 mg at week 0, 40 mg at week 1, then 40 mg every other week
Etanercept	50 mg twice weekly for 12 weeks, then 50 mg once weekly
Infliximab	5 mg/kg at weeks 0, 2, and 6, then every 8 weeks
Ustekinumab	45 mg at weeks 0 and 4, then every 12 weeks

Cost data

Economic evaluations should go beyond the acquisition cost of drugs in order to reflect real-life clinical practice. Costing in this way requires that all resources used by a particular program or treatment are identified and valued.

To health economists, cost refers to the sacrifice of benefits made when a given resource is consumed in a program or treatment – in other words, the opportunity cost. The value of opportunity forgone in the next-best alternative use of health resources does not necessarily equate to the market price of the resources used, because the total costs of treatment should be considered. The total costs comprise the sum of all expenditures during a given time frame, including the direct costs incurred by the health care provider and patient, as well as the indirect costs to society of productivity lost. It is important to assess the relative importance of a cost item to the overall outcome, since the inclusion of minor costs may not be justified in certain cases. An example is when the cost of drug acquisition (a direct cost) far outweighs the magnitude of other costs, such as productivity loss (an indirect cost). Thus, in this model, only direct costs expressed in euros (2009) were considered.

Costs incurred during the maintenance years of therapy were not discounted. The costs associated with the management of adverse events were not incorporated in the model, as they were assumed to be the same across the biologics compared.

Drug acquisition costs were calculated on an annual basis for both the induction and maintenance years for each drug. The doses and number of administrations for each product were taken from the respective European Medicines Agency summaries of product characteristics (Table 3). According to expert medical opinion in

Greece, for patients receiving ustekinumab, approximately 7% of patients weighing >100 kg receive 90 mg ustekinumab rather than the standard dose of 45 mg. This proportion was deemed to be too small to be incorporated in the model.

Prices of the biologics were taken from officially published price bulletins from the Ministry of Development (www.ypan.gr). Tariffs from the largest social health insurance fund (www.ika.gr) were used to assess monitoring (outpatient visits to dermatologist), administration (visits to nurse, day hospital, or dermatologist's private office), and inpatient costs.

In order to capture the total health care costs for the treatment of psoriasis, the type of costs considered in this analysis incorporated not only drug acquisition costs but also associated medical resource use costs, including resource costs for non-responders such as supportive care, outpatient visits, and hospitalization.

From a health care system perspective, office visits represent a substantial usage of health care infrastructure and are therefore an important component of fixed health care costs. For this reason, dispensing fees, administration costs, and office visits are commonly factored into economic analyses in the economic evaluation literature. This has been the preferred approach in numerous studies, even though the charges for administration costs may not necessarily differ between the therapies being compared (e.g., multivalent vaccines and infusion cancer therapies, in which office visits and administration costs are critical components of the economic analysis) [29,30]. This approach has been endorsed by the "Good Research Practices for Measuring Drug Costs in Cost Effectiveness Analyses" developed by the International Society for Pharmacoeconomics and Outcomes Research [31]. This document indicates that the administration cost of a medication is an integral part of the overall cost of treatment and, in fact, economic evaluations should go beyond the acquisition cost of drugs in order to reflect real-life clinical practice.

Sensitivity analysis

In order to assess the impact of uncertainty of various model inputs on the results of the study, univariate sensitivity analyses were conducted on three variables that contributed to the cost of treatment and that were derived

Table 4 Administration setting (%) for biologic agents

Agent	Hospital	Pharmacy	Dermatologist's private office	Nurse at home	Alone at home	Health center/private clinic
Adalimumab	9	12	2	8	60	8
Etanercept	11	12	4	9	58	7
Infliximab	99	0	1	0	0	0
Ustekinumab	68	3	2	16	12	0

Note: The percentages do not sum up to 100% across all rows because of rounding.

Table 5 Annual number of visits to health care professionals (excluding visits for administration)

Agent	Hospital	Dermatologist's private office	GP's private office
Adalimumab	6	5	2
Etanercept	6	5	2
Infliximab	5	2	0
Ustekinumab	6	4	1

from the expert panel: hospitalization for non-responders; supportive care costs for non-responders; and market share of ustekinumab. Non-responders' health care costs were varied, with the variation attributed to differences in resource use (i.e., the number of inpatient and outpatient visits). These costs were allowed to vary by ±10% in one-way sensitivity analyses, whereas the market share of ustekinumab for years 1–5 was allowed to vary by ±3% and ±6% (the latter being equally distributed to or withdrawn from all other biologic agents).

Results

Primary research results

Interviews with dermatologists and the expert panel validation that followed showed that 8% of patients with skin disease visiting a dermatologist are diagnosed with psoriasis. Of patients with psoriasis visiting a dermatologist, 63% have moderate to severe disease; of these, 28% are eligible for biologic therapies.

This primary research also showed that there is some variability in where patients receive their medicine, depending on the agent in question (Table 4).

The number of visits of patients with psoriasis to health care professionals for monitoring the progress of their psoriasis, outside the visits for treatment administration purposes, is presented in Table 5. For all the biologics, patients more commonly visit hospitals than dermatologists' private offices.

The annual number of visits to dermatologists increases with disease severity (Table 6). Non-responders to biologic agents have on average 6 additional visits to hospitals and 6 additional visits to dermatologists per year compared with responders (Table 7).

Finally, the expert panel provided estimates of the market share of ustekinumab and the other biologic

Table 6 Mean annual number of visits to dermatologists, by severity of disease and work location of the dermatologist

Work Location	Moderate psoriasis	Severe psoriasis
Office-based dermatologist	7	8
Hospital-based dermatologist	6	10

Table 7 Mean annual number of additional visits for non-responders to biologic agents

Visit Location	Mean number of additional visits
Hospital	6
Dermatologist's private office	6
GP private office	0

agents, after the introduction of the former for the treatment of moderate to severe psoriasis (Table 8). Ustekinumab's market share is expected to increase over a 5 year time horizon, starting from 9% in year 1 and reaching 26% in year 5.

Model results

Based on the model results, the inclusion of ustekinumab in the biologic treatment setting for moderate to severe psoriasis is predicted to lead to total per-patient savings of €443 and €900 in years 1 and 5 of its introduction, respectively (Figure 1).

These results are mainly driven by the low number of administrations required with ustekinumab over a 5-year treatment period (22 for ustekinumab, compared with 272 for etanercept, 131 for adalimumab, and 36 for infliximab; Table 9). The cost savings for ustekinumab are also attributable to reduced hospitalization costs for non-responders and improved efficacy.

Sensitivity analyses

Results of the sensitivity analyses confirmed the robustness of the model to wide variation in inputs. Variation of non-responders' outpatient costs by ±10% led to a minor change in the net budget impact of ustekinumab. Variation of non-responders' hospitalization costs brought greater changes to ustekinumab's budget impact, as hospitalization is an important cost driver of psoriasis. However, ustekinumab remained cost-saving at both ends of the range of inputs for hospitalization costs in the sensitivity analysis (Table 10).

In addition, even using the more conservative base-case market share assumption for ustekinumab (–10%), the introduction of ustekinumab as a treatment option for moderate to severe psoriasis is predicted to deliver substantial annual cost savings per patient, ranging from €254 in year 1 to €665 in year 5.

Table 8 Estimated market share (%) of biologic agents for the treatment of moderate to severe psoriasis

Agent	Base year	Year 1	Year 2	Year 3	Year 4	Year 5
Adalimumab	30	27	25	24	23	23
Etanercept	45	42	39	37	36	35
Infliximab	25	22	20	18	17	16
Ustekinumab	0	9	16	21	24	26

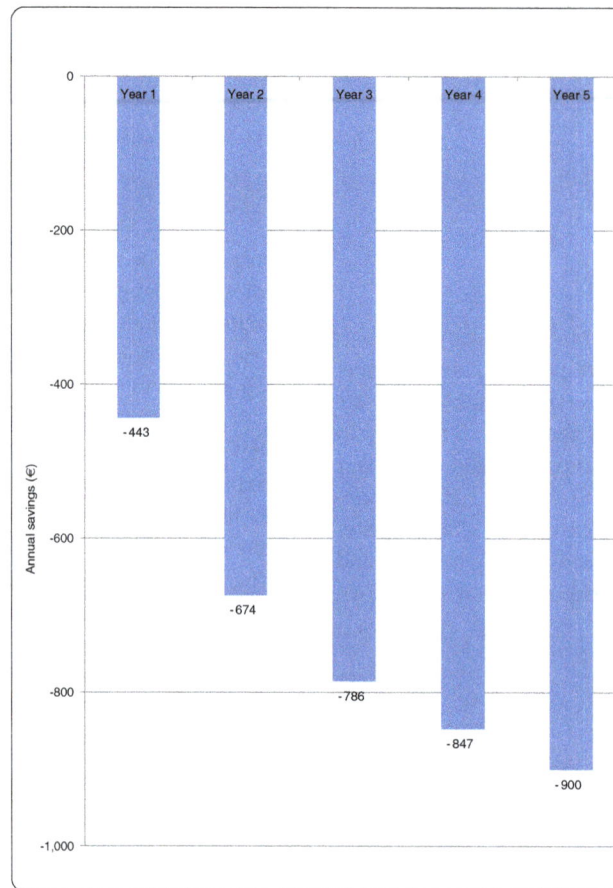

Figure 1 Net budget impact of ustekinumab (annual cost savings per patient in €).

Discussion

Moderate to severe psoriasis is a chronic, incurable disease, with substantial economic consequences for the health care budget. This is the first study to investigate the treatment patterns and resource utilization of psoriasis in Greece and the economic impact of the introduction of a new biologic treatment option.

The current study consisted of two parts: field work with questionnaires to dermatologists to identify resource use data; and a budget impact model to estimate the costs associated with adding ustekinumab to the current treatment options for psoriasis. The collection of resource use data through face-to-face interviews with

physicians, rather than being derived from clinical trials or observational studies, could be criticized on the grounds of subjectivity and be considered a limitation of this study. However, in order to strengthen the validity of the data collected, an expert panel consisting of key opinion leaders was set up to assess the primary results.

The selection of dermatologists to participate in the primary research was mainly based on the level of experience they had with psoriatic patients, the rationale being that physicians with more experience on psoriasis would be able to provide more robust estimates for the parameters investigated in the study. As a result, the estimated eligible patient population entering the model in year 1 is potentially shifted upwards compared to actual numbers, leading to a subsequent overestimate in the budget impact of the related biologic treatments. However, the results of the present study in terms of cost differences across treatments, are not affected, as the eligible population is the same for all treatments and therefore has a proportionate impact on respective budgets.

Table 9 Number of administrations for each product

Agent	Induction year	Maintenance year	5 year total
Adalimumab	27	26	131
Etanercept	64	52	272
Infliximab	8	7	36
Ustekinumab	5	4	22

Table 10 Sensitivity analysis of net budget impact of ustekinumab per patient (€)

	Year 1	Year 2	Year 3	Year 4	Year 5
Base case	−443	−674	−786	−847	−900
Non-responders' outpatient costs					
−10%	−443	−673	−785	−846	−899
+10%	−444	−674	−786	−848	−901
Non-responders' hospitalization costs					
−10%	−417	−647	−759	−820	−873
+10%	−470	−700	−812	−874	−927
Ustekinumab share					
−5%	−340	−559	−671	−732	−785
+5%	−547	−789	−901	−962	−1,015
−10%	−254	−441	−552	−614	−665
+10%	−648	−906	−1,018	−1,080	−1,133

Note: Negative values indicate budget savings.

The results reveal that etanercept is currently the preferred treatment option for moderate to severe psoriasis, followed by adalimumab and infliximab. An interesting finding is that although etanercept and adalimumab are administered at home for the majority of patients, patients more commonly visit hospital-based physicians than the private offices of dermatologists to monitor their treatment progress. This may be attributed to the fact that specialized psoriasis centers are located in some hospitals.

The results also show that resource utilization and related costs increase with disease severity, a finding confirmed by the literature [32]. Moreover, the investigation of the budget impact of adding ustekinumab as a treatment option for psoriasis shows that this would lead to substantial cost savings, even in the first year of its introduction.

The therapeutic benefits of ustekinumab have been confirmed in three large Phase 3 trials in patients with moderate to severe psoriasis [25,26,28]. These studies found that a significantly higher proportion of patients receiving ustekinumab compared with placebo or etanercept achieved PASI 75 at 12 weeks. Other efficacy measures, including the Physician's Global Assessment at week 12, also favored ustekinumab [25,26,28]. Moreover, subcutaneous ustekinumab was generally well tolerated [24-26,28]. Treatment with ustekinumab has also been found to result in significantly improved HRQoL (Dermatology Life Quality Index) [33,34], lowered depression and anxiety rates based on the Hospital Anxiety and Depression Scale [34], and improved employability and productivity [35].

A possible shortcoming of the present study is that hospitalization and outpatient costs may have been underestimated. Social health insurance fund tariffs, which have been used in this model, do not reflect actual costs; actual costs are higher than the amount reimbursed by insurance funds.

Another limitation is that indirect costs were not considered. Indirect costs related to psoriasis include lost work time (i.e., days missed from work) and reduced productivity. Indirect costs increase with disease severity and can be significant [32]. In a UK study, 59.3% of patients with psoriasis who were still working had lost an average of 26 days from work in the previous year because of their psoriasis, and of the 180 patients not working, 33.9% reported not working because of their psoriasis [36]. A study in Germany showed that the mean indirect costs and loss of productivity per patient with psoriasis were €1,310 per year, accounting for 19.5% of total psoriasis costs [37]. However, clinical trials of biologics, including ustekinumab, demonstrate that patients who respond to treatment experience improvements in productivity and reductions in work-day loss. Therefore, the omission of indirect costs in this analysis is unlikely to adversely affect the research findings.

An important finding of this study is that, based on expert opinion, 67.5% of ustekinumab-treated patients will initially be administered the product in hospital rather than at home or in their dermatologist's private office. This is probably due to physicians' reservations regarding a new biologic agent. According to the expert panel, reinforcement of ustekinumab's efficacy and safety data with local dermatologists' own experience is likely to lead to patients receiving the drug outside of the hospital setting. The expert panel's opinion was that similar treatment patterns as with etanercept and adalimumab (where 58% and 60% of patients, respectively, perform administration at home) are expected for ustekinumab users in the future.

Two Phase 3 studies of ustekinumab have shown that the drug has a comparable safety profile with self-administration versus administration by a health care professional [25,26]. A movement toward more frequent administration at home rather than in the hospital setting could further reduce the direct costs of ustekinumab use.

Overall, the present study investigated, for the first time in Greece, the treatment patterns and resource utilization of patients with moderate to severe psoriasis. These findings may be used to inform the development of national treatment guidelines in psoriasis and health policy resource allocation decisions.

Conclusions

Ustekinumab offers a promising alternative to currently approved biologic agents for psoriasis, with both short- and long-term economic benefits. Based on the present model calculation, the introduction of ustekinumab as an alternative treatment option for moderate to severe psoriasis in Greece is anticipated to bring substantial cost savings to the national health care budget.

Competing interests
HK has provided consultancy services to Janssen-Cilag Greece Pharmaceutical SACI. LX was a paid employee of Janssen-Cilag Greece Pharmaceutical SACI until December 2009. BS is a paid employee of Janssen Scientific Affairs, LLC, Horsham, PA, USA. IB, GC, AK, MK, AP, DS, TS, PS, and ET received honoraria from Janssen-Cilag Greece Pharmaceutical SACI for their participation in the expert panel.

Authors' contributions
HK and LX participated in the design and coordination of the study and the analysis and interpretation of the data, and drafted the manuscript. BS revised the manuscript critically for important intellectual content. GA, IB, GC, AK, MK, AP, DS, TS, PS and ET participated in the expert panel for the validation of the data on medical resource utilization and contributed to the manuscript preparation. All authors read and approved the final manuscript.

Author details
[1]Department of Skin and Venereal Diseases, University of Ioannina, Ioannina, Greece. [2]Department of Dermatology, Hospital for Skin and Venereal Diseases, Thessaloniki, Greece. [3]Department of Dermatology, University of Athens, Hospital "A. Syggros", Athens, Greece. [4]Department of Dermatology, Medical School, Aristotle University of Thessaloniki, Thessaloniki, Greece. [5]Department of Dermatology, University of Patras, Patras, Greece. [6]Department of Dermatology and Venereology, "Attikon" General University Hospital, Athens, Greece. [7]Janssen Cilag Pharmaceutical SACI, Athens, Greece. [8]PRMA Consulting Ltd, Hampshire, UK. [9]Janssen Scientific Affairs, LLC, Horsham, PA, USA.

References

1. Woolacott N, Hawkins N, Mason A, Kainth A, Khadjesari Z, Vergel YB, et al: Etanercept and efalizumab for the treatment of psoriasis: a systematic review. *Health Technol Assess* 2006, **10**:No 46.

2. Lebwohl M: Psoriasis. *Lancet* 2003, **361**:1197–1204.
3. Kyriakis KP, Palamaras I, Pagana G, Terzoudi S, Evangelou G: Lifetime prevalence fluctuations of chronic plaque psoriasis and other non-pustular clinical variants. *J Eur Acad Dermatol Venereol* 2008, **22**:1513–1514.
4. Stern RS: Psoriasis. *Lancet* 1997, **350**:349–353.
5. National Psoriasis Foundation: *The psoriasis and psoriatic arthritis pocket guide -Treatment algorithms and management options.* Portland; 2009.
6. Yu AP, Tang J, Xie J, Wu EQ, Gupta SR, Bao Y, Mulani P: Economic burden of psoriasis compared to the general population and stratified by disease severity. *Curr Med Res Opin* 2009, **25**:2429–2438.
7. Rapp SR, Feldman SR, Exum ML, Fleischer AB Jr, Reboussin DM: Psoriasis causes as much disability as other major medical diseases. *J Am Acad Dermatol* 1999, **41**:401–407.
8. Chen SC, Bayoumi AM, Soon SL, Aftergut K, Cruz P, Sexton SA, et al: A catalog of dermatology utilities: a measure of the burden of skin diseases. *J Investig Dermatol Symp Proc* 2004, **9**:160–168.
9. Zug KA, Littenberg B, Baughman RD, Kneeland T, Nease RF, Sumner W, et al: Assessing the preferences of patients with psoriasis. A quantitative, utility approach. *Arch Dermatol* 1995, **131**:561–568.
10. Schmitt JM, Ford DE: Role of depression in quality of life for patients with psoriasis. *Dermatology* 2007, **215**:17–27.
11. Fried RG, Friedman S, Paradis C, Hatch M, Lynfield Y, Duncanson C, et al: Trivial or terrible? The psychosocial impact of psoriasis. *Int J Dermatol* 1995, **34**:101–105.
12. Akay A, Pekcanlar A, Bozdag KE, Altintas L, Karaman A: Assessment of depression in subjects with psoriasis vulgaris and lichen planus. *J Eur Acad Dermatol Venereol* 2002, **16**:347–352.
13. Gupta MA, Schork NJ, Gupta AK, Kirkby S, Ellis CN: Suicidal ideation in psoriasis. *Int J Dermatol* 1993, **32**:188–190.
14. Bhosle MJ, Feldman SR, Camacho FT, Timothy WJ, Nahata MC, Balkrishnan R: Medication adherence and health care costs associated with biologics in Medicaid-enrolled patients with psoriasis. *J Dermatolog Treat* 2006, **17**:294–301.
15. Cockayne SE, Cork MJ, Gawkrodger DJ: Treatment of psoriasis: day care vs. inpatient therapy. *Br J Dermatol* 1999, **140**:375–376.
16. Colombo G, Altomare G, Peris K, Martini P, Quarta G, Congedo M, et al: Moderate and severe plaque psoriasis: cost-of-illness study in Italy. *Ther Clin Risk Manag* 2008, **4**:559–568.
17. Rich SJ, Bello-Quintero CE: Advancements in the treatment of psoriasis: role of biologic agents. *J Manag Care Pharm* 2004, **10**:318–325.
18. Finlay AY, Salek MS, Haney J: Intramuscular alefacept improves health-related quality of life in patients with chronic plaque psoriasis. *Dermatology* 2003, **206**:307–315.
19. Feldman SR, Menter A, Koo JY: Improved health-related quality of life following a randomized controlled trial of alefacept treatment in patients with chronic plaque psoriasis. *Br J Dermatol* 2004, **150**:317–326.
20. Farhi D, Dupin N: Biologic therapies in the treatment of psoriasis. *Presse Med* 2009, **38**:832–843.
21. Bongartz R, Sutton AJ, Sweeting MJ, et al: Anti-TNF antibody therapy in rheumatoid arthritis and the risk of serious infections and malignancies: systematic review and meta-analysis of rare harmful effects in randomized controlled trials. *JAMA* 2006, **295**:2275–2285.
22. Bissonnette R, Ho V, Langley RG: Safety of Conventional Systemic Agents and Biologic Agents in the treatment of Psoriasis. *Journal of Cutaneous Medicine and Surgery* 2009, **13**(2):S67–S76.
23. Chien AL, Elder JT, Ellis CN: Ustekinumab: a new option in psoriasis therapy. *Drugs* 2009, **69**:1141–1152.
24. Weber J, Keam SJ: Ustekinumab. *BioDrugs* 2009, **23**:53–61.
25. Leonardi CL, Kimball AB, Papp KA, Yeilding N, Guzzo C, Wang Y, et al: Efficacy and safety of ustekinumab, a human interleukin-12/23 monoclonal antibody, in patients with psoriasis: 76-week results from a randomised, double-blind, placebo-controlled trial (PHOENIX 1). *Lancet* 2008, **371**:1665–1674.
26. Papp KA, Langley RG, Lebwohl M, Krueger GG, Szapary P, Yeilding N, et al: Efficacy and safety of ustekinumab, a human interleukin-12/23 monoclonal antibody, in patients with psoriasis: 52-week results from a randomised, double-blind, placebo-controlled trial (PHOENIX 2). *Lancet* 2008, **371**:1675–1684.
27. Reich K, Burden AD, Eaton JN, Hawkins NS: Efficacy of biologics in the treatment of moderate to severe psoriasis. *Br J Dermatol* 2012, **166**:179–188.

28. Griffiths C, Strober BE, Van de Kerkhof P, Ho V, Fidelus-Gort H, Yeilding N, *et al*: Comparison of ustekinumab and etanercept for moderate-to-severe psoriasis. *N Engl J Med* 2010, **362**:118–128.
29. Chu E, Cartwright TH: Pharmacoeconomic benefits of capecitabine-based chemotherapy in metastatic colorectal cancer. *J Clin Oncol* 2008, **26**:2224–2226.
30. Tilson L, Thornton L, O'Flanagan D, Johnson H, Barry M: Cost effectiveness of hepatitis B vaccination strategies in Ireland: an economic evaluation. *Eur J Public Health* 2008, **18**:275–282.
31. ISPOR Drug Cost Task Force: *Good Research Practices for Measuring Drug Costs in Cost Effectiveness Analyses*. South Lawrenceville; 2010.
32. Feldman SR, Fleischer AB Jr, Reboussin DM, Rapp SR, Bradham DD, Exum ML, *et al*: The economic impact of psoriasis increases with psoriasis severity. *J Am Acad Dermatol* 1997, **37**:564–569.
33. Lebwohl M, Papp K, Han C, Schenkel B, Yeilding N, Wang Y, *et al*: Ustekinumab improves health-related quality of life in patients with moderate-to-severe psoriasis: results from the PHOENIX 1 trial. *Br J Dermatol* 2010, **162**:137–146.
34. Langley RG, Feldman SR, Han C, Schenkel B, Szapary P, Hsu M-C, *et al*: Ustekinumab significantly improves symptoms of anxiety, depression, and skin-related quality of life in patients with moderate-to-severe psoriasis: results from a randomized, double-blind, placebo-controlled Phase III trial. *J Am Acad Dermatol* 2010, **63**:457–465.
35. Reich K, Schenkel B, Zhao N, Szapary P, Augustin M, Borcier M, *et al*: Ustekinumab decreases work limitations, improves work productivity, and reduces work days missed in patients with moderate-to-severe psoriasis: results from PHOENIX 2. *J Derm Treat* 2011, **22**:337–347.
36. Finlay AY, Coles EC: The effect of severe psoriasis on the quality of life of 369 patients. *Br J Dermatol* 1995, **132**:236–244.
37. Schoffski O, Augustin M, Prinz J, Rauner K, Schubert E, Sohn S, *et al*: Costs and quality of life in patients with moderate to severe plaque-type psoriasis in Germany: a multi-center study. *J Dtsch Dermatol Ges* 2007, **5**:209–218.

Innate lymphoid cells and the skin

Maryam Salimi and Graham Ogg[*]

Abstract

Innate lymphoid cells are an emerging family of effector cells that contribute to lymphoid organogenesis, metabolism, tissue remodelling and protection against infections. They maintain homeostatic immunity at barrier surfaces such as lung, skin and gut (Nature 464:1367–1371, 2010, Nat Rev Immunol 13: 145–149, 2013). Several human and mouse studies suggest a role for innate lymphoid cells in inflammatory skin conditions including atopic eczema and psoriasis. Here we review the innate lymphoid cell family and discuss their function in the skin and during inflammation.

Keywords: Innate lymphoid cells, Atopic dermatitis, Psoriasis, IL-33, IL-25, TSLP, PGD2, KLRG1, E-cadherin

Introduction

Innate lymphoid cells

Recent advances in the field of immunology have identified a novel family of CD45 expressing haematopoietic effector cells. These cells have phenotypical features of lymphoid cells but lack rearranged antigen specific surface receptors of adaptive immune cells and are termed innate lymphoid cells (ILCs) [1]. ILCs are essential for lymphoid organogenesis, metabolism, tissue homeostasis and repair, protection against viral and helminth infections [2-4]. They reside in the blood, spleen, intestine, liver, fat associated lymphoid clusters (FALC), and mesenteric lymph nodes of humans and mice. Their development depends on the expression of the transcriptional repressor Id2 that regulates the activity of helix-loop-helix protein E47 and RORC. Cytokines that signal through the common γ chain of IL-2 receptor and Jak3 are essential for their maintenance.

ILCs are thought to be able to influence adaptive immune responses as they reside in the interface of T and B cell zones in the splenic follicles of mice and can express co-stimulatory molecules essential for T cell priming and survival, including CD40 ligand and CD30 ligand [5]. Each distinct functional subset produces cytokines that were previously thought to be specific to adaptive immune system lineages. Based on their cytokine profile and functional characteristics, they can be divided into three main groups [1], although recent studies on lineage relationships and common precursors of ILCs make this classification debatable [6].

Review

Group 1 ILCs

The most studied prototype of this family is group 1 ILCs including NK cells and group 1 innate lymphoid cells (ILC1) which were identified in 1975 and 2012, respectively [7-9]. They express transcription factors T-bet, Nfil3 (E4BP4) and Eomes [10], and IL-15 and IL-12 are required for their development and function. NK cell subsets include cytolytic effectors of the innate immune system and can produce IFN-γ, TNF-α, MIP1-α, MIP1-β and RANTES. They are believed to be responsible for defence against intracellular pathogens, tumours and viruses, but may contribute to aberrant inflammation in certain settings. Unlike NK cells, ILC1 lack granzyme B and perforin but express CD103 [11] and CXCR3 [9]. IL-7Rα+ IL-12Rβ2+ IL-1R+ group 1 ILCs produce IFN-γ in response to IL-12 and are enriched in inflamed mucosal tissue such as tonsils, intestine and in diseased tissue including the lamina propria of patients with Crohn's disease [11] and inflamed lungs of patients with chronic obstructive pulmonary disease (COPD) [12]. Interestingly group 1 ILCs are absent from foetal gut and develop after colonisation of the intestine with commensal bacteria [9]. These findings indicate their potential role in protection against certain bacteria in homeostatic conditions and their involvement in the pathogenesis of inflammatory bowel disease and COPD. The origin of group 1 ILC is not clear; however several studies have

* Correspondence: Graham.ogg@ndm.ox.ac.uk
Department of Medicine, MRC Human Immunology Unit, NIHR Biomedical Research Centre, Radcliffe University of Oxford, Oxford, UK

showed that RORγt– IFN-γ producing ILC1 can originate from NKp44[+] group 3 ILC under the influence of IL-12 and IL-15 [9,13].

Group 2 ILCs

The production of key type 2 cytokines, IL-13, IL-4 and IL-5 in response to epithelial cytokines IL-25 and IL-33 in Rag[−/−] mice led to the discovery of group 2 ILCs. In 2010, three separate groups reported lineage negative cells (CD3, CD4, CD8α, TCRαβ, TCRγδ, CD5, CD19, B220, NK1.1, Ter119 (Ly76), Gr-1 (Ly6g), Mac-1 (Itgam), CD11c (Itgax) and FcεRIα) that expressed c-Kit (CD117) and T1/ST2, CD90 (Thy-1), CD45 and IL-7Rα (CD127) in mice. They were designated nuocytes [2], innate helper type 2 (IHC) [14] and natural helper cells (NHC) [15] but demonstrated similar functional characteristics. Concurrently, Saenz described a similar population of multipotent progenitor type 2 (MPP type2) cells but unlike other populations, MPP type 2 cells exhibited progenitor capacity and could differentiate to myeloid and lymphoid lineage descendants [16]. Therefore, it has been speculated that they might be precursors of group 2 ILCs [17]. Recently the term ILC2 was proposed to group type 2 cytokine producing ILC in to a single family [1]. Lack of RORγt expression and IFN-γ production differentiate this group of innate cells from LTi cells and ILC1, respectively. ILC2s were described in fat associated lymphoid clusters (FALC), mesenteric lymph nodes (mLN), intestine and gut associated lymphoid tissues (GALT), liver and spleen. Bearing IL-17RB (IL-17BR, IL-25R), ST-2 (IL-33R) and TSLP receptors ILC2 cells respond to epithelial cytokines including IL-25 (IL-17E), IL-33 and TSLP, by producing type 2 cytokines as IL-13, IL-4, IL-5, IL-9.

Human ILC2s were discovered in healthy human lung parenchyma and broncho-alveolar lavage (BAL) fluid of patients receiving a lung transplant as lineage negative cells (CD3, TCRαβ, CD11c, CD11b, CD56, CD19) that express IL-7Rα and ST2 subunit of the IL-33 receptor [18]. Spits et al. reported lineage negative (CD3, CD4, CD11c, CD14, CD19, CD34, CD123, TCRαβ, TCRγδ, BDCA2, and FcεRI), CD45[hi], CD127[+] and CD117[+] cells in peripheral blood, foetal gut and inflamed nasal polyps of patients with rhinosinusitis. They also express prostaglandin D2 receptor (CRTH2), CD161 (KLRB1), CD7 and CD25. In response to epithelial cytokines and IL-2 the cells produce large amounts of IL-13 and IL-5 but not IL-17A or IL-22 [19,20].

ILC2 represent a vital source of IL-13 for expulsion of the gut helminth, Nippostrongylus brasiliensis [2,15,16] by inducing goblet cell hyperplasia, eosinophilia and intestinal smooth muscle cell contraction. ILC2 also contribute to homeostasis and allergic responses in the airways. Using IL-4[+/eGFP] IL-13[+/Tom] dual reporter mice, it was shown that ILC2s were the major source of type 2

cytokines in Ovalbumin induced allergy and after intranasal administration of IL-25 and IL-33 [21]. Moreover, depletion of lung resident ILC2 in mice after infection with H1N1 influenza virus A resulted in impaired airway epithelial integrity and lung function, with exaggerated thermodysregulation and higher total protein concentration in the broncho-alveolar lavage (BAL) fluid. Such function is predominantly mediated by amphiregulin production by ILC2, a wound-healing modulator of the epidermal growth factor family [18]. Recent studies demonstrated mutual interaction between ILC2 and T cells [22,23]. Activated T cells produce IL-2 that induces proliferation and cytokine production of ILC2 [23]. ILC2 in humans and mice express MHC-II and co-stimulatory molecules CD80 and CD86. Co-culture of ILC2s and T cells in the presence of antigen, induced TH2 differentiation and type 2 cytokine production in T cells [22,23]. In addition, ILC2 also enhance differentiation of polyclonally activated naïve T cells to a TH2 phenotype in an MHC-independent contact-dependent manner [23]. Furthermore, N. brasiliensis infection of two mouse models deficient in ILC2 showed delayed worm expulsion and a dramatic decrease in IL-13 and IL-5 producing CD4[+] T cells. Moreover, IL-2 released from T cells promotes ILC2 proliferation and cytokine production [22].

Group 3 ILCs

Group 3 ILCs include lymphoid tissue inducers (LTi cells), NCR[+] ILC3 (NK22, NCR22, ILC22) and NCR[−] ILC3 (ILC17) [24]. Group 3 ILCs are important in inflammation, anti-microbial protection, mucosal immunity and homeostasis. LTi cells express c-Kit, IL-7Rα, IL-1R, IL-23R and lymphotoxin-β (LTβ), CCR6, and aryl hydrocarbon receptor (AHR) [25]. They initiate lymphoid structure formation and induce expression of VCAM-1 and ICAM-1 on mesenchymal cells through LTβR and TNFR signalling during embryogenesis and produce IL-17A [26]. After birth, LTi cells contribute to the formation of solitary lymphoid follicles and Peyer's patches. After birth splenic LTi cells produce IL-22 and IL-17A [25] in response to yeast cell wall product zymosan which suggests that they contribute to host defence. Furthermore, they also support class switching to IgA and are thus important for adaptive immune responses [27].

Two phenotypically distinct RORγt dependent subsets of ILC3 were characterised recently, and based on the expression of natural cytotoxicity receptors, NKp46 in mice and NKp44 in human, they were divided into NCR[+] [24] and NCR[−] ILC3 [1]. Postnatal NCR[+] ILC3 derived from tonsils largely produce IL-22 and small amounts of IL-17. They are thymus independent and reside in the intestine, dermis, tonsils and mLNs. NKp44[+] RORγt[+] IL-22[+] are diminished in germ free mice which suggests that their maintenance and functional properties are largely dependent on commensal bacteria [28]. IL-22 produced by RORγt$^+$ ILCs is essential in protection against *Citrobacter rodentium* induced acute colitis in mice [28]. Recently it was shown that Notch-2-dependent CD103$^+$ CD11b$^+$ cDCs are a major source of IL-23 during early stages of infection with *Citrobacter rodentium*. The population expansion of these cells was mediated by LTβR signalling [29]. The expression of IL-22 in NCR$^+$ ILC3 is negatively regulated by the epithelial cytokine IL-25 as intestinal inflammation and epithelial damage by administration of dextran sodium sulfate (DSS) that concomitantly increased IL-23 and reduced IL-25, induced population expansion and IL-22 production by RORγt$^+$ ILCs [30]. The NCR$^-$ ILC3 population in mice expresses SCA-1, IL-23 receptor, transcription factor RORγt and high levels of Thy-1. The cells accumulate in the gut during *Helicobacter hepaticus* induced colitis. Stimulation of NCR$^-$ ILC3s with IL-23 induces production of IL-17 and IFN-γ [3].Recent studies showed that group 3 innate lymphoid cells can regulate adaptive immune responses. NCR$^-$ ILC3 express high levels of major histocompatibility complex class II (MHCII) whereas NKp46$^+$ ILC3 express minimal levels of MHCII. Although ILC3 can process and present antigen, they cannot induce T cell proliferation of naïve T cells as they lack co-stimulatory molecules, CD80, CD86, and CD40. Instead they appear to reduce T cell responses to commensal flora. Lack of MHC II on RORγt$^+$ ILCs induces spontaneous mild colitis, splenomegaly, shortened intestine and crypt elongation [31].

ILC2 origin and transcription factors

Group 2 innate lymphoid cells arise in bone marrow from common lymphoid progenitors (CLP) at the double-negative stage 1 (DN1) and stage 2 (DN2). Their presence in thymus deficient Foxn1$^{nu/nu}$ (nude) mice confirms that they do not require the thymus for their development [20,32]. Unlike most previous studies that categorized NK and LTi cells in group 1 and group 3 ILCs respectively, recent work by Constantinides *et al.* showed a common ILC progenitor (ILCP) in foetal liver and adult bone marrow that can differentiate into ILC1, ILC2 and ILC3 but not NK and LTi cells. ILCP were Lin$^-$ IL-7Rα$^+$ c-Kit$^+$ α4β7$^+$ and phenotypically similar to precursors of LTi cells. High levels of PLZF, a transcription factor associated with NKT cells, as well as high levels of Id2, GATA3 and TOX were found in ILCP. PLZF$^+$ ILCP arise from an α4β7 IL-7Rα$^+$ population from which NK and LTi progenitors are also known to develop. However, interestingly depletion of PLZF altered ILC development but did not affect NK and LTi cells, which shows that NK and LTi cells have distinct precursors [6].

ILC2s require IL-7, IL-33 and signalling through tyrosine kinase receptor Flt-3 [32]. Jak3$^{-/-}$ mice are deficient of ILC2 which confirms their requirement for signalling through common γ chain of IL-2 [20]. T cell factor-1 (TCF-1) essential for normal T cell lineage specification and is also required for development of ILC2. In Tcf7$^{-/-}$ mice the frequency of ILC2 is 5% of wild type mice, and the remaining ILC2 are functionally compromised. Transient Notch signalling is another vital requirement for ILC2 development that acts upstream of TCF-1 but does not require the HES-1 pathway [33]. Forced expression of TCF-1 can bypass Notch requirement by up-regulating GATA-3 expression. GATA-3 maintains the expression of IL-17RB, IL-2R, IL-1RL1 receptors and production of IL-13 and IL-5. Its effect is intrinsic and dose dependent [33,34]. Upon activation with IL-33 or a combination of IL-2 and IL-25, it binds to the IL-5 and IL-13 promoter in a p38 dependent manner [35]. GATA-3 induces the expression STAT-5 and increases responsiveness to IL-33 and TSLP [36]. Unlike TH2 cells, the expression of GATA3 and production of type 2 cytokines in the lung resident ILC2 in mice are STAT-6 and STAT-3 independent [37]. STAT-6 regulates the proliferation of these cells and induction of eosinophilia in response to Alternaria challenge.

Consistent with the lymphoid origin of ILC2, the transcription factor Ikaros is necessary for their development [20]. Although in one report a trace of RAG-1 expression was detected in these cells, mature ILC2s do not express any rearranged antigen receptors [38] and unlike other members of ILC family, their development is largely dependent on RORA but not RORC expression [32]. The precise interaction between GATA-3 and RORA is not clear; Mjösberg *et al.* showed that RORA is not regulated by GATA-3 and these two transcription factors possibly work in parallel during development of ILC2, whereas Wolterink *et al.* observed the lack of RORα expression in the absence of GATA-3 [34,36]. Although RORA and GATA-3 have a pivotal role in development of ILC2, RORA is not essential for cytokine production and maintenance of mature ILC2 [35]. Lung ILC2 were observed in germ free mice and therefore thought to be independent of commensal bacteria for their development [18]. Although a degree of plasticity has been shown in ILC3 and ILC1 populations as a proportion of RORγt$^+$ NKR$^+$ LTi cells can down regulate RORγt and produce IFN-γ [13], it has yet to be determined whether ILC2 have any plastic characteristics.

ILC2 and skin

Kim *et al.* provided the first evidence on the presence of an ILC2 population in mouse and human skin. In mice, they reported a population of Lin$^-$ CD25$^+$ ST2$^+$ c-Kit$^+$ CD127$^+$ ICOS$^+$ that did not express ILC3 associated markers CD4, NKp46 and RORγt. Although they found a similar population in healthy human skin (Lin$^-$ CD25$^+$ IL-33$^+$) these cells were negative for CRTH2 and CD161, previously described markers of ILC2 in humans [19], and they only acquired the expression of these markers in atopic dermatitis (AD) lesions. Therefore it raised the possibility that this population is either a distinct population of ILCs in human skin or is in a different stage of activation.

Later, the existence of ILC2 in human skin with the same morphology as described in other organs was confirmed [39-41]. Skin resident ILC2 did not express common lineage markers (CD3, CD8, CD14, CD19, CD56, CD11c, CD11b, FcεRI, TCR-αβ, TCR-γδ and CD123) but were positive for CD45, IL-7Rα, CRTH2, CD161, c-Kit, CD25 and ICOS [39,40]. They expressed transcription factors RORα and GATA-3 whereas no RORγt was detected [39]. ILC2 isolated from peripheral blood express skin homing markers cutaneous lymphocyte antigen (CLA), CCR10 [41] and the levels were further up regulated in the skin resident ILC2 [39] (16.7% to 37% and 0.9% to 84%, respectively) which suggests that similar to other organs, bone marrow derived ILC2 circulate in the blood and can migrate to the skin. ILC2 effector functions are at least partly mediated through cytokine receptors IL25R (IL-17RB), IL-33R (ST2) and TSLP-R [39-42] (Figure 1). In an activated state, these receptors are further up-regulated. IL-33 alone or in combination with IL-25 and TSLP could increase IL-13 and IL-5 production in human skin resident ILC2 [39].

In another report the combination of IL-2 and TSLP induced production of type 2 cytokines and addition of IL-25 to this cytokine mixture further enhanced IL-13 production, indicative of a synergistic effect. This synergy was not observed with IL-33 [41]. Activation of skin resident ILC2 promotes amphiregulin production, which is a ligand for epithelial growth factor receptor (EGFR) and regulates proliferation, apoptosis and migration of epithelial cells, and therefore contributes to wound healing and tissue repair [39].

Roediger et al. demonstrated potential immunosurveillance activity of ILC2 in mouse skin. They reported a unique and abundant population of CD45$^+$ CD11b$^-$ CD90^{hi} CD3$^-$ CD2$^-$ c-Kit$^-$ IL-17RB$^+$ ILC2s in the dermis of naïve mice and called them 'dermal ILC2' (dILC2). Dermal ILC2 expressed integrin αEβ7 (CD103) and comprised 5-10% of CD45$^+$ cells. Using 4C13R dual reporter mice in which single alleles of IL-13 and IL-4 were substituted with dsRed and AmCyan respectively, they showed that homeostasis of the skin in the steady state was mainly controlled by CD3$^-$ NK1.1$^-$ dermal ILC2 rather than TH2 cells as they were the main producers of IL-13. Although the dermal ILC2 population was unable to produce IL-4 under homeostatic conditions, the cells acquired this capacity upon stimulation with TSLP. Furthermore, intravital multiphoton microscopy showed that CXCR6$^+$ ILC2 are mainly aggregated in the close vicinity

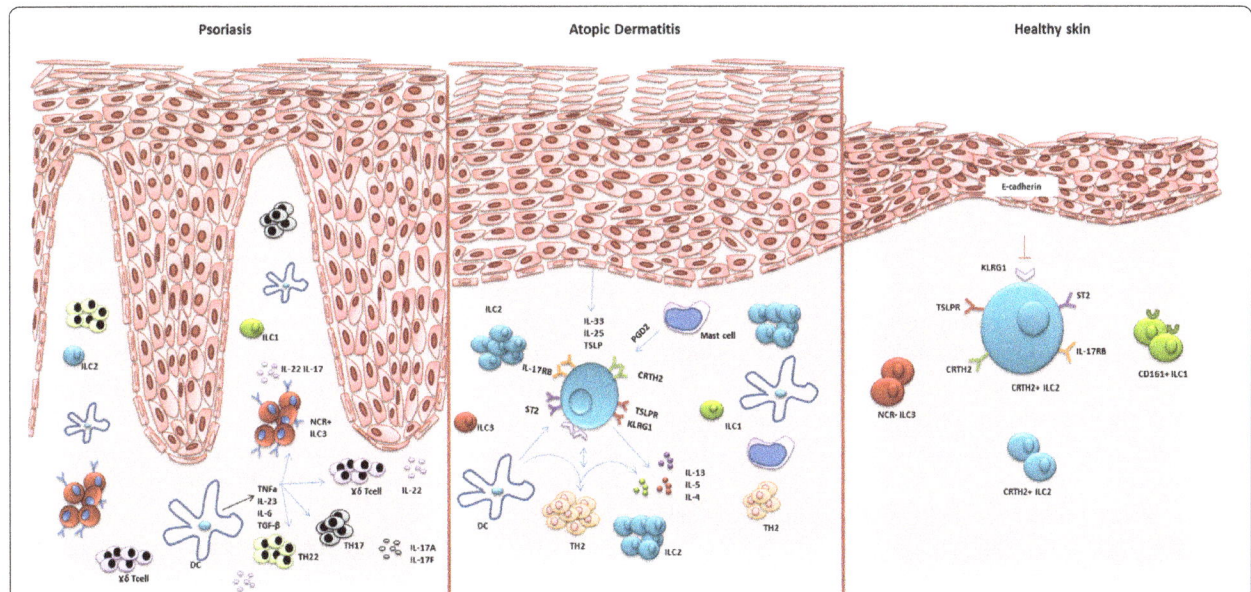

Figure 1 ILC1, ILC2 and ILC3 interactions in human skin. ILC1s express CD161. ILC2s express IL-17RB, ST2, CRTH2, TSLPR and an inhibitory receptor KLRG1. In homeostatic conditions, the expression of adhesion molecule E-cadherin on normal human keratinocytes inhibits the activation of ILC2s. NKp44$^-$ ILC3s are the main subset of ILC3 in healthy skin. ILC2s are enriched in atopic dermatitis lesions and show higher expression of ST2, IL-17RB and TSLP-R, probably an activated phenotype. They express IL-13, IL-5, and IL-4 in response to IL-33, IL-25 and TSLP produced by keratinocytes and PGD2 released by mast cells and other cells. Concurrently, the diminished expression of E-cadherin on keratinocytes is a novel mechanism of sensing a dysfunctional barrier. The frequency of ILC1 and ILC3 in AD lesions are similar to healthy skin. The frequency of NKp44$^+$ ILC3s is increased in psoriatic skin lesions. They produce IL-22 when stimulated with IL-23.

of blood vessels. They constantly patrol the skin local microenvironment with rapid migration (5 μm/min) but with intermittent long interactions with dermal mast cells that lasted 20 to 30 minutes. Interestingly mast cells were not essential for development and maintenance of dermal ILC2 as mast cell deficient mice (B6-Kit$^{W-sh/W-sh}$ and WBB6F1-Kit$^{W/W-v}$) had intact population of dermal ILC2, but in the presence of mast cells, dermal ILC2 were able to regulate them through IL-13.

Anti-CD90.2 antibody is routinely used to deplete ILC2 in mice. This method has been successfully used in the skin by Salimi et al. [39] and Kim et al. [42] although Roediger et al. [20] could not deplete CD103$^+$ dILC2 from the skin using this method and only the ILC2 population in the spleen was depleted, which suggests that CD103$^+$ dILC2 population might represent a distinct sub-population of ILC2 in the skin. Therefore instead of using a depletion strategy to study ILC2 function in the skin, they activated dILC2 in vivo using complexes of IL-2 and JES6-1. Consistent with their immunomodulatory function, dILC2 underwent proliferation and produced large amounts of IL-13 and IL-5. IL-13 suppressed the IgE dependent release of inflammatory cytokines by mast cells in a dose dependent manner [20].

The interaction between ILC2 and mast cells is important in regulating allergic type responses. Human ILC2 can respond to prostaglandin D2 (PGD2), a major metabolite produced by mast cells and other cells. This interaction is mediated through CRTH2 [40,43]. Activation of human ILC2 by PGD2 increased expression of type 2 cytokines as well as IL-3, IL-8, IL-9, IL-21, GM-CSF and CSF-1. Interestingly PGD2 can induce production of IL-4 in human ILC2 which was not observed following stimulation with IL-25 and IL-33 [39-41]. PGD2 stimulation can augment expression of IL-33 receptor (ST2) and the IL-17A subunit of IL-25 receptor [40] and enhance ILC2 responses to IL-33 and IL-25 [43]. Consistent with their quick effector function, both PGD2 and IL-33 induced rapid migration of ILC2. IgE activated mast cell supernatant which contained endogenously synthesized PGD2, mediated the same CRTH2-dependent effector functions such as cell migration and cytokine production in human ILC2 as exogenous PGD2.

Innate lymphoid cells, atopic dermatitis and psoriatic skin inflammation

Atopic dermatitis is a chronic, relapsing inflammatory skin condition characterized by hypersensitivity reactions to common environmental allergens. Given increased levels of type 2 cytokines, IL-13, IL-4 and IL-5, in acute atopic eczema lesions and enhanced production of epithelial cytokines IL-33, IL-25 and TSLP, it is plausible that group 2 innate lymphoid cells contribute to the pathogenesis of atopic dermatitis. Indeed, ILC2 were found in higher proportions in the lesions of patients with atopic dermatitis while the frequency of the cells was similar in the blood of both healthy and atopic individuals [39,42]. ILC2 in atopic lesions showed an activated phenotype with higher expression of cytokine receptors, IL-17B (IL-25R), ST2 (IL-33R) and TSLP receptor. Increased mRNA levels of IL-17RB, ST2, TSLPR, CRTH2, RORA and AREG were detected in lesional skin biopsies of AD patients [39]. Interestingly sampling the skin with or without intra epidermal delivery of house dust mite (HDM) using a suction blister technique in humans, showed that ILC2 infiltrate in to the skin in response to allergen challenge in allergic individuals. A similar effect was seen after subcutaneous administration of HDM extract in mice.

A possible mechanism of skin barrier sensing was described for activated ILC2 in atopic dermatitis lesions. ILC2 express the KLRG1 receptor that upon interaction with its ligand, E-cadherin, conveys inhibitory signals. KLRG1 is up-regulated in response to ILC2 stimulating cytokines. KLRG1 ligation to E-cadherin in a plate-bound assay reduced production of type 2 cytokines, IL-13 and IL-5, and diminished amphiregulin expression and decreased GATA-3 expression. It is speculated that in healthy tissues expressing E-cadherin, ligation to KLRG1 regulates ILC2 responses. There is known to be a significant down-regulation of E-cadherin on keratinocytes in AD lesions which may reduce inhibitory signals to ILC2 and lead to production of type 2 cytokines (Figure 1). The type 2 cytokines may contribute to cutaneous inflammation by down-regulating filaggrin and anti-microbial peptides [44].

Group 2 innate lymphoid cells contribute to inflammation in mouse models of AD-like inflammation. hK14mIL33tg mice in which IL-33 is expressed under the keratin 14 promoter developed spontaneous atopic dermatitis-like inflammation of the skin at 6–8 weeks of age in specific pathogen-free (SPF) conditions. Similar to AD lesions, the pattern of IL-33 expression in this model was confined to the epidermal cell nuclei. Dermatitis lesions in hK14mIL33tg mice were associated with a substantial increase in the concentration of IL-13, IL-5, RANTES/CCL5 and Eotoxin 1/CCL11, whereas the levels of TSLP, IFN-γ and TNF-α were not altered. Increased degranulating IgE$^+$ c-Kit$^+$ mast cells as well as a significant infiltration of eosinophils were observed in the lesions and blood of transgenic mice (7.4 and 4.5 fold higher expression compared to wild type mice respectively). Concurrently skin lesions and regional lymph nodes were enriched for Lin$^-$ ST2$^+$ Sca-1$^+$ ILC2 producing IL-5 and IL-13 [45].

Interestingly treatment of Rag1$^{-/-}$ mice with IL-2 and anti-IL-2 complex (JES6-1) for 2–3 weeks induced spontaneous skin inflammation around ears, eyes, mouth and tail. Extensive accumulation of neutrophils, eosinophils and increased degranulation of mast cells were observed in these lesions which were caused in part by dILC2. dILC2 showed an activated phenotype with higher expression of CD25, ICOS, CD69, ST2 and enhanced production of IL-13 and IL-5 [20].

Topical application of a form of vitamin D3, calcipotriol (MC903), induces ear thickening, xerosis and histopathological changes comparable to AD lesions and is recognized as an experimental murine model of atopic dermatitis. Coincident with ear thickening, increased infiltration of ILC2 was observed in the ear pinna and draining lymph nodes of treated mice [39,42] which was independent of adaptive immunity as Rag1$^{-/-}$ mice still developed AD-like inflammation. Treatment of Rorc$^{-/-}$ mice with calcipotriol induced the same level of inflammation which ruled out the involvement of RORγt dependent ILC3s [42]. Depleting ILC2 using anti-CD90.2 [39,42] or anti-CD25 antibodies [42] in Rag1$^{-/-}$ mice significantly ameliorated inflammation and histopathological changes observed in this model. To eliminate the possibility of involvement of other cell types that potentially express CD90.2 antigen, Salimi et al. used RORα$^{-/-}$ bone marrow chimera mice that had significantly lower numbers of ILC2s. Absence of ILC2s strongly correlated with reduced ear swelling in this model [39].

The hierarchal significance of ILC2 inducing epithelial cytokines IL-25, IL33 and TSLP was established using IL-17RB$^{-/-}$ IL-1RL1$^{-/-}$ and TSLPR$^{-/-}$ respectively backcrossed to BALB/c and C57BL/6 strain backgrounds. In cytokine receptor deficient mice generated on a BALB/c strain background, the greatest protection against calcipotriol induced inflammation was observed in mice lacking IL-25 signalling pathway followed by IL-1RL1 deficient mice. The reduction in ear swelling correlated with a decreased frequency of ILC2s in ear pinna and draining lymph nodes. TSLPR deficient BALB/c mice showed a modest reduction in ILC2 numbers and ear inflammation. Surprisingly, the C57BL/6 strain background showed greater dependency on TSLP signalling pathway with a lower but significant role for IL-25 and IL-33 signalling pathways in inducing AD-like inflammation compared to the BALB/c background [39].

It is noteworthy to mention that as well as ILC2s, populations of NCR$^-$ ILC3 (26.5 ± 8.6%) and CD161$^+$ ILC1 (24.8 ± 11.0% of CD45$^+$ Lin$^-$ CD127$^+$ ILC) were observed in normal human skin [41] (Figure 1). There is a noticeable population of NKp44$^+$ ILC3s in cultured dermal explants, although rare in freshly isolated cells. NCR$^+$ ILC3s differentiated from NCR$^-$ ILC3 upon culture with IL-23, IL-1β and express IL-22.

Blood and lesional skin biopsies of patients with psoriatic skin inflammation showed enrichment of NCR$^+$ ILC3 although similar frequencies of CD161$^+$ ILC1 and CRTH2$^+$ ILC2 were observed [41,46,47] (Figure 1). These cells were an innate source of IL-22. One report found that the frequency of NKp44$^+$ ILC3 correlated with disease severity using PASI score [41] whereas another report could not show a similar finding [46]. Treatment of one psoriatic patient using anti-TNF monoclonal antibody (adalimumab) showed substantial drop (75%) in frequency of NKp44$^+$ ILC3 and equivalent increase in population of NCR$^-$ ILC3s. This reduction inversely correlated with disease severity (PASI score 21.2 to 13.6) which shows the potential importance of NCR$^+$ ILC3 in the pathogenesis of psoriasis.

Conclusions

In the skin, innate lymphoid cells comprise ILC1, ILC2 and ILC3 populations [41,46,47]. Group 2 innate lymphoid cells express CD45, CRTH2 and IL-7Rα while negative for common lineage markers. Bearing receptors for epithelial cytokines and lipid mediators, they produce IL-13, IL-5, IL-4 and IL-9 in response to IL-33, IL-25, TSLP and PGD2 [39,40]. In the skin, ILC2s express skin homing markers and play a role in type 2 mediated inflammation. Indeed, a higher frequency of ILC2 with an activated phenotype was observed in the lesional skin biopsies of patients with atopic dermatitis and established mouse models of atopic dermatitis supported their contribution to the pathogenesis of this disease [39,42,45]. Therefore ILC2s and their activating cytokines or lipid mediators may be new targets for the treatment of atopic dermatitis.

Although research in the field of innate lymphoid cells is moving at a fast pace, many important questions regarding the role of ILC in health and disease still remain unanswered. Detailed interactions of ILC2 with other cell types, including epithelial cells, keratinocytes, fibroblasts, and other cells of the innate and adaptive immune systems would provide a better understanding of the extent of their contribution to homeostatic conditions and disease pathogenesis. Detailed evaluation of signals and mechanisms that regulate ILC activation and inhibition during and after the onset of inflammation and epithelial dysfunction, would help us to identify specific targets for therapeutic interventions.

Abbreviations

DC: Dendritic cell; NK: Natural killer; ILC: Innate lymphoid cells; TSLP: Thymic stromal lymphopoietin; FALC: Fat associated lymphoid clusters; KLRG1: Killer-cell lectin like receptor G1; COPD: Chronic obstructive pulmonary disease; TCR: T cell receptor; MLN: Mesenteric lymph nodes; GALT: Gut associated lymphoid tissues; ROR: Receptor tyrosine kinase-like orphan receptor.

Competing interests

The authors declare that they have no competing interests.

Authors' contributions

MS and GO wrote the manuscript and approved the final submitted version.

Acknowledgements
We are grateful for funding from the MRC, Barrie Trust and the NIHR
Biomedical Research Centre Programme for funding. We also acknowledge
the support of the National Institute for Health Research Clinical Research
Network.

References
1. Spits H, Artis D, Colonna M, Diefenbach A, Di Santo JP, Eberl G, Koyasu S,
    Locksley RM, McKenzie AN, Mebius RE, Powrie F, Vivier E: Innate lymphoid
    cells - a proposal for uniform nomenclature. *Nat Rev Immunol* 2013,
    13(2):145–149.
2. Neill DR, Wong H, Bellosi A, Flynn RJ, Daly M, Langford TKA, Bucks C, Kane
    CM, Fallon PJ, Pannell R, Jolin HE, McKenzie AN: Nuocytes represent a new
    innate effector leukocyte that mediates type-2 immunity. *Nature* 2010,
    464:1367–1371.
3. Buonocore S, Ahern PP, Uhlig HH, Ivanov II, Littman DR, Maloy KJ, Powrie F:
    Innate lymphoid cells drive interleukin-23-dependent innate intestinal
    pathology. *Nature* 2010, 464(7293):1371–1375.
4. Sawa S, Cherrier M, Lochner M, Satoh-Takayama N, Fehling HJ, Langa F, Di
    Santo JP, Eberl G: Lineage relationship analysis of RORgammat + innate
    lymphoid cells. *Science* 2010, 330(6004):665–669.
5. Spits H, Cupedo T: Innate lymphoid cells: emerging insights in
    development, lineage relationships, and function. *Annu Rev Immunol*
    2012, 30:647–675.
6. Constantinides MG, McDonald BD, Verhoef PA, Bendelac A: A committed
    precursor to innate lymphoid cells. *Nature* 2014, 508(7496):397–401.
7. Vivier E, Raulet DH, Moretta A, Caligiuri MA, Zitvogel L, Lanier LL, Yokoyama
    WM, Ugolini S: Innate or adaptive immunity? The example of natural
    killer cells. *Science* 2011, 331(6013):44–49.
8. Kiessling R, Klein E, Pross H, Wigzell H: "Natural" killer cells in the mouse. II.
    Cytotoxic cells with specificity for mouse Moloney leukemia cells.
    Characteristics of the killer cell. *Eur J Immunol* 1975, 5(2):117–121.
9. Bernink JH, Peters CP, Munneke M, te Velde AA, Meijer SL, Weijer K,
    Hreggvidsdottir HS, Heinsbroek SE, Legrand N, Buskens CJ, Bemelman WA,
    Mjosberg JM, Spits H: Human type 1 innate lymphoid cells accumulate in
    inflamed mucosal tissues. *Nat Immunol* 2013, 14(3):221–229.
10. Gordon SM, Chaix J, Rupp LJ, Wu J, Madera S, Sun JC, Lindsten T, Reiner SL:
    The transcription factors T-bet and Eomes control key checkpoints of
    natural killer cell maturation. *Immunity* 2012, 36(1):55–67.
11. Fuchs A, Vermi W, Lee JS, Lonardi S, Gilfillan S, Newberry RD, Cella M,
    Colonna M: Intraepithelial type 1 innate lymphoid cells are a unique
    subset of IL-12- and IL-15-responsive IFN-gamma-producing cells.
    Immunity 2013, 38(4):769–781.
12. Brusselle GG, Joos GF, Bracke KR: New insights into the immunology of
    chronic obstructive pulmonary disease. *Lancet* 2011, 378(9795):1015–1026.
13. Vonarbourg C, Mortha A, Bui VL, Hernandez PP, Kiss EA, Hoyler T, Flach M,
    Bengsch B, Thimme R, Holscher C, Honig M, Pannicke U, Schwarz K, Ware
    CF, Finke D, Diefenbach A: Regulated expression of nuclear receptor
    RORgammat confers distinct functional fates to NK cell receptor-
    expressing RORgammat(+) innate lymphocytes. *Immunity* 2010,
    33(5):736–751.
14. Price AE, Liang HE, Sullivan BM, Reinhardt RL, Eisley CJ, Erle DJ, Locksley RM:
    Systemically dispersed innate IL-13-expressing cells in type 2 immunity.
    Proc Natl Acad Sci U S A 2010, 107(25):11489–11494.
15. Moro K, Yamada T, Tanabe M, Takeuchi T, Ikawa T, Kawamoto H, Furusawa J,
    Ohtani M, Fujii H, Koyasu S: Innate production of T(H)2 cytokines by
    adipose tissue-associated c-Kit(+)Sca-1(+) lymphoid cells. *Nature* 2010,
    463(7280):540–544.
16. Saenz SA, Siracusa MC, Perrigoue JG, Spencer SP, Urban JF Jr, Tocker JE,
    Budelsky AL, Kleinschek MA, Kastelein RA, Kambayashi T, Bhandoola A, Artis
    D: IL25 elicits a multipotent progenitor cell population that promotes
    TH2 cytokine responses. *Nature* 2010, 464:1362–1366.
17. Saenz SA, Siracusa MC, Monticelli LA, Ziegler CG, Kim BS, Brestoff JR,
    Peterson LW, Wherry EJ, Goldrath AW, Bhandoola A, Artis D: IL-25
    simultaneously elicits distinct populations of innate lymphoid cells and
    multipotent progenitor type 2 (MPPtype2) cells. *J Exp Med* 2013,
    210(9):1823–1837.
18. Monticelli LA, Sonnenberg GF, Abt MC, Alenghat T, Ziegler CG, Doering TA,
    Angelosanto JM, Laidlaw BJ, Yang CY, Sathaliyawala T, Kubota M, Turner D,
    Diamond JM, Goldrath AW, Farber DL, Collman RG, Wherry EJ, Artis D:
    Innate lymphoid cells promote lung-tissue homeostasis after infection
    with influenza virus. *Nat Immunol* 2011, 12(11):1045–1054.
19. Mjosberg JM, Trifari S, Crellin NK, Peters CP, van Drunen CM, Piet B, Fokkens
    WJ, Cupedo T, Spits H: Human IL-25- and IL-33-responsive type 2 innate
    lymphoid cells are defined by expression of CRTH2 and CD161. *Nat
    Immunol* 2011, 12(11):1055–1062.
20. Roediger B, Kyle R, Yip KH, Sumaria N, Guy TV, Kim BS, Mitchell AJ, Tay SS,
    Jain R, Forbes-Blom E, Chen X, Tong PL, Bolton HA, Artis D, Paul WE, Fazekas
    de St Groth B, Grimbaldeston MA, Le Gros G, Weninger W: Cutaneous
    immunosurveillance and regulation of inflammation by group 2 innate
    lymphoid cells. *Nat Immunol* 2013, 14(6):564–573.
21. Barlow JL, Bellosi A, Hardman CS, Drynan LF, Wong H, Cruickshank JP,
    McKenzie AN: Innate IL-13–producing nuocytes arise during allergic lung
    inflammation and contribute to airways hyperreactivity. *J Allergy Clin
    Immunol* 2012, 129(1):191–198.
22. Oliphant CJ, Hwang YY, Walker JA, Salimi M, Wong SH, Brewer JM,
    Englezakis A, Barlow JL, Hams E, Scanlon ST, Ogg GS, Fallon PG, McKenzie
    AN: MHCII-mediated dialog between group 2 innate lymphoid cells and
    CD4+ T cells potentiates type 2 immunity and promotes parasitic
    helminth expulsion. *Immunity* 2014, 41(2):283–295.
23. Mirchandani AS, Besnard AG, Yip E, Scott C, Bain CC, Cerovic V, Salmond RJ,
    Liew FY: Type 2 innate lymphoid cells drive CD4+ Th2 cell responses.
    J Immunol 2014, 192(5):2442–2448.
24. Luci C, Reynders A, Ivanov II, Cognet C, Chiche L, Chasson L, Hardwigsen J,
    Anguiano E, Banchereau J, Chaussabel D, Dalod M, Littman DR, Vivier E, Tomasello
    E: Influence of the transcription factor RORgammat on the development of
    NKp46+ cell populations in gut and skin. *Nat Immunol* 2009, 10(1):75–82.
25. Takatori H, Kanno Y, Watford WT, Tato CM, Weiss G, Ivanov II, Littman DR,
    O'Shea JJ: Lymphoid tissue inducer-like cells are an innate source of
    IL-17 and IL-22. *J Exp Med* 2009, 206(1):35–41.
26. Cupedo T, Crellin NK, Papazian N, Rombouts EJ, Weijer K, Grogan JL, Fibbe
    WE, Cornelissen JJ, Spits H: Human fetal lymphoid tissue-inducer cells are
    interleukin 17-producing precursors to RORC+ CD127+ natural killer-like
    cells. *Nat Immunol* 2009, 10(1):66–74.
27. Tsuji M, Suzuki K, Kitamura H, Maruya M, Kinoshita K, Ivanov II, Itoh K,
    Littman DR, Fagarasan S: Requirement for lymphoid tissue-inducer cells in
    isolated follicle formation and T cell-independent immunoglobulin A
    generation in the gut. *Immunity* 2008, 29(2):261–271.
28. Satoh-Takayama N, Vosshenrich CA, Lesjean-Pottier S, Sawa S, Lochner M,
    Rattis F, Mention JJ, Thiam K, Cerf-Bensussan N, Mandelboim O, Eberl G, Di
    Santo JP: Microbial flora drives interleukin 22 production in intestinal
    NKp46+ cells that provide innate mucosal immune defense. *Immunity*
    2008, 29(6):958–970.
29. Satpathy AT, Briseno CG, Lee JS, Ng D, Manieri NA, Kc W, Wu X, Thomas SR,
    Lee WL, Turkoz M, McDonald KG, Meredith MM, Song C, Guidos CJ,
    Newberry RD, Ouyang W, Murphy TL, Stappenbeck TS, Gommerman JL,
    Nussenzweig MC, Colonna M, Kopan R, Murphy KM: Notch2-dependent
    classical dendritic cells orchestrate intestinal immunity to attaching-and-
    effacing bacterial pathogens. *Nat Immunol* 2013, 14(9):937–948.
30. Sawa S, Lochner M, Satoh-Takayama N, Dulauroy S, Berard M, Kleinschek M,
    Cua D, Di Santo JP, Eberl G: RORgammat + innate lymphoid cells regulate
    intestinal homeostasis by integrating negative signals from the
    symbiotic microbiota. *Nat Immunol* 2011, 12(4):320–326.
31. Hepworth MR, Monticelli LA, Fung TC, Ziegler CG, Grunberg S, Sinha R,
    Mantegazza AR, Ma HL, Crawford A, Angelosanto JM, Wherry EJ, Koni PA,
    Bushman FD, Elson CO, Eberl G, Artis D, Sonnenberg GF: Innate lymphoid
    cells regulate CD4+ T-cell responses to intestinal commensal bacteria.
    Nature 2013, 498(7452):113–117.
32. Wong SH, Walker JA, Jolin HE, Drynan LF, Hams E, Camelo A, Barlow JL, Neill
    DR, Panova V, Koch U, Radtke F, Hardman CS, Hwang YY, Fallon PG,
    McKenzie AN: Transcription factor RORα is critical for nuocyte
    development. *Nat Immunol* 2012, 13(3):229–236.
33. Yang Q, Monticelli LA, Saenz SA, Chi AW, Sonnenberg GF, Tang J, De
    Obaldia ME, Bailis W, Bryson JL, Toscano K, Huang J, Haczku A, Pear WS,
    Artis D, Bhandoola A: T cell factor 1 is required for group 2 innate
    lymphoid cell generation. *Immunity* 2013, 38(4):694–704.
34. Klein Wolterink RG, Serafini N, van Nimwegen M, Vosshenrich CA, de Bruijn
    MJ, Fonseca Pereira D, Veiga Fernandes H, Hendriks RW, Di Santo JP:

Essential, dose-dependent role for the transcription factor Gata3 in the development of IL-5+ and IL-13+ type 2 innate lymphoid cells. *Proc Natl Acad Sci U S A* 2013, **110**(25):10240–10245.

35. Furusawa J, Moro K, Motomura Y, Okamoto K, Zhu J, Takayanagi H, Kubo M, Koyasu S: Critical role of p38 and GATA3 in natural helper cell function. *J Immunol* 2013, **191**(4):1818–1826.

36. Mjösberg J, Bernink J, Golebski K, Karrich JJ, Peters CP, Blom B, te Velde AA, Fokkens WJ, van Drunen CM, Spits H: The transcription factor GATA3 is essential for the function of human type 2 innate lymphoid cells. *Immunity* 2012, **37**(4):649–659.

37. Doherty TA, Khorram N, Chang JE, Kim HK, Rosenthal P, Croft M, Broide DH: STAT6 regulates natural helper cell proliferation during lung inflammation initiated by Alternaria. *Am J Physiol Lung Cell Mol Physiol* 2012, **303**(7):L577–L588.

38. Yang Q, Saenz SA, Zlotoff DA, Artis D, Bhandoola A: Cutting edge: natural helper cells derive from lymphoid progenitors. *J Immunol* 2011, **187**(11):5505–5509.

39. Salimi M, Barlow JL, Saunders SP, Xue L, Gutowska-Owsiak D, Wang X, Huang LC, Johnson D, Scanlon ST, McKenzie AN, Fallon PG, Ogg GS: A role for IL-25 and IL-33-driven type-2 innate lymphoid cells in atopic dermatitis. *J Exp Med* 2013, **210**(13):2939–2950.

40. Xue L, Salimi M, Panse I, Mjosberg JM, McKenzie AN, Spits H, Klenerman P, Ogg G: Prostaglandin D2 activates group 2 innate lymphoid cells through chemoattractant receptor-homologous molecule expressed on TH2 cells. *J Allergy Clin Immunol* 2014, **133**(4):1184–1194.

41. Teunissen MB, Munneke JM, Bernink JH, Spuls PI, Res PC, Te Velde A, Cheuk S, Brouwer MW, Menting SP, Eidsmo L, Spits H, Hazenberg MD, Mjosberg J: Composition of innate lymphoid cell subsets in the human skin: enrichment of NCR ILC3 in lesional skin and blood of psoriasis patients. *J Invest Dermatol* 2014, **134**(9):2351–2360.

42. Kim BS, Siracusa MC, Saenz SA, Noti M, Monticelli LA, Sonnenberg GF, Hepworth MR, Van Voorhees AS, Comeau MR, Artis D: TSLP elicits IL-33-independent innate lymphoid cell responses to promote skin inflammation. *Sci Transl Med* 2013, **5**(170):170ra116.

43. Barnig C, Cernadas M, Dutile S, Liu X, Perrella MA, Kazani S, Wechsler ME, Israel E, Levy BD: Lipoxin A4 regulates natural killer cell and type 2 innate lymphoid cell activation in asthma. *Sci Transl Med* 2013, **5**(174):174ra126.

44. Leung DY, Boguniewicz M, Howell MD, Nomura I, Hamid QA: New insights into atopic dermatitis. *J Clin Invest* 2004, **113**(5):651–657.

45. Imai Y, Yasuda K, Sakaguchi Y, Haneda T, Mizutani H, Yoshimoto T, Nakanishi K, Yamanishi K: Skin-specific expression of IL-33 activates group 2 innate lymphoid cells and elicits atopic dermatitis-like inflammation in mice. *Proc Natl Acad Sci U S A* 2013, **110**(34):13921–13926.

46. Villanova F, Flutter B, Tosi I, Grys K, Sreeneebus H, Perera GK, Chapman A, Smith CH, Di Meglio P, Nestle FO: Characterization of innate lymphoid cells in human skin and blood demonstrates increase of NKp44+ ILC3 in psoriasis. *J Invest Dermatol* 2014, **134**(4):984–991.

47. Dyring-Andersen B, Geisler C, Agerbeck C, Lauritsen JP, Gudjonsdottir SD, Skov L, Bonefeld CM: Increased number and frequency of group 3 innate lymphoid cells in nonlesional psoriatic skin. *Br J Dermatol* 2014, **170**(3):609–616.

Longitudinal, mixed method study to look at the experiences and knowledge of non melanoma skin cancer from diagnosis to one year

Fiona Bath-Hextall[1*], Claire Jenkinson[5], Arun Kumar[1], Jo Leonardi-Bee[3], William Perkins[4], Karen Cox[1] and Cris Glazebrook[2]

Abstract

Background: Skin cancer is the most common type of cancer in humans and the incidence is increasing worldwide. Our objective was to understanding the needs, experiences and knowledge of individuals with Non Melanoma Skin Cancer (NMSC) from diagnosis up until one year.

Methods: Patients with NMSC completed questionnaires at diagnosis, treatment, 8 weeks post treatment and 12 months post diagnosis. Body image, psychological morbidity and Quality of Life (QOL) were assessed at each time point, with the exception of QOL that was not assessed at diagnosis. Knowledge of NMSC was assessed at baseline and 8 weeks. A sub-sample of participants was also interviewed to allow a more in-depth exploration of patients' experiences.

Results: 76 participants completed the initial questionnaire, of which 15 were interviewed. Patients were anxious about a diagnosis of skin cancer, however they were no more depressed or anxious than the general population. QOL significantly improved from diagnosis to 8 weeks and from diagnosis to one year. Knowledge of NMSC was poor and did not improve after treatment. Hairdressers were highlighted as playing an important role in raising awareness and encouraging individuals to seek medical help. Most participants were aware of the need to check their skin for suspicious lesions but were not sure what to look for. At one year participants had forgotten their experience and were not overly concerned about skin cancer.

Conclusion: There is a need to raise awareness of the signs and symptoms of NMSC. Information on skin cancer needs to be tailored to the individual both at the start of treatment and during the follow up months, ensuring that participants' needs and expectations are met. Targeting education at individuals in the community who regularly come into contact with skin should help in early identification of NMSC. This is important since skin cancer caught early is easily treatable and delay in presentation leads to larger and more complex lesions which impacts in terms of increased morbidity and increased health care costs.

Keywords: Skin cancer, Non melanoma skin cancer, NMSC, Needs, Experiences, Knowledge

Background

Skin cancer is the most common type of cancer in humans [1], accounting for 20% of all cancers diagnosed in the UK. Around 97% of skin cancers are epithelial in origin and are either basal cell carcinomas (BCCs) or squamous cell carcinomas (SCCs), collectively known as non-melanoma skin cancer (NMSC). A systematic review of the worldwide incidence of Non Melanoma Skin Cancer (NMSC) [2] has shown that the incidence of NMSC varies widely with highest rates in Australia (> 1000/ 100,000 person-years for BCC) and lowest rates in parts of Africa (< 1/100,000 person-years for BCC). The average incidence rates in England were 76.21/100,000 persons and 22.65/100,000 persons for BCC and SCC respectively. The incidence rates in the UK appear to be increasing at a greater rate when compared to the rest of Europe. NMSC is most common in older age groups but the incidence of BCC is increasing in the young [3-6]. There are many

* Correspondence: fiona.bath-hextall@nottingham.ac.uk
[1]School of Health Sciences, Faculty of Medicine & Health Sciences, University of Nottingham, Queen's Medical Centre, Nottingham NG7 2UH, UK
Full list of author information is available at the end of the article

options for the treatment of NMSC and these have been reviewed elsewhere [7-9].

The National Institute for Clinical Excellence (NICE) guidelines for improving care of people with skin tumours [10] highlighted a lack of research into the needs and experiences of people with skin cancer and the need for high quality patient information.

A systematic review looking at qualitative research alone [11] found only two papers that examined the needs and experiences of people with skin cancer (melanoma and/or non-melanoma skin cancer). The studies identified by the review focused mainly on melanoma skin cancer and did not investigate patients' perceptions of their information, support, and decision making needs over the course of their illness, or the extent to which these had been met. A study in 40 patients exploring patients' understanding of pigmented skin lesions and skin cancer concluded that changing moles were often perceived as trivial and not signifying possible skin cancer [12]. A recently published study looked at 982 consecutive American patients presenting for Mohs micrographic surgery for NMSC and found that 71% of people delayed going to their doctor with NMSC because they were in denial about the severity of their condition [13]. It is known that early diagnosis can dramatically improve prognosis and the patient experience since early lesions are treated more simply compared with larger or neglected lesions [13]. It has been shown that patients with melanoma, BCC and SCC experience similar levels of anxiety and depression after diagnosis and treatment [14], and surgery for skin cancer has been shown to impact on their appearance [15]. Health professionals working with skin cancer patients need to understand the psychosocial concerns of this patient group in order to design services appropriately and to provide patients with the support they need and information that they can easily understand. The patient experience is an important component in the evidence based cycle. Research in this area has predominantly focused on malignant melanoma. This study combines both quantitative and qualitative methods to follow skin cancer patients on their journey from diagnosis to one year post diagnosis.

Methods

A mixed method study, using postal questionnaires and semi structured interviews. Our objective was to understand the needs, experiences and knowledge of individuals with Non Melanoma Skin Cancer (NMSC) from diagnosis up until one year.

Consecutive patients, referred from primary care, attending a skin cancer clinic in a large teaching hospital in the East Midlands over an 8 month period in 2008/9 with a new clinical diagnosis of NMSC, were invited to take part in the study. No recurrent cases were included however patients with previous skin cancer were not excluded.

Ethical approval was obtained from the Nottingham Research Ethics Committee 1 (08/H0403/83) and signed consent was obtained from all participants.

Questionnaires (Additional files 1 and 2) were sent to patients at four time points: baseline (just after diagnosis, usually the next day), treatment (same day or next day), 8 weeks post-treatment and 12 months from baseline. Body image and psychological morbidity were assessed at each time point using the *Derriford Appearance Scale 24 (DAS24)* [16] and the *Hospital Anxiety and Depression Scale (HADS)* [17]. Knowledge of NMSC was assessed at baseline and 8 weeks post-treatment. This instrument was adapted from the melanoma knowledge questionnaire [18] in consultation with dermatologists and piloted prior to use. Demographics and sun exposure data were collected at baseline and participants' concerns about how NMSC affected their quality of life were assessed after treatment, 8 weeks post-treatment and at 12 months from baseline using the *Skin Cancer Index (SCI)* [19]. See study flow chart, Figure 1. SCI was not assessed at baseline as the questions were deemed inappropriate for patients who had just received a diagnosis of NMSC.

We invited all participants to take part in an interview. Purposive sampling ensured we captured a proportion of younger people (< 60 yrs). Interviews were designed to elicit in-depth views, perceptions and descriptions of the experience of being treated for NMSC, recovery from treatment and feelings 12 months after diagnosis. A flexible interview guide (Additional file 3) was used to ensure consistency across the interviews while allowing interviewees to express their ideas, understanding and concerns freely.

Anxiety and Depression were measured using the Hospital Anxiety and Depression Scale (HADS), a 14-item self-rating scale, with questions pertaining to the past week, in medical outpatients, primary care and community settings, which have been validated for cancer patients. The HADS was answered by the participant on a four-point (0–3) response category with a possible score of 0 to 21 for anxiety (7 items) and for depression (7 items). For each construct, a score below 8 was classified as 'normal', 8–10 as 'borderline' and above 10 as 'caseness' (probable presence of disorder).

The Derriford Appearance Scale (DAS24) is a 24-item scale designed to measure distress and dysfunction in relation to problems of appearance. Some of the items request a response about the intensity of emotional response, using response categories of 'extremely' to 'not at all' (e.g. 'How distressed do you get when you see yourself in the mirror/window?'). Other items ask about the frequency of particular behaviours indicative of a self-conscious response (e.g. 'I avoid going out of the house'), using an 'almost always' to 'never/almost never' set of response categories. Where appropriate, a response of 'not applicable' is allowed. There is no threshold score or cut-off point to indicate 'caseness'.

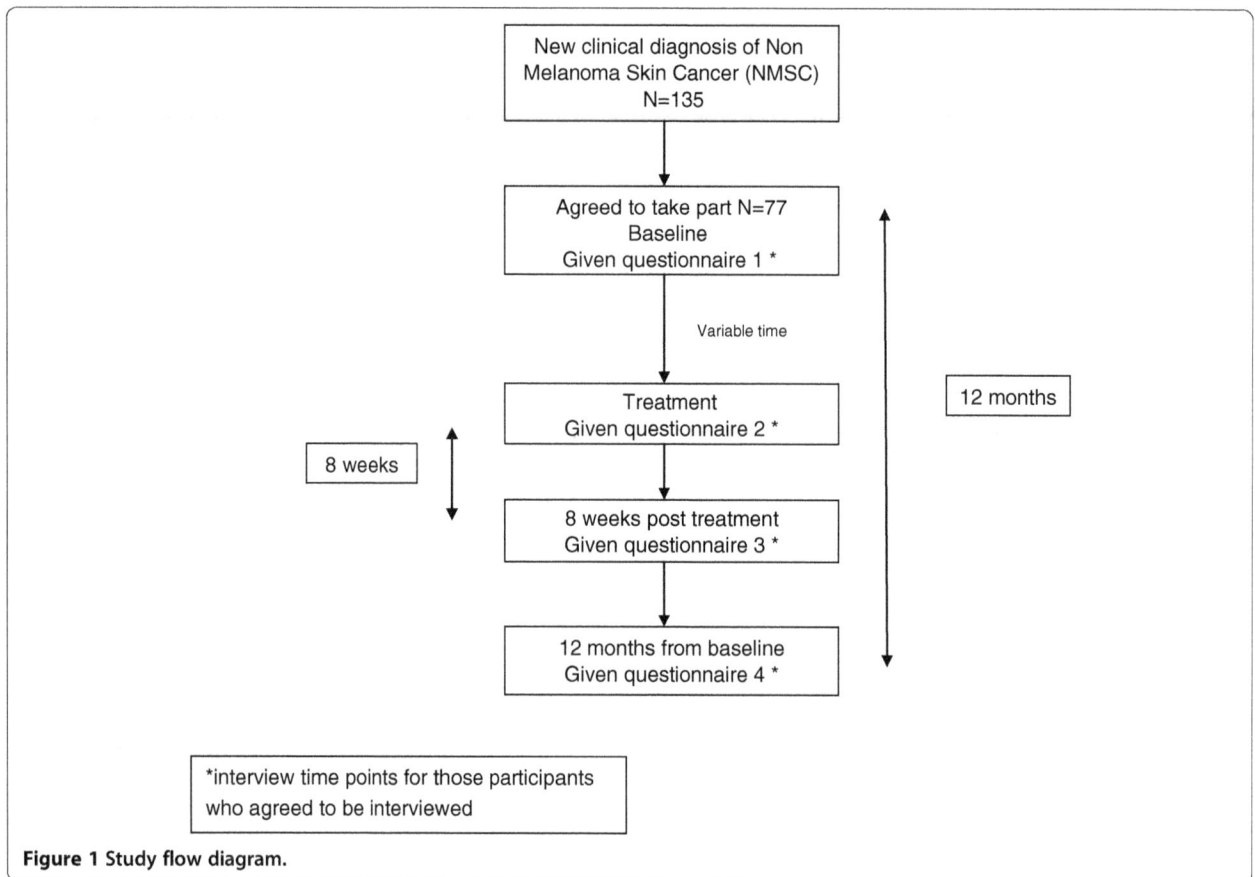

Figure 1 Study flow diagram.

The minimum score is 11 and the maximum is 96 (highest distress/dysfunction).

Knowledge of NMSC was ascertained using three free-response questions to assess knowledge about how to reduce risk from NMSC (one mark for each of avoiding sunburn, not using sun beds, checking skin frequently), what type of people are at risk of NMSC (one mark for each of fair skin, sunbather, work outdoors, use of sun beds, previous skin cancer/family history of skin cancer, older age), and early skin signs of NMSC (one mark for stating any of the following: lump/pearly lump/change in lump/sore/unusual area/new area/recently grown plus one mark for mentioning a surface change that is non-healing : crusting, scabbing, bleeding plus half a mark for using the word raised). The maximum possible score is 11.5.

The Skin Cancer Index (SCI) is a 15 item, validated, disease-specific QOL instrument with 3 distinct subscales, Emotion, Social, and Appearance. Higher scores reflect better quality of life [20]. Summary statistics were computed for each SCI question, the three SCI subscale totals, and the overall SCI total. The subscales were transformed so that each subscale, and the total, was between 0 and 100.

All quantitative analyses was performed using SPSS version 16.0. Summary statistics were computed for the HADS anxiety and depression, DAS24, Knowledge of

NMSC, and total SCI. 95% confidence intervals for the means of each outcome were calculated at various time points and for the change over time windows. We used paired t test for examining the HADS, DAS24 and also the SCI index. We calculated the mean change in HADS anxiety and depression and DAS24 across three different time windows: baseline – 12 months post baseline, treatment – eight weeks post treatment, and treatment – 12 months post baseline. We also calculated the mean change in SCI across 2 different time windows: treatment - 8 weeks post treatment and treatment - 12 months post baseline.

Interviews were transcribed and analysed using thematic content analysis [21]. The qualitative data analysis package NVivo8 was used to deductively and inductively derive codes and check that these harmonized with the context of the interview statement. Codes were grouped into clusters and categorised into major themes. Members of the team collectively analysed and discussed the emerging themes.

Results

One hundred and thirty five patients with an initial clinical diagnosis of NMSC were referred to the researcher by the clinician of whom 77 (57%) agreed to take part in the study and returned a consent form. The clinical diagnosis was confirmed in all but one person who was then excluded. The mean age of the group was 70 years (range 35–89), 40 (53%) were male and a quarter reported having had a previous skin cancer. BCC was the most common (80%), the majority of which were on the head or neck, Table 1. Twenty nine percent of the participants had outdoor occupations and 20% of participants had lived abroad. Over half of the participants had sunburn (causing pain/discomfort/peeling) as a child (32% had 1–2 episodes and 25% had > = 3 episodes). Seventeen percent had sunburn in the last two years (38% were under 60 years of age and 12% were over 60 years of age). Seventy seven percent of participants spent between 1–4 weeks on holiday and 11% spent between 5–12 weeks on holiday. Seven percent of participants aged > 60 yrs frequently sunbathed compared to 14% in the 40–60 year olds and 33% of those < 40 yrs. Of the participants who sunbathed, 78% used sunscreen although most participants were unsure as to the SPF.

The time from first clinic visit to treatment varied from 0 to 159 days (median 41 days, IQR 23.5 - 57.5 days). Sixty-eight participants were treated by excision, one was treated by excision followed by radiotherapy and 8 were treated by Mohs micrographic surgery. The mean time from diagnosis to treatment for Mohs micrographic surgery was 101 days (SD 33.33, range 47–159 days). The mean time from diagnosis to treatment for excision was 37.18 days. Two patients received diagnosis and treatment on the same day and resultant histology confirmed their clinical diagnosis. Participants' demographics and disease characteristics are shown in Table 1.

The mean age of the interviewees was 66 (range 39–88). Four were aged ≤ 60 years. Thirteen were clinically diagnosed with BCC and 2 with SCC. Six participants (40%) were male and 3 (20%) reported having had a previous skin cancer. The site of skin cancer was located on the head for all but one interviewee whose lesion was on the torso. Ten of the participants sunbathed regularly, five had used sun beds, four had been sunburnt in the past 2 years, five spent more than 50% of their holidays abroad, three had lived abroad in hot countries and two remembered getting sunburnt as a child.

Quantitative results

Baseline, treatment, 8 weeks post-treatment and 12 months post-baseline questionnaires were returned by 76, 67, 67, and 66 participants respectively. A number of participants did not return the questionnaires at various time points but no reasons were given. A number of participants withdrew (one due to broken ankle, three due to a broken limb, one lesion was not a NMSC, one gave no reason and one died (not related to NMSC) 8 weeks post treatment.

Baseline scores for HADS anxiety and depression were classified as normal for 84% (anxiety) and 93% (depression) of the participants respectively. The DAS24 scores

were consistent with those reported by a general (non-patient) population (Table 1). Knowledge of NMSC was low (range 0–7.5) with a mean total score of 3.28/11.5 (SD 1.61). There were no significant gender differences with respect to anxiety (p = 0.087), depression (p = 0.274), DAS24 (p = 0.213), or knowledge (p = 0.371). Knowledge was no better in participants who had previously had a skin cancer. A significant positive correlation was found between age and depression with older people having higher depression scores (Rs = 0.374, p = 0.001). A significant positive correlation was seen between the HADS Anxiety score and DAS24 score (Rs = 0.454, p < 0.001), with those with higher DAS24 scores (poorer body image) having a higher anxiety score.

Quality of life significantly improved from treatment to 8 weeks post treatment (p = 0.034) and from treatment to 12 months post baseline (p = 0.001) (Table 2). There was no significant change in body image from baseline to 12 months post baseline or from treatment to 8 weeks post treatment (Table 2). There was no significant change in knowledge of NMSC from baseline to 8 weeks post treatment (Table 3).

Although mean anxiety and depression scores were in the normal range (≤ 8.0) at each time point (Table 2), we found that patients became even less anxious (p = 0.003) and depressed (p = 0.003) 12 months post diagnosis (Table 2).

Qualitative results

Forty one participants (53%) consented to be interviewed. Of these 15 were interviewed. These 15 were selected to give us a broad a range of views and experiences as possible covering gender, age (above and below 60). The interviews were conducted over the telephone with the exception of one interviewee who was interviewed face to face. The interviews were audio-taped and fully transcribed. There were no significant differences in demographics between the participants interviewed and those comprising the whole study.

At baseline (just after diagnosis) four major themes emerged from analysis of the 15 interviewees : *Chance and cue to action*; *Rationalisation for delay in seeking medical help*; *Reaction to clinical diagnosis* and *I'm quite aware now*. The themes and their variations are described below and highlighted by comments from interviewees.

Chance and cue to action

Participants were asked what prompted them to go to their doctor. Reasons included the inability of their skin condition to heal completely and the persistent cycle of bleeding, scab formation and re-emergence. Others recalled visiting their general practitioner for some other reason and just mentioning in passing a skin condition that they were not particularly concerned about. A number of participants

Table 1 Demographic characteristic of participants

Characteristics	No (%) of participants
Age, yrs	
30-49	5 (7)
50-59	11 (15)
60-69	15 (20)
70-79	28 (37)
80-89	17 (22)
Sex	
Male	40 (53)
Female	36 (47)
Marital status	
Single	5 (7)
Married	47 (62)
Living with partner	5 (7)
Widowed	14 (8)
Divorced	5 (7)
Previous skin cancer	
No	56 (74)
Yes	19 (25)
Missing	1 (1)
Histology	
BCC	61 (80)
SCC	14 (18)
Missing	1 (1)
Site	
Head/neck	60 (79)
Rest of body	15 (20)
Missing	1 (1)
Diameter (mm)	
1-4	12 (16)
5-9	36 (47)
> = 10	19 (25)
Missing	9 (12)
HADS	Median (IQR) 6.0 (1–11)
Anxiety	
0-7	63 (84)
8-10	8 (11)
> = 11	4 (5)
	Median (IQR) 3.0 (1–6)
Depression	
0-7	70 (93)
8-10	2 (3)

Table 1 Demographic characteristic of participants *(Continued)*

> = 11	3 (4)
	Median (IQR) 2.0 (0–5)
DAS-24 (N = 69)	Mean (SD) 23.7 (8.8)

SD standard deviation.
BCC Basal Cell Carcinoma.
SCC Squamous Cell Carcinoma.

said that their hairdresser (13%) had drawn their attention to the skin lesion and suggested they went to see their general practitioner. Other individuals who encouraged participants to seek advice included a community skin cancer specialist (7%), a dentist (7%) and a friend (7%). A number of participants (some of whom had a previous experience of skin cancer), visited their general practitioner without prompting (66%).

> *"My hairdresser said to me, a few weeks ago, "The next time you go to the doctor's mention the mark on your temple," he said, "because I don't like the looks of it"… and it wasn't until I went to the doctor's about three weeks ago when I thought, "Oh", I said, "can you just have a look at this mark on my temple, the hairdresser told me to mention it to you." And he looked at it, and then he got a magnifying glass and he said, "I don't think it's anything to worry about but I'll refer you to a dermatologist…"*

F, 74, BCC

Rationalisation for delay in seeking medical help

Most participants found it difficult to remember exactly when they first noticed the lesion. A lack of awareness that it could be skin cancer was the main reason for delay. The majority were aware of the skin lesion and that it sometimes caused physical discomfort such as irritation or bleeding and failed to heal. The lesion was often attributed to being a minor skin condition, a symptom of old age that might heal on its own and nothing to worry about.

> *"I'd got a spot that was reoccurring and didn't know whether it was just old age or whether it was something that was untoward… I didn't really see it as a priority. I wish I'd have gone earlier but at the time didn't think it was anything."*

F, 39, BCC

> *"It's over five years because I'd had had this tiny red patch…I mean I'm saying five years, it could have been ten years… I just assumed it was definitely a*

Table 2 Changes in quantitative outcomes over time

Scale	Comparison Mean (95% CI)	P value
DAS-24	Baseline to 12 months post diagnosis (N = 59)	0.289
	23.9 (21.5,26.3) to 23.0 (20.9,25.2)	
	Treatment to 8 week post treatment (N = 61)	0.306
	23.0 (20.8,25.3) to 22.2 (20.2,24.2)	
HADS		
Anxiety	Baseline to 12 months post diagnosis (N = 62)	0.003
	3.6 (2.7,4.4) to 2.5 (1.8,3.3)	
	Treatment to 8 week post treatment (N = 59)	0.026
	3.1 (2.2,3.9) to 2.5 (1.7,3.2)	
Depression	Baseline to 12 months post diagnosis (N = 59)	0.003
	2.9 (2.0,3.7) to 1.9 (1.2,2.6)	
	Treatment to 8 week post treatment (N = 59)	0.848
	2.2 (1.5,2.9) to 2.2 (1.4,2.9)	
SCI	Treatment to 8 weeks post treatment (N = 63)	0.034
	78.21 (73.8, 82.6) to 82.3 (78.6, 85.9)	
	Treatment to 12 months post diagnosis (N = 57)	0.001
	78.4 (73.8, 83.0) to 85.5 (82.0, 89.0)	

little patch of eczema, so it never occurred to me that it could be skin cancer."

F, 67, BCC

Reaction to clinical diagnosis

The mention of the word 'cancer' caused alarm and concern for most participants. Concern was mainly about how long they had had the cancer and if it could have spread and if they had other undetected skin cancers. Appearance and potential disfigurement following treatment was another concern. All patients felt they had a good rapport with the dermatologist, however some participants felt their information needs had not been met and thought they should have received more information especially when some patients compared the information given to them with that given to patients with other types of cancer.

"You know, to the person who has actually got it it's not relatively minor... it's that big C word again, and while it's there it can spread. But that's a personal feeling of mine and I don't know how many people are diagnosed with this type of thing yearly but I bet most people feel the same."

M, 55, SCC

'I'm quite aware now'

Several participants felt that having experienced a NMSC they would generally know what to look for in future and would have the confidence to act more quickly in presenting to a general practitioner. Others were aware of the need to check the skin but were not sure what to look for. Some participants remained unaware that they needed to check their skin but some participants changed their behaviour.

"Well, I mean, yeah, if anything, I got a scab and I were picking it well I'd be straight to the doctors"

F, 69, BCC

"I wear cream all the time. I wear a hat all the time now as well. I don't sit in the sun, I used to years ago, I used to sit in the sun a lot, but I don't do that anymore."

F, 70, BCC

Immediately post treatment the themes to emerge were: *Treatment satisfaction; Appearance and information needs; Recurrence and new lesions; Increased awareness.*

Treatment satisfaction

All patients were satisfied with their care. For most, treatment satisfaction was associated with the knowledge that their skin cancer had been completely removed.

"The good thing is the bad stuff's gone and I'm not that vain, if you know what I mean."

M, 45, BCC

Table 3 Knowledge of Non Melanoma Skin Cancer (NMSC)

	Baseline	8 weeks after treatment	Mean difference (95% CI)*	P value for difference
Knowledge Category	n, Mean (SD)	n, Mean (SD)		
Reduce Risk	76, 1.00 (0.40)	67, 1.02 (0.41)	0.03 (−0.07-0.13)	0.57
Risk Type	76, 1.39 (0.97)	67, 1.30 (0.80)	−0.10 (−0.36-0.15)	0.42
Signs of NMSC	76, 0.89 (0.78)	67, 0.72 (0.70)	−0.19 (−0.41-0.04)	0.10
Total Knowledge	76, 3.28 (1.61)	67, 3.03 (1.28)	−0.32 (−0.69-0.05)	0.09

*Difference in scores based on 67 participants with baseline and 8 weeks after treatment scores.

Appearance and information needs

Potential disfigurement and scarring was a concern for many patients. Participants were concerned that they had no information about what was happening after the treatments.

"I was a little anxious because I didn't quite know what I was going to look like when I was finished."

F, 62, BCC

"Maybe a little bit more information about what the scar would feel like and look like and, you know, I'm not sure whether this lumpiness and the hardness of the scar is going to soften and go away or whether it's permanent".

F,67, BCC

Recurrence and new lesions

Patients were concerned that although the lesion had been removed, it might come back and they worried about further lumps and bumps.

"Well, it's just that, you know, I just hope that it's all gone and that it's not going to flare up again. I mean, I'm touching wood, I don't think it will do because I don't think it was that sort of thing, but there's bound to be doubts, small doubts, you know, even though people do try and reassure you. But hopefully everything will be okay."

F, 74, BCC

Increased awareness

Patients were more aware of skin cancer and were taking steps to avoid getting another lesion. They were checking for new lesions, although some were not sure what they were looking for. Participants also said they were spreading the word to others about the need to check their skin.

"... it has raised awareness significantly in our family now, yeah....I've been into town today and bought a moisturiser with SPF25 or something or other, so yeah. So I'll wear that constantly now rather than general moisturisers."

F, 39, BCC

"I am [checking], yes, but I'm not too sure what to look for.... Now if I see anything that's not, I'll be, instead of waiting I shall be straight to the doctor's and see what it is."

M, 45, BCC

8 weeks post treatment the main themes to emerge were: *Information needs about checking skin; Spreading the word.*

Patients understood the need to continue to check for further skin lesions although most were not sure what they were looking for. Many participants continued to spread the word about skin cancer advising others to seek medical advice regarding suspicious lesions.

Information needs about checking skin

"Well I mean in my experience the problem has not known what to look for. I mean if all these things were identical in appearance, then I would feel a lot easier. But by and large they've taken different forms, and it is a question of knowing what to look for ...."

M, 78, BCC

Speading the word

"One or two people I have spoken to and I've said, I did say look out for dubious looking spots and things that won't go away with ointments and things."

F, 79, BCC

12 months post baseline the main themes to emerge at one year post diagnosis were *Satisfaction* and *Not sure what to look for?*

One year on, most people were satisfied with the treatment and care they had received. They were happy that their NMSC had been completely removed and that any scaring had healed. Some participants continue to check their skin but were still not sure what to look for. Interestingly, when they spoke about skin cancer they spoke about moles despite having had a non melanoma skin cancer.

Satisfaction

"I'm fine, absolutely fine, I don't really think about it at all. I had this spot and they took it off and its fine. It doesn't worry me at all."

F, 64, BCC

Not sure what to look for?

"I wasn't really given any advice on checking it at all. You know, I was just told that it was sun damage on my face and on my nose but I wasn't given any advice on how to check it. I mean I know, I've read up a lot about it, so I know that I check

and then if there's things I can't see like my back, I get my husband to check, and I always check his regularly as well."

F, 70, BCC

Discussion

Although not a life threatening disease, a diagnosis of NMSC caused concern for many participants, and whilst this was not evident from the total quantitative data this was evident from those we interviewed. At diagnosis our participants were neither clinically anxious nor depressed; however, levels of anxiety were higher than levels of depression and 16% of our participants experienced significant levels of psychological distress. These results are similar to another study that found 19% of NMSC patient experienced significant levels of psychological distress [22]. Participants who were most anxious had a poorer body image although body image scores were not high and were representative of the general population who are not concerned about their appearance [16]. A review of psychological distress in patients with melanoma also found participants more anxious than depressed [23]. Our study participants were anxious at diagnosis when they heard the word cancer. They were concerned about how long they had had the cancer, whether it had spread and possible disfigurement. Eight weeks after treatment participants were significantly less anxious and when interviewed, said that the concerns they had at treatment no longer existed. By 12 months, participants had forgotten any concerns that they may have had. Anxiety, depression and quality of life all significantly improved post diagnosis.

Knowledge of NMSC was very poor, even among those who had skin cancer previously.

A telephone survey in recently treated Squamous Cell Carcinoma patients in Italy also found skin cancer knowledge to be low [24]. We found no significant difference in knowledge from diagnosis to 8 weeks post treatment. Participants told us that information given at diagnosis was not really considered as they were so shocked at hearing the word 'cancer' that everything went out of their head and they couldn't think of anything else. Lack of knowledge of NMSC most likely contributed to the delay in presentation for many of the participants with some not consulting a doctor for up to 2–5 years. Our study found lack of awareness to be one of the main reasons for delay. Despite participants being aware of their skin lesion for many years, most thought it was a sign of ageing or something that would go away despite in many cases the lesion repeatedly bleeding and failing to heal and despite self-treating with various creams. A recent study [13] in patients presenting for Mohs micrographic surgery for NMSC found similar reasons for delay in presentation, however they did not look at what prompted people to eventually seek advice. We found many participants only consulted a doctor after others such as hairdressers, dentist, or friends had encouraged them to do so. Knowledge is a necessary prerequisite for anyone to be able to interpret a symptom as a signal of cancer or to judge it as serious and requiring medical attention [25].

Hairdressers were highlighted in this study as playing an important role in raising awareness and encouraging their clients to seek medical help. A recent study that surveyed hair professionals provides evidence that hair professionals would be receptive to skin cancer education especially as they are already looking for suspicious lesions on customers' scalp, neck, and face and are acting as lay skin cancer educators [26]. The regular contact hairdressers have with their clients ensures familiarity with their clients' skin and therefore they are in a good position to see unusual changes on the head and neck. These findings add to the evidence that educating people about skin cancer is crucial in identifying and thus appropriately treating the disease [27]. Two recently published commentaries have considered the possibility of utilizing hairdressers for early detection of head and neck melanoma [28] and have suggested that hair salon operators should perform opportunistic surveillance of their clients to recognise suspicious lesions and then advise that they see their doctor [29].

The main concern of our patients at 12 months after diagnosis was that they were still not sure if they would recognise skin changes that might be skin cancer. It is interesting to note that whilst most of our participants at 12 months were still aware of the need to be cautious in the sun, they talked about checking skin for moles with no mention of Non Melanoma Skin Cancer. Knowledge of the risk factors for skin cancer has been found to increase skin surveillance, which in turn is associated with thinner melanoma tumours [30].

Despite there being no change in body image over the course of the study, participants continued to be concerned about their appearance at 8 weeks post treatment.

Quality of life of our participants improved significantly over time and like those in the SCI validation study by Rhee et al., [19] were skewed to the upper range. Our 8 week post-treatment mean total SCI of 82.2 is 6% higher than the 16 week post-surgery score (77.3) in Rhee's study of 183 patients with a biopsy proven NMSC of the face or neck referred to a dermatological Mohs micrographic surgery clinic. Our group was older, had a higher percentage of men and relatively few patients underwent Mohs micrographic surgery, factors which may account for our relatively high quality of life scores.

Strengths and limitations

A strength of our study was that we were able to follow participants over time from diagnosis through treatment and a year following diagnosis. A limitation of this study may be that we recruited from only one out-patient clinic; patients are, however, referred to this large teaching hospital from a very wide area and are representative of the general population. Another limitation may be that we adapted the knowledge questionnaire from a melanoma knowledge questionnaire, although upmost care was taken in doing this in close consultation with clinicians.

Conclusions

Information on skin cancer needs to be tailored to the individual both at the start of treatment and during the follow up months, ensuring that the participants' needs and expectations are met. There is a real need to raise awareness of the signs and symptoms of NMSC especially in elderly populations. Knowledge about recognising the signs of skin cancer is particularly important since 44% of patients will develop additional lesions within 3 years [31]. Targeting education at individuals in the community who regularly come into contact with skin should help in early identification of NMSC. This is important since skin cancers caught early are easily treatable and delay in presentation leads to larger and more complex lesions which in turn may increase patient morbidity and increased health care costs.

Abbreviations
NMSC: Non melanoma skin cancer; QOL: Quality of life; BCC: Basal cell carcinoma; SCC: Squamous cell carcinoma; DAS24: Derriford appearance scale 24; HADS: Hospital anxiety and depression scale; SCI: Skin cancer index.

Competing interest
All authors declare that they have no competing interest.

Authors' contributions
FB-H conceived the study, participated in its design and coordination, was involved in the acquisition of data, analysis, drafting of the initial paper and critically revised the manuscript for important intellectual content. WP contributed to the design of the study, acquisition of data and revised the manuscript critically for important intellectual and clinical content. CJ participated in acquisition of data, analysis, and initial draft of paper and critically revised the manuscript for important intellectual content. AK participated in acquisition of data, analysis and critically revised the manuscript for important intellectual content. JL-B participated in the quantitative data analysis and critically revised the manuscript for important intellectual content. KC participated in the design of the study, the qualitative analysis and revised the manuscript critically for important intellectual content. All authors approved the final version to be published.

Acknowledgements
We thank all the staff at the Treatment Centre and we especially thank all the participants. We also thank our citizen participant, Mrs J Foster, for her invaluable contribution to the design of the study.
Funded by: The Burdett Trust for Nursing: 41 Tower Hill, London, EC3N 4SG.

Author details
[1]School of Health Sciences, Faculty of Medicine & Health Sciences, University of Nottingham, Queen's Medical Centre, Nottingham NG7 2UH, UK. [2]Division of Psychiatry, School of Community Health Sciences, Queen's Medical Centre, Nottingham NG7 2UH, UK. [3]Division of Epidemiology and Public Health, Clinical Sciences Building, City Hospital, Nottingham NG5 1PB, UK. [4]Department of Dermatology, Queen's Medical Centre, University Hospital, Nottingham NG7 2UH, UK. [5]Nottingham Clinical Trials Unit, University of Nottingham, Queen's Medical Centre, Nottingham NG7 2UH, UK.

References
1. Martinez J, Otey C: The management of melanoma and nonmelanoma skin cancer: a review for the primary care physician. *Mayo Clin Proc* 2001, **76**(12):1253–1265.
2. Lomas A: A systematic Review of worldwide incidence of Non-melanoma skin cancer. *British Journal Dermatology* 2012, **166**(5):1069–1080.
3. Bath-Hextall F, Leonardi-Bee J, Smith C, Meal A, Hubbard R: Trends in incidence of basal cell carcinoma; Additional evidence from a UK-primary care database study. *Int J Cancer* 2007, **121**:2105–2108.
4. Christenson L, Borrowman T, Vachon C, Tellefson M, Otley C, Weaver A, Roenigk R: Incidence of basal cell and squamous cell carcinomas in a population younger than 40 years. *JAMA* 2005, **294**:681–690.
5. de Vries E, van de Poll-Franse L, Louwman W, de Gruijl F, Coebergh J: Predictions of skin cancer incidence in the Netherlands up to 2015. *Br J Dermatol* 2005, **152**:481–488.
6. Skellett A, Hafiji J, Greenberg D, Wright K, Levell N: The incidence of basal cell carcinoma in the under-30s in the UK. *Clin Exp Dermatol* 2012, **37**:227–229.
7. Bath-Hextall F, Perkins W, Bong J, Williams H: Interventions for basal cell carcinoma of the skin. *Cochrane Database Syst Rev* 2007(1). Art.No.: CD003412.DOI:10.1002/14651858.CD003412.pub2.
8. Lansbury L, Leonardi-Bee J, Perkins W, Goodacre T, Tweed JA, Bath-Hextall FJ: Interventions for non-metastatic squamous cell carcinoma of the skin. *Cochrane Database Syst Rev* 2010(4). Art. No.: CD007869. DOI: 10.1002/14651858.CD007869.pub2.
9. Bath-Hextall F, PERKINS W: Skin Cancer Awareness. *Geriatric Medicine* 2009, **39**(7):364–400.
10. National Institute for Health and Clinical Excellence: *Improving Outcomes for people with Skin Tumours including Melanoma*. London: NICE; 2006.
11. Barker J, Kumar A, Stanton W, Bath-Hextall F: The needs and experiences of people with a diagnosis of skin cancer: a systematic review. *The JBI Library of Systematic Reviews* 2011, **9**(4):104–121.
12. Walter F, Humphrys E, Tso S, Johnson M, Cohn S: Patient understanding of moles and skin cancer, and factors influencing presentation in primary care: a qualitative study. *BMC Fam Pract* 2010, **11**:62.
13. Alam M, Goldberg L, Silapunt S, Gardner E, Strom S, Rademaker A, Margolis D: Delayed treatment and continued growth of nonmelanoma skin cancer. *J Am Acad Dermatol* 2011, **64**:839–848.
14. Winterbottom A, Harcourt D: Patients experiences of the diagnosis and treatment of skin cancer. *J Adv Nurs* 2004, **48**(3):226–233.
15. Cassileth B, Lusk E, Tenaglia A: Patients' perceptions of the cosmetic impact of melanom resection. *Plastic Reconstructive Surgery* 1983, **71**(1):73–75.
16. Carr T, Moss T, Harris D: The DAS24: a short form of the Derriford Appearance Scale DAS59 to measure individual responses to living with problems of appearance. *Br J Health Psychol* 2005, **10**(2):285–298.
17. Zigmond A, Snaith R: The hospital anxiety and drpression scale. *Acta Psychiatr Scand* 1983, **67**:361–370.
18. GLAZEBROOK C, Garrud P, Avery A, Coupland C, Williams H: Impact of multimedia intervention"Skinsafe" on patients' knowledge and protective behaviours. *Preventative Medicine* 2006, **42**(6):449–454.
19. Rhee JSMB, Neuburg M, Logan BR, Burzynski M, Nattinger AB: Validation of a quality-of-life instrument for patients with Nonmelanoma skin cancer. *Arch Facial Plast Surg* 2006, **8**:314–318.
20. Rhee JSMB, Neuburg M, Logan BR, Burzynski M, Nattinger AB: The skin cancer index: clinical responsiveness and predictors of quality of life. *Laryngoscope* 2007, **117**(3):399–405.

21. Braun V, Clarke V: **Using thematic analysis in psychology.** *Qual Res Psychol* 2006, **3**(2):77–101.
22. Roberts N, Czajkowska Z, Radiotis G, Korner A: **Distress and coping strategies among patients with skin cancer.** *J Clin Psychol Med Settings* 2013, **20**(2):209–214. doi: 10.1007/s10880-012-9319-y.
23. Kasparian N, McLoone J, Butow P: **Psychological responses and coping stategies among patients with malignant melanoma.** *Arch Dermatol* 2009, **145**(12):1415–1426.
24. Renzi C, Mastroeni S, Mannooranparampil T, Passarelli F, Caggiati A, Potenza C, Pasquini P: **Delay in diagnosis and treatment of squamous cell carcinoma of the skin.** *Acta Derm Venereol* 2010, **90**:595–601.
25. De Nooijer J, Lechner L, De Vries H: **A qualitative study on detecting cancer symptoms and seeking medical help: an application of Andersen's model of total patient delay.** *Patient Educ Couns* 2001, **42**:145–157.
26. Bailey E, Marghoob A, Orengo I, Testa M, White V, Geller A: **Skin cancer knowledge, attitudes, and behaviours in the salon.** *Arch Dermatol* 2011, **147**(10):1159–1165.
27. Schofield P, Freeman J, Dixon H, Borland R, Hill D: **Trends in sun protection ehaviour among Australian young adults.** *Health Promot* 2001, **25**(1):62–65.
28. Roosta N, Wong M, Woodley D: **Utilizing hairdressers for early detection of head and neck melanoma: an untapped resource.** *J Am Acad Dermatol* 2012, **66**:687–688.
29. Mostow E: **Practice gaps. Skin cancer detection in hair salons: opportunity knocking:comment on "skin cancer knowledge, attitudes, and behaviours in the salon'.** *Arch Dermatol* 2011, **147**(10):1159–1165.
30. Oliveria S, Christos P: **Patient knowledge, awareness, and delay in seeking medical attention for malignant melanoma.** *J Clin Epidemiol* 1999, **52**(11):1111–1116.
31. Marcil I, Stern R: **Risk of developing a subsequent nonmelanoma skin cancer in patients with a history of nonmelanoma skin cancer.** *Arch Dermatol* 2000, **136**:1524–1530.

miR-125b induces cellular senescence in malignant melanoma

Anne Marie Nyholm[1], Catharina M Lerche[1], Valentina Manfé[1], Edyta Biskup[1], Peter Johansen[2], Niels Morling[2], Birthe Mørk Thomsen[3], Martin Glud[1] and Robert Gniadecki[1*]

Abstract

Background: Micro RNAs (miRs) have emerged as key regulators during oncogenesis. They have been found to regulate cell proliferation, differentiation, and apoptosis. Mir-125b has been identified as an oncomir in various forms of tumours, but we have previously proposed that miR-125b is a suppressor of lymph node metastasis in cutaneous malignant melanoma. Our goal was therefore to further examine this theory.

Methods: We used in-situ-hybridization to visualise miR-125b expression in primary tumours and in lymph node metastasis. Then using a miRVector plasmid containing a miR-125b-1 insert we transfected melanoma cell line Mel-Juso and then investigated the effect of the presence of a stable overexpression of miR-125b on growth by western blotting, flow cytometry and β-galactosidase staining. The tumourogenicity of the transfected cells was tested using a murine model and the tumours were further examined with in-situ-hybridization.

Results: In primary human tumours and in lymph node metastases increased expression of miR-125b was found in single, large tumour cells with abundant cytoplasm. A stable overexpression of miR-125b in human melanoma cell line Mel-Juso resulted in a G0/G1 cell cycle block and emergence of large cells expressing senescence markers: senescence-associated beta-galactosidase, p21, p27 and p53. Mel-Juso cells overexpressing miR-125b were tumourigenic in mice, but the tumours exhibited higher level of cell senescence and decreased expression of proliferation markers, cyclin D1 and Ki67 than the control tumours.

Conclusions: Our results confirm the theory that miR-125b functions as a tumour supressor in cutaneous malignant melanoma by regulating cellular senescence, which is one of the central mechanisms protecting against the development and progression of malignant melanoma.

Keywords: hsa-miR-125b, Melanoma, Senescence, In-situ-hybridization, Mel-Juso

Background

Replicative cellular senescence is the principal mechanism limiting proliferation of normal human cells [1,2]. After approximately 40–60 cell divisions (the Hayflick limit) the cells enter a senescence-associated, irreversible mitotic arrest and exhibit characteristic features comprising flattened morphology with abundant cytoplasm and biochemical markers such as senescence-associated beta-galactosidase (SA-beta-gal), p53 and cell cycle Inhibitors (p16, p21, p27) [3]. Telomere shortening is the primary mechanism of replicative senescence in normal diploid cells [4].

It has recently been discovered that various forms of DNA and cellular damage may cause premature cellular senescence before achieving the Hayflick limit. Interestingly, activation of oncogenes provides a potent senescence signal (oncogene-induced-senescence, OIS) which is considered to be an early protective mechanism against development of cancer [3,5-7]. Increased SA-beta-gal staining is seen in a variety of pre-malignant conditions, such as lung adenomas, congenital naevi, benign prostatic hyperplasia and premalignant prostatic intraepithelial neoplasia supporting the role of OIS in early control of malignancy [3,5,8,9]. It has also been observed that progression to the invasive tumour stage is associated with a suppression of

* Correspondence: r.gniadecki@gmail.com
[1]Department of Dermatology, Faculty of Health and Medical Sciences, University of Copenhagen, Bispebjerg Hospital, Copenhagen, Denmark
Full list of author information is available at the end of the article

OIS [5,6,9-11]. Cellular senescence may also be a mechanism inhibiting cancer progression, since senescence-like state can be induced in established tumours and cancer cell lines by a variety of mechanisms including chemotherapeutic agents or radiation (therapy-induced senescence, TIS) [11,12].

Cutaneous malignant melanoma (MM) is a common, highly aggressive cancer derived from the melanocytes in the skin. MM is an area of high medical need since the metastasis occurs early despite a very low primary tumour mass and metastatic disease is highly resistant to chemotherapy and radiotherapy. MM cells are resistant to apoptosis and the induction of cellular senescence could be explored as a novel approach to therapy [13].

MicroRNAs (miRNA) are 21–25 nt non-coding RNA molecules, which bind to the 3′UTR of mRNAs conferring translational inhibition or degradation [14]. MiRNAs have been found to regulate cell proliferation, differentiation, and apoptosis [15-17] and they have also been implicated in the regulation of senescence (miR-29, miR-30, miR-34a, miR-34b, miR-34c, miR122 miR-203, miR-205 and miR-217) [18-23] mostly by interfering with either the p53 pathway or the retinoblastoma RB1/E2F function. By an extensive analysis and comparison of miRNA expression levels Kozubek et al. showed that it was possible to distinguish melanoma speciments from benign neavi based on the miRNA signature [24]. This supports the theory that miRNA level may influence the development MM.

Two independent research groups have reported a miRNA-dependent induction of senescence in MM cell lines with a focus on miR-205/miR-203-E2F axis [23,25].

By comparing miR expression profiles in metastasizing and non-metastasizing MM we proposed that miR-125b is implicated in the progression of human MM [26]. MiR-125b expression is decreased in the primary cutaneous MM producing sentinel node metastasis comparing to the T-stage-matched non-metastasizing tumours [26]. This has later been confirmed by other groups [27,28]. Mir-125b is a known oncomir and has been implicated in the pathogenesis of leukemias and B-cell lymphomas, breast cancer, squamous cell carcinoma, urothelial carcinoma, prostate carcinoma and colon cancer [29-35]. In MM it has been shown to be related to the pigmentation level [27]. Kappelmann et al. showed that treatment of MM cells with pre-mir-125b resulted in a strong suppression of cellular proliferation [28].

We have gathered preliminary evidence that miR-125b may be involved in the regulation of senescence in MM [36]. In this paper we show that upregulation of miR-125b induces senescence and might constitute one of the possible mechanisms of the suppressive effect of miR-125b in MM.

Methods

Cell culture

Human MM cell line Mel-Juso (DSMZ, Braunschweig, Germany) was grown in DMEM Glutamax (Invitrogen, Carlsbad, CA) with 10% FBS (Life Technologies, LT) in 37°C and 5% CO_2. Transfected Mel-Juso cells were cultured in selection medium, which was the same medium supplemented with 10-μg/mL blasticidin (Invitrogen).

Plasmid transfection

Mel-Juso cells were transfected with a miRVector plasmid containing a miR-125b-1 [UCSC Genome Bioinformatics: uc010rzr.1] [37] insert and a blasticidin resistance gene (miRVec-125b) [38] or the control miRNA Vector plasmid with a blasticidin resistance gene but without any insert (miRVec-control) (Source BioScience, LifeSciences, Nottingham, UK) (map and sequence of miR-125b, see Additional file 1: Figure S1). 300.000 cells were seeded out 24 h before transfection to reach a confluency of 70–90%. 1 μg of the plasmid was mixed with 400 μl OPTI-MEM (Invitrogen) and 5 μl Lipofectamine RNAiMax (Invitrogen). The mixture was incubated at room temperature (RT) for 20 min and added to freshly washed Mel-Juso cells in 1600 μl culture medium for 24 h followed by a 14-day-culture in the selection medium in 37°C/5% CO_2. miR-125b expression was confirmed using PCR in each clone. Optimisation in the beginning of the study showed that the transfection efficacy in Mel-Juso cells was higher with Lipofectamine RNAiMax than any other transfection reagents. Transfection procedure was done in four replicates for each plasmid and each evaluated using PCR.

Flow cytometry

For the measurement of BrdU incorporation, Mel-Juso cells transfected with miRVec-125b or the miRVec-control were pulsed for 20 min with 10 μM BrdU, fixed in 70% ethanol for at least 2 h, washed with phosphate-buffered saline (PBS), incubated in 2 N HCl for 30 min, washed in neutralizing buffer (0.2 M $Na_2B_4O_7$, pH 8.5) and resuspended in dilution buffer (0.5% Tween 20 and 0.5% bovine serum albumin in PBS) prior to the addition of anti-BrdU mouse antibodies (Becton Dickinson, Franklin Lakes, NJ). Goat anti-mouse antibodies labeled with Alexa-Fluor 488 (1:1000; Invitrogen, Carlsbad, CA) were applied as secondary antibodies. DNA was stained with 0.0003% (30–40 μl per samlpe) 7-amino-actinomycin D solution (7AAD; Beckman Coulter, Brea, CA). Samples were analyzed by means of flow cytometry (Beckman-Coulter, Fullerton, CA). BrdU-positive events (FL1) were plotted versus cellular DNA content (FL3).

Tumour formation in mice

Mice experiments were performed in accordance with the national law for the experiments on animals of 14 Jun

2011 (full text available on https://www.retsinformation. dk/Forms/r0710.aspx?id=145380) and supervised by an authorised researcher (CML). All mice work is approved by Dyreforsoegstilsynet (generel permit for our laboratory work in mice, permit number 2012-15-2934-00419). All surgery was performed under sodium pentobarbital anesthesia, and every effort was made to minimize suffering.

Six Male BALB/C nude mice (Taconic, Rye, Denmark), 7 weeks of age, were housed in separate boxes with free access to water and standard laboratory food, in an animal facility at a 12 h light/dark cycle and the temperature 23°-24°C. Mice were acclimatized for one week before the experiments. Subsequently they were anesthetized with 0.05 ml HypDorm given subcutaneously and 5×10^6 Mel-Juso cells transfected with miRVec-125b vector or the control vector in 0.2 ml PBS were injected subcutaneously into the left or right flank, respectively. Tumours with a diameter of at least 1 mm were mapped separately for each animal and followed until these reached a diameter of 12 mm or for a maximum time of 4 weeks. Animals were killed and tumours were weighed and cut into three parts, which were fixed in RNA Later (for RNA isolation), 4% formalin (for standard histology, immunohistochemistry and in situ hybridization) or were frozen at –80°C (for SA-beta-gal staining). Formalin fixed samples were embedded in paraffin and serial sections were stained with hematoxylin and eosin, Ki-67 and cyclin D1, according to standard histopathology protocols. The quantification of Ki-67 and cyclin D1 expression was done semiquantitatively in each tumour using the following ordinal scale: grade 1 (0%-25% positive tumour cells), grade 2 (26%-50% positive cells), grade 3 (51%-75% positive cells), grade 4 (76%-100% positive cells). Lungs and liver were taken out and cut in to three parts each, which were treated as the tumour samples and checked for distance metastases.

In situ hybridization (ISH) for miR-125b

Formalin-fixed and paraffin-embedded human tissue samples from the archives of the Department of Pathology (Rigshospitalet, Copenhagen, Denmark) were stage T1-T4 cutaneous MM and matched lymph node metastases (14 males and 3 females; mean age 52 years, range 24 to 83 years); mean Breslow depth 1.53 mm (range 0.37 to 4.00 mm); 15 superficial spreading MM and 2 nodular MM. Mouse tumour samples were prepared as described above. Paraffin sections (6 μm) were mounted on SuperFrost®Plus slides (Dako, Glostrup, Denmark) and air-dried for 1–2 h at RT. Sections were deparaffinized in xylene and hydrated through decreasing ethanol concentrations into PBS. Proteinase-K treatment 15 μg/ml in PK-buffer (5 mM Tris–HCl, pH 7.4, 1 mM EDTA, 1 mM NaCl) was performed at 37°C for 8 min

in a volume of 300 μL in a Dako hybridizer (Dako). Sections were washed twice in sterile PBS and immediately dehydrated through an increasing gradient of ethanol solutions. Aliquots of 3 different Mercury LNA miRNA Detection Probes; hsa-miR-125b, scrambled probe, and U6 snRNA (Exiqon, Vedbaek, Denmark) were then denatured by heating to 90°C for 4 min and diluted to 40 nM, 40 nM, and 1 nM, respectively, in a formamide-free ISH buffer (Exiqon). 50 μL probe mixture was hybridized with the tissue sections in the hybridizer at 55°C for 60 min. The slides were placed at RT in 5× saline-sodium citrate (SSC) (Invitrogen) and stringency washes were performed for 5 min each at 55°C in 5× SSC (one wash), 1× SSC (two washes) and 0.2× SSC (two washes). The sections were then washed in PBS and blocked with DIG Wash and Block Buffer Set (Roche, Mannheim, Germany). Alkaline phosphatase (AP)-conjugated anti-DIG (Roche) was diluted 1:800 in the blocking solution and incubated for 60 min at RT. Slides were washed twice with PBS containing 0.1% Tween-20. Ready to use tablets (Roche) of 4-nitro-blue tetrazolium chloride (NBT) and 5-brom-4-chloro-3′-indolyl-phosphate (BCIP) substrate were dissolved in aqueous 0.2 mM levamisole. Slides were incubated for 120 min at 30°C to develop the dark-blue NBT-formazan precipitate. Sections were washed twice for 5 min in KTBT buffer (50 mM Tris–HCl, 150 mM NaCl, 10 mM KCl), and then twice in water, dehydrated in the ethanol gradient and mounted.

SA-beta-gal staining

Monolayers of Mel-Juso cells transfected with miRVec-125b or the miRVec-control after a 24-h culture in 4-chamber glass (Nunc, Rochester, NY) or cryostat tissue sections from mice mounted on SuperFrost®Plus slides were washed twice in PBS and fixed in 0.5% glutaraldehyde (pH = 7.0) for 15 min at RT. The samples were washed twice with 20 ml 1 mM $MgCl_2$ in PBS (pH = 6.0) and stained with the SA-beta-gal staining solution containing 1 mg/ml of 5-bromo-4-chloro-3-indolyl beta-galactopyranocid, 4% dimethylformamide, 0.0012 mM potassium ferrocyanide and 1 mM $MgCl_2$ in PBS (pH = 6.0) for 4 h (Mel-Juso) or overnight (melanocytes) at 37°C [3,5]. Percentage of positive cells was evaluated blindely by one of the investigators (RG).

Western blotting

Cells were washed in PBS and lysed in the sample buffer 0.5 M Tris–HCl pH 6.8; 5% glycerol; 10% SDS; DTT 0.2 M) supplemented with protease inhibitor cocktail (Roche). Equal amounts of protein were separated by a 4-8% and 12% Bis-Tris gel electrophoresis at 200 V followed by electrophoretic transfer to a nitrocellulose membrane (Bio-Rad Laboratories, Hercules, CA). Membranes were blocked for 1 h at 4°C with Li-Cor blocking agent (Li-Cor, Lincoln, NE) before incubation with the primary antibodies against β-actin (mouse) (Sigma Aldrich, St. Louis, MO), p16 (mouse) (BD Pharmingen, San Diego, CA), p21 (mouse) (Dako), p27 (mouse) (Santa Cruz Biotechnology, Santa Cruz, CA) or p53 (rabbit) (Dako) overnight at 4°C. Subsequently, they were incubated for 1 h with the appropriate secondary antibodies labeled with 800IR dye (anti-rabbit) (Li-Cor), Alexa Fluor 680 (anti-mouse or anti-rat) both from Molecular Probes (Invitrogen). Protein bands were detected and quantified with the infrared Odyssey imaging System (Li-Cor). Quantified intensities were adjusted to the relevant actin intensity and control and sample was then compaired.

Clonogenic assay

10.000 Mel-Juso cells transfected with miRVec-125b or the miRVec-control were seeded in 10 cm petri dishes containing 10 ml selection medium and cultured for 10–14 days until the appearance of macroscopically visible colonies. The plates were washed, fixed in paraformaldehyde for 24 h and stained with crystal violet 0.05% (Sigma Aldrich) for 20 min before washing in water. Plates were photographed (microscope Olympus IX 70 and camera Nikon D60) and colonies were counted manually.

Cell viability and apoptosis assessment

1.500.000 Mel-Juso cells transfected with miRVec-125b or the miRVec-control were seeded in 10 cm Petri dishes containing 10 ml selection medium, the medium changed after 24 h and all (floating and adherent) cells collected after another 24 h. Unfixed cells were stained simultaneously with FITC-Annexin-V and PI, according to the manufacturer's protocol (Beckman-Coulter, Fullerton, CA) and analyzed by means of flow cytometry (Beckman-Coulter, Fullerton, CA) as described previously [39].

RNA isolation and real-time q-PCR (RT-qPCR)

Mel-Juso cells transfected with miRVec-125b or the miRVec-control were collected and washed twice in PBS. Murine tumour tissue samples were homogenized using a TissueLyzer II (Qiagen, Valencia, CA, USA) and processed as previously described [40]. Small RNAs were purified using the mirVana Isolation Kit (Ambion, Foster City, CA) and the PureLink RNA Micro to Midi Kit (Invitrogen) according to the manufacturer's instructions. The concentration of RNA was measured spectrophotometrically using NanoDrop ND-1000 (Thermo Scientific, Wilmington, DE), and RNA integrity was confirmed with Agilent 2100 Bioanalyzer using Agilent Nano RNA kit (Agilent Technologies, Santa Clara, CA). miR-125b expression was measured in the samples containing the same amount of RNA with quantitative qRT-PCR

assay (TaqMan TM microRNA Reverse Transcription kit-4366596, and TaqMan Universal PCR Master mix-4324018, Applied Biosystems, Foster City, CA) and validated primer sets (Applied Biosystems) according to the manufacturer's instructions. MiR-191 was used as a reference for the normalization of qRT-PCR-data. The q-PCR was performed in triplicates using a 7900HT Fast Real-Time PCR System (Applied Biosystems).

Sequencing

DNA was extracted from transfected Mel-Juso cell lines containing either miRVec-125b or miRVec-control using QIAamp DNA mini-Kit (Qiagen) in accordance with the manufacturer's protocol. PCR was made with reagents from Life Technologies as follows: Master mix (10% Gene amp PCR buffer II, 2.5 mM MgCl$_2$, 400 μM dNTP, 0.2 μM of each primer and 1U Ampli Taq gold) was prepared and 7.2 μL was mixed with 16.8 μL of ddH$_2$O and 1 μL of 5 ng/μL DNA (template). PCR was setup on an Eppendorf MasterCycler gradient cycler (Hamburg, Germany) with the following program: 95°C 10 min, then 35 cycles of: 95°C 30 s, 62°C 30 s and 72°C 1.5 min; ended with 72°C 10 min and 4°C hold. The PCR product was visually inspected on a 2.2% agarose gel on the Flashgel system (Lonza, Basel, Switzerland). The remaining PCR product was purified on Qiaquick columns (Qiagen) according to manufacturer's specifications and eluted in 50 μL buffer. Four μL of purified PCR product were used as template in the sequencing reaction.

Sequencing was performed in duplicates with the BigDye V.1.1 cycling sequencing kit (Life Technologies) Samples consisted of 4 μL of Ready reaction mix, 2 μL of BigDye buffer, 3.2 pmol of primer (forward-GCGTTT AAACTTAAGCTTGGTACCGAGC, reverse-CATTCC CCCCTTTTTCTGGAGAC), 4 μL of template and 20 μL of ddH$_2$O. Reactions were performed with forward and reverse primers in duplicate with the following program: 96°C 1 min, then 25 cycles of: 96°C 10s, 50°C 5 s and 60°C 4 min, ending with 4°C hold. PCR products were purified with Centrisep columns (Princeton Separations, Adelphia, NJ) according to the manufacturer's recommendations. Two μL of purified sequencing product were mixed with 8 μL of HiDi formamide and run on an ABI3130xl DNA Sequencer (Life Technologies) with the following specifications: Array 36 cm, polymer POP4, injection voltage 3 kV, injection time 7 s, run voltage 15 kV and run time 1700 sec. One of the reverse duplicates was removed due to low quality. Results were analyzed and assembled with Sequencher v.5 (Gene Codes Corporation, Ann Arbor, MI, USA). Differences in the chromatograms were visually inspected. Low quality regions resulting in differences were removed. Sequence ends had to be cropped due to low reaction quality.

Statistics

All numeric results are given as mean ± SD unless stated otherwise. *t*-test was used for intergroup comparison. P < 0.05 was considered significant.

Results

miR-125b is expressed in human primary cutaneous MM and lymph node metastases

We have previously shown by miRNA array approach that miR-125b is expressed in primary cutaneous MM [26,41]. By comparing metastasizing and non-metastasizing stage T2 cutaneous MM we detected an overall decrease in miR-125b expression in metastasizing tumours [26]. Here we employed ISH to further define the expression pattern of miR-125b in MM. As shown in Figure 1 miR-125b is expressed in MM cells both in the primary tumours and in the sentinel node metastases. The staining of miR-125b seems to be located predominantly to the nuclei. We noted that the expression was not homogenous and some cells characterized by large size and abundant cytoplasm expressed higher amounts of miR-125b than other cells (arrows in Figure 1A,B). These larger cells could represent a more malignant, highly atypical tumour cell population, but could also comprise the population of cells undergoing spontaneous cellular senescence. Since SA-beta-gal staining is not possible on paraffin-embedded material and fresh samples from primary cutaneous MM are not available due to ethical considerations, we decided to examine the potential functional involvement of miR-125b in MM cell proliferation and senescence in vitro.

miR-125b inhibits proliferation and induces senescence in human melanoma line Mel-Juso

Mel-Juso cell line is established from the primary tumour of a 58-year-old woman with MM in 1977. This line has wildtype BRAF, is poorly differentiated [42] and exhibits intermediate invasiveness [43]. Transfection with miRVec-125b resulted in an 8.0 ± 1.13-fold upregulation of miR-125b by RT-qPCR compared to the miRVec-control transfected cells. After the experiments were completed, the miR-125b insert was sequenced to confirm that no mutation had occurred in the miR-125b sequence of the insert throughout the experimental period. For full insert consensus sequence, see Additional file 1: Figure S2.

As shown in Figure 2A,B and E the miRVec-125b transfected cells formed smaller and fewer colonies than the control cells (930 ± 105.2, n = 4 replicates vs. 1207.5 ± 218.8, n = 4 replicates, p-value 0.011). The miRVec-125b transfected cells showed a G0/G1 cell cycle arrest, demonstrated in Figure 2 (F, G) by a significantly increased proportion of G0/G1 cells (p < 0.05) and a significant decrease in BrdU incorporation (p < 0.05).

Microscopic examination of the colonies (Figure 2C,D) revealed that the miRVec-125b-transfected cells were enlarged, flattened, and had abundant cytoplasm, consistent with cellular senescence, in contrast with the normal spindle-shaped cell morphology in the control group. SA-beta-gal staining showed increased expression of SA-beta-gal in estimated 60-70% of the miRVec-125b transfected compared to estimated 5-10% of the control cells (Figure 3A,B). Western blot analysis of the miRVec-125b cells showed an up regulation of the expected

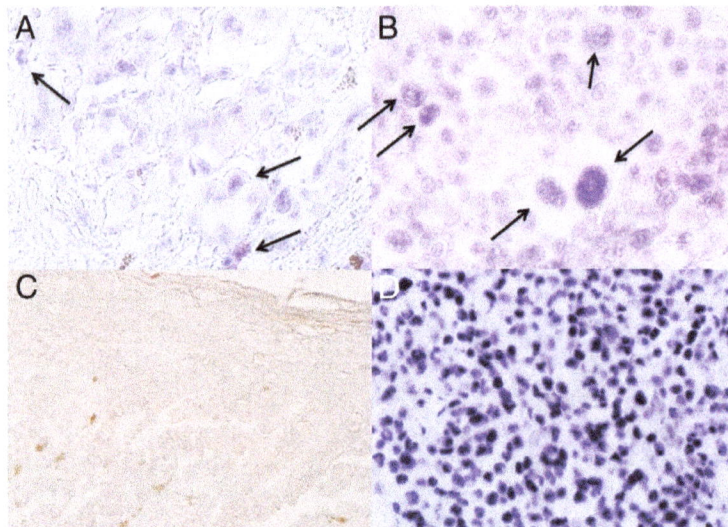

Figure 1 Expression of miR-125b in primary cutaneous malignant melanoma and lymph node metastases shown with ISH. Primary cutaneous MM (stage T2; **A, C**) and a sentinel node with micrometastases **(B)** were hybridized with the probe for miR-125b **(A, B)** or with the control, scrambled probe **(C)**. Arrows show the cells with prominent staining for miR-125b. **(D)** U6 probe (positive control). Magnification: **A** x60, **B** x40, **C** x20, **D** x20.

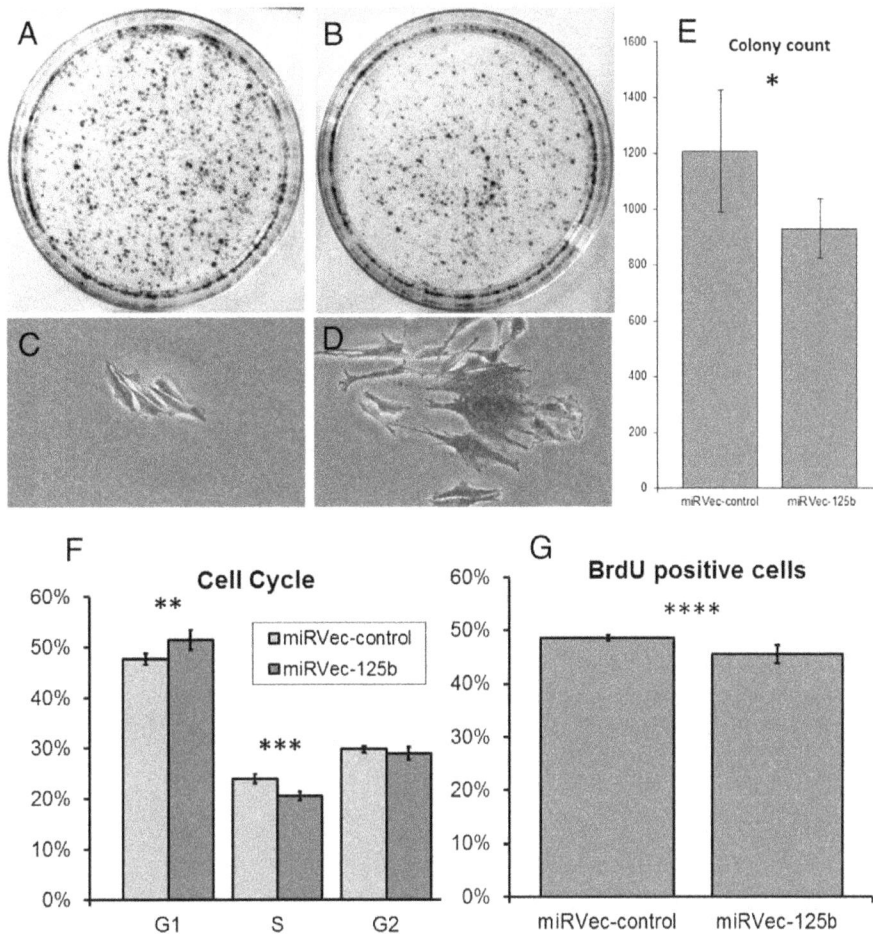

Figure 2 miR-125b inhibits the proliferation rate in cell line Mel-Juso. Transfected cells with miRVec-125b vector **(B, D)** or miRVec-control plasmid **(A, C)**. Colony formation **(A, B)**, morphology of the colonies **(C, D)**. **(E)** Quantification of colonies from the colony formation assay. * p = 0,011. **(F)**: Cell cycle analysis. The percentages of cells in G0/G1, S and G2/M phases are plotted for each group. ** p = 0,044, *** p = 0,01 **(G)** Cell proliferation measured by BrdU incorporation **** p = 0.039.

markers of senescence: p53, p21 and p27 compaired to the control. p16 was not expressed in the Mel-Juso cell line. (Figure 3C).

To evaluate whether apoptosis was responsible for the apparent lesser growth observed in the colony forming assay we compared the proportions of annexin-positive cells in the miRVec-125b transfected cells with the controls. We found no evidence of apoptosis in either group (95.5% ±0.7% annexin-negative, viable cells in the miRVec-125b transfected cell line versus 94.7% ±1.2% in the control; p = 0.46).

miR-125b expression in Mel-Juso cells induces senescence and reduces proliferation in a murine tumour model

To further investigate the significance of miR-125b in the regulation of MM growth we established an in vivo model of tumour formation from Mel-Juso cells injected subcutaneously into immunodeficient, nude BALB/c mice.

In this model the Mel-Juso cells formed subcutaneous tumours within a time span of 4 weeks, but did not produce distant metastases (confirmed by macroscopic and histological examination of lung and liver tissue). ISH revealed considerable expression of miR-125b in the tumours originating from the miRVec-125b vector-transfected cells, in contrast to a negligible expression in the tumours emerging from the miRVec-control cells. The tumours were very homogeny in their appearances which was consistent with the fact that they were developed from a clone rather than the normal progression from normal tissue to tumour with the following heterogeneity otherwise known from Melanoma tumours [44,45]. The stability of miR-125b overexpression was confirmed by RT-q-PCR quantification of miR-125b in the tumour tissue showing an 11.6 ± 6.0 fold increased expression in the miRVec-125b transfected tumours. As could be expected from the in vitro experiment, SA-beta-gal staining revealed a focal increase in the

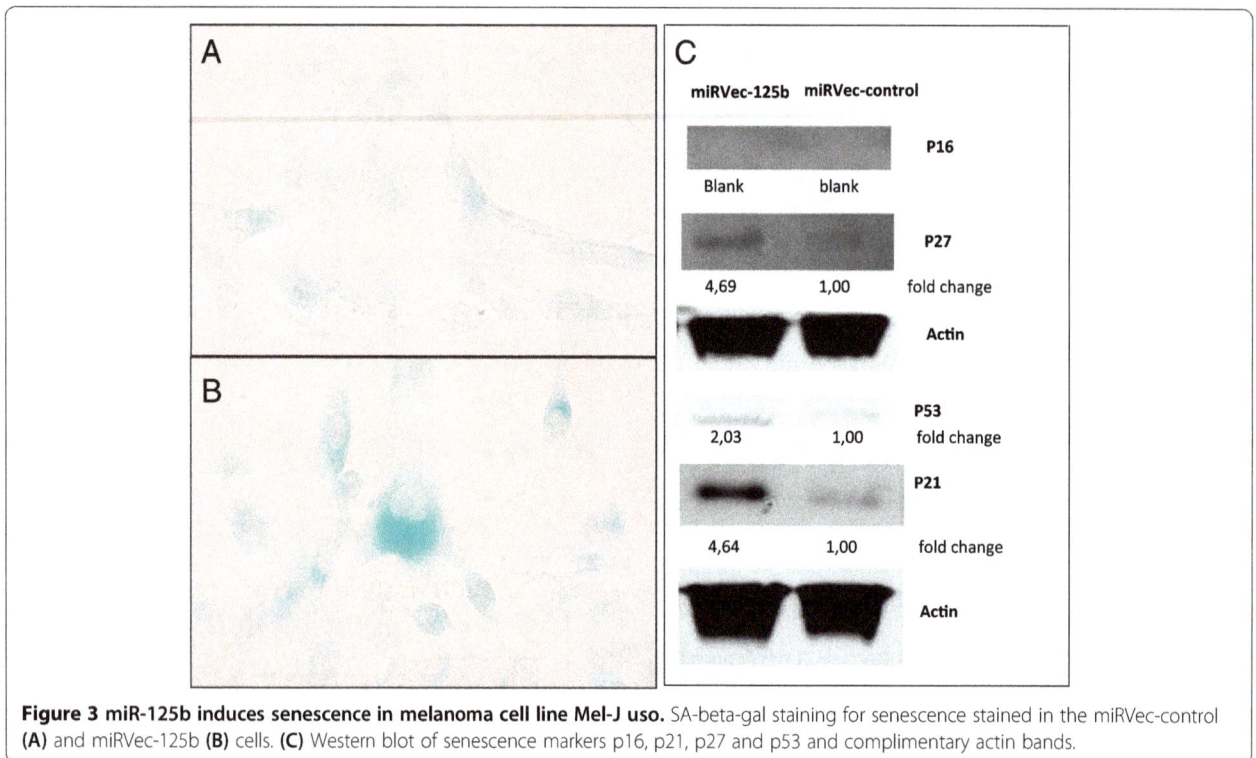

Figure 3 miR-125b induces senescence in melanoma cell line Mel-J uso. SA-beta-gal staining for senescence stained in the miRVec-control **(A)** and miRVec-125b **(B)** cells. **(C)** Western blot of senescence markers p16, p21, p27 and p53 and complimentary actin bands.

staining suggesting accelerated senescence in the tumours originating from miRVec-125b -transfected cells. This was paralleled by the marked decrease in the expression of proliferation markers Ki67 and cyclin D1 (Figure 4). However, we did not detect any difference in weight between the tumours originating from miRVec-125b -transfected cells and the control, miRVec-control transfected cells (mean weight miR-125b: 0.021 g ± 0.003, control: 0.023 g ± 0.004).

Discussion

This study documented that stable, ectopic expression of miR-125b induced cellular senescence in a MM cell line Mel-Juso, both in vitro and in a xenotransplantation model in mice in vivo. The results were surprising, since miR-125b is generally considered to be an oncogene and in a transgenic mouse model miR-125b overexpression causes myeloid leukemia and B-cell malignancies [46,47]. However, our and other's preliminary evidence suggested that miR-125b has an anticancer effect in MM [26,28,36,41] and its decreased expression correlated with the metastatic potential of primary cutaneous MM. In the present study we substantiated this hypothesis using a model of stably transfected Mel-Juso cell line with the miRVec-125b vector previously developed by Voorhoeve et al. [38]. We were able to demonstrate an increase in senescence markers (SA-beta-gal, p27, p21, p53) and decreased proliferation with a G0/G1 arrest in miRVec-125b-transfected cells as compared with the control.

miRVec-125b -transfected cells were tumourigenic in vivo, but the tumours showed an increased rate of senescence and decreased amount of proliferating cells, as measured by Ki67 and cyclin D1 staining. Together with the results of ISH showing that miR-125b is expressed in primary human MM and lymph node metastases, the data indicate that miR-125b is implicated in the regulation of senescence in human MM.

The mechanism by which miR-125b overexpression promotes cellular senescence is unknown. MiR-125b may negatively regulate the p53 tumour suppressor gene and Bak1 [48] but such a downregulation has not been seen in Mel-Juso cells in our experiments (data not shown). Other known targets are BMF and Lin28a [49] but they are unlikely to be involved in cellular senescence in MM. In general, the functional role of miR-125b seems to be cell specific, since in some types of cancer (e.g. urothelial carcinoma) this miR seems to acts as a tumour suppressor [34].

MiR-dependent induction of cellular senescence in MM has recently and independently been demonstrated by other researchers for miR-203 and miR-205 in cutaneous MM and for miR-34a in uveal MM [23,25,50]. A common biochemical pathway in these cases seems to be mediated by E2F and downregulation of Akt. This is an unlikely mechanism in the case of miR-125b since the screening for the effect of miR-125b overexpression on Akt, Stat, mTOR did not show any changes in the

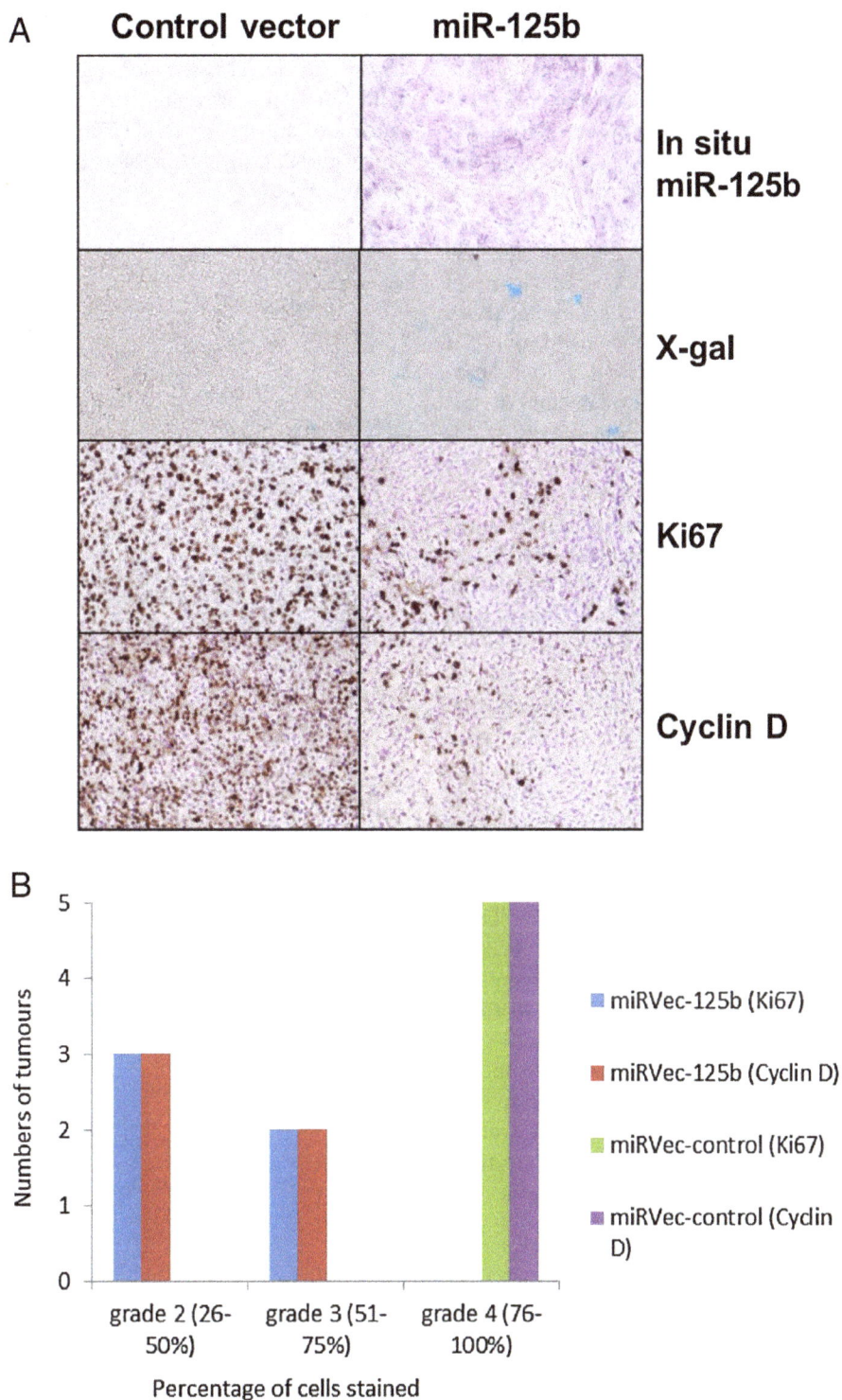

Figure 4 Reduced mitotic activity and increased senescence in tumours emerging from miRVec-125b transfected Mel-Juso cells shown by (A) ISH with miR-125b (In situ miR-125b), SA-beta-galactosidase staining (X-gal), Ki67 and Cyclin D. The different stainings were not made in paralelle. **(B)** Quantification of Ki67 and cyclin D expression in murine tumours by visual grading of the proportion of positive cells. In one case the control and experimental tumours were too small for microscopic analysis and therefore the graph shows data for 5 tumours.

expression level in MM cell lines and E2F2 and E2F3 proteins are not expressed in Mel-Juso cells (data not shown).

In this study we used ISH to evaluate the miR-125b expression locally in the tissue. We observed that the ISH on human tissue samples showed a strong nucleic concentration of miR-125b. This has been surprising since the conventional theory requires the cytoplasmic presence of miRNA for its proper function [51-53]. However, the studies on the compartmentalization of miR-125b have been done with cell lines and not tissue samples, like in our study. On the other hand, our ISH staining on the murine tumours showed a more pronounced cytoplasmic staining. One explanation of this could be that the miR-125b distribution in the cell is different between cells from a cultivated cell line and cells from tissue samples. Kobuzek et al. [24] showed that the miR-125b signal in MM is different in tissue and cell lines. Another explanation could be that the specific distribution varies from tissue to tissue. This is supported by the fact that ISH staining for miR-125b on other tissues have showed that in some tissues there is a clear staining of the nuclei [54-56] while in others the staining is mainly cytoplasmatic [57,58]. This will have to be validated in further studies. It is finally possible, that nuclear miR-125b have a distinct biological role, as previously suggested for other miRNA species.

Another limitation of this study is that the functional role of miR-125b has only been investigated in Mel-Juso cells and it remains to be seen whether the same is valid for other MM cell lines and primary melanocytes. These experiments were attempted but failed due to massive apoptotic response caused by miRVec-125b plasmid. It is known that Mel-Juso cells are very resistant to apoptosis, which enabled us to achieve a stable miR-125b overexpression. Second, we focused primarily on the effect of the sustained overexpression of miR-125b in MM cells. The use of inducible miR-125b vectors will be helpful to elucidate the effect of acute changes in miR-125b levels.

Conclusion

Our results confirm the theory that miR-125b function as a tumour supressor in cutaneous malignant melanoma by regulating cellular senescence, which is one of the central mechanisms protecting against the development and progression of malignant melanoma.

In view of the recent developments in the use of miRNA mimics and inhibitors for therapy, it is conceivable that miR-125b would be utilized for the treatment of MM by inducing senescence of cancer cells. However, as exemplified by our murine MM model, miR-125b induces senescence focally in the tumours and the effect on tumour mass is negligible. It is known that miRNAs

act primarily as switches and amplifiers of the cellular signaling pathways and their physiological effect is rarely very strong [21]. It is therefore our goal for future research to identify which signaling pathways of therapeutic relevance are targeted by miR-125b and devise strategies by which mir-125b overexpression may amplify the effect of anticancer drug.

Abbreviations

ISH: In situ hybridization; miR-125b: MicroRNA 125b; miRNA: MicroRNA; MM: Malignant melanoma; OIS: Oncogene-induced-senescence; PBS: Phosphate-buffered saline; TIS: Therapy-induced senescence.

Competing interests

The authors declare that they have no competing interests.

Authors' contributions

AMN helped design the study and coordinated the in vitro experiment, made all transfections and western blots, RNA-extractions, participated in the flow studies and the PCR-work, performed the statistical analysis and drafted the manuscript. CML carried out the in vivo studies and the in-situ-hybridizations. VM carried out the PCR-work. EB carried out most flow studies. PJ carries out all sequencing work. NM supervised the sequencing work. BMT processed the tissuesamples for parafine embedment and made the HE, Ki67 and Cyclin D stainings. MG helped with study design. RG designed the study, helped drafting the manuscript and helped with the statistical analysis. All authors read and approved the final manuscript.

Acknowledgement

We thank Eva Hoffman, Omid Niazi and Pia Eriksen for their technical help with the experiments. miRVectors were kindly donated by prof. Anders Lund, Biotech Research and Innovation Centre, University of Copenhagen, Denmark. The study was supported by research grants from the following foundations: Aage Bang Foundation, Birgit and Svend Igor Pock-Steens Foundation and The Danish Cancer Society.

Author details

[1]Department of Dermatology, Faculty of Health and Medical Sciences, University of Copenhagen, Bispebjerg Hospital, Copenhagen, Denmark. [2]Department of Forensic Medicine, Section of Forensic Genetics, Faculty of Health and Medical Sciences, University of Copenhagen, Copenhagen, Denmark. [3]Department of Pathology, University of Copenhagen, Faculty of Health and Medical Sciences, Bispebjerg Hospital, Copenhagen, Denmark.

References

1. Hayflick L, MOORHEAD PS: The serial cultivation of human diploid cell strains. Exp Cell Res 1961, 25:585–621.
2. Hayflick L: The cell biology of aging. J Invest Dermatol 1979, 73:8–14.
3. Michalogou C, Vredeveld LC, Soengas MS, Denoyelle C, Kuilman T, van der Horst CM, Majoor DM, Shay JW, Mooi WJ, Peeper DS: BRAFE600-associated senescence-like cell cycle arrest of human naevi. Nature 2005, 436:720–724.
4. Harley CB, Futcher AB, Greider CW: Telomeres shorten during ageing of human fibroblasts. Nature 1990, 345:458–460.
5. Collado M, Gil J, Efeyan A, Guerra C, Schuhmacher AJ, Barradas M, Benguria A, Zaballos A, Flores JM, Barbacid M, Beach D, Serrano M: Tumour biology: senescence in premalignant tumours. Nature 2005, 436:642.
6. Collado M, Serrano M: The power and the promise of oncogene-induced senescence markers. Nat Rev Cancer 2006, 6:472–476.

7. Collado M, Serrano M: **Senescence in tumours: evidence from mice and humans.** *Nat Rev Cancer* 2010, **10**:51–57.

8. Choi J, Shendrik I, Peacocke M, Peehl D, Buttyan R, Ikeguchi EF, Katz AE, Benson MC: **Expression of senescence-associated beta-galactosidase in enlarged prostates from men with benign prostatic hyperplasia.** *Urology* 2000, **56**:160–166.

9. Majumder PK, Grisanzio C, O'Connell F, Barry M, Brito JM, Xu Q, Guney I, Berger R, Herman P, Bikoff R, Fedele G, Baek WK, Wang S, Ellwood-Yen K, Wu H, Sawyers CL, Signoretti S, Hahn WC, Loda M, Sellers WR: **A prostatic intraepithelial neoplasia-dependent p27 Kip1 checkpoint induces senescence and inhibits cell proliferation and cancer progression.** *Cancer Cell* 2008, **14**:146–155.

10. Braig M, Lee S, Loddenkemper C, Rudolph C, Peters AH, Schlegelberger B, Stein H, Dorken B, Jenuwein T, Schmitt CA: **Oncogene-induced senescence as an initial barrier in lymphoma development.** *Nature* 2005, **436**:660–665.

11. Serrano M: **Shifting senescence into quiescence by turning up p53.** *Cell Cycle* 2010, **9**:4256–4257.

12. Gewirtz DA, Holt SE, Elmore LW: **Accelerated senescence: an emerging role in tumor cell response to chemotherapy and radiation.** *Biochem Pharmacol* 2008, **76**:947–957.

13. Giuliano S, Ohanna M, Ballotto R, Bertolotto C: **Advances in melanoma senescence and potential clinical application.** *Pigment Cell Melanoma Res* 2010, **24**:295–308.

14. Pasquinelli AE: **MicroRNAs and their targets: recognition, regulation and an emerging reciprocal relationship.** *Nat Rev Genet* 2012, **13**:271–282.

15. Bartel DP: **MicroRNAs: genomics, biogenesis, mechanism, and function.** *Cell* 2004, **116**:281–297.

16. Farh KK, Grimson A, Jan C, Lewis BP, Johnston WK, Lim LP, Burge CB, Bartel DP: **The widespread impact of mammalian MicroRNAs on mRNA repression and evolution.** *Science* 2005, **310**:1817–1821.

17. Kato M, Slack FJ: **microRNAs: small molecules with big roles - C. elegans to human cancer.** *Biol Cell* 2008, **100**:71–81.

18. He X, He L, Hannon GJ: **The guardian's little helper: microRNAs in the p53 tumor suppressor network.** *Cancer Res* 2007, **67**:11099–11101.

19. Martinez I, Cazalla D, Almstead LL, Steitz JA, DiMaio D: **miR-29 and miR-30 regulate B-Myb expression during cellular senescence.** *Proc Natl Acad Sci U S A* 2011, **108**:522–527.

20. Menghini R, Casagrande V, Cardellini M, Martelli E, Terrinoni A, Amati F, Vasa-Nicotera M, Ippoliti A, Novelli G, Melino G, Lauro R, Federici M: **MicroRNA 217 modulates endothelial cell senescence via silent information regulator 1.** *Circulation* 2009, **120**:1524–1532.

21. Inui M, Martello G, Piccolo S: **MicroRNA control of signal transduction.** *Nat Rev Mol Cell Biol* 2010, **11**:252–263.

22. Benhamed M, Herbig U, Ye T, Dejean A, Bischof O: **Senescence is an endogenous trigger for microRNA-directed transcriptional gene silencing in human cells.** *Nat Cell Biol* 2012, **14**:266–275.

23. Noguchi S, Mori T, Otsuka Y, Yamada N, Yasui I, Iwasaki J, Kumazaki M, Maruo K, Akao Y: **Anti-oncogenic microRNA-203 induces senescence by targeting E2F3 in human melanoma cells.** *J Biol Chem* 2012, **287**:11769–11777.

24. Kozubek J, Ma Z, Fleming E, Duggan T, Wu R, Shin DG, Dadras SS: **In-depth characterization of microRNA transcriptome in melanoma.** *PLoS One* 2013, **8**:e72699.

25. Dar AA, Majid S, De SD, Nosrati M, Bezrookove V, Kashani-Sabet M: **miRNA-205 suppresses melanoma cell proliferation and induces senescence via regulation of E2F1 protein.** *J Biol Chem* 2011, **286**:16606–16614.

26. Glud M, Rossing M, Hother C, Holst L, Hastrup N, Nielsen FC, Gniadecki R, Drzewiecki KT: **Downregulation of miR-125b in metastatic cutaneous malignant melanoma.** *Melanoma Res* 2010, **20**:479–484.

27. Kim KH, Bin BH, Kim J, Son ED, Park PJ, Choi H, Kim BJ, Yu SJ, Kang H, Kang HH, Cho EG, Lee TR: **Novel inhibitory function of miR-125b in Melanogenesis.** *Pigment Cell Melanoma Res* 2013, **27**:140–144.

28. Kappelmann M, Kuphal S, Meister G, Vardimon L, Bosserhoff AK: **MicroRNA miR-125b controls melanoma progression by direct regulation of c-Jun protein expression.** *Oncogene* 2013, **32**:2984–2991.

29. Guan Y, Yao H, Zheng Z, Qiu G, Sun K: **MiR-125b targets BCL3 and suppresses ovarian cancer proliferation.** *Int J Cancer* 2010, **128**:2274–2283.

30. Huang L, Luo J, Cai Q, Pan Q, Zeng H, Guo Z, Dong W, Huang J, Lin T: **MicroRNA-125b suppresses the development of bladder cancer by targeting E2F3.** *Int J Cancer* 2010, **128**:1758–1769.

31. Hui AB, Lenarduzzi M, Krushel T, Waldron L, Pintilie M, Shi W, Perez-Ordonez B, Jurisica I, O'Sullivan B, Waldron J, Gullane P, Cummings B, Liu FF: **Comprehensive MicroRNA profiling for head and neck squamous cell carcinomas.** *Clin Cancer Res* 2010, **16**:1129–1139.

32. Baffa R, Fassan M, Volinia S, O'Hara B, Liu CG, Palazzo JP, Gardiman M, Rugge M, Gomella LG, Croce CM, Rosenberg A: **MicroRNA expression profiling of human metastatic cancers identifies cancer gene targets.** *J Pathol* 2009, **219**:214–221.

33. Schaefer A, Jung M, Mollenkopf HJ, Wagner I, Stephan C, Jentzmik F, Miller K, Lein H, Kristiansen G, Jung K: **Diagnostic and prognostic implications of microRNA profiling in prostate carcinoma.** *Int J Cancer* 2010, **126**:1166–1176.

34. Veerla S, Lindgren D, Kvist A, Frigyesi A, Staaf J, Persson H, Liedberg F, Chebil G, Gudjonsson S, Borg A, Mansson W, Rovira C, Hoglund M: **MiRNA expression in urothelial carcinomas: important roles of miR-10a, miR-222, miR-125b, miR-7 and miR-452 for tumor stage and metastasis, and frequent homozygous losses of miR-31.** *Int J Cancer* 2009, **124**:2236–2242.

35. Calin GA, Sevignani C, Dumitru CD, Hyslop T, Noch E, Yendamuri S, Shimizu M, Rattan S, Bullrich F, Negrini M, Croce CM: **Human microRNA genes are frequently located at fragile sites and genomic regions involved in cancers.** *Proc Natl Acad Sci U S A* 2004, **101**:2999–3004.

36. Glud M, Manfe V, Biskup E, Holst L, Dirksen AM, Hastrup N, Nielsen FC, Drzewiecki KT, Gniadecki R: **MicroRNA miR-125b induces senescence in human melanoma cells.** *Melanoma Res* 2011, **21**:253–256.

37. *UCSC genoma bioinfromatics.* 2013. http://genome-euro.ucsc.edu/.

38. Voorhoeve PM, le SC, Schrier M, Gillis AJ, Stoop H, Nagel R, Liu YP, van DJ, Drost J, Griekspoor A, Zlotorynski E, Yabuta N, De VG, Nojima H, Looijenga LH, Agami R: **A genetic screen implicates miRNA-372 and miRNA-373 as oncogenes in testicular germ cell tumors.** *Cell* 2006, **124**:1169–1181.

39. Kamstrup MR, Gjerdrum LM, Biskup E, Lauenborg BT, Ralfkiaer E, Woetmann A, Odum N, Gniadecki R: **Notch1 as a potential therapeutic target in cutaneous T-cell lymphoma.** *Blood* 2010, **116**:2504–2512.

40. Holst LM, Kaczkowski B, Gniadecki R: **Reproducible pattern of microRNA in normal human skin.** *Exp Dermatol* 2010, **19**:e201–e205.

41. Holst LM, Kaczkowski B, Glud M, Futoma-Kazmierczak E, Hansen LF, Gniadecki R: **The microRNA molecular signature of atypic and common acquired melanocytic nevi: differential expression of miR-125b and let-7c.** *Exp Dermatol* 2011, **20**:278–280.

42. Ziegler-Heitbrock HW, Munker R, Johnson J, Petersmann I, Schmoeckel C, Riethmuller G: **In vitro differentiation of human melanoma cells analyzed with monoclonal antibodies.** *Cancer Res* 1985, **45**:1344–1350.

43. Wach F, Eyrich AM, Wustrow T, Krieg T, Hein R: **Comparison of migration and invasiveness of epithelial tumor and melanoma cells in vitro.** *J Dermatol Sci* 1996, **12**:118–126.

44. Fidler IJ: **Tumor heterogeneity and the biology of cancer invasion and metastasis.** *Cancer Res* 1978, **38**:2651–2660.

45. Hoek KS, Schlegel NC, Brafford P, Sucker A, Ugurel S, Kumar R, Weber BL, Nathanson KL, Phillips DJ, Herlyn M, Schadendorf D, Dummer R: **Metastatic potential of melanomas defined by specific gene expression profiles with no BRAF signature.** *Pigment Cell Res* 2006, **19**:290–302.

46. Enomoto Y, Kitaura J, Hatakeyama K, Watanuki J, Akasaka T, Kato N, Shimanuki M, Nishimura K, Takahashi M, Taniwaki M, Haferlach C, Siebert R, Dyer MJ, Asou N, Aburatani H, Nakakuma H, Kitamura T, Sonoki T: **Emu/miR-125b transgenic mice develop lethal B-cell malignancies.** *Leukemia* 2011, **25**:1849–1856.

47. Bousquet M, Harris MH, Zhou B, Lodish HF: **MicroRNA miR-125b causes leukemia.** *Proc Natl Acad Sci U S A* 2010, **107**:21558–21563.

48. Le MT, Teh C, Shyh-Chang N, Xie H, Zhou B, Korzh V, Lodish HF, Lim B: **MicroRNA-125b is a novel negative regulator of p53.** *Genes Dev* 2009, **23**:862–876.

49. Chaudhuri AA, So AY, Mehta A, Minisandram A, Sinha N, Jonsson VD, Rao DS, O'Connell RM, Baltimore D: **Oncomir miR-125b regulates hematopoiesis by targeting the gene Lin28A.** *Proc Natl Acad Sci U S A* 2012, **109**:4233–4238.

50. Yan D, Zhou X, Chen X, Hu DN, Dong XD, Wang J, Lu F, Tu L, Qu J: **MicroRNA-34a inhibits uveal melanoma cell proliferation and migration through downregulation of c-Met.** *Invest Ophthalmol Vis Sci* 2009, **50**:1559–1565.

51. Jeffries CD, Fried HM, Perkins DO: **Nuclear and cytoplasmic localization of neural stem cell microRNAs.** *RNA* 2011, **17**:675–686.

52. Ohrt T, Muetze J, Svoboda P, Schwille P: **Intracellular localization and routing of miRNA and RNAi pathway components.** *Curr Top Med Chem* 2012, **12**:79–88.

53. Liao JY, Ma LM, Guo YH, Zhang YC, Zhou H, Shao P, Chen YQ, Qu LH: **Deep sequencing of human nuclear and cytoplasmic small RNAs reveals an unexpectedly complex subcellular distribution of miRNAs and tRNA 3' trailers.** *PLoS One* 2010, **5:**e10563.

54. Gu Y, Sun J, Groome LJ, Wang Y: **Differential miRNA expression profiles between the first and third trimester human placentas.** *Am J Physiol Endocrinol Metab* 2013, **304:**E836–E843.

55. Vacchi-Suzzi C, Hahne F, Scheubel P, Marcellin M, Dubost V, Westphal M, Boeglen C, Buchmann-Moller S, Cheung MS, Cordier A, De BC, Deurinck M, Frei M, Moulin P, Oakeley E, Grenet O, Grevot A, Stull R, Theil D, Moggs JG, Marrer E, Couttet P: **Heart structure-specific transcriptomic atlas reveals conserved microRNA-mRNA interactions.** *PLoS One* 2013, **8:**e52442.

56. Manfe V, Biskup E, Willumsgaard A, Skov AG, Palmieri D, Gasparini P, Lagana A, Woetmann A, Odum N, Croce CM, Gniadecki R: **cMyc/miR-125b-5p signalling determines sensitivity to bortezomib in preclinical model of cutaneous T-cell lymphomas.** *PLoS One* 2013, **8:**e59390.

57. Xu N, Zhang L, Meisgen F, Harada M, Heilborn J, Homey B, Grander D, Stahle M, Sonkoly E, Pivarcsi A: **MicroRNA-125b down-regulates matrix metallopeptidase 13 and inhibits cutaneous squamous cell carcinoma cell proliferation, migration, and invasion.** *J Biol Chem* 2012, **287:**29899–29908.

58. Arora A, Guduric-Fuchs J, Harwood L, Dellett M, Cogliati T, Simpson DA: **Prediction of microRNAs affecting mRNA expression during retinal development.** *BMC Dev Biol* 2010, **10:**1.

Survey and online discussion groups to develop a patient-rated outcome measure on acceptability of treatment response in vitiligo

Selina K Tour[1], Kim S Thomas[1*], Dawn-Marie Walker[2], Paul Leighton[2], Adrian SW Yong[3] and Jonathan M Batchelor[1]

Abstract

Background: Vitiligo is a chronic depigmenting skin disorder which affects around 0.5-1% of the world's population. The outcome measures used most commonly in trials to judge treatment success focus on repigmentation. Patient-reported outcome measures of treatment success are rarely used, although recommendations have been made for their inclusion in vitiligo trials. This study aimed to evaluate the face validity of a new patient-reported outcome measure of treatment response, for use in future trials and clinical practice.

Method: An online survey to gather initial views on what constitutes treatment success for people with vitiligo or their parents/carers, followed by online discussion groups with patients to reach consensus on what constitutes treatment success for individuals with vitiligo, and how this can be assessed in the context of trials. Participants were recruited from an existing database of vitiligo patients and through posts on the social network sites Facebook and Twitter.

Results: A total of 202 survey responses were received, of which 37 were excluded and 165 analysed. Three main themes emerged as important in assessing treatment response: a) the match between vitiligo and normal skin (how well it blends in); b) how noticeable the vitiligo is and c) a reduction in the size of the white patches. The majority of respondents said they would consider 80% or more repigmentation to be a worthwhile treatment response after 9 months of treatment. Three online discussion groups involving 12 participants led to consensus that treatment success is best measured by asking patients how noticeable their vitiligo is after treatment. This was judged to be best answered using a 5-point Likert scale, on which a score of 4 or 5 represents treatment success.

Conclusions: This study represents the first step in developing a patient reported measure of treatment success in vitiligo trials. Further work is now needed to assess its construct validity and responsiveness to change.

Keywords: Vitiligo, Outcome measure, Patient-reported outcome, Randomised controlled trial

Background

Vitiligo is a chronic depigmenting skin disease characterised by loss of skin colour in patches [1]. It affects people of all ages, ethnic groups and skin types [2,3] and around 0.5%-1% of the world's population [1,2] although estimates are higher in countries and cultures where the stigma of the skin disease may be higher [1].

There is no cure for vitiligo but there are numerous treatment options. These include topical and oral preparations, light therapy, surgical procedures, psychological and complementary therapies [1]. The only licensed treatment for vitiligo in the UK is cosmetic camouflage [3], although many other treatments are used in clinical practice.

Physical symptoms in vitiligo are usually mild, but the unpredictable nature of the disease and its tendency to progress in the majority of cases can be psychologically and cosmetically overwhelming [1,2,4]. Living with vitiligo can be a continuous struggle, with the psychological characteristics of each individual determining their ability to adjust to and cope with disfigurement [5].

Although clinical studies have assessed many treatments for vitiligo, the heterogeneity of these studies makes comparison of the effectiveness of treatments – alone or

* Correspondence: kim.thomas@nottingham.ac.uk
[1]Centre of Evidence Based Dermatology, The University of Nottingham, Nottingham, UK
Full list of author information is available at the end of the article

combined – very difficult [1,2,6]. The updated Cochrane systematic review of interventions for vitiligo published in 2010 [1] and other reviews have highlighted problems such as variance in design and a lack of standardised outcome measures and scales used in clinical trials [1,2,6,7]. There is a pressing need to develop core outcome measures, so that effectiveness of treatments can be compared and combined more easily across trials 2].

It is important that outcomes used in trials are relevant to patients as well as clinicians [2]. Repigmentation is the most frequently used outcome measure and is typically captured using either clinical assessments or through digital images [2]. Vitiligo results in patches of depigmented skin, so intuitively it would seem to be a simple matter of recording treatment success or failure based on changes in the amount of repigmented skin. However, repigmentation of vitiligo can often be uneven, resulting in a poor cosmetic result from a patient's perspective.

Despite recommendations for the inclusion of patients' views when evaluating interventions [1,6], patient-reported outcomes have not been commonly used in trial to date [2], and validated tools are lacking.

The aim of the study was to develop and provide preliminary data on the face validity of a patient-reported outcome measure of the acceptability of treatment response.

Specific objectives were:

- To conduct patient surveys and online discussion groups to establish the most appropriate form of wording and scale to use.
- To ensure that the wording of the question assessing satisfaction with treatment response is relevant to, and easily understood by, vitiligo patients (face validity).
- To establish what represents clinically worthwhile treatment response from a patient's perspective.

In addition to improving our understanding of what constitutes a successful treatment response from a patient perspective, it is anticipated that the resulting outcome measure will be useful for use in future vitiligo trials and clinical practice. The results will also be used to inform an ongoing international initiative to establish a core outcome set for use in vitiligo trials [8].

Methods
This project was conducted in two stages. First, an online survey was used to identify which aspects of treatment response are most important to patients.

The online survey was followed by three separate online discussion groups, in which the results of the survey were explored with patients, and consensus was reached regarding the most appropriate form of wording for the proposed patient-reported outcome measure.

The project was approved by the University of Nottingham's Medical School Research Ethics committee (Ethics Reference No. LTg15082013 SoM Dermatol).

Online survey
Participants
Participants were recruited from an existing mailing list held at the Centre of Evidence-Based Dermatology at the University of Nottingham. This list consisted of individuals who had participated in a previous Vitiligo Priority Setting Partnership [7] and those who had contacted us expressing interest in being involved in vitiligo research. In addition, participants were recruited through the UK Vitiligo Society Facebook Page, and details of the survey were 'tweeted' under the UK Dermatology Clinical Trials Network Twitter feed. Participants in the survey included both those who had sought treatment for their vitiligo and those who had not, and included parents/guardians of children with vitiligo as well as those with vitiligo themselves. We did not include clinicians and healthcare professionals who had participated in the previous Priority Setting Partnership. Efforts were made to ensure broad representation across all age and ethnic groups. Although recruitment was targeted largely at participants in the UK, there were no exclusions based on country of residence and details of nationality were recorded.

Survey distribution
The survey, which took approximately 5minutes to complete was created using Survey Monkey software [9] and consisted of 14 questions. No incentives were offered for participation. Prior to distribution, we piloted it by asking a group of clinicians, researchers and members of the Centre of Evidence-Based Dermatology (CEBD) Patient Panel to review the survey and comment on the relevance of the survey content and how easy it was to understand and complete.

Details of the survey and information sheets were emailed to 188 potential participants from an existing mailing list held at the CEBD that included patients who had previously expressed an interest in finding out more about vitiligo research. The survey was open from 29th July 2013 until the 19th August 2013. Two reminders were emailed to all on the mailing list, and additional posts were placed on the Vitiligo Society's Facebook page and the UK Dermatology Clinical Trials Network Twitter feed in order to broaden recruitment. Completion of more than 1 survey question implied consent to participate.

Data collection included demographic details; the extent of the vitiligo and previous treatments used; opinions on what a 'cosmetically acceptable response' to treatment meant to the participant and whether they felt it was the same as 'satisfaction with the result'. A selection of 11 words and phrases to describe treatment response were also presented, from which participants chose the most meaningful to them (see Results section).

Participants were also asked to look at a series of images featuring a young boy with dark skin with a vitiliginous lesion. Using image manipulation software (Adobe® Photoshop® CS2, Adobe Systems Incorporated; San Jose, California, USA) the lesion was gradually reduced in the sequential images to simulate repigmentation at different percentages. Participants were asked to indicate the degree of repigmentation that they considered worthwhile after 9 months of treatment, followed by the minimum level of repigmentation they would be prepared to accept.

Online discussion groups
Participants
Survey participants who indicated interest in further involvement in research were invited to participate in an online discussion groups. All participants received a £10 amazon e-voucher.

Invitations were sent by email, with an information sheet attached. In total, 57 initial invitations were sent. Reminder emails and further invitations were sent if necessary, to ensure that 6–8 people were confirmed for each of the three discussion groups [9]. To aid participation, two groups were held in the evening. We used online discussion groups to make it easier for participants to join the discussion (rather than having to travel) and to make it easier for them to talk about more personal aspects of their experience with vitiligo (which might have been more difficult if they had attended in person).

To ensure familiarity with the concepts involved and the context in which the patient assessment of treatment response would be placed, confirmed participants were sent reading material on clinical research methods and primary outcome measures (see Additional file 1). Participants were also advised to read information on vitiligo from the NHS Choices web pages [10] and to watch a short video explaining clinical trials from the Medical Research Council via YouTube [11].

Hosting the online discussion groups
Online discussion groups were used in favour of face-to-face focus group discussions in order to facilitate engagement with a broad range of participants from throughout the UK [12-14].

The online discussion groups were hosted in a private chat room based within the Vitiligo Society's web pages. All participants followed an email link, registered for the group and, once approved by the moderator (ST), were given access to the chat room for the time of their online discussion. Prior to the groups taking place, participants

were sent information about the objectives of the groups, and about consent to participate. Participants gave consent at time of registration and were encouraged to use an alias if they wished to remain anonymous.

Each group lasted for approximately 90minutes, to allow adequate time for discussion whilst avoiding participant fatigue. Participants were able to type text and send emoticons as in a standard chat room. Groups were facilitated by two to three members of the research team.

The discussion groups were semi-structured; a list of prompts was prepared in advance and these were inserted into the discussion thread at relevant time points. This ensured similarity between the questions asked of each group. Page links were created for images and inserted into the discussion thread at relevant times during the discussion to allow participants to view images of vitiligo before and after treatment and a selection of measurement scales.

Examples of prompts used in online discussion groups:
Discussion prompts were used to direct participants' attention to relevant points. Here are examples of prompts used under various themes covered by the online discussion groups:

Prompt number and details

Theme: Most important concepts when assessing treatment success

The survey results showed that the three main areas of importance to people with regards to judging treatment success were (in order of frequency):

1. Colour match between their vitiligo and normal skin i.e. how well it blends in
2. How noticeable the vitiligo is
3. A reduction in the size of the white patches.

Which of these do you think is the most important if we are trying to capture a measure of treatment success?

Theme: Wording of questions about how noticeable vitiligo is

Let's try some example questions that ask about how noticeable your vitiligo is. These questions can be used at the end of a trial to ask people about how successful their treatment is. What do people think about these possible questions? Does the wording seem right?

Q1 How noticeable do you feel your vitiligo is, compared with the start of treatment?
Q2 How successful do you feel the treatment has been, in terms of how noticeable the vitiligo is?
Q3 How satisfied are you with how noticeable the vitiligo is?
Q4 Compared to before treatment, how noticeable is your vitiligo now?

Theme: Using the agreed question format to assess treatment response for whole body versus individual lesions

If some areas of vitiligo respond well to treatment and some do not, do you think that this question is useful to measure how noticeable the vitiligo is on all body sites affected? Or do you think that the question is only useful for assessing individual patches of vitiligo?

Adequate time was allowed after insertion of each prompt to allow participants to respond and discuss with each other freely. The facilitators guided discussion with the aim of trying to achieve consensus, and summarised the discussion findings at various intervals to check that all participants were in agreement.

At the end of the discussion group, a copy of the entire discussion thread was downloaded and saved.

Sample size and participant selection

The sample size for this study was dictated by the time and resources available. However, we aimed to include at least 100 participants in the survey (assuming a confidence interval of 95%, and an accuracy rate or +/− 10%) and 18 − 20 participants in the discussion groups, in order to gather a broad selection of views.

For the discussion groups, purposive sampling was used to ensure diversity in terms of ethnicity and age within the groups. Using SPSS 21 Software, potential participants who had responded to the online survey were split into three groups – parents/carers of those with vitiligo (n = 13), people with vitiligo aged 17–45 (n = 45) and those aged 46 and above (n = 76). We tried to take participants' ages into consideration when forming the discussion groups given the potentially greater familiarity with technology and "text speak" in younger participants [13]. Invitations were sent to all parents/carers, plus a random selection from other age groups. All potential participants from non-white ethnic backgrounds were invited, as well as a random selection of those from white backgrounds. This was to enable discussion of treatment for vitiligo in the context of different skin types.

Statistical analysis

Survey results were analysed using SPSS Statistics 21 software. Results were presented descriptively. Responses to open questions were analysed thematically by a researcher (ST) and checked by a second researcher (JB) for agreement. This allowed for comparison between themes emerging from open and closed questions to be made, as well as allowing for ranking of themes by popularity overall for use in the discussion groups.

The main objective of the discussion groups was to seek consensus regarding the most appropriate wording of the question to ask people about the response of vitiligo to treatment. Whilst more formal methods of consensus development (e.g. Delphi and Nominal Group Technique) are the focus of much academic consideration, informal consensus groups such as those employed here are commonly employed in health care settings [15]. To counter some of those criticisms that informal mechanisms for consensus reaching lack 'control', 'focus' and 'scientific credibility' [15] here data is handled and analysed systematically following an adapted version of Template Analysis [16,17]. Template analysis utilises a hierarchical model to organise text in order to aid interpretation. In this case each point of consensus was taken as a higher-level organising code within which to summarise and consider the group discussion. So for each point of agreement the discussion which led toward this was considered and coded to reflect those factors which contributed towards the consensus and those which were a barrier. This process was completed for each discussion group with a final template constructed to include all statements where agreement spanned the different groups. This mode of analysis provides greater depth in understanding consensus, both mapping where agreement occurred and charting the process and factors which generated it. Two researchers independently checked the copy of each discussion group thread to ensure that all relevant points had been adequately identified and extracted with any discrepancies discussed with a third researcher. Consensus points are summarised below, with examples of key comments made by participants. The qualitative aspect of this study adhered to the RATS guidelines for reporting qualitative research modified for BioMed Central [18].

Results

Participants

In total, 202 survey responses were received. Of these, 165 (82%) were included in analyses, and of these, 154 (76%) were fully completed surveys (Figure 1).

Responses were excluded for the following reasons:

- If the survey had been completed from the same Internet Protocol (IP) address more than once:
  - The first completely filled survey was included, and the rest excluded.
  - If multiple surveys were completed fully, only the first was included.
- The same two rules applied for duplicate email addresses given
- If the survey had not been completed past question 1, it was excluded.

The only exception to these exclusion criteria was where email addresses and demographic responses indicated that two different individuals had responded from the same IP address, so both sets of responses were included.

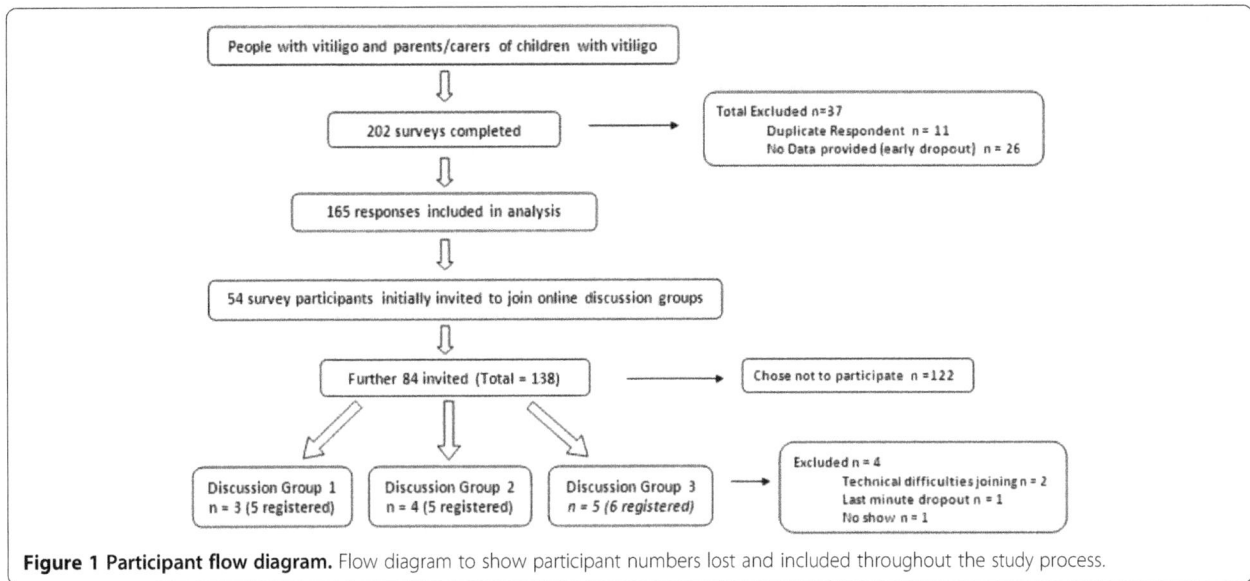

Figure 1 Participant flow diagram. Flow diagram to show participant numbers lost and included throughout the study process.

Baseline characteristics of the survey participants are summarised in Table 1.

The majority of participants were aged between 31 and 65 years of age and had had vitiligo for more than 10 years. One hundred and thirty three (80.6%) of those completing the survey were from white ethnic backgrounds, and 135 (81.8%) were from the UK.

Results of survey

Question 1: "When thinking about repigmentation of vitiligo after treatment, what does a 'cosmetically acceptable result' mean to you?"

There were 143 responses to this open question. Multiple themes per response were allowed, yielding a total of 237 items of information coded from the 143 responses. The three most common themes related to the concept of the skin returning to normal and the vitiligo patches being less visible or noticeable. Reduction in the size of the lesion was ranked 4th and was mentioned in just 12.2% of responses. The main themes to emerge are summarised in Table 2.

Six responses were not relevant to the question, such as "I have given up on treatment after various unsuccessful attempts". Four respondents (1.7%) stated specifically that a 'cosmetically acceptable result' was not meaningful to them and not an encouraging phrase.

Question 2: "The list below gives some possible words or phrases used to describe treatment results in vitiligo. Please tell us the words/phrases that best reflect how you would judge whether or not a vitiligo treatment has worked (please tick up to THREE options)"

This question received 157 responses. The most popular words/phrases are summarised in Table 3. Eighteen responses (4.3%) were given under the category 'Other', and most were not relevant to treatment response, such as "Never had treatment".

Question 3: "When thinking about the repigmentation of vitiligo after treatment, do you think that 'cosmetic acceptability of result' and 'satisfaction with the result' mean the same thing?"

In total, 159 responses were given for this question, with 88 (55.3%) answering 'No', 46 (28.9%) answering 'Yes' and 25 (15.7%) 'Not sure'.

An open comment box allowed respondents to give further details, which suggested that participants felt that 'cosmetic acceptability' was a medical view or that of someone else and that 'satisfaction with the result' was a more personal and patient-led view. An example response was "The second statement suggests that the person is happy with the result whereas the first statement sounds more medical...". In addition, negative views about the term 'cosmetic acceptability' were given, such as "rather vague", "impersonal" and "implies vitiligo only affects skin".

Question 4: "Please give us any other suggestions on the questions we should ask people about the result of vitiligo treatment."

The main theme that emerged was asking questions regarding psychological factors, (36 responses; 34.6%) such as individual feelings, confidence, and comfort in wearing fewer clothes. The next emerging themes were

Table 1 Demographic/other characteristics of survey respondents

Characteristic	Online survey	Online discussion groups
	N = 165	N = 12
Responses completed on behalf of – n (%)		
Themselves	149 (90.3)	12 (100)
Other	14 (8.5)	
Child with vitiligo	13(92.9)	0 (0)
Spouse with vitiligo	1 (7.1)	
Themselves and other(s)	2 (1.2)	0 (0)
Unknown	0 (0)	0 (0)
Age – n (%)		
<5 years	1 (0.6)	0 (0)
5-16 years	10 (6.1)	1 (8.3)
17-30 years	17 (10.3)	2 (16.7)
31-45 years	43 (26)	3 (25)
46-65 years	55 (33.3)	3 (25)
> 65years	29 (17.6)	3 (25)
Unknown	10 (6.1)	0 (0)
Ethnicity- n (%)		
White British	117 (70.9)	9 (75)
White Irish	1 (0.6)	0 (0)
Other White Background	15 (9.1)	0 (0)
Any Other Mixed Background	1 (0.6)	0 (0)
Indian/British Indian	9 (5.5)	1 (8.3)
Pakistani/British Pakistani	1 (0.6)	0 (0)
Bangladeshi/British Bangladeshi	2 (1.2)	1 (8.3)
Caribbean/British Caribbean	1 (0.6)	1 (8.3)
African/British African	1 (0.6)	0 (0)
Other	7 (4.2)	0 (0)
Unknown	10 (6.1)	0 (0)
Country of residence – n (%)		
UK	135 (81.8)	11 (91.7)
USA	12 (7.3)	1 (8.3)
Europe (excluding UK)	3 (1.8)	0 (0)
Australia	1 (0.6)	0 (0)
Asia	1 (0.6)	0 (0)
Dual – UK and Other	2 (1.2)	0 (0)
Unknown	11 (6.7)	0 (0)
Duration of Diagnosis- n (%)		
6-12 months	3 (1.9)	0 (0)
1-2 years	3 (1.9)	0 (0)
2-5 years	12 (7.7)	2 (16.7)
5-10 years	26 (16.8)	1 (8.3)
> 10 years	111 (71.6)	9 (75)

Table 1 Demographic/other characteristics of survey respondents *(Continued)*

Percentage of skin affected (estimate) - n (%)		
0-10%	37 (23.3)	1 (8.3)
10-25%	49 (30.8)	4 (33.3)
25-50%	33 (20.8)	5 (41.7)
50-80%	24 (15.1)	2 (16.7)
>80%	16 (10.1)	0 (0)
Unknown	6 (3.6)	0 (0)
Area (s) of skin affected – n (%) NB: More than one response could be given		
Face/Neck	129 (78.2)	10 (83.3)
Body	110 (66.7)	7 (58.3)
Arms	113 (68.5)	8 (66.7)
Legs	109 (66.1)	8 (66.7)
Hands	127 (77)	10 (83.3)
Feet	113 (68.5)	9 (75)
I'd rather not say	2 (1.2)	0 (0)
Other (responses included: under arms, genitalia and hair)	35 (21.2)	2 (16.7)
Treatments used previously – n (%) NB: More than one response could be given		
No treatment	57 (34.5)	2 (16.7)
Topical corticosteroid	41 (24.8)	3 (25)
Protopic (Tacrolimus)	46 (27.9)	6 (50)
Elidel (Pimecrolimus)	6 (3.6)	0 (0)
Vitamin D derived cream or ointment (e.g. calcipotriol)	5 (3)	2 (16.7)
UVB	33 (20)	5 (41.7)
PUVA	20 (12.1)	2 (16.7)
Not Sure	1 (0.6)	0 (0)
Other (Responses included diet changes and alternative therapies)	28 (17)	3 (25)

details about the treatment (19 responses; 18.3%) and the duration of the improvement (14 responses; 13.5%). Other results are summarised in Table 4.

Question 5: "After 9 months of vitiligo treatment, which of the pictures below shows a level of treatment response that you feel would be worthwhile to you? Please choose the letter associated with the chosen image."

The 158 responses are summarised in Table 5. Almost 80% of participants said that they would consider at least an 80% improvement to be a worthwhile result after 9 months of treatment (equating to images G H and I).

Question 6: "After 9 months of vitiligo treatment, which of the pictures below represents the MINIMUM treatment response that you would be prepared to accept?"

Table 2 'When thinking about repigmentation of vitiligo after treatment, what does a "cosmetically acceptable result" mean to you?' (Themes in descending order of popularity)

Theme	Number of responses	Percent
Blends well with skin	45	19%
Less noticeable	35	14.8%
Skin back to normal	31	13.1%
Reduction in white patches	29	12.2%
Confident/Comfortable	25	10.5%
Repigment visible sites	19	8%
Any Improvement	17	7.2%
Mostly repigmented	14	5.9%
Cosmetics	9	3.8%
Unaffected by tanning	5	2.1%
Means nothing	4	1.7%
Lasting repigmentation	3	1.3%
Completely depigmented	1	0.4%

The 156 responses are summarised in Table 5. Similar to Question 5, when asked to identify the MINIMUM acceptable treatment response, the results were heavily skewed towards high levels of repigmentation. Sixty four percent of participants wanted to see at least a 70% improvement after 9 months of treatment (images F, G, H and I), although improvement of as little as 50% was also considered worthwhile for some.

Key messages to be explored in discussion groups
The survey revealed some key messages, which were taken forward to the online discussion groups for further exploration.

Table 3 Popularity of Words/Phrases to describe treatment results for vitiligo

Words/Phrases	Number of votes	Percent
Good colour match between treated vitiligo patches and normal skin	72	17%
Skin is back to normal	66	15.6%
Feel better about appearance of skin	58	13.7%
Reduction in area of skin affected by vitiligo	48	11.3%
Even pattern of repigmentation	43	10.2%
Cosmetically acceptable result	26	6.1%
Satisfied with result	23	5.4%
Worth continuing with treatment	21	5%
Other	18	4.3%
Worthwhile result	17	4%
Result of treatment is acceptable	9	2.1%

Table 4 Themes emerging from "other suggested questions"

Theme	Number of Responses	Percent
Psychological	36	34.6%
Treatment details	19	18.3%
Improvement duration	14	13.5%
Was the treatment worth the results	8	7.7%
Adverse effects	6	5.8%
Satisfaction	6	5.8%
Back to normal	4	3.8%
Has colour returned	3	2.9%
Reduction in white patches	3	2.9%
Sun protection	2	1.9%
Would they do it again	2	1.9%
Make it simple	1	1%

The first of these was that there were three main areas of importance to people when judging treatment success, namely: colour match between their vitiligo and normal skin, i.e. how well it blends in; how noticeable the vitiligo is; and a reduction in the size of the white patches.

Another key message for further exploration was that the majority of respondents said they would consider 80% or more repigmentation to be worthwhile treatment response after 9months and that the minimum they would be prepared to accept would be 70% repigmentation.

Results of discussion groups
Three online discussion groups were held, involving a total of 12 participants (n = 4; n = 3 and n = 5 respectively). Participants ranged in age from 16 to over 65 years old, and

Table 5 Worthwhile treatment response and minimum level of response acceptable for after 9 months

Treatment response image (Approximate% repigmentation)	Worthwhile treatment response	Minimum treatment response acceptable
	Number of votes (cumulative %)	Number of votes (cumulative %)
A (20)	2 (1.3)	8 (5.1)
B (30)	0 (1.3)	8 (10.2)
C (40)	3 (3.2)	7 (14.7)
D (50)	7 (7.6)	17 (25.6)
E (60)	8 (12.1)	16 (35.9)
F (70)	12 (19.8)	26 (52.6)
G (80)	18 (31.6)	43 (80.2)
H (95)	57 (77.7)	22 (94.3)
I (100)	51(100)	9 (100)

had been affected by vitiligo for between four and 27 years. An additional four participants were registered to join the groups, but did not participate because they had technical difficulties in accessing the chat room, or were unavailable at the last minute. Due to participant availability, we were not able to run separate discussion groups for participants of different age groups, as we had planned. However, this did not seem to have an adverse effect on any participants' ability to contribute to discussions. A total of 50 pages (approximately 16,000 words) of text were obtained from the three groups and analysed as described above.

Summary of areas of consensus

All three groups achieved consensus both within and between the individual discussion groups in several areas.

Points for which there was consensus across the groups included:

i. The most important concept when asking about success of treatment response is "how noticeable the vitiligo is after treatment".

ii. A scale with five response options (both words and numbers) is the best scale to use when answering the question
   Question: Compared to before treatment, how noticeable is the vitiligo now?
   a. More noticeable (1)
   b. As noticeable (2)
   c. Slightly less noticeable (3)
   d. A lot less noticeable (4)
   e. No longer noticeable (5)

iii. A score of 4 or 5 on the above five-point scale would represent a successful treatment response

iv. The question should only be used to assess individual vitiligo lesions, rather than all areas affected by vitiligo

These areas of consensus are discussed in more detail below.

Most important concept: How noticeable vitiligo is after treatment

In response to the question regarding the most important concept when judging treatment success, all three groups were unanimous that the most important concept was how 'noticeable' the vitiligo is after treatment. Although some participants initially felt that other concepts were important, after further discussion with other participants, consensus was soon reached, with minimal input from the facilitators. Moreover, several participants commented that the 'noticeability' of the vitiligo was a useful 'catch-all' phrase which

covered elements of the other two concepts (colour match/blending and a decrease in size of the lesions). For example:

'Of the three you have written, I think 1 and 3 are covered by 2'

'I would say, most noticeable first, as 1 and 3 determine this'

Participants in all groups acknowledged that for people with paler skin tones, 'noticeability' may be less of an issue than for people with darker skin:

Participant: *I am lucky in that I have very fair skin so my condition is not that easy to notice......... but I imagine it is a big issue if it can be seen.*

Facilitator: *Do you think that if your vitiligo was in visible areas, that how noticeable it was would be the most important to you?*

Participant: *Yes*

Having established that the 'noticeability' of the vitiligo was the most important concept, participants then decided on the best wording of the question to ask trial participants in order to establish the 'noticeability'. Prompts used for this discussion are shown in the 'examples of prompts used in online discussion groups' subsection.

There was agreement that asking about "satisfaction" alongside the notion of "noticeability" was confusing for patients, as the two terms have contradictory implications.

'Because noticeable to me, denotes it is noticeable- which is a negative and yet I am being asked how satisfied I am-which is a bit confusing'

There was rapid development of consensus in the first two groups that Q4 ('Compared to before treatment, how noticeable is your vitiligo now?') was the most appropriate and easy to understand, and the third group agreed with this:

'Love it- uncomplicated and to the point'

What scale to use when answering the question

When groups were asked about the best scale with which to measure responses to the question, a preference was expressed for a linear scale, as opposed to a scale made up of images such as pictograms or emoticons.

However, participants felt that the linear scale needed to contain a reasonable number of choices:

'I think it's sometimes more difficult to make a judgement when there are fewer parameters'

Although the first group expressed a provisional preference for a linear scale with 10 divisions, time was limited for discussion of this point and so the discussion was developed further in groups 2 and 3. The subsequent groups felt that a 5-point scale with adjectival markers was best.

Having agreed on the question 'Compared to before treatment, how noticeable is your vitiligo now?' in group 1, further discussion with the participants in groups 2 and 3 showed support for the response options shown in the left-hand column of Table 6. The final wording of two responses was amended slightly after the discussion groups had been completed (so that all responses consistently included the word 'noticeable'). The amended wording, shown in the right-hand column of Table 6, was circulated amongst all participants and there was unanimous support for it.

What score on the scale constitutes treatment 'success?'

The groups were unanimous that a 'successful' treatment would need to score at least a '4' on this scale (a lot less noticeable [4] or no longer noticeable [5]).

In particular, participants expressed a preference for having both numbers and words on the scale, and for the option of ticking a box to give an answer.

Participants in all groups agreed that the question and scale were suitable when assessing vitiligo lesions that have partially repigmented but which, due to hyperpigmentation or uneven repigmentation, are actually more noticeable after treatment. Here is a summary of a discussion when participants in one group were shown some 'before and after' images that included hyperpigmentation (Figure 2 for images):

Participant 1: *That is interesting. There is a reduction in vitiligo area but the patchiness makes it look more obvious. In spite of the partial repigmentation, I would answer 1.*

Table 6 Wording of response options

Wording agreed during discussion groups	Amended wording, approved after discussion group by participants
Worse than before (1)	More noticeable (1)
About the same (2)	As noticeable (2)
Slightly less noticeable (3)	Slightly less noticeable (3)
A lot less noticeable (4)	A lot less noticeable (4)
Hardly noticeable (5)	No longer noticeable (5)

Participant 2: *On balance I think I would say 2, because the area near to the eye has responded well but the chin seems more noticeable now that it is not such a large block*

Participant 3: *To me it is more blotchy so 1*

Facilitator: *So if this was your vitiligo, would you say that treatment was successful or unsuccessful?*

Participant 2: *Unsuccessful I think*

Participant 1: *Partly successful, but if I had to opt for successful or unsuccessful, I would go for unsuccessful as it has made the vitiligo more obvious.*

Participant 3: *Unsuccessful.*

Use of the question to refer to individual treated vitiligo lesions or all affected areas of vitiligo

In the final discussion group, participants were asked to comment specifically on whether the question could be used to ask about all areas affected by vitiligo or whether it was best used to assess specific patches (see 'examples of prompts used in online discussion groups' subsection for prompts). Participants were unanimous that the question should be specific to target areas, and that this was particularly important for visible sites.

Use of the question with children and their parents/carers

The third group was also asked about the suitability of the question if the trial participant was a child, and a proxy response from a parent or carer was required:

'I feel that parents could answer for their child as they would be fully aware of the child's feelings'

'I think the questions would be suitable for children, although their responses might be a bit more optimistic than adults'

'For a child, I think noticeability will be determined by their peers - a parent may or may not have good insight into this'

Discussion
Summary of main findings

This work has provided valuable insight into how patients with vitiligo evaluate treatment success and has laid the foundation for creating a validated patient-rated outcome measure for use in future trials of vitiligo treatments.

Although the concept of a 'cosmetically acceptable result' had previously been identified as an important measure of treatment success amongst people with vitiligo [2], our

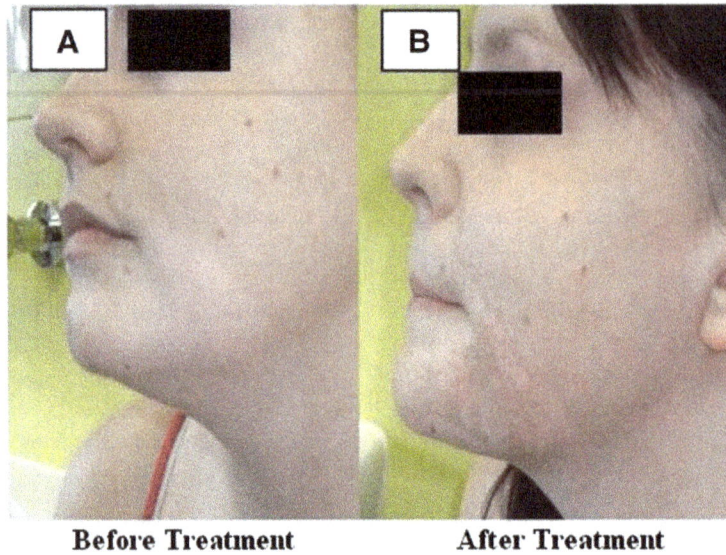

Figure 2 A set of 'before' and 'after' images showing hyperpigmentation used in the online discussion groups. A set of 'before' and 'after' images showing hyperpigmentation used in the online discussion groups. This set of images consent was gained from the individual seen in Figure 2 for use of their images in research publications as well as was obtained from images held at the Centre of Evidence Based Dermatology of before and after treatment. Full future studies.

initial survey work showed that this term was rather unhelpful to patients, who felt that it was vague, impersonal and rather 'medical'; or it implied that vitiligo was just something to be covered up (using cosmetic camouflage).

There was good agreement between the open and closed responses to survey questions. Common themes including 'blends well with skin', 'less noticeable' and 'reduction in white patches', were mentioned most frequently in response to an open question. While the most popular phrases in response to a more closed question were: 'good colour match', 'reduction in area of skin affected' and 'even pattern of repigmentation'.

'Feel better about appearance of skin' was another popular theme, and although this is a highly important concept, we did not pursue it further in the discussion groups because psychological response to treatment was beyond the remit of this study. Specific validated scales to assess the impact of vitiligo on psychological wellbeing have been described elsewhere [19,20] as have quality of life scales regarding physical appearance and cosmetic products [21].

Another main theme to emerge from the survey results was that many respondents equated a cosmetically acceptable result with 'skin is back to normal'. Although this is of course the ideal result for people with vitiligo, the likelihood of vitiliginous skin fully returning to normal after treatment is low. In addition, responses to a question about the skin being 'back to normal' would be in a binary 'Yes/No' form and would not allow for a scale of more gradual increments,

which is more likely to be useful when measuring the partial repigmentation expected after treatment. 'Skin back to normal' would also be covered by the top rating on any scale used to judge treatment success. For these reasons, we decided not to pursue this theme further during the discussion groups, focusing instead on the other three key themes that had emerged (colour match between their vitiligo and normal skin; how noticeable the vitiligo is; and a reduction in the size of the white patches).

Responses to survey questions about the minimum level of repigmentation considered to be worthwhile after a 9-month period of treatment showed that people with vitiligo generally hope for very high degrees of repigmentation; nearly 80% of respondents said they would consider 80% or more repigmentation to be worthwhile and 64% said that the minimum they would be prepared to accept would be 70% or more repigmentation. This was helpful in guiding our understanding of what patients might consider to be a clinically meaningful treatment response and corresponds with the quartile of >75% repigmentation being taken to represent treatment success in many previous vitiligo trials [2].

The online discussion groups used in the second stage of this work were very successful and popular amongst the participants. Due to the widespread availability of internet access and increasing familiarity with online means of communication, online discussion groups are emerging as a useful medium for conducting health research [12,13,22]. The study also reflects an increasing use of electronic communication to support group decision making and consensus making [22].

It was striking that the members of the online discussion groups quickly reached consensus in a number of areas. The first area of consensus was that the 'noticeability' of vitiligo was the most important concept when assessing treatment success, and that the 'noticeability' of vitiligo is a useful 'catch-all' concept that reflects the other two main concepts to emerge from the survey (colour match/blending and a decrease in size of the lesions).

Consensus was also reached rapidly regarding the use of a 5-point scale of responses, including words and numbers, when answering the question: 'Compared to before treatment, how noticeable is the vitiligo now?' Participants were happy that this scale was suitable for assessing lesions with different percentages and patterns of repigmentation, and there was strong consensus that a score of 4 or 5 on the scale equated with treatment success. Participants also agreed unanimously that if individual vitiligo lesions are treated, the noticeability of the lesions should be assessed individually, as opposed to assessing noticeability of vitiligo as a global measure for all affected areas of skin.

Conclusions
Strengths and limitations of the study
Limitations of this research work include the fact that the participants involved in the survey and discussion groups were almost entirely based in the UK. It is possible that the views of people with vitiligo in other countries may be quite different from those in the UK, and this may limit the external validity of the patient-rated measure. Another limitation was the absence of parents/carers of children with vitiligo from the discussion groups. We tried hard to recruit such individuals to the groups, by offering to host the groups at times that would be convenient for them, but none of the parents/carers who had participated in the survey were willing, or able, to join the discussion groups. We did, however, obtain positive feedback from parents/carers about the outcome measure after the discussion groups had taken place. Because it is not possible to know the characteristics of those who chose not to respond to the survey, it is possible that a degree of bias may have arisen due to a particular cohort of participants choosing to respond.

Given the potentially disproportionate impact of vitiligo on people with darker skin types, it was possibly disappointing that only 4.2% of study participants were from black and ethnic groups. However, this figure is representative of the mix of ethnicities in the UK population. For example, 85.8% of survey participants were white, and the Office of National Statistics estimates that 87.9% of the population are white; 7.7% of participants were Indian, Pakistani or other of Asian ethnicity, compared to the ONS estimate of 5.8% of the UK population [7].

In this work, we did not explore participants' views on the impact of vitiligo on their quality of life. There is already and extensive literature on this subject, and there are validated vitiligo-specific quality of life scales available for assessing this [19]. Once fully validated, the outcome measure we are developing can be used in parallel with vitiligo-specific quality of life scales, to assess both the visual and psychological aspects of treatment 'success' from the patient's perspective.

Qualitative research such as this can be prone to biases if carried out by one particular group (e.g. clinicians). Our group included two clinicians, a psychology student, a non-clinical Professor of applied dermatology research, and two qualitative researchers. We believe this is a suitable mix to avoid some of the potential for bias in the design and interpretation of the study.

Implications for research
This work has demonstrated for the first time that percentage repigmentation may not be the best measure of vitiligo treatment success from a patient's perspective. Instead, how noticeable the vitiligo patches are is a key concept for patients. Greater awareness of patients' perspectives in judging treatment response in future clinical trials is essential. Additional work is now required to validate this measure further; in particular with respect to construct validity. We will ensure that these findings are incorporated into future international discussions regarding the most appropriate core outcome measure for inclusion in future vitiligo trials.

Abbreviations
UVB: Ultraviolet B; PUVA: Psoralen plus ultraviolet A.

Competing interests
The authors declare that they have no competing interests and are not in personal receipt of any funding for this or any other work.

Authors' contributions
SKT, JMB and KST made substantial contributions to the acquisition of data, analysis and interpretation of the data as well as making major contributions to the draft manuscript. DMW made substantial contributions to the study design of the online discussion groups and PL contributed to the analysis and interpretation of qualitative data analysis. ASWY contributed to the creation of repigmentation images to be used in online survey work. All authors read, redrafted and approved the final manuscript.

Authors' information

SKT BSc (Hons). Research Associate, Centre of Evidence-based Dermatology, University of Nottingham. KST BSc, PhD. Professor of Applied Dermatology Research, Centre of Evidence-based Dermatology, University of Nottingham. DMW BSc (Hons), MA, MSc, PhD. Lecturer, School of Medicine, Research Design Service, University of Nottingham. PL PhD. Lecturer, School of Medicine, University of Nottingham. ASWY BSc (Hons), MB BS, MRCP. Specialty Registrar in Dermatology, Norfolk and Norwich University Hospitals NHS Foundation Trust, Norwich, UK. JMB B MedSci, BM BS, FRCP. Consultant Dermatologist and Honorary Consultant Lecturer, Centre of Evidence-based Dermatology, University of Nottingham.

Acknowledgments

This publication presents independent research commissioned by the National Institute for Health Research (NIHR) under its Programme Grants for Applied Research funding scheme ("Setting Priorities and Reducing Uncertainties for the Prevention and Treatment of Skin Disease 2008 – 2013", RP-PG-0407-10177). The views expressed in this publication are those of the author (s) and not necessarily those of the NHS, the NIHR or the Department of Health. The NIHR provided funding for this work and gave final approval of the manuscript but was not involved in any other part of the design, data collection, analyses or writing. We are extremely grateful to the Vitiligo Society, in particular Fred Fredriksen, for their help in setting up the secure online discussion groups, which were hosted through the Vitiligo Society's website. We are also grateful to the Vitiligo Society for giving us permission to publicise this work through their Facebook page, and to the UK Dermatology Clinical Trials Network for publicising the work through their Twitter feed. We would like to thank all of the people with vitiligo who responded to the survey and participated in the discussion groups. We are grateful to Mrs Maxine Whitton, Dr Joanne Chalmers, Dr Viktoria Eleftheriadou, and Dr Jane Ravenscroft for their help in reviewing the survey and the discussion group prompts.

Author details

[1]Centre of Evidence Based Dermatology, The University of Nottingham, Nottingham, UK. [2]Faculty of Medicine and Health Sciences, University of Nottingham, Nottingham, UK. [3]Norfolk and Norwich University Hospitals NHS Foundation Trust, Norwich, UK.

References

1. Whitton ME, Pinart M, Batchelor J, Lushey C, Leonardi-Bee J, Gonzalez U: **Interventions for vitiligo.** *Cochrane Database Syst Rev* 2010, **1**:CD003263.
2. Eleftheriadou V, Thomas KS, Whitton ME, Batchelor JM, Ravenscroft JC: **Which outcomes should we measure in vitiligo? Results of a systematic review and a survey among patients and clinicians on outcomes in vitiligo trials.** *Br J Dermatol* 2012, **167**(4):804–814.
3. Joint Formulary Committee: *British National Formulary (BNF) 66.* London: Pharmaceutical Press; 2013.
4. Hann SK, Chun WH, Park YK: **Clinical characteristics of progressive vitiligo.** *Int J Dermatol* 1997, **36**(5):353–355.
5. Thompson AR, Kent G, Smith JA: **Living with vitiligo: Dealing with difference.** *Br J Health Psychol* 2002, **7**(2):213–225.
6. Gonzalez U, Whitton M, Eleftheriadou V, Pinart M, Batchelor J, Leonardi-Bee J: **Guidelines for designing and reporting clinical trials in vitiligo.** *Arch Dermatol* 2011, **147**(12):1428–1436.
7. Eleftheriadou V, Whitton ME, Gawkrodger DJ, Batchelor J, Corne J, Lamb B, Ersser S, Ravenscroft J, Thomas KS: **Future research into the treatment of vitiligo: where should our priorities lie? Results of the vitiligo priority setting partnership.** *Br J Dermatol* 2011, **164**(3):530–536.
8. Comet Initiative: **International outcomes Consensus for Vitiligo.** http://www.comet-initiative.org/studies/details/357 (accessed November 2013).
9. McNally NJ, Phillips DR, Williams HC: **Focus groups in dermatology.** *Clin Exp Dermatol* 1998, **23**(5):195–200.
10. NHS Choices: **Vitiligo.** Available from: http://www.nhs.uk/Conditions/Vitiligo/Pages/Introduction.aspx.
11. Medical Research Council: **The Gold Standard: What are randomised controlled trials and why are they important?** 2013. https://www.youtube.com/watch?v=U6kVlRn6G0w (accessed August 2013).
12. Walker DM: **The internet as a medium for health service research. Part 1.** *Nurse Res* 2013, **20**(4):18–21.
13. Walker DM: **The internet as a medium for health services research. Part 2.** *Nurse Res* 2013, **20**(5):33–37.
14. Baltes BB, Dickson MW, Sherman MP, Bauer CC, LaGanke JS: **Computer-Mediated Communication and Group Decision Making: A Meta-Analysis.** *Organ Behav Hum Decis Process* 2002, **87**(1):156–179.
15. Murphy M, Black N, Lamping D, McKee C, Sanderson CF, Askham J, Marteau T: **Consensus development methods and their use in clinical guideline development.** *Health Technol Assess* 1998, **2**:3.
16. Brooks J, King N: *Qualitative Psychology in the Real World: The Utility of Template Analysis.* London, UK: British Psychological Society Annual Conference; 2012.
17. King N: **Doing Template Analysis.** In *Qualitative Organizational Research: Core Methods and Current Challenges.* Edited by Symon G, Cassell C. London: Sage; 2012.
18. BioMedCentral: **Qualitative research review guidelines – RATS.** 2003. Available from: http://www.biomedcentral.com/authors/rats.
19. Lilly E, Lu PD, Borovicka JH, Victorson D, Kwasny MJ, West DP, Kundu RV: **Development and validation of a vitiligo-specific quality-of-life instrument (VitiQoL).** *J Am Acad Dermatol* 2013, **69**(1):e11–8.
20. Krishna GS, Ramam M, Mehta M, Sreenivas V, Sharma VK, Khandpur S: **Vitiligo impact scale: An instrument to assess the psychosocial burden of vitiligo.** *Indian J Dermatol Venereol Leprol* 2013, **79**(2):205–210.
21. Beresniak A, de Linares Y, Krueger GG, Talarico S, Tsutani K, Duru G, Berger G: **Validation of a new international quality-of-life instrument specific to cosmetics and physical appearance: Beautyqol questionnaire.** *Arch Dermatol* 2012, **148**(11):1275–1782.
22. Benford P, Walker DM: **The Internet as a Research Medium.** In *An Introduction to Health Services Research: a practical guide.* Edited by Walker DM. London: Sage; 2014.

What determines patient preferences for treating low risk basal cell carcinoma when comparing surgery vs imiquimod? A discrete choice experiment survey from the SINS trial

Michela Tinelli[1], Mara Ozolins[2]*, Fiona Bath-Hextall[2] and Hywel C Williams[2]

Abstract

Background: The SINS trial (Controlled Clinical Trials ISRCTN48755084; Eudract No. 2004-004506-24) is a randomised controlled trial evaluating long term success of excisional surgery vs. imiquimod 5% cream for low risk nodular and superficial basal cell carcinoma (BCC). The trial included a discrete choice experiment questionnaire to explore patient preferences of a cream versus surgery for the treatment of their skin cancer.

Methods: The self-completed questionnaire was administered at baseline to 183 participants, measuring patients' strength of preferences when choosing either alternative 'surgery' or 'imiquimod cream' instead of a fixed 'current situation' option (of surgical excision as standard practice in UK). The treatments were described according to: cost, chance of complete clearance, side effects and appearance. Participants had to choose between various scenarios. Analysis was performed using a mixed logit model, which took into account the impact of previous BCC treatment and sample preference variability.

Results: The analysis showed that respondents preferred 'imiquimod cream' to their 'current situation' or 'surgery', regardless of previous experience of BCC symptoms and treatment. Respondents were more likely to be worried about their cosmetic outcomes and side effects they might experience over and above their chance of clearance and cost. Those with *no experience* of surgery (compared *with experience*) valued more the choice of 'imiquimod cream' (£1013 vs £781). All treatment characteristics were significant determinants of treatment choice, and there was significant variability in the population preferences for all of them.

Conclusions: Patients with BCC valued more 'imiquimod cream' than alternative 'surgery' options, and all treatment characteristics were important for their choice of care. Understanding how people with a BCC value alternative interventions may better inform the development of health care interventions.

Keywords: Patient preferences, Discrete choice, Willingness to pay, Nodular and superficial basal cell carcinoma, Surgery, Imiquimod cream

Background

To make an informed choice when choosing between surgery and imiquimod cream treatments for low risk basal cell carcinomas (BCCs) such as superficial BCC or small nodular BCC not located on the central face (as specified by the British Association of Dermatology BCC treatment guidelines [1]), patients need to balance trade-offs between different aspects (e.g. risk of scarring, clearance, and out-of-pocket costs) attached to these alternative treatments (Weston and Fitzgerald [2]; Essers et al. [3]). Our aim was to investigate patient preferences for 'surgery' or 'imiquimod cream' for the treatment of BCC using a discrete choice experiment (DCE; Ryan et al. [4]) approach in a sample of patients participating in a randomised controlled trial of surgery vs. imiquimod for low risk nodular and superficial BCC (Ozolins et al.

* Correspondence: Mara.Ozolins@Nottingham.ac.uk
[2]Centre of Evidence Based Dermatology, University of Nottingham, A103, King's Meadow Campus, Lenton Lane, Nottingham NG7 2NR, UK
Full list of author information is available at the end of the article

[5]). We chose the Discrete Choice Experiments (DCEs) technique as it has been previously used in health care to evaluate different cancer screening strategies (Wordsworth et al. [6]; Marshall et al. [7]; Kruijshaar et al. [8]; van Dam et al. [9]; Hol et al. [10]); and willingness to pay (WTP) for methyl aminolevulinate photodynamic therapy vs surgery in BCC (Weston and Fitzgerald [2]) and for Mohs micrographic surgery vs surgery (Essers et al. [3]). Patient experience with previous treatment has been shown to influence the utility (benefit) patients derive from health care interventions (Salkeld et al. [11]; Ryan and Ubach [12]; Cheraghi-Sohi et al. [13]). We are also aware that information from such experiments can help health professionals to understand individual preferences for treatment, and, indeed, inform policy (Eberth et al. [14]; De Bekker-Grob et al. [15]). To our knowledge there is no evidence of research investigating: i) *how* patients with a BCC value alternative treatments on offer ii) the extent of preference variability or heterogeneity in the sample and iii) bearing in mind that BCCs are often asymptomatic and multiple, whether patients *with experience* of tumour symptoms and previous treatments may have better informed preferences. This study investigates how patients with a low risk BCC participating in a randomized controlled trial of excisional surgery versus topical imiquimod value the choice between the two treatment modalities.

Methods
The Discrete Choice Experiment (DCE) questionnaire
The Discrete Choice Experiment (DCE) technique is an attribute based approach that quantifies strength of patients' preferences for the health care services or interventions. Respondents choose between alternative hypothetical interventions described in terms of their characteristics and associated levels. Results from the regression model identify which attributes, such as chance of clearance, side effects or convenience, are significant in the decision to choose, and their relative importance across treatments (i.e. magnitude of the attributes). Money as an attribute can also be used to estimate trade-off or Willingness To Pay (WTP, a monetary measure of benefit) for changes in attribute levels (e.g. WTP for improving by 1% their chance of clearance). The DCE technique, and its application to health care, is extensively discussed elsewhere (Ryan et al. [4]; de Bekker-Grob et al. [15]).

In this experiment, a list of attributes, their levels, and *status quo* alternative (see below) were derived from a previous DCE exercise applied to BCC (Weston et al. [2]), and from systematic discussion with the research team plus advice provided by a panel of experts. They were chosen to be general aspects of treatment that best described the alternative interventions on offer within the SINS trial i.e. 'surgery' vs.

'imiquimod cream' (Table 1). The "cost to you" attribute was added to find out how much patients valued the treatment. How the treatments and attributes were presented to the participants can be seen in the questionnaire (see Additional file 1).

A DCE labelled ('surgery' vs. 'imiquimod cream') experiment was created from design catalogues [16] using a fold-over approach (Louviere et al. [17]; Rose and Bliemer [18]), as a commonly used technique to inform experimental design creation (de Bekker-Grob et al. [15]). Employing such a design minimised the number of choices for each respondent, from 135 ($5^1 * 3^3$) to 16 choices. To the 16-choice design, a third *status quo* alternative was added, representing surgical excision as current (standard) practice in UK hospitals (i.e. 'current situation'). It defined an average surgical excision in a hospital setting with a 4 mm clear excision margin, use of a local anaesthetic injection, closure with sutures and removal of sutures on a separate visit. The 'current situation' was characterised by the following fixed levels: 96% chance of complete clearance; mild pain (that does not disturb sleep); a noticeable (but easy to cover) scar after treatment; and £0 cost to the patient (the procedure was undertaken free at the point of care in the UK National Health Service). An example of a choice is reported in Figure 1.

Participants, sample size, setting and data collection
Our study sample included men and women of any age with low risk [1] nodular or superficial BCC participating in the SINS (Surgery vs Imiquimod in Nodular and Superficial basal cell carcinoma) study [5]. The SINS study is a randomized controlled trial to compare excision 'surgery' and 'imiquimod cream' for nodular and superficial basal cell carcinoma presenting in low risk areas. The study (ISRCTN48755084) received full ethical and hospital approval, and is conducted according to the declaration of Helsinki; all participants gave informed written consent.

Since size, type of experimental design, and the number of independent variables were unknown in advance, a minimum estimate of 50–100 responses per subgroup of interest was stipulated. The questionnaire was distributed to 183 of 501 consecutive patients participating in the trial (18th to 200th), during their baseline visit (August 2003-January 2005). A minimum target response of 170 (response rate of 85%), allowing for comparison between two subgroups *with experience* and *with no experience* of BCC and treatment, was felt appropriate compared with similar studies (Pearmain et al. [19]).

Analysis
Response rates, patient characteristics, and questionnaire completion: Descriptive statistics were presented as

Table 1 Summary of coding for discrete choice experiment attributes and their levels

Attributes	Attribute levels			Variable names
	Surgery	*Imiquimod cream*	*Current situation*	
1) Cost [cost to you]	£0	£0	£0	COST
	£150	£150		
	£300	£300		
	£500	£500		
	£750	£750		
2) Chance [Chance of complete clearance]	94%	50%	96%	CHANCE
	96%	70%		
	98%	90%		
3) Side effects	MILD	MILD	MILD	MILD SIDE EFFECTS
	(mild pain that does not disturb sleep)	(Mild irritation, burning or redness)	(mild pain that does not disturb sleep)	
	MODERATE	MODERATE		MODERATE SIDE EFFECTS
	(pain that sometimes might disturb sleep)	(Moderate irritation, burning, redness or weeping)		
	SEVERE	SEVERE		(compared with severe)
	(pain that disturbs sleep)	(Severe irritation, burning, redness or ulceration)		
4) Appearance	NORMAL	NORMAL	MODERATE CHANGE	NORMAL APPEARANCE
	(Barely visible scar)	(Not discoloured skin)	(noticeable scar)	
	MODERATE CHANGE	MODERATE CHANGE		MODERATE CHANGE IN APPEARANCE
	(Noticeable scar)	(Slight lightening skin)		
	SEVERE CHANGE	SEVERE CHANGE		(compared with severe change)
	(Slightly raised scar)	(Discoloured skin)		
ALTERNATIVES	SURGERY	IMIQUIMOD CREAM	CURRENT SITUATION	SURGERY
			(fixed surgery option from their experience alternative to an hypothetical 'surgery')	CREAM (compared with current situation)

	SURGERY	**CREAM**	**CURRENT SITUATION**
Chance of complete clearance (%)	96	90	96
Side Effects	Moderate pain	Severe irritation, burning, redness or ulceration	Mild pain
Appearance after treatment	Slightly raised permanent scar	Skin as normal	Noticeable scar
Cost to you (£)	150	300	0
Which situation would you prefer? (*Tick one box only*)	**SURGERY** ☐	**CREAM** ☐	**CURRENT SITUATION** ✔

Figure 1 Example of Choice Set.

frequencies and percentages (binary variables) and median and inter-quartile range (continuous variables). Differences in patient characteristics between subgroups *with experience* and *with no experience* were reported and tested using the non parametric Mann–Whitney test and Chi square tests (where appropriate). SPSS software version 16 [20] was used to analyse the data.

Patient preferences: DCE modelling, its theoretical validity and subgroup analysis. Patient preference data were analysed using the mixed logit model (MLM, largely applied to multiple choice health care data, de Bekker-Grob et al. [15]). The Biogeme package [21] was used to support this analysis. Theoretical validity of responses was checked by testing the direction and significance of the model attributes. *A priori* we expected respondents to prefer: a decreased cost (a negative sign for 'COST'); an increased chance of complete clearance (positive sign for 'CHANCE'); a decreased severity of side effects (positive signs for 'MILD SIDE EFFECTS' and 'MODERATE SIDE EFFECTS'); and improved appearance (positive signs for 'NORMAL APPEARANCE', and 'MODERATE CHANGE IN APPEARANCE'). No *a-priori* assumptions were made concerning their preferred alternative (represented by the alternative specific constants (ASCs) for 'surgery' and 'imiquimod cream' options, 'ASC$_{SURGERY}$' and 'ASC$_{CREAM}$').

Subgroup analysis was undertaken to test whether different choices may result if respondents had experience of BCC and treatment. This follows current evidence in health care, reporting that respondents usually ascribe more value to the things they have experienced, (i.e. *status quo* bias: see Salkeld et al. [11]). The MLM model was presented considering all valid respondents (*whole sample*) and subgroups of those *with experience* and *with no experience* of BCC and treatment.

Estimated preferences were compared between experience subgroups. Difference in i) incremental WTP or ii) in proportion of respondents with preferences for a particular change in treatment characteristics (described by their mean and standard deviation) were reported and tested using independent *t* test statistics.

Results and discussion
Response rates, patient characteristics, and questionnaire completion
The DCE questionnaire was completed by 174/183 (95%) consecutive SINS trial participants. Overall 22% considered the questionnaire difficult/very difficult to complete (Table 2). The median age of the respondents was 65 years, 61% were men, 80% had a weekly income less than £300, and about 32% had previous experience of symptoms and treatment for BCC. Both subgroups *with experience* and *with no experience* presented socioeconomic characteristics similar to the *whole DCE sample* (See Table 2).

Patient preferences
Specifications of the MLM model, its output for analysing the *whole sample* and subgroups with and without previous BCC are presented in Tables 3, 4. Figures 2, 3 display mean utility values and marginal WTP attached to the alternative treatments and their characteristics. The proportion of respondents for whom a particular characteristic had a positive effect is illustrated in Figure 4.

In the *whole group* and subgroups with and without previous BCC, all treatment choice attributes are statistically significant at 95% and therefore significant in the decision to choose. There is also evidence that individuals valued these characteristics differently. Overall, all characteristics have the expected directions supporting theoretical validity of the findings (see above). The positive signs on the alternative specific constants (ASCs) indicate that, everything else being equal, respondents preferred alternative treatments to their 'current situation', and, when choosing an alternative to their 'current situation', the 'imiquimod cream' was preferred overall to the 'surgery' (as indicated by the higher positive value). See Tables 3, 4 for further details.

Whole sample
Across all treatment characteristics choosing mild instead of severe side effects was the most valued aspect (as indicated by the largest significant coefficient of 'MILD SIDE EFFECTS' with a mean value of 1.38), whilst an increase in cost was the least preferred ('COST' with a mean value of –0.0031; see Figure 2).

Figure 3 and Table 3 also show respondents' marginal WTP for a unit change in each treatment characteristic. For example, marginal WTP for choosing mild instead of severe side effects is £445.16 (standard deviation £541.94).

The proportion of respondents for whom a particular characteristic had a positive effect is reported in Figure 4, Table 3. For example, 79% of the sample preferred a change from severe to mild side effects, while the others did not value this change so highly.

Subgroup with experience of BCC and treatment
For those with previous BCC experience, the movement from severe change to normal appearance was the most important marginal change in an attribute (having the largest significant coefficient with a mean value of 1.31), and 'COST' remained the least preferred characteristic (see Figure 2, Table 4). The marginal WTP for choosing normal instead of severe change to appearance is £392.22 (standard deviation £377.25; Figure 3, Table 4). Ninety seven percent of the sample preferred normal appearance where as the others did not value this change so highly (Figure 4, Table 4).

Table 2 Patient characteristics (*whole sample* and subgroups relating to experience of BCC symptoms and treatment)

	Whole sample N=174	With no experience N=118	With experience N=56	With no vs. with experience
	% (n)	% (n)	% (n)	P value
Gender				0.3
Male	60.9 (106)	63.6 (75)	55.4 (31)	
Female	39.1 (68)	36.4 (43)	44.6 (25)	
Age				0.1
Median [IQR]	65 [57–72]	63 [55–72]	68 [60–72]	
Employment status				N.A. [1]
Employed	35.6 (62)	39.8 (47)	26.8 (15)	
Retired	63.2 (110)	59.3 (70)	71.4 (40)	
Unemployed	1.2 (2)	0.9 (1)	1.8 (1)	
Weekly income[2]				0.21
<£299	50.0 (80)	44.9 (53)	48.2 (27)	
£300-499	19.5 (34)	20.3 (24)	17.9 (10)	
£>=500	19.5 (34)	19.5 (23)	19.6 (11)	
(Not recorded to be excluded from analysis)	14.9 (26)	15.3 (18)	14.3 (8)	
Previous experience of BCC symptoms and treatment				
Yes	32.2 (56)	0 (0)	100 (56)	
No	67.8 (118)	100 (118)	0 (0)	
Difficulties in completing the questionnaire				N.A. [1]
Extremely easy	13.2 (23)	9.3 (11)	21.4 (12)	
Easy	28.7 (50)	26.3 (31)	33.9 (19)	
Moderate	35.6 (62)	39.8 (47)	26.8 (15)	
Difficult	16.1 (28)	16.1 (19)	16.1 (9)	
Extremely difficult	6.3 (11)	8.5 (10)	1.8 (1)	

[1] Cells have expected count less than 5. [2]Some respondents presented not recorded data, as the question was not asked (dropped from assessments) or they did not complete it.

Subgroup with no experience of a previous BCC and treatment

With *no BCC experience*, the movement from severe to mild side effects was the most important marginal change in an attribute (having largest significant coefficient with a mean value of 1.37), and 'COST' remained the least preferred characteristic (see Figure 2, Table 4). The marginal WTP when choosing mild instead of severe side effects was £455.15 (Figure 3, Table 4). Of the sample 80% preferred mild instead of severe side effects, while the others did not value this change so highly (Figure 1, Table 4).

Comparison between subgroups

Respondents preferred a change from the 'current situation' to alternative treatments and they mostly preferred moving to the 'imiquimod cream', regardless of their experience of a previous BCC and treatment. The subgroup with *no experience* valued more such change compared with the subgroup *with experience* ('ASC$_{CREAM}$'; £1013 vs. £781). The subgroup with *no experience* valued best

choosing mild instead of severe side effects, and their willingness to pay for this choice was similar to the other subgroup ('MILD SIDE EFFECTS'; £455 vs. £344, p=0.23). In the subgroups *with experience* the most valued characteristic was an improvement in their appearance from severe changes to normal appearance and they valued it more than the subgroup *with no experience* ('NORMAL APPEARANCE'; £392 vs. £299, p=0.02). More details are presented in Figure 3 and Table 4.

When considering the difference in preference distribution across groups a greater proportion of participants *with experience* compared *with no experience* preferred the idea of a change from severe to moderate side effects ('MODERATE SIDE EFFECTS'; 99% vs. 87%, p<0.01), or from severe change to normal appearance ('NORMAL APPEARANCE'; 97% vs. 85%, p<0.01; see Table 4). Other random coefficient distributions did not present statistically significant differences between groups ('CHANCE' p=0.13; 'MILD SIDE EFFECTS' p=0.45; 'MODERATE CHANGE IN APPEARANCE' p=0.11).

Table 3 Patient preferences for the *whole sample* (n=174)

		Whole sample				
		Regression[1]		Incremental WTP[2] (£)		Their preference is for:
		Value	(SD)	Value	(SD)	
ASC SURGERY	Coefficient	**1.4200**	(0.253)	**458.06**	-	Surgery (compared with current situation)
ASC CREAM	Coefficient	**2.8700**	(0.398)	**925.81**	-	Imiquimod cream (compared with current situation)
COST	Coefficient	**−0.0031**	(0.000)	-	-	Decreased cost
CHANCE	Mean	**0.1090**	(0.018)	**35.16**	(38.71)	increased chance, 82% of respondents
	SD	**0.1200**	(0.022)			
MILD SIDE EFFECTS	Mean	**1.3800**	(0.314)	**445.16**	(541.94)	mild side effects (compared with severe, 79% of respondents)
	SD	**1.6800**	(0.282)			
MODERATE SIDE EFFECTS	Mean	**0.8390**	(0.265)	**270.65**	(199.68)	moderate side effects (compared with severe, 91% of respondents)
	SD	**0.6190**	(0.396)			
NORMAL APPEARANCE	Mean	**1.0200**	(0.265)	**329.03**	(267.74)	normal appearance (compared with severe change, 89% of respondents)
	SD	**0.8300**	(0.333)			
MODERATE CHANGE IN APPEARANCE	Mean	**0.5400**	(0.345)	**174.19**	(548.39)	moderate change (compared with severe change, 62% of respondents)
	SD	**1.7000**	(0.274)			
Number of respondents		174				
Number of observations		2765 (=171 respondents *16 choices +1respondents*14 choices+1 respondent*8 choices+ 1 respondent*7 choices)				
Log-likelihood		−2013.9				
Adjusted Rho-square		0.333				
LR statistic		2047.47				

[1]The preferred model is a MLM and presents all characteristics (apart from 'COST', 'ASC_SURGERY', 'ASC_CREAM') as random and independently normally distributed. The simulation process is based on 500 draws. All coefficients (either fixed or random) and the standard deviations of the random coefficients are statistically significant at 95%. [2]WTP estimates are based on the regression results in column 3 and rounded to 2 decimal places. The standard deviations are in parentheses. Marginal WTP for a unit change in a treatment characteristic = (mean coefficient of characteristic)/-(coefficient 'COST'), with SD = (SD of characteristic coefficient)/ -(coefficient 'COST').

Note: Alternative specific constants (ASC) for surgery (ASC _SURGERY) and for cream (ASC _CREAM) show the preferences of these alternatives relative to the current situation, everything else being equal.

Key: SD = standard deviation, WTP = Willingness to Pay, LR = Likelihood Ratio.

Summary of preference findings

This Discrete Choice Experiment (DCE) exercise was embedded within a wider randomised controlled trial. This provided the main trial with new empirical evidence of strength of patient preferences for alternative treatments on offer for low risk BCC, the impact of previous experience of a BCC and treatment on their preferences, and a measure of the spread or heterogeneity of preferences in the sample.

To our surprise, respondents preferred the 'imiquimod cream' treatment to their 'current situation' or alternative 'surgery', regardless of their experience of a previous BCC and treatment, though it might be questioned whether respondents *with no experience* of a condition or treatment are in a position to inform decision making (Gafni [22]).

Our study showed that regardless of their experience, respondents valued all aspects of treatment, but they were more likely to be worried about their cosmetic outcomes and side effects they might experience over and above their chance of clearance and cost. A cream option with better cosmetic outcomes was more appealing to them than a surgery intervention with better clearance outcomes.

Respondents *with experience* of a previous BCC and treatment (usually surgical) valued the 'imiquimod cream' option less than those without such experience, a finding supported in the literature of *status quo* bias, where people are more likely to adopt a conservative response to health services innovations (Salkeld et al. [11]; Ryan and Ubach [12]; Tinelli et al. [23]). In this particular case respondents' experience for a surgery intervention might have limited

Table 4 Patient preferences according to experience of BCC and treatment

		With experience					With no experience				
		Regression[1]		Incremental WTP (£)		Their preference is for:	Regression[1]		Incremental WTP (£)		Their preferences is for:
		Value	(SD)	Value	(SD)		Value	(SD)	Value	(SD)	
ASC SURGERY	Coefficient	1.6300	(0.457)	488.02	-	Surgery (compared with current situation)	1.3400	(0.310)	445.18	-	Surgery (compared with current situation)
ASC CREAM	Coefficient	2.6100	(0.719)	781.44	-	Imiquimod cream (compared with current situation)	3.0500	(0.488)	1013.29	-	Imiquimod cream (compared with current situation)
COST	Coefficient	−0.0033	(0.001)			Decreased cost	−0.0030	(0.001)			Decreased cost
CHANCE[2]	Mean	0.0898	(0.033)	26.89	(44.61)	Increased chance (compared with deceased; 73% of respondents)	0.1210	(0.026)	40.20	(37.54)	Increased chance (compared with decreased; 86% of respondents)
	SD	0.1490	(0.058)				0.1130	(0.023)			
MILD SIDE EFFECTS	Mean	1.1500	(0.553)	344.31	(616.77)	Mild side effects (compared with severe; 71% of respondents)	1.3700	(0.390)	455.15	(541.53)	Mild side effects (compared with severe; 80% of respondents)
	SD	2.0600	(0.474)				1.6300	(0.327)			
MODERATE SIDE EFFECTS[2-3]	Mean	1.1600	(0.480)	347.31	(−153.89)	Moderate side effects (compared with severe; 99% of respondents)	0.6710	(0.312)	222.92	(−199.67)	Moderate side effects (compared with severe; 87% of respondents)
	SD	0.5140	(0.519)				0.6010	(0.423)			
NORMAL APPEARANCE[2-3]	Mean	1.3100	(0.531)	392.22	(377.25)	Normal appearance (compared with severe change; 97% of respondents)	0.9000	(0.304)	299.00	(158.80)	Normal appearance (compared with severe change, 85% of respondents)
	SD	1.2600	(0.633)				0.4780	(0.498)			
MODERATE CHANGE IN APPEARANCE	Mean	0.9230	(0.564)	276.35	(407.19)	Moderate change (compared with severe; 75% of respondents)	0.4630	(0.433)	153.82	(634.55)	Moderate change (compared with severe; 60% of respondents)
	SD	1.3600	(0.539)				1.9100	(0.408)			
No. respondents		56					118				
No. observations		896 (=56 respondents*16 choices)					1869 (=115 respondents*16 choices+ 1 respondent*14 choices+1 respondent* 8 choices+1 respondent*7 choices)				
Log-likelihood		−649.27					−1350.8				
Adj Rho-square		0.327					0.336				
LR statistic		670.18					1405.08				

Note: Alternative specific constants (ASC) for surgery (ASC$_{SURGERY}$) and for cream (ASC$_{CREAM}$) show the preferences of these alternatives relative to the current situation, everything else being equal. WTP estimates are based on the regression results in column 3 and rounded to 2 decimal places. The standard deviations are in parentheses. [1] The preferred model is a MLM and presents all characteristics (apart from 'COST', 'ASC$_{SURGERY}$', 'ASC$_{CREAM}$') as random and independently normally distributed. The simulation process is based on 500 draws. All coefficients (either fixed or random) and the standard deviations of the random coefficients are statistically significant at 95% [2] Differences in marginal WTP between groups are significant at the 95% level. [3] Differences in preference distribution between groups are significant at the 99% level. Key: SD = standard deviation, WTP = Willingness to Pay, LR = Likelihood Ratio, No. = Number of.

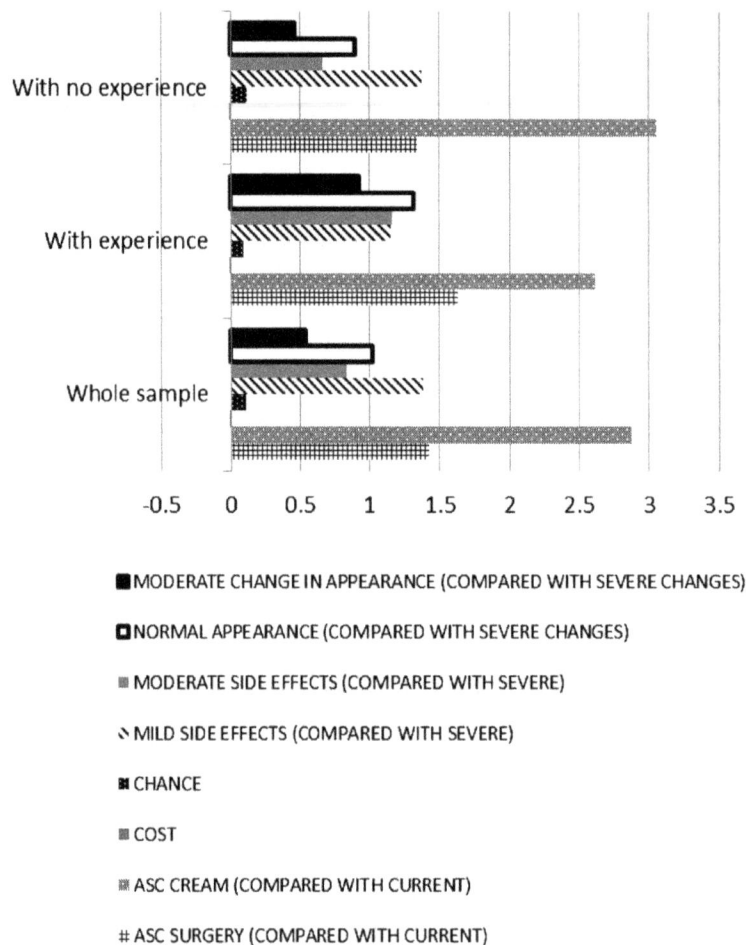

Figure 2 Modelling patient preferences: Utility values. Note: This Figure reports on average values only, whilst the complete output from the logistic regression model is presented in Tables 3 (*whole sample*) and 4 (subgroups *with experience* and *with no experience* of BCC symptoms and treatment). Alternative specific constants (ASC) for surgery (ASC _SURGERY_) and for cream (ASC _CREAM_) show the preferences of these alternatives relative to the current situation, everything else being equal. The cost attribute reported a mean value of −0.0031, and therefore it is less noticeable than the other attributes. Due to differences in scale factors across data sets, utility values from different subgroups are not directly comparable. For comparison between subgroups *with experience* and *with no experience* of BCC symptoms and treatment please see marginal WTP (Figure 3) and proportion of respondents (Figure 4). Overall findings from subgroup analyses are also presented in Table 4.

their shift of preferences from their *status quo* to an innovative 'imiquimod cream' intervention on offer.

With experience of a previous BCC and surgical intervention (with risk of permanent scar), the movement from severe change to normal appearance was the most important marginal change; this subgroup were more likely to value a treatment with the best cosmetic outcomes, regardless of other characteristics, compared with those with no previous BCC.

How people differed

Evidence of significant variation (heterogeneity) of preferences was found in the chance of clearance, side effects and appearance characteristics. Preferences for treatment characteristics were not specific to one particular improvement in their cosmetic outcomes or chance of clearance, though some changes might be regarded as not sufficient e.g. only 62% preferring moderate change vs. severe change. The distributions of preference were statistically different across experience subgroups. Results confirmed that respondents with experience of a BCC were more likely to value a treatment with the best cosmetic outcomes, whilst respondents with no past BCC might value less highly such improved characteristics.

Study strengths and limitations

A particular strength was using a multiple choice design with inclusion of a *status quo* option; forcing a

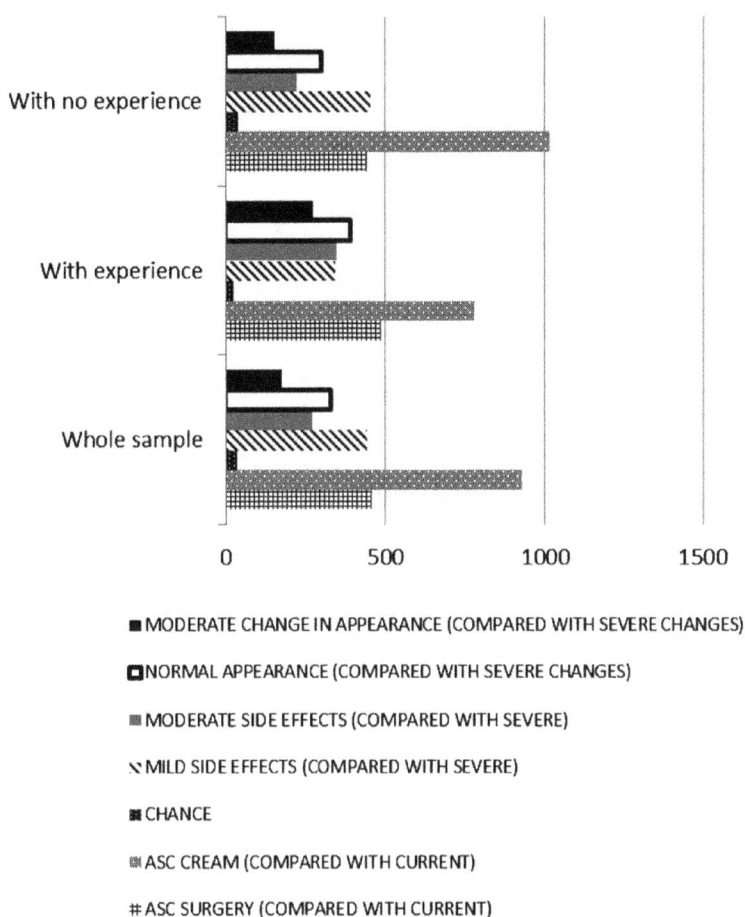

Figure 3 Modelling patient preferences: Marginal WTP values (£). Note: This Figure reports on mean values only, whilst the complete output from the logistic regression model, marginal WTP calculations (mean and standard deviation values), and their comparison between subgroups is presented in Tables 3 (*whole sample*) and 4 (subgroups with *experience* and *with no experience* of BCC symptoms and treatment). For 'CHANCE', 'MODERATE SIDE EFFECTS' and 'NORMAL APPEARANCE' differences in marginal WTP between subgroups (*with experience* vs. *with no experience* of BCC symptoms and treatment) are significant at the 95% level.

choice i.e. no *status quo* alternative when this reflects the reality may result in an overestimation of responses (Boyle et al. [24]).

Other strengths included exploring heterogeneity of responses, and the mixed logit model (MLM) allowed statistical investigation of how preferences varied across groups. Information on variation (heterogeneity) of preferences is recognised as an important aspect when integrating patient views into decision making (de Bekker-Grob et al. [15]). A MLM was applied to the data as it is commonly used to analyse multiple choice health care data (de Bekker-Grob et al. [15]), although alternative models, such as the latent class model, could also be adopted (Hensher et al. [25] Hensher and Greene [26]). Our modelling study also confirmed the importance of exploring preference variation across groups to better understand and implement innovative services on offer. Patient knowledge of the condition and treatment experience might provide more informed choice.

A limitation is that participants in this study are unlikely to have experienced topical imiquimod, thus we could not assess how previous imiquimod experience influenced their preferences (including the risk of possible reactions/side effects to the treatment), whereas we could at least partly with surgical excision as some had already experienced it for a previous BCC. It would have been informative to analyse the DCE further, for example, comparing any changes in patient preferences later in the study after experiencing surgery or imiquimod cream. Also, patients with both nodular and superficial BCC were included in the current analysis. Future studies could aim to collect larger sample sizes to perform a subgroup analysis according to the type of BCC affecting the patients. Time constraints did

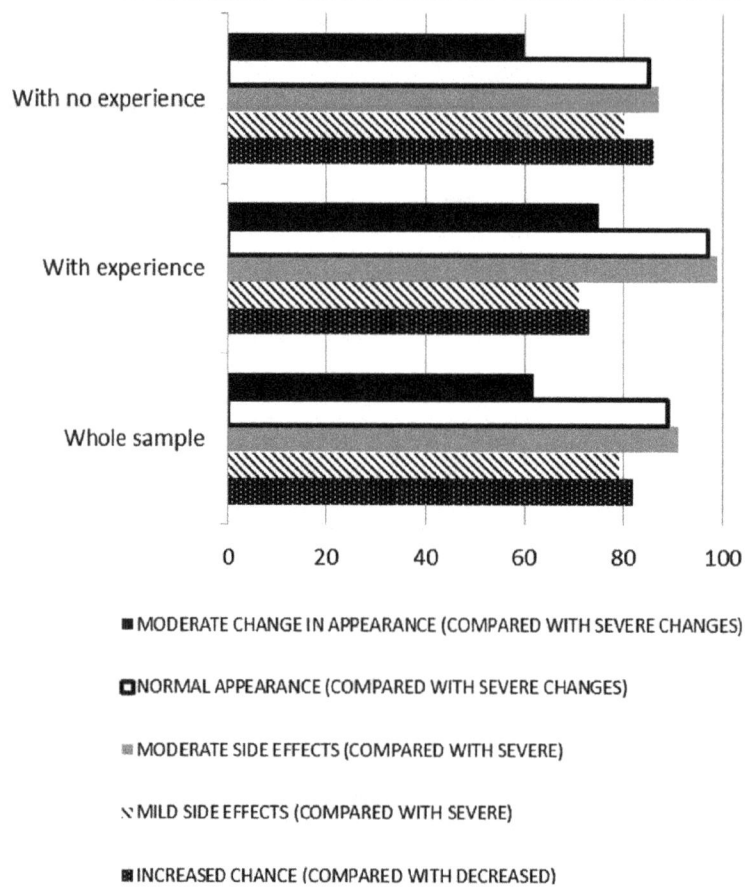

Figure 4 Modelling patient preferences: the proportion of respondents (%) with positive effect of particular characteristic. Note: The output from the logistic regression model used to inform these estimates is presented in Tables 3 (*whole sample*) and 4 (subgroups *with experience* and *with no experience* of BCC symptoms and treatment, and their comparison). For 'MODERATE SIDE EFFECTS' and 'NORMAL APPEARANCE' differences in preference distribution between subgroups (*with experience* vs. *with no experience* of BCC symptoms and treatment) are significant at the 95% level.

not allow us to further inform the decision on the choice of the attributes and their levels with patient interviews and focus groups. Other attribute levels (e.g. different levels for the cost attributes pending on the specific treatment compared) could be considered for future exercises and informed by trial economic evaluation.

Although our 95% overall response rate was high, respondents in this DCE survey might not have been representative of all BCC patients because they are all participants in the SINS trial, who by definition are more equipoise and willing to consider both options of 'imiquimod cream' and alternative 'surgery' intervention; also it is not a random sample. Most patients (with or without previous surgical experience) who had a strong preference for a *status quo* approach with surgical excision would probably not have chosen to participate in the SINS trial, and therefore their preferences were not captured by this DCE survey. Of those choosing not to take part in the study 48% (126/265) gave the reason as wanting to have surgery.

A further seven dropped out of the study after randomisation because they did not want surgery.

The DCE can provide very useful information, but the completion difficulties and time taken in this elderly population (median age 68, up to a maximum of 92 years) are not to be underestimated – many found it difficult to understand the concept of choosing between hypothetical situations and hence took up to an hour to complete. The research nurse helped them to understand what they had to do. The results showed, however, consistency of answers, suggesting that participants were not just making random choices. DCE surveys will benefit from providing participants with help and support from experienced research staff during questionnaire completion if needed.

Although this research refers to a representative group of mainly elderly patients in the UK with low risk BCC, our findings of attitudes and preference to treatment options may not be generalisable to other countries and ethnic groups. It is also important to emphasise the low risk nature of this BCC population. The trade-off between clearance and cosmetic results in recurrences of aggressive tumours for example is likely to be different from those observed in this study population.

Conclusions

Understanding how people with BCC value alternative interventions using the DCE technique may better inform the development of health care interventions, although this particular application proved data collection to be challenging and time consuming; elderly participants are likely to need help and support.

Abbreviations

ASC: Alternative specific constant; BCC: Basal cell carcinoma; DCE: Discrete choice experiment; MLM: Mixed logit model; SINS study: Surgery vs. imiquimod in nodular and superficial basal cell carcinoma; WTP: Willingness to pay; vs: Versus or compared with.

Competing interests

The authors declare they have no competing interests.

Authors' contributions

MT designed the discrete choice experiment, analysed the data, wrote the first draft of the manuscript, and revised the manuscript. MO provided input to the design of the experiment, entered and processed the data, revised the manuscript, and coordinated submission. FB-H provided input to the design of the experiment, and revised the manuscript. HCW provided input to the design of the experiment, and revised the manuscript. All authors read and approved the final manuscript.

Acknowledgements

Many thanks to Cancer Research UK for providing the grant (C7484/A2869) from which the DCE was funded. Cancer Research UK did not have any part in study design or the writing of the manuscript, or the decision to submit the manuscript for publication.
We wish to thank Prof. Mandy Ryan for her initial advice on the Discrete Choice Experiment (DCE) approach, and providing our contact with Dr Tinelli. Thanks also to Dr Paul Miller for the idea of evaluating patient treatment preferences in BCC using conjoint analysis (later changed to the DCE approach), and to the SINS team for their input to the SINS clinical trial which this experiment was part of.

Author details

[1]Centre of Academic Primary Care and Health Economics Research Unit, University of Aberdeen, Aberdeen, UK. [2]Centre of Evidence Based Dermatology, University of Nottingham, A103, King's Meadow Campus, Lenton Lane, Nottingham NG7 2NR, UK.

References

1. Telfer N, Colver G, Morton C: Guidelines for the management of basal cell carcinoma. Br J Dermatol 2008, 159:35–48.
2. Weston A, FitzGerald P: Discrete choice experiment to derive willingness-to-pay for methyl aminolevulinate photodynamic therapy versus simple excision surgery in the treatment of basal cell carcinoma. PharmacoEconomics 2004, 22:1195–1208.
3. Essers BAB, Van Helvoort-Postulart D, Prins MH, et al: Does the Inclusion of a Cost Attribute Result in Different Preferences for the Surgical Treatment of Primary Basal Cell Carcinoma?: A Comparison of Two Discrete-Choice Experiments. PharmacoEconomics 2010, 28:507–520.
4. Ryan M, Gerard K, Amaya-Amaya M: Using Discrete Choice Experiments to Value Health and Health Care. New York: Springer Berlin Heidelberg; 2008.
5. Ozolins M, Williams HC, Armstrong SJ, Bath-Hextall FJ: The SINS trial: A randomised controlled trial of excisional surgery versus imiquimod 5% cream for nodular and superficial basal cell carcinoma. Trials 2010, 11:42.
6. Wordsworth S, Ryan M, Skåtun D, Waugh N: Women's preferences for cervical cancer screening: A study using a discrete choice experiment. Int J of Technol Assess in Health Care 2006, 22(3):344–350.
7. Marshall DA, Johnson FR, Phillips KA, et al: Measuring Patient Preferences for Colorectal Cancer Screening Using a Choice-Format Survey. Value in Health 2007, 10:415–430.
8. Kruijshaar ME, Essink-Bot ML, Donkers B, et al: A labelled discrete choice experiment adds realism to the choices presented: preferences for surveillance tests for Barrett esophagus. BMC Medical Research Methodology 2009, 9:31.
9. Van Dam L, Hol L, De Bekker-Grob EW, et al: What determines individuals' preferences for colorectal cancer screening programmes? A discrete choice experiment. Eur J Cancer 2010, 46:150–159.
10. Hol L, De Bekker-Grob EW, vanDam L, et al: Preferences for colorectal cancer screening strategies: a discrete choice experiment. Br J Cancer 2010, 102:972–980.
11. Salkeld G, Ryan M, Short L: The veil of experience: do consumers prefer what they know best? Health Econ Letters 2000, 9:267–270.
12. Ryan M, Ubach C: Testing for an experience endowment effect in health care. Appl Econ Letters 2003, 10:407–410.
13. Cheraghi-Sohi S, Bower PJ, Mead NJ, et al: Making sense of patient priorities: applying discrete choice methods in primary care using 'think aloud' technique. Fam Pract 2007, 24:276–282.
14. Eberth B, Watson V, Ryan M, et al: Does one size fit all? Investigating heterogeneity in men's preferences for benign prostatic hyperplasia treatment using mixed logit analysis. Med Decis Making 2009, 29:707–717.
15. De Bekker-Grob EW, Ryan M, Gerard K: Discrete choice experiments in health economics: a review of the literature. In Health Economics: published online in Wiley online library (wileyonlinelibrary.com); 2010. doi:10.1002/hec.1697.
16. Sloane NJA. A library of orthogonal arrays. [http://www.research.att.com/~njas/oadir/] [accessed 14/05/12]
17. Louviere JJ, Hensher DA, Swait JD: Stated Choice Methods, Analysis and Application. Cambridge University Press; 2000.
18. Rose JM, Bliemer MCJ: Constructing Efficient Stated Choice Experimental Designs. Transp Rev 2009, 29:587–617.
19. Pearmain D, Swanson J, Kroes E, Bradley M: Stated preferences techniques: a guide to practice. Steer Davis Gleave and Hague Consulting Group: The Hague, 1991.
20. SPSS software. [URL http://www-01.ibm.com/software/analytics/spss/] [accessed 14/05/12]
21. Biogeme software for discrete choice models. [http://biogeme.epfl.ch/ accessed 14/05/12]
22. Gafni A: Willingness-to-pay as a measure of benefits: relevant questions in the context of public decision making about health care programs. Med Care 1991, 29:1246–1252.
23. Tinelli M, Ryan M, Bond C: Patient preferences for an increased pharmacist role in the management of drug therapy. Int J Pharm Pract 2009, 17:275–282.
24. Boyle KL, Holmes TP, Teisl MF, Roe B: A comparison of conjoint analysis response formats. Am J Agric Econ 2001, 83:441–454.
25. Hensher D, Rose J, Greene W: Applied choice analysis: A primer. Cambridge: Cambridge University Press; 2005:744pp.
26. Hensher D, Greene W: A latent class model for discrete choice analysis: contrasts with mixed logit. Working paper Institute of Transport Studies, Sydney University, 2002.

Effects of tofacitinib on lymphocyte sub-populations, CMV and EBV viral load in patients with plaque psoriasis

Fernando Valenzuela[1], Kim A Papp[2], David Pariser[3], Stephen K Tyring[4], Robert Wolk[5], Marjorie Buonanno[5], Jeff Wang[6,8], Huaming Tan[5] and Hernan Valdez[7,9*]

Abstract

Background: Plaque psoriasis is a debilitating skin condition that affects approximately 2% of the adult population and for which there is currently no cure. Tofacitinib is an oral Janus kinase inhibitor that is being investigated for psoriasis.

Methods: The design of this study has been reported previously (NCT00678210). Patients with moderate to severe chronic plaque psoriasis received tofacitinib (2 mg, 5 mg, or 15 mg) or placebo, twice daily, for 12 weeks. Lymphocyte sub-populations, cytomegalovirus (CMV) and Epstein-Barr virus (EBV) DNA were measured at baseline and up to Week 12.

Results: Tofacitinib was associated with modest, dose-dependent percentage increases from baseline in median B cell count at Week 4 (24–68%) and Week 12 (18–43%) and percentage reductions from baseline in median natural killer cell count at Week 4 (11–40%). The proportion of patients with detectable CMV and EBV DNA (defined as >0 copies/500 ng total DNA) increased post-baseline in tofacitinib-treated patients. However, multivariate analyses found no relationship between changes in CMV or EBV viral load and changes in lymphocyte sub-populations or tofacitinib treatment.

Conclusions: Twelve weeks of treatment with tofacitinib had no clinically significant effects on CMV or EBV viral load, suggesting that lymphocyte sub-populations critical to the response to chronic viral infections and viral reactivation were not significantly affected. Replication of these findings during long-term use of tofacitinib will allow confirmation of this observation.

Keywords: Cytomegalovirus, Epstein-Barr virus, Janus kinase inhibition, Lymphocyte, Plaque psoriasis, Tofacitinib, Viral reactivation

Background

Psoriasis is a debilitating and recurring immune-mediated inflammatory disease that affects 0.91–8.5% of the adult population according to geographic region [1]. Plaque psoriasis is by far the most prevalent form, accounting for approximately 80% of cases [2]. Tofacitinib is an oral Janus kinase (JAK) inhibitor that is being investigated for psoriasis. Oral tofacitinib has been evaluated in a Phase I study in patients with active psoriasis [3], and in Phase II and Phase III studies in patients with chronic plaque psoriasis [4-6] (see also NCT01276639 and NCT01309737). Tofacitinib binds to and inhibits JAK1 and JAK3, thereby blocking pro-inflammatory cytokine signaling, in particular interleukin (IL)-6 and interferon γ [7,8]. C-reactive protein (CRP), a marker of inflammation, is under the transcriptional control of IL-6 [9] and, thus, may be modulated by tofacitinib. Tofacitinib also modulates the activity of several other interleukins (including IL-2, –4, –7, –9, –15, and –21) that have roles in mediating immune response to viral infection/reactivation, lymphocyte development, and effector function [10,11]. Owing to the chronic nature of

* Correspondence: hernan.valdez@pfizer.com
[7]Pfizer Inc, New York, NY, USA
[9]Specialty Care Medicines Development Group, Pfizer Inc, 219 E 42nd Street, 7th Floor Room 50, NYO 219/07/01, New York, NY 10017, USA
Full list of author information is available at the end of the article

psoriasis and consequent prolonged and repeated periods of exposure to systemic immunomodulatory therapies, it is important to evaluate the potential effects of new therapies, such as tofacitinib, on immunosurveillance.

This exploratory analysis investigated the effect of oral tofacitinib on lymphocyte sub-populations to identify any impact of tofacitinib on immunosurveillance during a Phase IIb, 12-week, placebo-controlled study in patients with moderate to severe plaque psoriasis [4]. The potential for reactivation of latent viruses (eg cytomegalovirus [CMV], John Cunningham virus, Epstein-Barr virus [EBV], hepatitis B virus, and varicella zoster virus) has been described with other immunosuppressive agents [12-17]. Recurrence of CMV infection in immunocompromised patients can cause damage to the digestive system, lungs, and eyes [18]. CMV infections have been reported in patients with psoriasis receiving biologic therapies including the tumor necrosis factor inhibitor (TNFi) etanercept, and efalizumab, an anti-CD11a antibody [12,13]. Efalizumab was found to be associated with increased risk of John Cunningham virus-related progressive multifocal leukoencephalopathy, a potentially fatal infection of the central nervous system and, consequently, was withdrawn from the market in 2009 [19]. Reactivation of EBV is associated with development of lymphoproliferative malignancies including non-Hodgkin lymphoma, and has been reported in patients receiving biologic and nonbiologic treatment for psoriasis [14,15]. Reactivation of hepatitis B virus can lead to severe hepatitis, liver failure, and death [20]. A need for hepatitis B virus screening and pre-emptive therapy has been highlighted in patients receiving TNFi therapy [21]. Reactivation of latent varicella zoster virus causes shingles, the main complication of which is chronic pain, and is a long-term challenge in patients receiving immunosuppressive therapy [17].

In the present study, potential for viral reactivation in general was evaluated using CMV and EBV DNA copy numbers as surrogates of viral-specific immune surveillance. To complement evaluation of lymphocyte sub-populations during tofacitinib treatment, changes in inflammatory activity during tofacitinib treatment were assessed using serum levels of CRP as a marker.

Methods

This was a Phase IIb, randomized, double-blind, parallel-group, placebo-controlled study conducted in 42 centers in the United States and Canada (NCT00678210). Patients were aged ≥18 years with moderate to severe chronic plaque-type psoriasis covering ≥15% of the total body surface area, had stable disease for ≥6 months, a Psoriasis Area and Severity Index (PASI) score ≥13 and were eligible for phototherapy or systemic treatment of psoriasis [4]. Patients were excluded if they had received

any prior lymphocyte-depleting therapy (eg alemtuzumab, cyclophosphamide, chlorambucil) or had received rituximab/other selective B lymphocyte-depleting therapy within the preceding 12 months.

The study design has been reported elsewhere [4]. Briefly, patients were randomized 1:1:1:1 to receive oral tofacitinib (2 mg, 5 mg, or 15 mg twice daily [BID]), or placebo, for 12 weeks. Follow-up continued for 4 weeks after study completion or withdrawal. The safety population (all patients who received at least one dose of tofacitinib or placebo) was used in this exploratory analysis. The study was performed in compliance with the International Conference on Harmonization Good Clinical Practice Guidelines. All patients provided written informed consent, and both consent documentation and the final protocol were reviewed and approved by the institutional review board and/or the independent ethics committee at each of the investigational centers participating in the study.

Cell and viral quantification

Whole blood and serum were collected and analyzed. Lymphocyte populations were identified and quantified by fluorescence-activated cell sorting (FACS) analysis at baseline, Weeks 4 and 12, or early termination. Lymphocyte subset markers analyzed included: $CD3^+$ (total T cells), $CD3^+/CD4^+$ (T helper cells; T_H), $CD3^+/CD8^+$ (cytotoxic T cells; T_C), $CD19^+$ (B cells), and $CD16^+/CD56^+$ (natural killer cells; NK).

Serum CRP levels were measured at baseline and Week 12 or early termination. Blood CMV and EBV DNA was measured at baseline, Weeks 4 and 8 (CMV only), and Week 12 or early termination. Viral loads were quantified by real-time polymerase chain reaction (PCR) using DNA isolated directly from peripheral blood leukocytes and expressed as viral DNA copies/500 ng of total DNA. CMV or EBV DNA levels >0 copies/500 ng total DNA were defined as detectable.

Statistical analysis

For continuous endpoints measured longitudinally, a repeated mixed-effect model was used to analyze change from baseline, where treatment, visit week, and interaction between treatment and visit week were included as fixed factors, along with baseline value as the covariate. For continuous endpoints evaluated at a single time point, analysis of covariance (ANCOVA) was used to analyze change from baseline, and the baseline value was included as covariate. For categorical data, comparisons between groups were performed using a Chi-squared test. Missing values were not imputed in any of these analyses.

Spearman's correlation analyses, based on the ranks of variables, were performed between change in viral load or CRP level, and change in lymphocyte sub-population cell counts. A linear model was used to assess potential relationships between change in viral load or CRP level, and change in lymphocyte sub-population cell counts, and doses of tofacitinib.

Results

Baseline demographics, disease characteristics, and laboratory values (including lymphocyte sub-population cell counts, CRP, CMV, and EBV viral load) were similar between groups (Table 1).

Effects on T cells

In patients receiving tofacitinib, there was a dose-dependent percentage increase from baseline in median total T (CD3$^+$) cell count at Week 4, returning to near baseline levels by Week 12 (Table 2, Figure 1). Such a trend was not observed in patients receiving placebo.

A similar pattern of dose-dependent percentage increases at Week 4, followed by a return to near baseline levels at Week 12, was observed in median T_H (CD3$^+$/CD4$^+$) cell counts (Table 2, Figure 1). No patient had a T_H cell count <200 cells/mm^3. Among patients with a T_H cell count of ≥500 cells/mm^3 at baseline (n = 170), two, two, one, and three patients receiving placebo, tofacitinib 2 mg, 5 mg, or 15 mg BID, respectively, had a single post-baseline

measurement of <500 cells/mm^3. Only one patient had two consecutive T_H cell counts <500 cells/mm^3 (Week 4 and Week 12). This patient received tofacitinib 2 mg BID. While there was some variability in T_C (CD3$^+$/CD8$^+$) cell counts, these changes did not appear to be dose dependent (Table 2, Figure 1).

Overall, there was a good correlation between total lymphocyte count and sub-population cell counts (T cells, T_H cells, and T_C cells) across groups, ranging from 0.62–0.93 at baseline, 0.58–0.94 at Week 4, and 0.56–0.92 at Week 12.

Effects on B cells

Tofacitinib treatment resulted in dose-dependent percentage increases from baseline in B cell counts that were sustained throughout the study (Table 2, Figure 1). At Week 12, five (13.2%), two (5.4%), and four (10.3%) patients receiving tofacitinib 2 mg, 5 mg, and 15 mg BID, respectively, had B cell counts above the normal range, compared with one patient (3.0%) in the placebo group.

Effects on natural killer cells

Treatment with tofacitinib resulted in dose-dependent percentage reductions from baseline in median NK cell count at Week 4. At Week 12 the median NK cell count reduced further in the tofacitinib 2 mg BID group,

Table 1 Patient demographics, disease characteristics, cell counts, CMV and EBV DNA count at baseline

	Placebo (n = 50)	Tofacitinib 2 mg BID (n = 49)	Tofacitinib 5 mg BID (n = 49)	Tofacitinib 15 mg BID (n = 49)
Mean age, years (SD)	43.9 (13.0)	45.7 (13.8)	44.0 (12.6)	43.6 (15.6)
Male, n (%)	36 (72.0)	29 (59.2)	29 (59.2)	31 (63.2)
White, n (%)	41 (82.0)	36 (73.5)	42 (85.7)	40 (81.6)
Mean weight, kg (SD)	89.6 (23.9)	89.6 (23.0)	92.2 (23.5)	93.1 (29.7)
Mean PASI score (SD)	21.5 (7.1)	21.5 (6.7)	21.2 (8.1)	22.6 (10.3)
Mean BSA, % (SD)	29.8 (13.5)	29.8 (13.4)	30.1 (17.0)	31.9 (18.8)
PGA, n (%):				
Mild	6 (12.0)	8 (16.3)	11 (22.4)	9 (18.8)
Moderate	41 (82.0)	39 (79.6)	33 (67.3)	33 (68.8)
Severe	3 (6.0)	2 (4.1)	5 (10.2)	6 (12.5)
Median cell counts, cells/mm^3 (Q25, Q75):				
T (CD3$^+$)	1310 (982, 1517)	1115 (894, 1455)	1206 (1047, 1578)	1162 (935, 1510)
T_H (CD3$^+$/CD4$^+$)	802 (615, 975)	730 (572, 931)	868 (637, 998)	744 (597, 950)
T_C (CD3$^+$/CD8$^+$)	431 (287, 570)	331 (246, 498)	392 (264, 501)	386 (292, 539)
B (CD19$^+$)	195 (134, 304)	241 (136, 322)	198 (163, 300)	247 (143, 343)
NK (CD16$^+$/CD56$^+$)	159 (93, 188)	135 (91, 214)	130 (95, 207)	152 (97, 216)
Median CMV viral load, copies/500 ng total DNA (Q25, Q75)	0 (0.00, 0.00)	0 (0.00, 0.00)	0 (0.00, 0.00)	0 (0.00, 0.00)
Median EBV viral load, copies/500 ng total DNA (Q25, Q75)	0 (0.00, 1.30)	0 (0.00, 0.95)	0 (0.00, 1.00)	0 (0.00, 0.85)
Median CRP, mg/L (Q25, Q75)	1.84 (0.83, 4.41)	2.54 (1.13, 7.79)	1.92 (1.02, 5.84)	3.14 (0.92, 7.86)

B, B cells; BSA, body surface area; BID, twice daily; CMV, cytomegalovirus; CRP, C-reactive protein; DNA, deoxyribonucleic acid; EBV, Epstein-Barr virus; n, number; NK, natural killer cells; PASI, Psoriasis Area and Severity Index; PGA, Physician's Global Assessment (scored on a five-point severity scale); Q, quartile; SD, standard deviation; T, total T cells; T_C, cytotoxic T cells; T_H, T helper cells.

Table 2 Change from baseline in lymphocyte sub-populations, EBV and CMV DNA counts, and CRP[a]

Median percent change in lymphocyte sub-population cell counts, cells/mm^3 (Q25, Q75)

	Time point	Placebo	Tofacitinib 2 mg BID	Tofacitinib 5 mg BID	Tofacitinib 15 mg BID
T (CD3$^+$)	Week 4	−0.39 (−14.03, 9.75)	4.79 (−7.45, 17.57)	6.36 (−4.05, 24.24)	8.38 (−9.07, 42.80)
	Week 12	2.28 (−8.31, 11.10)	0.10 (−17.18, 15.87)	3.73 (−11.75, 17.54)	0.65 (−23.86, 17.64)
T$_H$ (CD3$^+$/CD4$^+$)	Week 4	−0.14 (−10.71, 12.20)	5.52 (−6.73, 18.12)	9.56 (0, 30.24)	15.09 (−5.39, 56.12)
	Week 12	0.89 (−7.00, 15.95)	−0.90 (−12.29, 15.42)	3.82 (−9.54, 17.99)	−0.82 (−22.29, 32.57)
T$_C$ (CD3$^+$/CD8$^+$)	Week 4	−4.79 (−12.42, 15.01)	5.13 (−13.33, 19.62)	0.29 (−9.45, 27.35)	−0.23 (−19.05, 47.92)
	Week 12	3.74 (−11.43, 18.42)	−5.58 (−16.27, 11.29)	−1.48 (−12.46, 14.07)	−0.33 (−28.53, 24.61)
B (CD19$^+$)	Week 4	−6.87 (−19.05, 11.40)	23.88 (6.60, 43.13)	45.17 (16.28, 56.84)	67.90 (32.64, 103.79)
	Week 12	−0.67 (−12.93, 18.09)	18.03 (0.94, 47.37)	35.32 (9.66, 66.32)	42.86 (16.74, 67.50)
NK (CD16$^+$/CD56$^+$)	Week 4	0 (−27.68, 37.60)	−10.94 (−28.17, 8.28)	−26.11 (−46.71, 4.35)	−40.80 (−52.50, −10.06)
	Week 12	13.87 (−21.43, 26.67)	−20.00 (−34.17, 3.97)	−22.76 (−51.38, −1.59)	−34.31 (−57.07, −16.57)
Median change in viral load, copies/500 ng total DNA (Q25, Q75)					
CMV	Week 4	0 (0.00, 0.00)	0 (0.00, 0.00)	0 (0.00, 0.00)	0 (0.00, 0.00)
	Week 8	0 (0.00, 0.00)	0 (0.00, 0.00)	0 (0.00, 0.00)	0 (0.00, 0.90)
	Week 12	0 (0.00, 0.00)	0 (0.00, 0.00)	0 (0.00, 0.00)	0 (0.00, 0.00)
EBV	Week 12	0 (−1.10, 0.00)	0 (0.00, 1.25)	0 (0.00, 0.60)	0.70 (0.00, 2.90)
Median percent change in CRP, % (Q25, Q75)					
CRP	Week 12	9.42 (−52.41, 61.08)	−24.71 (−47.43, 5.49)	−36.31 (−74.62, 5.49)	−69.17 (−82.20, −34.38)

[a]Safety set, no imputation.

B, B cells; BID, twice daily; CMV, cytomegalovirus; CRP, C-reactive protein; DNA, deoxyribonucleic acid; EBV, Epstein-Barr virus; NK, natural killer cells; Q, quartile; T, total T cells; T$_H$, T helper cells; T$_C$, cytotoxic T cells.

remained similar in the tofacitinib 5 mg BID group, and increased in the tofacitinib 15 mg BID group (Table 2, Figure 1).

Changes in C-reactive protein levels
Median CRP values at baseline are shown in Table 1. At Week 12, there were dose-dependent percentage reductions from baseline in median CRP levels in the tofacitinib groups, whereas CRP increased in the placebo group (Table 2).

Cytomegalovirus and Epstein-Barr virus DNA
The median (quartile [Q]25, Q75) CMV viral load at baseline was 0 copies/500 ng total DNA (0.0, 0.0) in all groups. The median change from baseline in CMV DNA was 0 copies/500 ng total DNA at Week 4, Week 8, and Week 12 (the Q25 and Q75 were 0.0 for all groups and time points except for the tofacitinib 15 mg BID group at Week 8, in which the Q75 value was 0.9) (Table 2, Figure 2).

CMV DNA was detected in three patients at baseline: one each in the placebo, tofacitinib 2 mg, and tofacitinib 5 mg BID groups. In all three patients, the CMV viral load was <1 copy/500 ng total DNA. Only one patient, a 78-year-old white male receiving tofacitinib 15 mg BID, had post-baseline incidences of CMV DNA >10 copies/

500 ng total DNA, which were as follows. This patient had a positive test for CMV on Day 57 (150 copies/500 ng total DNA), which was reported as a mild adverse event. He reported no other adverse signs or symptoms at this time and continued study treatment. CMV levels subsequently reduced to 92 copies/500 ng total DNA at Day 70 while on treatment. Once the initial positive test was relayed to the investigator site, study treatment was discontinued on Day 86, and on Day 87 his CMV level was 19 copies/500 ng total DNA. The event subsequently resolved. Another patient had a single incidence of CMV DNA ≥5 copies/500 ng total DNA. This patient received tofacitinib 15 mg BID, and had a CMV viral load of 7 copies/500 ng total DNA at Week 8, with no adverse events reported. The patient discontinued treatment and the elevated CMV levels resolved.

No comparison of baseline vs post-baseline CMV detectability was possible for patients with detectable CMV at baseline, due to limited sample size (Tables 1 and 3). In patients with undetectable CMV at baseline, tofacitinib was associated with detectable CMV at one or more time points post-baseline (Chi-squared test, p = 0.0001; Table 3). When individual tofacitinib groups were evaluated, the number of patients in whom CMV became detectable post-baseline was significant in the tofacitinib 15 mg BID group only (p = 0.004 vs placebo).

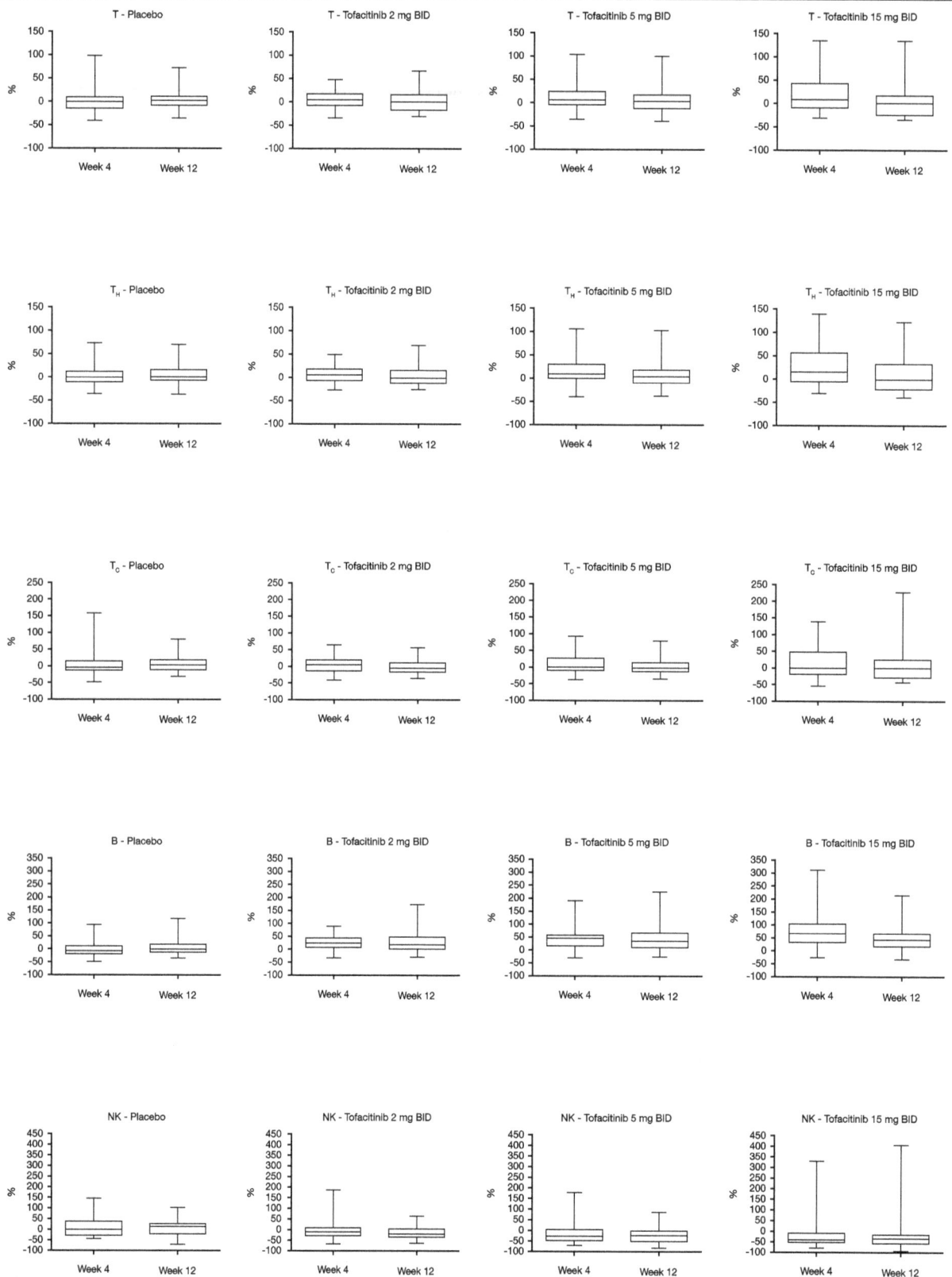

Figure 1 Median percent change from baseline in lymphocyte sub-population cell counts. The horizontal line within each box represents median, with the bottom and top of each box representing the 1st and 3rd quartiles, respectively. Error bars represent minimum and maximum values. B, B cells; BID, twice daily; NK, natural killer cells; T, total T cells; T_H, T helper cells; T_C, cytotoxic T cells.

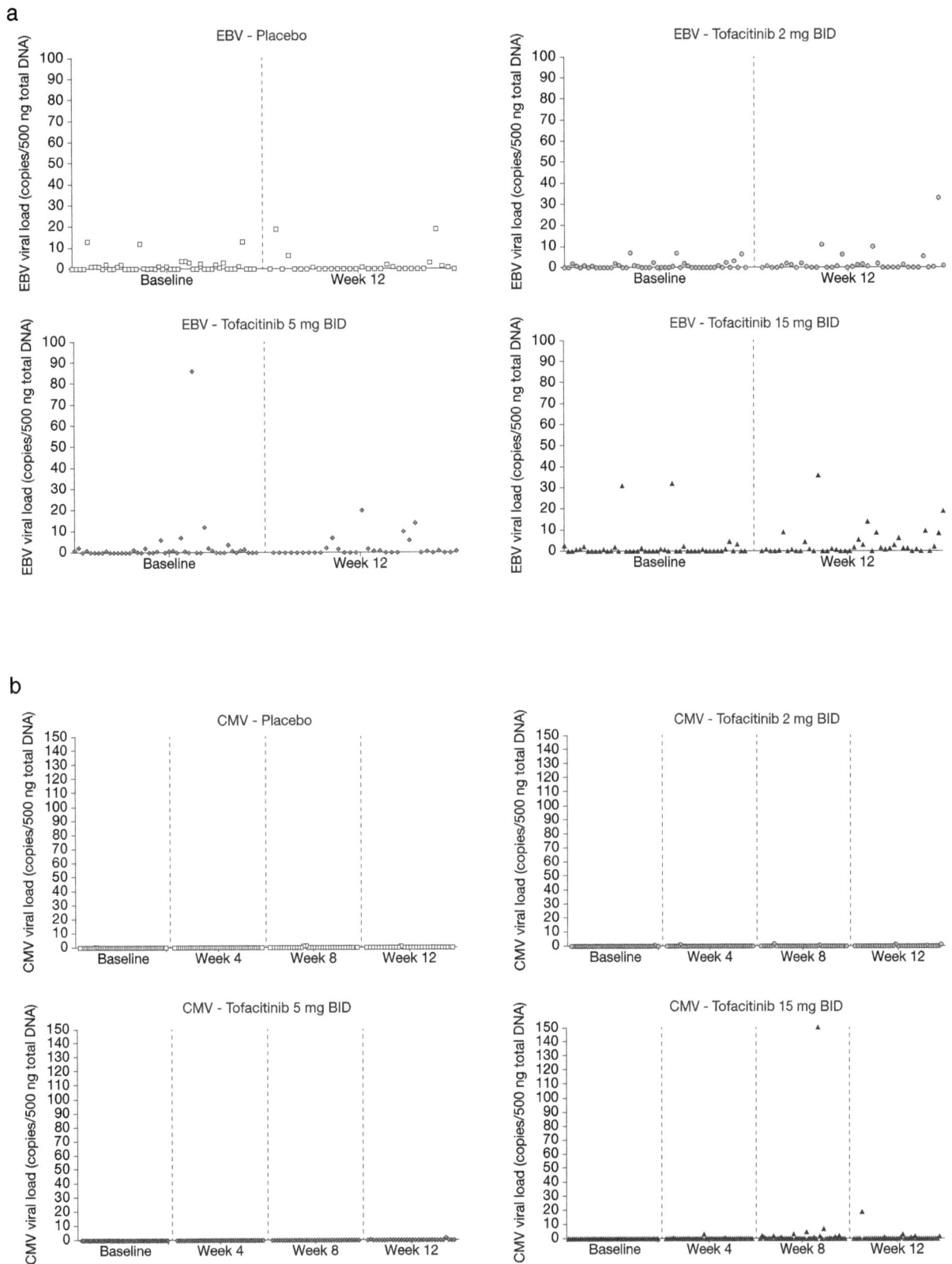

Figure 2 Viral DNA count at baseline and post-baseline in patients receiving tofacitinib or placebo. For: **a)** CMV and **b)** EBV; each data point represents a measurement for an individual patient. BID, twice daily; CMV, cytomegalovirus; EBV, Epstein-Barr virus.

Table 3 Changes from baseline in CMV and EBV viral load in patients receiving placebo or tofacitinib 2 mg, 5 mg or 15 mg BID

	Baseline status	Post-baseline status		Chi-squared p value (vs placebo)	Overall p value (vs baseline)
Patients with CMV undetectable at baseline	Undetectable N (n)	Remained undetectable n (%)	Became detectable n (%)		
Placebo	49 (46)	44 (95.7)	2 (4.3)	N/A	0.0001
Tofacitinib 2 mg BID	48 (46)	41 (89.1)	5 (10.9)	0.2381	
Tofacitinib 5 mg BID	48 (45)	42 (93.3)	3 (6.7)	0.6274	
Tofacitinib 15 mg BID	49 (48)	32 (66.7)	16 (33.3)	0.0004	
Patients with CMV detectable at baseline[a]	Detectable N (n)	Remained detectable n (%)	Became undetectable n (%)		
Placebo	1 (1)	0 (0)	1 (100.0)	N/A	–
Tofacitinib 2 mg BID	1 (1)	0 (0)	1 (100.0)	–	
Tofacitinib 5 mg BID	1 (1)	0 (0)	1 (100.0)	–	
Tofacitinib 15 mg BID	0 (0)	0 (0)	0 (0)	–	
Patients with EBV undetectable at baseline	Undetectable N (n)	Remained undetectable n (%)	Became detectable n (%)		
Placebo	28 (20)	18 (90.0)	2 (10.0)	N/A	0.0122
Tofacitinib 2 mg BID	30 (25)	14 (56.0)	11 (44.0)	0.0124	
Tofacitinib 5 mg BID	26 (19)	15 (78.9)	4 (21.1)	0.3390	
Tofacitinib 15 mg BID	31 (28)	14 (50.0)	14 (50.0)	0.0038	
Patients with EBV detectable at baseline	Detectable N (n)	Remained detectable n (%)	Became undetectable n (%)		
Placebo	21 (19)	9 (47.4)	10 (52.6)	N/A	0.1299
Tofacitinib 2 mg BID	18 (13)	9 (69.2)	4 (30.8)	0.2208	
Tofacitinib 5 mg BID	21 (14)	10 (71.4)	4 (28.6)	0.1669	
Tofacitinib 15 mg BID	17 (14)	12 (85.7)	2 (14.3)	0.0236	

[a]A statistical comparison of change in CMV detectability from detectable at baseline to undetectable post-baseline was not possible due to limited sample size.
BID, twice daily; CMV, cytomegalovirus; EBV, Epstein-Barr virus; N, number of patients with baseline values; n, number of patients with baseline and post-baseline values; N/A, not applicable.

The median (Q25, Q75) EBV viral load at baseline was 0.0 copies/500 ng total DNA (0.0, 1.3) in all groups (Table 1). Twelve patients had baseline EBV DNA ≥5 copies/500 ng total DNA: three receiving placebo, and three, four, and two patients receiving tofacitinib 2 mg, 5 mg, and 15 mg BID, respectively. Of these, seven patients (three in the placebo group, and two each in the tofacitinib 5 mg and 15 mg BID groups) had EBV DNA >10 copies/500 ng total DNA. The highest EBV DNA value at baseline (86 copies/500 ng total DNA) was reported for a patient in the tofacitinib 5 mg BID group. This patient had a mild, upper respiratory tract infection at study entry, which began 12 days before treatment and resolved on Day 15.

At Week 12, the median (Q25, Q75) change from baseline in EBV viral load was 0 (–1.1, 1.3) for all groups except for the tofacitinib 15 mg BID group, in which the median EBV DNA count increased by 0.7 copies/500 ng total DNA (0.0, 2.9) (Table 2). Twenty-two patients had EBV DNA ≥5 copies/500 ng total DNA at Week 12:

three receiving placebo, and five, five, and nine patients receiving tofacitinib 2 mg, 5 mg, and 15 mg BID, respectively. Of these, nine patients (two each in the placebo, tofacitinib 2 mg, and 5 mg BID groups, and three in the tofacitinib 15 mg BID group) had EBV DNA >10 copies/500 ng total DNA. The highest EBV DNA values at Week 12 were reported for a patient receiving tofacitinib 2 mg BID and a patient receiving tofacitinib 15 mg BID (33 copies and 36 copies/500 ng total DNA, respectively). Both had EBV levels ≥5 copies/500 ng total DNA at baseline. The patient with EBV levels of 33 copies/500 ng total DNA had adverse events of increased low-density lipoprotein and increased blood cholesterol reported at that time point. The patient with EBV DNA 36 copies/500 ng total DNA had no adverse events reported.

Overall, in patients with undetectable EBV at baseline, tofacitinib was associated with detectable EBV at Week 12 (Chi-squared test, p = 0.0122). The number of patients in whom EBV became detectable post-baseline was significant vs placebo in the tofacitinib 2 mg BID (p = 0.0124) and 15 mg BID (p = 0.0038) groups (Table 3). However, there was also a significant proportion of patients in the tofacitinib 15 mg BID group who had detectable EBV at baseline and undetectable EBV at Week 12 (p = 0.0236 vs placebo) (Table 3).

Correlation analyses

Spearman's rank correlation coefficient (rho) analyses of pooled patient data showed that EBV viral load, but not CMV viral load, was weakly correlated with larger changes in total T cell, T_H cell, T_C cell, and B cell counts after 12 weeks of treatment (rho: 0.19, 0.20, 0.17, and 0.25, respectively). Changes in CRP level showed a weak inverse correlation with larger changes in total T cell, T_H cell, T_C cell, and B cell counts after 12 weeks of treatment (rho: −0.28, −0.26, −0.20, and −0.40, respectively) (Table 4).

Potential correlations between tofacitinib dose, lymphocyte sub-population cell counts, CMV and EBV viral load, and CRP level were evaluated. Multivariate analyses using a general linear model detected no correlation between change in CMV or EBV viral load and lymphocyte sub-populations or dose of tofacitinib (Table 5). However, there was strong and significant correlation between change in CRP levels and change in T_C cell count (p = 0.043) or dose of tofacitinib (p = 0.026) (Table 5).

Discussion

Clinical data describing the impact of immunosuppressive therapies on the overall risk of infection and serious infection are limited in patients with psoriasis compared with rheumatoid arthritis (RA). However, there is emerging evidence to suggest that the infection risk associated with various therapies used in the RA setting may not be replicated in the psoriasis setting [22-24]. Moreover, effects of psoriasis therapies on immunosurveillance may vary according to the mechanism of action for each agent.

In this investigation, there was no clinically significant relationship between changes in CMV or EBV viral load and changes in lymphocyte sub-populations. Minimal and transient effects on T cell counts were identified in patients receiving tofacitinib, which may be related to modulation of cytokines, resultant modulation of adhesion molecules, and consequent trafficking of T cells. This is supported by dose-dependent percent changes from baseline in median total T cell (CD3⁺) count at Week 4, which appeared to normalize across all doses by Week 12. Dose-dependent percentage changes in median B cell and NK cell count were observed with tofacitinib treatment, with B cell count increased from baseline and NK cell count decreased from baseline at Week 12. Overall, changes in lymphocyte sub-populations observed in this study appear consistent with observations in patients receiving tofacitinib for RA [25].

T_H cell counts correlated well with total lymphocyte counts over time, suggesting that tofacitinib does not change the T_H cell distribution. A T_H cell count <200 cells/mm³, which is a known risk factor for opportunistic infections in patients with human immunodeficiency virus (HIV) [26] was not observed in any patient in the present study. In addition, excluding those patients with a T_H cell count <500 cells/mm³ at baseline, fewer than 5% of patients in each group had a post-baseline T_H cell count <500 cells/mm³. In other settings in which patients may be immunocompromised, including bone marrow transplantation, a significant correlation with the occurrence of opportunistic infection has been observed only in patients with a T_H cell count below 115 cells/mm³ [27,28]. Based on data collected during this study, there is no need to routinely monitor levels of lymphocyte sub-populations in patients receiving tofacitinib therapy for plaque psoriasis. However, longer-term observation would be needed to confirm these findings.

In the present study, mean baseline CRP levels for each group ranged from 3.10 to 5.47 mg/L, which is above the 3.0 mg/L threshold for high relative risk of cardiovascular disease [29]. Tofacitinib therapy was associated with dose-dependent reductions in CRP at Week 12, reflecting the anti-inflammatory activity of tofacitinib. This is supported by the significant correlation between tofacitinib dose and changes in CRP. Furthermore, the observed, transient increase from baseline in peripheral lymphocytes in patients receiving tofacitinib, and the inverse correlation between changes in CRP level and larger changes in T cell, T_H cell,

Table 4 Spearman's rank correlation coefficients between change from baseline to week 12 in CMV or EBV viral load, or CRP level, and change in lymphocyte sub-populations

Change in outcome variables, rho (p value)	Lymphocyte sub-populations				
	T (CD3⁺)	T_H (CD3⁺/CD4⁺)	T_C (CD3⁺/CD8⁺)	B (CD19⁺)	NK (CD16⁺/CD56⁺)
CMV viral load, copies/500 ng total DNA	−0.0499 (0.5742)	−0.0889 (0.3164)	0.0020 (0.9817)	−0.0530 (0.5505)	−0.0148 (0.8674)
EBV viral load, copies/500 ng total DNA	0.1872 (0.0351)	0.1970 (0.0264)	0.1711 (0.0544)	0.2491 (0.0047)	0.0033 (0.9709)
CRP level, mg/L	−0.2832 (0.0008)	−0.2644 (0.0017)	−0.2009 (0.0181)	−0.3996 (0.0000)	0.0699 (0.4152)

The correlation analyses presented above were performed using pooled data from the placebo and tofacitinib groups.
B, B cells; CMV, cytomegalovirus; CRP, C-reactive protein; DNA, deoxyribonucleic acid; EBV, Epstein-Barr virus; NK, natural killer cells; rho, Spearman's rank correlation coefficient; T, total T cells; T_H, T helper cells; T_C, cytotoxic T cells.

Table 5 Correlation analysis results from a general linear model with change from baseline to week 12 in CMV or EBV viral load or change in CRP level as the response variable, and dose of tofacitinib and change in lymphocyte sub-populations as explanatory variables

Change in response variables		Explanatory variables					
		Dose of tofacitinib[a]	Lymphocyte sub-populations				
			T (CD3$^+$)	T$_H$ (CD3$^+$/CD4$^+$)	T$_C$ (CD3$^+$/CD8$^+$)	B (CD19$^+$)	NK (CD16$^+$/CD56$^+$)
CMV viral load, copies/500 ng total DNA	df	3	1	1	1	1	1
	F value	1.26	0.14	0.04	0.68	0.00	0.03
	p value	0.2926	0.7047	0.8411	0.4112	0.9925	0.8592
EBV viral load, copies/500 ng total DNA	df	3	1	1	1	1	1
	F value	0.50	0.54	1.69	0.11	0.02	0.57
	p value	0.6807	0.4627	0.1955	0.7430	0.8906	0.4501
CRP level, mg/L	df	3	1	1	1	1	1
	F value	3.18	1.45	1.84	4.18	0.11	1.83
	p value	0.0262	0.2315	0.1775	0.0430	0.7450	0.1784

[a]Doses of tofacitinib considered in this analysis were 0 mg, 2 mg, 5 mg, and 15 mg BID.
B, B cells; BID, twice daily; CMV, cytomegalovirus; CRP, C-reactive protein; df, degrees of freedom; DNA, deoxyribonucleic acid; EBV, Epstein-Barr virus; NK, natural killer cells; T, total T cells; T$_H$, T helper cells; T$_C$, cytotoxic T cells.

T$_C$ cell, and B cell counts after 12 weeks of treatment, is consistent with the recruitment of lymphocytes to sites of inflammation and release of lymphocytes as inflammation resolves.

There is published evidence to suggest an association between active plaque psoriasis and reactivation of CMV, with one study identifying a correlation between psoriasis disease activity in CMV seropositive patients and severity of CMV-antigenemia [30]. In the present study, there was an overall association between tofacitinib and post-baseline detectability of CMV and EBV DNA, and significant changes in CMV and EBV detectability in the tofacitinib 2 mg and 15 mg BID groups (vs placebo). When considered alongside viral load measurements for individual patients, in most cases, changes in CMV and EBV detectability are likely to reflect only subtle differences in viral load. Indeed, a multivariate analysis showed no correlation between viral load and dose of tofacitinib. Considering the important role of T cells and NK cells in the response to viral infection [31,32], this finding implies that the modest changes in lymphocyte sub-populations observed during 12 weeks of tofacitinib therapy did not translate into clinically significant changes in effective immunosurveillance. Moreover, the lack of changes in viral load also suggests that T cell function, critical for control of viral infections [33], is preserved in patients treated with tofacitinib, at least over the course of 12 weeks. This conclusion is supported by the case of one patient with a treatment-emergent adverse event of elevated CMV, whose CMV levels reduced before stopping treatment and who did not develop any clinical symptoms.

In the HIV setting, a CMV viral load of >200 copies/mL predicts the future occurrence of CMV end organ disease [34]. There is no single treatment threshold for CMV in the transplant setting. However, a CMV viral load cut-off of 5000 copies/mL for pre-emptive therapy was described in a recent study investigating CMV reactivation in 161 liver transplant patients [35]. In another study involving 28 liver transplant patients, the median viral load associated with symptomatic CMV disease was 230,000 copies/mL [36]. These levels are substantially in excess of the maximum CMV level reported in any patient in this study.

There are few published studies describing the effects of other therapies for RA or psoriasis on CMV or EBV viral load. A study with 62 patients, aged 2–28 years, receiving biologic (including infliximab and etanercept) or nonbiologic treatment for juvenile RA, Crohn's disease, or ulcerative rectocolitis detected CMV DNA in 1.6% of patients and EBV in 4.8% of patients [37]. All but one patient with detectable CMV or EBV had received non-biologic therapy in the preceding year. Neither CMV nor EBV DNA was detected in the control group, which comprised 62 healthy volunteers. However, the extent to which viral load was related to the underlying disease or the treatment received was unclear [37]. A study of EBV viral load in 122 patients receiving biologic agents, including TNFi, for inflammatory arthritis found that 90% of patients receiving active treatment (and 98% of biologic-naïve controls) had a positive antibody test for EBV during treatment, although subsequent PCR testing revealed no evidence of viral activation [38]. In addition, Niemann and colleagues detected no EBV DNA in 26 patients with psoriasis who received at least eight weeks of treatment with various nonbiologic and biologic agents (methotrexate, cyclosporine, etanercept, or alefacept) [39]. It should be noted that our investigation, and the above studies by McKeown and Niemann et al., measured viral load in patients who were asymptomatic for infection with CMV or EBV. In other indications where immunosuppressive therapy is used, such as RA and transplantation, an associated risk of viral infections has been observed [40], although the duration of treatment in that study was substantially longer than the 12-week duration of tofacitinib therapy in this study. Thus, the available evidence suggests that, while CMV or EBV DNA may become detectable in some patients during treatment with biologic or nonbiologic therapy for inflammatory diseases such as plaque psoriasis, viral reactivation and symptomatic clinical infections are rare.

Potential limitations of this analysis were the duration of exposure to tofacitinib (12 weeks) and the use of lymphocyte subsets (CD4 and CD8) as surrogates of virus-specific CD4+ and CD8+ cells. While no effect of tofacitinib exposure on viral load was observed over the 12-week study period, one cannot be certain that such an effect would not be observed over a more prolonged period of exposure. With regard to lymphocyte subsets it is possible, albeit unlikely, that tofacitinib treatment could affect the number or function of virus-specific cells without markedly affecting the total number of cells. The absence of an observed increase in viral load suggests that the number and function of these virus-specific cells was sufficient to control viral replication.

Conclusions

In patients with psoriasis, 12 weeks of tofacitinib treatment had no clinically significant effects on CMV or EBV viral load, suggesting that lymphocyte sub-populations critical to the response to chronic viral infections and viral reactivation were not significantly affected. Replication of these findings during long-term use of tofacitinib will allow confirmation of this observation.

Abbreviations

ANCOVA: Analysis of covariance; B: B cells; BID: Twice daily; BSA: Body surface area; CMV: Cytomegalovirus; CRP: C-reactive protein; df: Degrees of freedom; DNA: Deoxyribonucleic acid; EBV: Epstein-Barr virus; HIV: Human immunodeficiency virus; IL: Interleukin; JAK: Janus kinase; N/A: Not applicable; NK: Natural killer cell; PASI: Psoriasis Area and Severity Index; PGA: Physician's Global Assessment; Q: Quartile; RA: Rheumatoid arthritis; rho: Spearman's rank correlation coefficient; SD: Standard deviation; T: Total T cells; T_C: Cytotoxic T cell; T_H: T helper cell; TNFi: Tumor necrosis factor inhibitor.

Competing interests

Fernando Valenzuela has been a principal investigator, member of a scientific advisory board or speaker for AbbVie, Eli Lilly, Janssen, Merck, Novartis, and Pfizer Inc. Kim A Papp has been a principal investigator, an advisor or consultant, a Scientific Officer, member of a Scientific Advisory Board and a speaker for Abbott, Amgen, Astellas, Celgene, Centocor-Ortho Biotech, Incyte, Isotechnika, Janssen, Lilly, Medimmune, Merck, Novartis, and Pfizer Inc. David Pariser has been a principal investigator, advisor or consultant for Abbott/AbbVie, Amgen, Astellas, Celgene, Eli Lilly, Janssen-Ortho, Novartis, Pfizer Inc, and Valeant. Stephen K Tyring has conducted research funded by Pfizer Inc. At the time of this analysis, Jeff Wang was an employee of Quintiles, and acted as a paid consultant to Pfizer Inc in connection with

the analysis of study data. Robert Wolk, Marjorie Buonanno, Huaming Tan, and Hernan Valdez are employees and stockholders of Pfizer Inc.

Authors' contributions

KAP enrolled and examined patients during the course of the study. The data analysis was planned by HV and HT, and executed by HT and JW. FV, DP, SKT, RW and MB contributed to the interpretation of data. All authors contributed to the development of the manuscript and provided critical input at all stages of development. All authors read and approved the final manuscript.

Acknowledgments

This work was supported by Pfizer Inc. Medical writing support was provided by Claire Cridland at Complete Medical Communications and was funded by Pfizer Inc. The authors would like to thank the patients who were involved in this study, as well as the investigators and study teams.

Previous presentations of the data contained in this manuscript

Sociedad Latinoamericana de Psoriasis (SOLAPSO) 2012. Valenzuela F, Papp K, Pariser D, Tyring S, Wolk R, Buonanno M, Valdez H. Effects of Tofacitinib on Lymphocyte Subpopulations, and CMV and EBV Viral Load, in Patients with Plaque Psoriasis. Buenos Aires; November 30–December 2, 2012, Abstract and Poster #81.
Congress of International Investigative Dermatology (IID), 2013. Valenzuela F, Papp K, Pariser D, Tyring S, Wolk R, Buonanno M, Valdez H. Tofacitinib has no clinically significant effects on cells controlling chronic viral infection and reactivation. Journal of International Investigative Dermatology 2013; 133(Supplement 1):S17; Abstract 102. Poster #102.

Author details

[1]Department of Dermatology, Faculty of Medicine, University of Chile and Probity Medical Research, Santiago, Chile. [2]Clinical Research and Probity Medical Research, Waterloo, ON, Canada. [3]Department of Dermatology, Eastern Virginia Medical School and Virginia Clinical Research Inc., Norfolk, VA, USA. [4]Department of Dermatology, University of Texas Medical School, Houston, TX, USA. [5]Pfizer Inc, Groton, CT, USA. [6]Quintiles, Cambridge, MA, USA. [7]Pfizer Inc, New York, NY, USA. [8]Present address: Statistical Consulting & Solutions, LLC, Brookline, MA, USA. [9]Specialty Care Medicines Development Group, Pfizer Inc, 219 E 42nd Street, 7th Floor Room 50, NYO 219/07/01, New York, NY 10017, USA.

References

1. Parisi R, Symmons DP, Griffiths CE, Ashcroft DM. Global epidemiology of psoriasis: a systematic review of incidence and prevalence. J Invest Dermatol. 2013;133:377–85.
2. Griffiths CE, Iaccarino L, Naldi L, Olivieri I, Pipitone N, Salvarini C, et al. Psoriasis and psoriatic arthritis: immunological aspects and therapeutic guidelines. Clin Exp Rheumatol. 2014;24(1 Suppl 40):S72–8.
3. Boy MG, Wang C, Wilkinson BE, Chow VF, Clucas AT, Krueger JG, et al. Double-blind, placebo-controlled, dose-escalation study to evaluate the pharmacologic effect of CP-690,550 in patients with psoriasis. J Invest Dermatol. 2009;129:2299–302.
4. Papp KA, Menter A, Strober B, Langley RG, Buonanno M, Wolk R, et al. Efficacy and safety of tofacitinib, an oral Janus kinase inhibitor, in the treatment of psoriasis: a Phase 2b randomized placebo-controlled dose-ranging study. Br J Dermatol. 2012;167:668–77.
5. Bissonnette R, Iversen L, Sofen H, Griffiths CE, Foley P, Romiti R, et al. Tofacitinib withdrawal and re-treatment in moderate-to-severe chronic plaque psoriasis: a randomised controlled trial. Br J Dermatol. 2014. Epub ahead of print.
6. Bachelez H, van de Kerkof PCM, Strohal R, Kubanov A, Valenzuela F, Lee JH, et al. Comparison of tofacitinib versus etanercept or placebo in moderate-to-severe chronic plaque psoriasis: a Phase 3 randomized trial [abstract]. Presented at the American Academy of Dermatology - 72nd Annual Meeting. 2014.
7. Ghoreschi K, Laurence A, O'Shea JJ. Janus kinases in immune cell signaling. Immunol Rev. 2009;228:273–87.
8. Li DQ, Chen Z, Song XJ, Luo L, Pflugfelder SC. Stimulation of matrix metalloproteinases by hyperosmolarity via a JNK pathway in human corneal epithelial cells. Invest Ophthalmol Vis Sci. 2004;45:4302–11.

9. Pepys MB, Hirschfield GM. C-reactive protein: a critical update. J Clin Invest. 2003;111:1805–12.
10. O'Shea JJ. Targeting the Jak/STAT pathway for immunosuppression. Ann Rheum Dis. 2004;63 Suppl 2:ii67–71.
11. Ghoreschi K, Jesson MI, Li X, Lee JL, Ghosh S, Alsup JW, et al. Modulation of innate and adaptive immune responses by tofacitinib (CP-690,550). J Immunol. 2011;186:4234–43.
12. Miquel FJ, Colomina J, Marli JI, Ortega C. Cytomegalovirus infection in a patient treated with efalizumab for psoriasis. Arch Dermatol. 2009;145:961–2.
13. Petersen B, Lorentzen H. Cytomegalovirus complicating biological immunosuppressive therapy in two patients with psoriasis receiving treatment with etanercept or efalizumab. Acta Derm Venereol. 2008;88:523–4.
14. Kikuchi K, Miyazaki Y, Tanaka A, Shigematu H, Kojima M, Sakashita H, et al. Methotrexate-related Epstein-Barr virus (EBV)-associated lymphoproliferative disorder–so-called "Hodgkin-like lesion"–of the oral cavity in a patient with rheumatoid arthritis. Head Neck Pathol. 2010;4:305–11.
15. Mahé E, Descamps V, Grossin M, Fraitag S, Crickx B. CD30+ T-cell lymphoma in a patient with psoriasis treated with ciclosporin and infliximab. Br J Dermatol. 2003;149:170–3.
16. Oh MJ, Lee HJ. A study of hepatitis B virus reactivation associated with rituximab therapy in real-world clinical practice: a single-center experience. Clin Mol Hepatol. 2013;19:51–9.
17. Erard V, Guthrie KA, Varley C, Heugel J, Wald A, Flowers ME, et al. One-year acyclovir prophylaxis for preventing varicella-zoster virus disease after hematopoietic cell transplantation: no evidence of rebound varicella-zoster virus disease after drug discontinuation. Blood. 2007;110:3071–7.
18. NHS. Cytomegalovirus (CMV) – Symptoms [http://www.nhs.uk/Conditions/Cytomegalovirus/Pages/Symptoms.aspx].
19. Talamonti M, Spallone G, Di Stefani A, Costanzo A, Chimenti S. Efalizumab. Expert Opin Drug Saf. 2011;10:239–51.
20. Shouval D, Shibolet O. Immunosuppression and HBV reactivation. Semin Liver Dis. 2013;33:167–77.
21. Nathan DM, Angus PW, Gibson PR. Hepatitis B and C virus infections and anti-tumor necrosis factor-alpha therapy: guidelines for clinical approach. J Gastroenterol Hepatol. 2006;21:1366–71.
22. Tan X, Balkrishnan R, Feldman SR. Infections associated with the use of tumor necrosis factor-α inhibitors in psoriasis. J Drugs Dermatol. 2013;12:e41–5.
23. Ortigosa LC, Silva LC, Duarte AJ, Takahashi MD, Benard G. Infliximab does not lead to reduction in the interferon-gamma and lymphoproliferative responses of patients with moderate to severe psoriasis. Acta Derm Venereol. 2014;94:26–31.
24. Burmester GR, Mease P, Dijkmans BA, Gordon K, Lovell D, Panaccione R, et al. Adalimumab safety and mortality rates from global clinical trials of six immune-mediated inflammatory diseases. Ann Rheum Dis. 2009;68:1863–9.
25. Pfizer Inc. Xeljanz prescribing information [http://labeling.pfizer.com/ShowLabeling.aspx?id=959].
26. Mocroft A, Furrer HJ, Miro JM, Reiss P, Mussini C, Kirk O, et al. The incidence of AIDS-defining illnesses at a current CD4 count ≥ 200 cells/muL in the post-combination antiretroviral therapy era. Clin Infect Dis. 2013;57:1038–47.
27. Izadi M, Jonaidi-Jafari N, Saburi A, Eyni H, Rezaiemanesh MR, Ranjbar R. Prevalence, molecular characteristics and risk factors for cryptosporidiosis among Iranian immunocompromised patients. Microbiol Immunol. 2012;56:836–42.
28. Fedele R, Martino M, Garreffa C, Messina G, Console G, Princi D, et al. The impact of early CD4+ lymphocyte recovery on the outcome of patients who undergo allogeneic bone marrow or peripheral blood stem cell transplantation. Blood Transfus. 2012;10:174–80.
29. Pearson TA, Mensah GA, Alexander RW, Anderson JL, Cannon III RO, Criqui M, et al. Markers of inflammation and cardiovascular disease: application to clinical and public health practice: A statement for healthcare professionals from the Centers for Disease Control and Prevention and the American Heart Association. Circulation. 2003;107:499–511.
30. Weitz M, Kiessling C, Friedrich M, Prösch S, Höflich C, Kern F, et al. Persistent CMV infection correlates with disease activity and dominates the phenotype of peripheral CD8+ T cells in psoriasis. Exp Dermatol. 2011;20:561–7.
31. Marcenaro E, Carlomagno S, Pesce S, Della Chiesa M, Parolini S, Moretta A, et al. NK cells and their receptors during viral infections. Immunotherapy. 2011;3:1075–86.
32. Moseman EA, Iannacone M, Bosurgi L, Tonti E, Chevrier N, Tumanov A, et al. B cell maintenance of subcapsular sinus macrophages protects against a fatal viral infection independent of adaptive immunity. Immunity. 2012;36:415–26.
33. Zinkernagel RM, Hengartner H. Protective 'immunity' by pre-existent neutralizing antibody titers and preactivated T cells but not by so-called 'immunological memory'. Immunol Rev. 2006;211:310–9.
34. Erice A, Tierney C, Hirsch M, Caliendo AM, Weinberg A, Kendall MA, et al. Cytomegalovirus (CMV) and human immunodeficiency virus (HIV) burden, CMV end-organ disease, and survival in subjects with advanced HIV infection (AIDS Clinical Trials Group Protocol 360). Clin Infect Dis. 2003;37:567–78.
35. Lautenschlager I, Loginov R, Mäkisalo H, Hockerstedt K. Prospective study on CMV-reactivations under preemptive strategy in CMV-seropositive adult liver transplant recipients. J Clin Virol. 2013;57:50–3.
36. Levitsky J, Freifeld AG, Puumala S, Bargenquast K, Hardiman P, Gebhart C, et al. Cytomegalovirus viremia in solid organ transplantation: does the initial viral load correlate with risk factors and outcomes? Clin Transplant. 2008;22:222–8.
37. Comar M, Delbue S, Lepore L, Martelossi S, Radillo O, Ronfani L, et al. Latent viral infections in young patients with inflammatory diseases treated with biological agents: prevalence of JC virus genotype 2. J Med Virol. 2013;85:716–22.
38. McKeown E, Pope JE, Leaf S. Epstein-Barr virus (EBV) prevalence and the risk of reactivation in patients with inflammatory arthritis using anti-TNF agents and in those who are biologic naive. Open Rheumatol J. 2009;3:30–4.
39. Neimann AL, Hodinka RL, Joshi YB, Elkan M, Van Voorhees AS, Gelfand JM. Epstein-Barr virus and human herpesvirus type 6 infection in patients with psoriasis. Eur J Dermatol. 2006;16:548–52.
40. Kim SY, Solomon DH. Tumor necrosis factor blockade and the risk of viral infection. Nat Rev Rheumatol. 2010;6:165–74.

HLA class II alleles may influence susceptibility to adult dermatomyositis and polymyositis in a Han Chinese population

Xiang Gao[1,2†], Lei Han[2†], Lan Yuan[3,4†], Yongchen Yang[5], Guimei Gou[5], Hengjuan Sun[5], Ling Lu[2*] and Liming Bao[3,4,6*]

Abstract

Background: Polymyositis (PM) and dermatomyositis (DM) are idiopathic inflammatory myopathies. Genetic variability in human leukocyte antigen (*HLA*) genes plays an important role in the pathogenesis of PM and DM. However, few studies on the subject in Chinese populations have been reported thus far.

Methods: We studied the influence of *HLA* polymorphisms on DM and PM susceptibility by analyzing *HLA-DRB1*, *HLA-DQA1*, and *HLA-DQB1* alleles in 71 adult DM patients, 20 adult PM patients, and 113 controls in a Han Chinese population.

Results: A positive association was found between *HLA-DQA1*0104* and DM ($p = 0.01$; corrected p (p_{corr}) NS; odds ratio (OR) = 2.58; 95% confidence interval (CI): 1.18–5.64), while an inverse correlation was noted between *HLA-DQB1*0303* and myositis patients with interstitial lung inflammation ($p = 0.01$; p_{corr} NS; OR = 0.25; 95% CI: 0.07–0.73). A positive relationship was also observed between *HLA-DRB1*07* and DM ($p = 0.01$; p_{corr} NS; OR = 2.26; 95% CI: 1.12–4.59), while *HLA-DRB1*03* seems to be protective against DM ($p = 0.01$; p_{corr} NS; OR = 0.26; 95% CI: 0.06–0.81). The lung complication was closely associated with *HLA-DRB1*04* ($p = 0.01$; p_{corr} NS; OR = 2.82; 95% CI: 1.15–6.76) and *HLA-DRB1*12* ($p = 0.02$; p_{corr} NS; OR = 2.52; 95% CI: 1.02–6.07). The frequency of *HLA-DRB1*07* was significantly higher among myositis patients with dysphagia than among controls ($p = 0.01$; p_{corr} NS; OR = 4.78; 95% CI: 1.03–24.42). The putative haplotype *DRB1*07-DQA1*01-DQB1*02* was positively correlated with DM ($p = 0.03$; p_{corr} NS; OR = 2.90; 95% CI: 1.02–8.93) and the lung complication ($p = 0.02$; p_{corr} NS; OR = 3.45; 95% CI: 1.04–11.58).

Conclusions: Our results demonstrate that *HLA* alleles may be involved in susceptibility to adult DM and PM in the Han Chinese population.

Keywords: Polymyositis, Dermatomyositis, *HLA*, Susceptibility, Chinese

Background

Polymyositis (PM) and dermatomyositis (DM) are idiopathic inflammatory myopathies (IIM), a group of autoimmune disorders characterized by inflammation present predominantly in muscle tissues. The chief clinical presentations include symmetric proximal muscle weakness, other organ involvement, and presence of autoantibodies [1]. Although the underlying pathogenesis for PM and DM remains unclear, evidence has suggested that, like many other autoimmune conditions, these disorders likely result from a combination of environmental exposure and genetic susceptibility [2]. Genetic variability in the human leukocyte antigen (*HLA*) genes is thought to play an important role in DM and PM pathogenesis [3,4]. This may be partly attributed to the influence of HLA molecules on T-cell receptor development, peripheral tolerance, and immune response to environmental agents. It has been established that geographic locations and ethnicities may affect susceptibility to autoimmune diseases [5,6]. The

* Correspondence: huashanlvling@sina.com; liming.bao@dartmouth.edu
†Equal contributors
²Departments of Rheumatology and Occupational Medicine, Huashan Hospital of Fudan University, Shanghai, China
³Center for Clinical Molecular Medicine; Ministry of Education Key Laboratory of Child Development and Disorders, Key Laboratory of Pediatrics in Chongqing, Chongqing, China
Full list of author information is available at the end of the article

HLA-DRB1*0301 and *HLA-DQA1*0501* alleles have been reported as risk factors for myositis in Western populations [7,8], whereas *DRB1*0803* may increase PM susceptibility among the Japanese population [9]. In studies of 52 DM and PM patients from Northern China, Han *et al.* reported positive associations between the *HLA-DRB1*04*, *HLA-DRB1*07*, and *HLA-DRB1*12* alleles and DM development [10]. They also observed that *HLA-DQB1*0401* is a risk factor for DM and PM [11]. However, the sample sizes of these studies were small; therefore, the possible role of *HLA* class II alleles in myopathies in Chinese patients requires further investigation.

To assess the effect of polymorphisms in *HLA-DRB1*, *HLA-DQA1*, and *HLA-DQB1* on DM and PM susceptibility, we conducted a study of 91 adult patients with DM or PM and 113 healthy controls in a Han Chinese population. Our results demonstrate that *HLA* class II alleles may influence adult DM and PM susceptibility in the Han Chinese population.

Methods
Study subjects
Between August 2009 and March 2012, 71 and 20 patients were diagnosed with DM and PM, respectively, at the Huashan Hospital of Fudan University in Shanghai, China. The patients met probable or definite diagnosis of DM or PM according to the Bohan and Peter [12] criteria [12,13]. Lung lesions were examined by chest computed tomography, and a diagnosis of interstitial lung disease (ILD) or idiopathic interstitial pneumonitis was made by a pulmonologist. All patients were ethnic Han Chinese (25 males and 66 females, median age of 51 ± 15.8 years). One hundred and thirteen healthy Han Chinese subjects (36 males and 77 females, median age of 40.0 ± 8.6 years) with no history of autoimmune disease were enrolled in the study as controls. The study followed protocols set by the Declaration of Helsinki and was approved by the ethics committee of Huashan Hospital. All patients and controls provided written informed consent prior to the study.

Experiments
DNA was extracted from blood using the Qiagen DNA extraction kit (Qiagen; Hilden, Germany). Low- and high-resolution typing of the *HLA-DRB1*, *HLA-DQA1*, and *HLA-DQB1* alleles were performed using the polymerase chain reaction (PCR)-sequence-specific primed (SSP) procedure described by Olerup *et al.* [14,15]. Serum was obtained from all patients for detection of myositis-specific antibodies (MSA; anti-Jo-1 autoantibodies) and myositis-associated antibodies (MAA; anti-Ro and anti-La autoantibodies). Autoantibodies were analyzed by an indirect immunofluorescence method using the kits from EUROIMMUN AG (Lubeck, Germany).

Statistical analysis
The allele, genotype, and haplotype frequencies of the *HLA* loci were compared between the patients and controls using the Fisher exact test or chi-square test, as appropriate. Data were expressed as odds ratios (ORs) with 95% confidence intervals (CIs). A p-value ≤ 0.05 was considered statistically significant. In multiple comparisons, p-values were adjusted using the Bonferroni correction to give a corrected p-value (p_{corr}). A p-value ≤ 0.05 before correction for multiple comparisons was considered as possibly statistically significant. The Hardy–Weinberg equilibrium constant in the control group was confirmed using a chi-square test. Putative haplotypes were inferred from unphased genotype data using the Bayesian statistical method available in the PHASE program v2.1.1 [16]. Putative haplotypes with a frequency higher than 3% among the controls were selected for further comparisons between the patients and controls. Unless otherwise stated, Stata (version 7.0; Stata Corp.; College Station, TX, USA) statistical software was used to perform the statistical analyses.

Results
Of the 91 patients, 71 had been diagnosed with DM and 20 with PM (66 female and 25 male [2.64:1]). Although most of the patients were positive for antinuclear antibodies, few were positive for either MSA or MAA. The frequencies of MSA and MAA were higher in the PM group than in the DM group (10% vs. 1.4%, $p = 0.06$ for MSA; 20% vs. 5.63%, $p = 0.05$ for MAA). As expected, cutaneous involvement such as rash or cuticular overgrowth was present only in DM patients. Approximately half of the patients had ILD, with a higher prevalence among patients with PM than those with DM (76.5% vs. 37.7%, $p = 0.04$). No significant differences in other clinical features were observed between the two groups (Table 1).

Genotyping analyses of the *HLA-DQA1* and *HLA-DQB1* loci were performed to study the relationship between the *HLA* class II alleles and susceptibility to DM and PM. Because there are several lines of evidence to suggest that DM and PM may be distinct diseases with different genetic backgrounds [17], we analyzed the influence of the *HLA* alleles on susceptibility to DM and PM individually rather than analyzing the combined DM/PM group (Table 2). Compared with the controls, the frequency of *HLA-DQA1*0104* was significantly higher in the DM group than in the PM group (16.42% vs. 8.18%, $p = 0.01$, p_{corr} NS; OR = 2.58; 95% CI: 1.18–5.74), implying a possible positive correlation between *HLA-DQA1*0104* and the risk of DM. Of the *HLA-DQB1* alleles analyzed, only the *HLA-DQB1*0303* frequency was lower in patients with ILD than in the controls (6.76% vs. 19.03%, $p = 0.01$, p_{corr} NS; OR = 0.25; 95% CI: 0.07 – 0.73), implying that

Table 1 Clinical features of patients with DM and PM

	DM n (%) (N = 71)	PM n (%) (N = 20)	p (DM vs. PM)
Serologic group			
MSA (anti-Jo-1)	1 (1.4)	2 (10)	0.06
MAA (SSA, SSB or Scl)	4 (5.63)	4 (20)	0.05
Clinical presentations			
Fever	4 (5.6)	1 (5)	0.92
Raynaud's disease	0.00	1 (5)	0.06
Arthritis	1 (1.4)	0.00	0.59
Interstitial lung disease	26[1] (37.7)	13[2] (76.5)	0.04
Palpitations	1 (1.4)	0.00	0.59
Dysphagia	10 (14.1)	4 (20)	0.51
V-sign	26 (36.6)	0.00	n/a
Gottron papules	24 (33.8)	0.00	n/a
Periorbital edematous rash	11 (15.5)	0.00	n/a
Shawl sign	13 (18.3)	0.00	n/a
Cuticular overgrowth	3 (4.2)	0.00	n/a

MSA: myositosis-specific autoantiboides; MAA: myositosis associated autoantibodies;
[1]69 DM patients evaluated; [2]17 PM patients evaluated; n/a: not applicable.

patients with this allele are less likely to develop the lung complication. This was further confirmed by the fact that the HLA-DQB1*0303 frequency was lower among those who developed ILD ($p < 0.01$; OR = 0.19; 95% CI: 0.038–0.37) than those who did not develop ILD. HLA-DRB1 typing analysis showed that compared to controls, DM patients had a considerably lower prevalence of HLA-DRB1*03 (3.08% vs. 11.27%, $p = 0.01$, p_{corr} NS; OR = 0.26; 95% CI: 0.06–0.81) and a higher frequency of HLA-DRB1*07 (20.77% vs. 13.24%, $p = 0.01$, p_{corr} NS, OR = 2.26, 95% CI, 1.12–4.59). Both HLA-DRB1*04 and HLA-DRB1*12 alleles are likely linked to the lung disease ($p = 0.01$, p_{corr} NS; OR = 2.82; 95% CI: 1.15–6.76 and $p = 0.02$, p_{corr} NS; OR = 2.52; 95% CI: 1.02–6.07, respectively). A similar effect of HLA-DRB1*04 on ILD development was also observed when the allele frequencies between patients with and without the lung complication were compared ($p = 0.026$; OR = 3.32; 95% CI: 1.22–9.08). Comparison of HLA-DRB1*12 allele frequencies between myositis patients with and without ILD showed a similar trend of being higher among those with ILD than among those without, although the difference between the two groups was not statistically significant ($p = 0.35$; OR = 1.59; 95% CI: 0.63–4.00). This is likely attributable to the small numbers in the groups examined. Moreover, the HLA-DRB1*07 allele showed a possible influence on the development of esophageal/muscle complications (30.00% vs. 13.24%, $p = 0.01$, p_{corr} NS; OR = 4.78; 95% CI: 1.03–24.42). A similar trend for a higher HLA-DRB1*07 allele frequency was also noted among patients who had

dysphagia as compared to those who did not ($p = 0.057$; OR = 3.55; 95% CI: 0.91–13.82).

We then examined the association between putative haplotypes involving the DRB1-DQA1-DQB1 loci and susceptibility to DM, PM, lung, and esophageal complications. In this analysis, only the putative haplotypes present in at least 3% of the controls were selected for further study. Of the 12 putative haplotypes selected, the frequency of DRB1*07-DQA1*01-DQB1*02 was higher in the DM group ($p = 0.03$, p_{corr} NS; OR = 2.90; 95% CI: 1.02–8.93) and in patients with ILD ($p = 0.02$, p_{corr} NS; OR = 3.45; 95% CI: 1.04–11.58) than in the controls, indicating that this putative haplotype might increase the risk of DM and the lung complication (Table 3). A further comparison of the DRB1*07-DQA1*01-DQB1*02 frequency in patients who developed dysphagia with those who did not showed a trend for a higher frequency of this haplotype among patients with dysphagia, although the difference between the groups was not statistically significant ($p = 0.23$; OR = 2.27; 95% CI: 0.68–7.72). Again, we consider that this result is likely due to the small sample sizes in both groups.

Discussion

There are differences in the clinical features of DM and PM between our cohort of Han Chinese patients and Western patients [1,18]. There are more DM cases in our cohort and among Mesoamerican patients, whereas PM is the major subtype among Caucasian patients [19]. Compared to Caucasian patients, our cohort had a higher prevalence of the lung complication [20]. The frequencies of dysphagia were comparable between our cohort and those reported in the West [1,21]. Approximately 30–40% of Caucasian and African American IIM patients are positive for MSA/MAA autoantibodies [19,22]. Although the proportion of patients who were positive for autoantibodies was relatively low in our cohort, it is nonetheless comparable to findings from other studies in Chinese patients [23,24].

There is a growing body of evidence to suggest that differences in the impact of HLA class II alleles on the susceptibility to DM and PM may exist among different ethnic groups and geographic locations [19,20,25-27]. It has been well documented that HLA class II alleles that form the 8.1 ancestral haplotype (8.1 AH), DRB1*03-DQA1*05-DQB1*02, are closely linked to DM and PM in Western populations [4,7,28]. Previous studies suggest that HLA-DQA1*0501 and HLA-DRB1*0301 may be risk factors for PM, whereas HLA-DQA1*0201 and HLA-DRB1*0401 confer protection against the disease in Caucasians [4,28-30]. Moreover, HLA-DRB1*07 has been reported to protect against PM and IIM in Caucasians and African Americans [4,22,28]. In their study of African American patients with IIM, O'Hanlon et al. [22]

Table 2 *HLA-DQA1, HLA-DQB1,* and *HLA-DRB1* allele frequencies in PM and DM patients and controls

Loci/ alleles	DM	PM	Myositis with ILD	Myositis with dysphagia	Control	Control vs. indicated patients (*p*; OR (95% CI))			
	n (%)	n (%)	n (%)	n (%)	n (%)	DM	PM	Myositis with ILD	Myositis with dysphagia
HLA-DRB1	N = 65	N = 19	N = 37	N = 10	N = 113				
*01	1 (0.77)	0 (0.00)	1 (1.35)	0 (0.00)	5 (2.45)	n/s	n/a	n/s	n/a
*03	4 (3.08)	4 (10.53)	4 (5.41)	1 (5.00)	23 (11.27)	0.01[1]; 0.26 (0.06–0.81)	n/s	n/s	n/s
*04	17 (13.08)	6 (15.79)	15 (20.27)	2 (10.00)	22 (10.78)	n/s	n/s	0.01[1]; 2.82 (1.15–6.76)	n/s
*07	27 (20.77)	1 (2.63)	14 (18.92)	6 (30.00)	27 (13.24)	0.01[1]; 2.26 (1.12–4.59)	n/s	n/s	0.01[1]; 4.78 (1.03–24.42)
*08	13 (10.00)	4 (10.53)	7 (9.46)	2 (10.00)	17 (8.33)	n/s	n/s	n/s	n/s
*09	20 (15.38)	2 (5.26)	3 (4.05)	3 (15.00)	26 (12.75)	n/s	n/s	n/s	n/s
*10	2 (1.54)	1 (2.63)	2 (2.70)	0 (0.00)	3 (1.47)	n/s	n/s	n/s	n/a
*11	3 (2.31)	3 (7.89)	2 (2.70)	0 (0.00)	9 (4.41)	n/s	n/s	n/s	n/a
*12	20 (15.38)	7 (18.42)	14 (18.92)	1 (5.00)	22 (10.78)	n/s	n/s	0.02[1]; 2.52 (1.02–6.07)	n/s
*13	7 (5.38)	1 (2.63)	2 (2.70)	1 (5.00)	8 (3.92)	n/s	n/s	n/s	n/s
*14	2 (1.54)	3 (7.89)	1 (1.35)	2 (10.00)	9 (4.41)	n/s	n/s	n/s	n/s
*15	10 (7.69)	4 (10.53)	7 (9.46)	1 (5.00)	29 (14.22)	n/s	n/s	n/s	n/s
*16	4 (3.08)	2 (5.26)	2 (2.70)	1 (5.00)	4 (1.96)	n/s	n/s	n/s	n/s
HLA-DQA1	N = 67	N = 20	N = 39	N = 12	N = 110				
*0101	9 (6.72)	0 (0.00)	5 (6.41)	1 (4.17)	11 (5.00)	n/s	n/a	n/s	n/s
*0102	18 (13.43)	10 (25.00)	16 (20.51)	4 (16.67)	44 (20.00)	n/s	n/s	n/s	n/s
*0103	26 (19.40)	6 (15.00)	10 (12.82)	6 (25.00)	28 (12.73)	n/s	n/s	n/s	n/s
*0104	22 (16.42)	4 (10.00)	11 (14.10)	4 (16.67)	18 (8.18)	0.01[1]; 2.58 1.18–5.64)	n/s	n/s	n/s
*0201	1 (0.75)	2 (5.00)	1 (1.28)	0 (0.00)	1 (0.45)	n/s	n/s	n/s	n/a
*0301	44 (32.84)	9 (22.50)	26 (33.33)	9 (37.50)	85 (38.64)	n/s	n/s	n/s	n/s
*0302	1 (0.75)	0 (0.00)	0 (0.00)	0 (0.00)	1 (0.45)	n/s	n/a	n/a	n/a
*0401	1 (0.75)	2 (5.00)	2 (2.56)	0 (0.00)	3 (1.36)	n/s	n/s	n/s	n/a
*0501	11 (8.21)	6 (15.00)	6 (7.69)	0 (0.00)	28 (12.73)	n/s	n/s	n/s	n/a
*0507	1 (0.75)	0 (0.00)	0 (0.00)	0 (0.00)	0 (0.00)	n/a	n/a	n/a	n/a
*0601	0 (0.00)	1 (2.50)	1 (1.28)	0 (0.00)	1 (0.45)	n/a	n/s		
HLA-DQB1	N = 67	N = 17	N = 37	N = 10	N = 113				
*0201	31 (23.48)	6 (16.67)	16 (21.62)	5 (25.00)	44 (19.47)	n/s	n/s	n/s	n/s
*0301	20 (15.15)	9 (25.00)	15 (20.27)	0 (0.00)	35 (15.49)	n/s	n/s	n/s	n/a
*0302	9 (6.82)	2 (5.56)	7 (9.46)	1 (5.00)	12 (5.31)	n/s	n/s	n/s	n/s
*0303	24 (18.18)	2 (5.56)	5 (6.76)	5 (25.00)	43 (19.03)	n/s	n/s	0.01[1]; 0.25 (0.07–0.73)	n/s
*0401	6 (4.55)	2 (5.56)	6 (8.11)	1 (5.00)	7 (3.10)	n/s	n/s	n/s	n/s
*0402	0 (0.00)	1 (2.78)	1 (1.35)	0 (0.00)	1 (0.44)	n.a.	n/s	n/s	n/a
*0501	1 (0.76)	2 (5.56)	3 (4.05)	0 (0.00)	8 (3.54)	n/s	n/s	n/s	n/a
*0502	5 (3.79)	2 (5.56)	5 (6.76)	0 (0.00)	7 (3.10)	n/s	n/s	n/s	n/a
*0503	4 (3.03)	1 (2.78)	0 (0.00)	2 (10.00)	8 (3.54)	n/s	n/s	n/a	n/s

Table 2 *HLA-DQA1, HLA-DQB1,* and *HLA-DRB1* **allele frequencies in PM and DM patients and controls** *(Continued)*

*0601	20 (15.15)	7 (19.44)	11 (14.86)	3 (15.00)	33 (14.60)	n/s	n/s	n/s	n/s
*0602	4 (3.03)	2 (5.56)	2 (2.70)	2 (10.00)	16 (7.08)	n/s	n/s	n/s	n/s
*0604	5 (3.79)	0 (0.00)	2 (2.70)	0 (0.00)	5 (2.21)	n/s	n/a	n/s	n/a
*0608	3 (2.27)	0 (0.00)	1 (1.35)	1 (5.00)	7 (3.10)	n/s	n/a	n/s	n/s

n/s: not significant; n/a: not applicable; [1]pcorr greater than 0.05; ILD: interstitial lung disease.

demonstrated that *HLA-DRB1*14* and *HLA-DRB1*0301* increase the risk of DM, while *HLA-DRB1*0301* influences PM susceptibility. Furuya *et al.* [9,26] found that both *HLA-DRB1*0803* and *HLA-DQA1*0501* provide an increased risk of DM but a reduced risk of PM in a Japanese population. In a study of 25 Korean patients with IIM, Rider *et al.* [27] reported that *HLA-DRB1*14* as a protective factor for DM and PM. To date, most studies on the subject have been focused on Western populations. In their studies of 52 DM and PM patients from Northern China, Han *et al.* reported that *HLA-DRB1*04, HLA-DRB1*07,* and *HLA-DRB1*12* may render an increased risk of DM [10], while *HLA-DQB1*0401* may have an impact on IIM susceptibility [11]. Our data demonstrate that the *HLA-DQA1*0104* and *HLA-DRB1*07* alleles are likely associated with an increased risk of DM, whereas *HLA-DRB1*03* may provide protection against DM. Although 8.1 AH is known as a risk factor for IIM among individuals of Northwestern European descent [4,7,28], such an association has not been established in other ethnic groups [25]. *DRB1*03-DQA1*05-DQB1*02* is not a major haplotype in our cohort and does not influence DM and PM susceptibility. Our results suggest that the *HLA-*

*DRB1*07-DQA1*01-DQB1*02* haplotype may be associated with DM and ILD.

It is interesting to note that *HLA-DRB1*07* influences IIM susceptibility among various ethnic groups. In our study of Han Chinese patients, the *HLA-DRB1*07* allele in the putative haplotype *DRB1*07-DQA1*01-DQB1*02* was found to be a risk factor for DM, but the same allele present in the *DRB1*07-DQA1*02-DQB1*02* haplotype was reported to be a protector against IIM in Caucasians and African Americans [4,22,25,28]. These findings imply that *HLA-DRB1*07* might have opposite effects on the diseases in different ethnic groups. Similar phenomena have been observed for the effect of *HLA-DQA1*0501* on IIM. This allele was reported as a protective factor against IIM in a Japanese population [9] but as a risk factor for IIM among US Caucasians [29]. Although it is unclear what might cause such different effects, possible explanations include referral bias, small sample sizes resulting in nonrepresentative populations, different pathogeneses, various environmental risk triggers around the world, and unidentified genetic loci responsible for disease development.

Furuya *et al.* [26] reported a positive relationship between *HLA-DRB1*0405* and anti-aminoacyl-tRNA synthetase

Table 3 Comparisons of frequencies of *HLA* class II putative haplotypes between DM and PM and controls

Haplotypes	DM (N =63)	PM (N = 18)	Myositis with ILD	Myositis with dysphagia	Control (N =100)	Controls vs. indicated patients (*p*; OR [95% CI])			
DRB1-DQA1-DQB1	n (%)	n (%)	n (%) N = 36	n (%), N = 9	n (%)	DM	PM	Myositis with ILD	Myositis with dysphagia
03-05-02	2 (1.59)	2 (5.56)	2 (2.78)	0 (0.00)	11 (5.50)	n/s	n/s	n/s	n/s
04-03-03	6 (4.36)	1 (2.78)	5 (6.94)	1 (5.56)	9 (4.50)	n/s	n/s	n/s	n/s
04-03-04	5 (3.97)	2 (5.56)	5 (6.94)	1 (5.56)	6 (3.00)	n/s	n/s	n/s	n/s
07-01-02	12 (9.52)	1 (2.78)	8 (11.11)	2 (11.11)	7 (3.50)	0.03[1]; 2.90 (1.02–8.93)	n/s	0.02[1]; 3.45 (1.04–11.58)	n/s
07-03-02	6 (4.76)	0 (0.00)	3 (4.17)	2 (11.11)	11 (5.50)	n/s	n/s	n/s	n/s
08-01-06	13 (10.32)	3 (8.33)	6 (8.33)	2 (11.11)	13 (6.50)	n/s	n/s	n/s	n/s
09-03-03	17 (13.49)	2 (5.56)	3 (4.17)	3 (16.67)	20 (10.00)	n/s	n/s	n/s	n/s
11-05-03	3 (2.38)	1 (2.78)	1 (1.39)	0 (0.00)	7 (3.50)	n/s	n/s	n/s	n/s
12-01-03	11 (8.73)	2 (5.56)	8 (11.11)	0 (0.00)	11 (5.50)	n/s	n/s	n/s	n/s
13-01-06	7 (5.56)	0 (0.00)	2 (2.78)	1 (5.56)	7 (3.50)	n/s	n/s	n/s	n/s
14-01-05	2 (1.59)	1 (2.78)	0 (0.00)	2 (11.11)	7 (3.50)	n/s	n/s	n/s	n/s
15-01-06	7 (5.56)	3 (8.33)	3 (4.17)	1 (5.56)	19 (9.50)	n/s	n/s	n/s	n/s

n/s: not significant; n/a: not applicable; [1]pcorr greater than 0.05; ILD: interstitial lung disease.

autoantibodies in Japanese IIM patients. In addition, O'Hanlon *et al.* found that the *HLA-DRB1*0302* allele is closely linked to myositis-specific anti-Mi-2 autoantibodies in DM [4]. In our study, the numbers of patients with MSA and MAA were too small to have sufficient statistical power for further analysis of the relationship between *HLA* alleles and MSA/MAA autoantibodies. It is also noteworthy that a greater frequency of myositis autoantibodies was found among PM patients from our cohort and the cohort reported by Chinoy and colleagues [20]. However, both cohorts were small in size, and in our study we analyzed only a limited number of autoantibodies.

Previous studies suggest that DM and PM may have different pathogeneses. It has been proposed that DM is likely the result of an autoimmune process induced by a humoral response, whereas PM may be caused by a cell-mediated autoimmune process [17]. Thus, it is plausible that DM and PM might have distinctive genetic susceptibilities. Further investigation is warranted to better understand the pathogeneses of these two diseases.

Possible explanations for the differences between the results from our study and those from other studies include the fact that the studies were conducted in different geographic locations with various environmental exposures, the heterogeneity in genetic backgrounds among the different ethnic groups and populations, the number of *HLA* polymorphic alleles analyzed, the different study methodologies used, referral bias, and the age and sex composition of the different study cohorts. The differences in the clinical and immunogenetic features between adult and childhood DM and PM are well documented [8,31].

Our study has some limitations. Although DM and PM are rare conditions and the number of patients in our cohort is the largest compared with similar studies in Chinese patients, it is still a relatively small cohort. It is likely that there are many genes and genetic polymorphisms that may influence DM and PM susceptibility, and we analyzed only a few of them. The data from our study should be validated by further analysis of multiple genes and alleles and their combined impacts on disease susceptibility. Nevertheless, our data shed some light on the genetic susceptibility of adult DM and PM, and may aid in stratifying disease subtypes according to genetic and ethnic backgrounds.

Conclusions

Our study of adult DM and PM in a Chinese population demonstrated that the putative haplotype *DRB1*07-DQA1*01-DQB1*02* and the *DRB1*07* and *DQA1*0104* alleles are associated with an increased risk of DM, while *DRB1*03* is associated with a reduced risk of DM. *DQB1*0303* may confer protection against the lung complication, and *DRB1*04*, *DRB1*12*, and *DRB1*07-DQA1*01-DQB1*02* are associated with an increased risk of developing the lung complication. Furthermore, *DRB1*07* is associated with an increased risk of developing dysphagia.

Abbreviations
PM: Polymyositis; DM: Dermatomyositis; HLA: Human leukocyte antigen; IIM: Idiopathic inflammatory myopathies.

Competing interests
The authors declare that they have no competing interests.

Authors' contributions
LB, LL and XG conceived the study design and manuscript preparation; LB, LL, XG, LY, LH, HS, and YY participated in data interpretation; XG, YY, LH, LY, HS, and GG collected data and conducted experiments and data analysis. All authors read and approved the final manuscript.

Acknowledgements
We are grateful to the patients and physicians for their participation in the study. This study was supported in part by Shanghai Nature and Sciences Fund (No. 11ZR1404900).

Author details
[1]The First Department of Health Care, Weifang People's Hospital, Shandong, China. [2]Departments of Rheumatology and Occupational Medicine, Huashan Hospital of Fudan University, Shanghai, China. [3]Center for Clinical Molecular Medicine; Ministry of Education Key Laboratory of Child Development and Disorders, Key Laboratory of Pediatrics in Chongqing, Chongqing, China. [4]Chongqing International Science and Technology Cooperation Center for Child Development and Disorders, Children's Hospital of Chongqing Medical University, Chongqing, China. [5]Shanghai Children's Hospital, Shanghai Children's Hospital Affiliated to Shanghai Jiao Tong University School of Medicine, Shanghai, China. [6]Department of Pathology, Geisel School of Medicine at Dartmouth College, Lebanon, New Hampshire, USA.

References
1. Mammen AL: **Dermatomyositis and polymyositis: Clinical presentation, autoantibodies, and pathogenesis.** *Ann N Y Acad Sci* 2010, **1184**:134–153.
2. Luppi P, Rossiello MR, Faas S, Trucco M: **Genetic background and environment contribute synergistically to the onset of autoimmune diseases.** *J Mol Med (Berl)* 1995, **73**(8):381–393.
3. Thorsby E, Lie BA: **HLA associated genetic predisposition to autoimmune diseases: Genes involved and possible mechanisms.** *Transpl Immunol* 2005, **14**(3–4):175–182.
4. O'Hanlon TP, Carrick DM, Targoff IN, Arnett FC, Reveille JD, Carrington M, Gao X, Oddis CV, Morel PA, Malley JD, Malley K, Shamim EA, Rider LG, Chanock SJ, Foster CB, Bunch T, Blackshear PJ, Plotz PH, Love LA, Miller FW: **Immunogenetic risk and protective factors for the idiopathic inflammatory myopathies: distinct HLA-A, -B, -Cw, -DRB1, and -DQA1 allelic profiles distinguish European American patients with different myositis autoantibodies.** *Medicine (Baltimore)* 2006, **85**(2):111–127.
5. Seldin MF, Amos CI, Ward R, Gregersen PK: **The genetics revolution and the assault on rheumatoid arthritis.** *Arthritis Rheum* 1999, **42**(6):1071–1079.
6. McLeod R, Buschman E, Arbuckle LD, Skamene E: **Immunogenetics in the analysis of resistance to intracellular pathogens.** *Curr Opin Immunol* 1995, **7**(4):539–552.
7. Arnett FC, Targoff IN, Mimori T, Goldstein R, Warner NB, Reveille JD: **Interrelationship of major histocompatibility complex class II alleles and autoantibodies in four ethnic groups with various forms of myositis.** *Arthritis Rheum* 1996, **39**(9):1507–1518.
8. Reed AM, Pachman LM, Hayford J, Ober C: **Immunogenetic studies in families of children with juvenile dermatomyositis.** *J Rheumatol* 1998, **25**(5):1000–1002.

9. Furuya T, Hakoda M, Higami K, Ueda H, Tsuchiya N, Tokunaga K, Kamatani N, Kashiwazaki S: Association of HLA class I and class II alleles with myositis in Japanese patients. *J Rheumatol* 1998, **25**(6):1109–1114.

10. Han X, Zhai N, Zhang Y, LI J, Liu J, Song F, Cehn H: Association of HLA-DRB1 alleles and polymyositis/dermatomyositis in northen Chinese. *Chin J Microbiol Immunol* 2003, **23**(3):225–227.

11. Han X, Zhai N, Zhang Q, Li J, Liu J, Du J, Song F: Association of HLA-DQB1 alleles and dermatomyositis/ polymyositis. *Chin J Med Genet* 2002, **19**(4):322–323.

12. Bohan A, Peter JB: Polymyositis and dermatomyositis (second of two parts). *N Engl J Med* 1975, **292**(8):403–407.

13. Bohan A, Peter JB: Polymyositis and dermatomyositis (first of two parts). *N Engl J Med* 1975, **292**(7):344–347.

14. Olerup O, Aldener A, Fogdell A: HLA-DQB1 and -DQA1 typing by PCR amplification with sequence-specific primers (PCR-SSP) in 2 hours. *Tissue Antigens* 1993, **41**(3):119–134.

15. Olerup O, Zetterquist H: HLA-DR typing by PCR amplification with sequence-specific primers (PCR-SSP) in 2 hours: an alternative to serological DR typing in clinical practice including donor-recipient matching in cadaveric transplantation. *Tissue Antigens* 1992, **39**(5):225–235.

16. Stephens M, Smith NJ, Donnelly P: A new statistical method for haplotype reconstruction from population data. *Am J Hum Genet* 2001, **68**(4):978–989.

17. Engel AG, Arahata K, Emslie-Smith A: Immune effector mechanisms in inflammatory myopathies. *Res Publ Assoc Res Nerv Ment Dis* 1990, **68**:141–157.

18. Robinson AB, Reed AM: Clinical features, pathogenesis and treatment of juvenile and adult dermatomyositis. *Nat Rev Rheumatol* 2011, **7**(11):664–675.

19. Shamim EA, Rider LG, Pandey JP, O'Hanlon TP, Jara LJ, Samayoa EA, Burgos-Vargas R, Vazquez-Mellado J, Alcocer-Varela J, Salazar-Paramo M, Kutzbach AG, Malley JD, Targoff IN, Garcia-De la Torre I, Miller FW: Differences in idiopathic inflammatory myopathy phenotypes and genotypes between Mesoamerican Mestizos and North American Caucasians: ethnogeographic influences in the genetics and clinical expression of myositis. *Arthritis Rheum* 2002, **46**(7):1885–1893.

20. Chinoy H, Salway F, Fertig N, Oddis CV, Ollier WE, Cooper RG: Clinical, serological and HLA profiles in non-Caucasian UK idiopathic inflammatory myopathy. *Rheumatology (Oxford)* 2009, **48**(5):591–592.

21. Marie I, Hachulla E, Levesque H, Reumont G, Ducrotte P, Cailleux N, Hatron PY, Devulder B, Courtois H: Intravenous immunoglobulins as treatment of life threatening esophageal involvement in polymyositis and dermatomyositis. *J Rheumatol* 1999, **26**(12):2706–2709.

22. O'Hanlon TP, Rider LG, Mamyrova G, Targoff IN, Arnett FC, Reveille JD, Carrington M, Gao X, Oddis CV, Morel PA, Malley JD, Malley K, Shamim EA, Chanock SJ, Foster CB, Bunch T, Reed AM, Love LA, Miller FW: HLA polymorphisms in African Americans with idiopathic inflammatory myopathy: allelic profiles distinguish patients with different clinical phenotypes and myositis autoantibodies. *Arthritis Rheum* 2006, **54**(11):3670–3681.

23. Yu KH, Wu YJ, Kuo CF, See LC, Shen YM, Chang HC, Luo SF, Ho HH, Chen IJ: Survival analysis of patients with dermatomyositis and polymyositis: analysis of 192 Chinese cases. *Clin Rheumatol* 2011, **30**(12):1595–1601.

24. Kuo CF, See LC, Yu KH, Chou IJ, Chang HC, Chiou MJ, Luo SF: Incidence, cancer risk and mortality of dermatomyositis and polymyositis in Taiwan: a nationwide population study. *Br J Dermatol* 2011, **165**(6):1273–1279.

25. Chinoy H, Lamb JA, Ollier WE, Cooper RG: Recent advances in the immunogenetics of idiopathic inflammatory myopathy. *Arthritis Res Ther* 2011, **13**(3):216.

26. Furuya T, Hakoda M, Tsuchiya N, Kotake S, Ichikawa N, Nanke Y, Nakajima A, Takeuchi M, Nishinarita M, Kondo H, Kawasaki A, Kobayashi S, Mimori T, Tokunaga K, Kamatani N: Immunogenetic features in 120 Japanese patients with idiopathic inflammatory myopathy. *J Rheumatol* 2004, **31**(9):1768–1774.

27. Rider LG, Shamim E, Okada S, Pandey JP, Targoff IN, O'Hanlon TP, Kim HA, Lim YS, Han H, Song YW, Miller FW: Genetic risk and protective factors for idiopathic inflammatory myopathy in Koreans and American whites: a tale of two loci. *Arthritis Rheum* 1999, **42**(6):1285–1290.

28. Chinoy H, Salway F, Fertig N, Shephard N, Tait BD, Thomson W, Isenberg DA, Oddis CV, Silman AJ, Ollier WE, Cooper RG: In adult onset myositis, the presence of interstitial lung disease and myositis specific/associated antibodies are governed by HLA class II haplotype, rather than by myositis subtype. *Arthritis Res Ther* 2006, **8**(1):R13.

29. Love LA, Leff RL, Fraser DD, Targoff IN, Dalakas M, Plotz PH, Miller FW: A new approach to the classification of idiopathic inflammatory myopathy: myositis-specific autoantibodies define useful homogeneous patient groups. *Medicine (Baltimore)* 1991, **70**(6):360–374.

30. Hausmanowa-Petrusewicz I, Kowalska-Oledzka E, Miller FW, Jarzabek-Chorzelska M, Targoff IN, Blaszczyk-Kostanecka M, Jablonska S: Clinical, serologic, and immunogenetic features in Polish patients with idiopathic inflammatory myopathies. *Arthritis Rheum* 1997, **40**(7):1257–1266.

31. Feldman BM, Rider LG, Reed AM, Pachman LM: Juvenile dermatomyositis and other idiopathic inflammatory myopathies of childhood. *Lancet* 2008, **371**(9631):2201–2212.

Subjective stress reactivity in psoriasis – a cross sectional study of associated psychological traits

Charlotta Remröd[1*], Karin Sjöström[2] and Åke Svensson[1]

Abstract

Background: Stress or psychological distress is often described as a causative or maintaining factor in psoriasis. Psychological traits may influence the appraisal, interpretation and coping ability regarding stressful situations. Detailed investigations of psychological traits in relation to stress reactivity in psoriasis are rare. The aim of this study was to examine whether patients with psoriasis who report an association between psychological distress and exacerbation, "stress reactors" (SRs), differ psychologically from those with no stress reactivity "non-stress reactors" (NSRs).

Methods: This cross-sectional study was conducted among 101 consecutively recruited outpatients with plaque psoriasis. A psychosocial interview was performed including questions concerning stress reactivity in relation to onset and exacerbation. Three validated self-rating scales were used: Spielberger State-Trait Anxiety Inventory (STAI, Form-Y), Beck Depression Inventory (BDI-II) and Swedish Universities Scales of Personality (SSP). Independent samples t-tests, Chi-square tests and one-way ANOVA analyses were used for group comparisons when appropriate. A logistic regression model was designed with SR as the dependent variable.

Results: Sixty-four patients (63%) reported a subjective association between disease exacerbation and stress (SRs). Patients defined as SRs reported significantly higher mean scores regarding state and trait anxiety, depression, and also five SSP scale personality traits, i.e. somatic trait anxiety, psychic trait anxiety, stress susceptibility, lack of assertiveness and mistrust, compared with NSRs. In multivariate analysis, SSP-stress susceptibility was the strongest explanatory variable for SR, i.e. OR (95% CI) = 1.13 (1.02 – 1.24), p = 0.018.

Conclusion: According to our results, patients who perceive stress as a causal factor in their psoriasis might have a more vulnerable psychological constitution. This finding suggests important opportunities for clinicians to identify patients who may benefit from additional psychological exploration and support.

Keywords: Plaque psoriasis, Psychology, Stress, Anxiety, Depression, Personality assessment

Background

Psoriasis is one of the most common immune-mediated skin diseases and is known to have a systemic inflammatory involvement [1]. The estimated prevalence of psoriasis is 1.5 – 3% in Scandinavia and Northern Europe [2,3]. A genetic–environmental interaction seems to offer a plausible aetiological explanation of psoriasis [1], and psychological distress has often been suggested as an important trigger [4,5]. Only a few prospective studies of stress and psoriasis exist [4,6,7], and the associations

and mechanisms involved remains unclear. Despite the lack of strong aetiological evidence for the association between psychological distress and psoriasis, between 37% and 71% of patients report psychological distress as one of the major causative agents for onset, exacerbation and maintenance of their psoriasis [8-15]. These patients may be defined as stress reactors. Psychological distress has also been found to reduce efficacy of treatment in psoriasis [16], and improvement of clinical parameters as a result of psychological interventions adds further evidence for the association between psychological distress and psoriasis [17,18].

Nevertheless, research has shown that focusing solely on stressors from the environment is too simplistic [19,20].

* Correspondence: charlotta.remrod@med.lu.se
[1]Department of Dermatology and Venereology, University of Lund, Hudkliniken, Skåne University Hospital, Jan Waldenströmsg. 16, Malmö 205 02, Sweden
Full list of author information is available at the end of the article

Almost no single life event would be regarded as a stressor by all individuals with such exposure, because individual responses are highly influenced by perceptions and interpretation of events. Genetic, personal, emotional and social factors will determine whether an individual can tolerate and overcome the effects of stressors [19,20]. Consequently, psychological traits are of significant importance in stress theory and research. Personality influences both the exposure to, and appraisal of stressful situations, and also the individual's interpretation of stressors and coping ability [19]. Some psychological traits can possibly predict increased emotional and physiological reactivity under stressful conditions [19-22].

Although stress has been recognised as an important factor within the field of psoriasis research, detailed investigations of psychological traits and clinical characteristics in relation to perceived stress-reactivity are rare. One of the few larger studies to elucidate this subject was conducted by Zachariae et al., [8] who found an association between subjective stress-reactivity and indicators of psychological vulnerability. Some smaller studies have reported subjective stress-reactivity to be associated with poorer levels of psychosocial well-being [13], pathological worrying [7,23], difficulties with assertion of anger, and dependency upon approval [9]. Devrimci-Ozguven et al. [14] showed conflicting results with no association between stress-reactivity and psychological morbidity. To the best of our knowledge, no previous study has as yet used a larger structured personality inventory in an investigation of stress reactivity in psoriasis.

The aim of this study was to examine the subjective influence of stress on psoriasis onset and exacerbations. Furthermore, we wanted to compare persons characterised as "stress reactors" (SRs) and "non-stress reactors" (NSRs) with respect to psychological variables, clinical- and socio-demographic factors and psoriasis-related distress. We hypothesise that stress-reactors have a more psychologically vulnerable constitution, as compared with non-stress reactors. By psychological vulnerability, we refer to an individual's inability to withstand the effects of a potentially stressful environment, due to psychological sensitivity and lack of adequate coping mechanisms.

Method
Subjects
All subjects were recruited consecutively from planned visits at the out-patient clinic of the Department of Dermatology and Venereology at the Skåne University Hospital in Malmö, Sweden. Inclusion criteria were: plaque psoriasis diagnosed by dermatologist, men and women aged 18 – 65 years, good command of the Swedish language, and no serious mental or cognitive disturbances.

A total of 109 patients were approached during early autumn 2008 (53%) and autumn 2009 (47%). Of them, 102 agreed to participate (94%) and gave their oral and written informed consent. One patient dropped out of the study, due to personal considerations. All of the 101 (93%) remaining patients were unpaid volunteers. A comparison of the two cohorts from 2008 and 2009 showed no statistically significant differences regarding any socio-demographic and clinical variables. The subjects were accordingly regarded as one cohort in statistical analyses.

No statistically significant differences were found between men and women regarding socio-demographic and clinical variables, psychosocial-, psychological-, and psoriasis-related variables.

Methods
A psychosocial semi-structured 25-item interview was conducted in a quiet room at the out-patient clinic. All subjects were interviewed by the same researcher (CR). The interview was designed by two of the authors (KS and CR), with the purpose of assessing (i) socio-demographic variables, (ii) social situation and close relationships, and (iii) psoriasis-related distress. Answers were rated on a 5-point Likert scale. Regarding (ii) social situation and close relationships, patients were asked about satisfaction with living conditions, working conditions, private economy and satisfaction with relationships with mother, father, partner, children, friends and colleagues. Answers were dichotomised as "satisfied" (1–3) and "not satisfied" (4–5). Regarding (iii) psoriasis-related distress, patients were asked about their psoriasis impact on daily life and on sexual relations. Answers were dichotomised as "low impact" (1–3) and "high impact" (4–5).

At the end of the interview, patients were asked: (A) "Do you relate the onset of your psoriasis to a particular stressful life situation?" (Answers were given as "yes", "no", "don't know"), and (B) "Do you experience that your psoriasis is aggravated during times of stress?" (Answers were given as "yes", "no", "sometimes" or "don't know"). For question (B), two groups were created for group comparisons, i.e. "stress reactors" (SRs) = (yes) and "non-stress reactors" (NSRs) = (no).

All patients were asked to rate their general degree of pruritus on a Visual Analogue Scale (VAS). The scale consisted of a 10 cm straight line without numbers or sections. The left end was labelled "no pruritus", and the right end was labelled "severe pruritus".

After the interview, each patient was given privacy to complete three psychometric self-rating scales in a quiet room, with the researcher readily available for questions in a room nearby.

Spielberger state-trait anxiety inventory (STAI)

The STAI (Form-Y) is a well-established self-rating scale with high stability and validity, often used in clinical research [24]. The first 20 statements assess state anxiety, i.e. anxiety at a particular moment or at a chosen period of time. (The subjects were asked to rate their state anxiety during the last week). The subsequent 20 statements assess trait anxiety, i.e. the relatively stable anxiety proneness. Answers are given on a 4-point Likert scale, and scores on the state and trait scales, respectively, range from 20 to 80 points. In large normative samples of working adults and college students, the mean values of state and trait anxiety for men range from 35.7 to 36.5 and 34.9 to 38.3, respectively, and for women from 35.2 to 38.8 and 34.8 to 40.4, respectively [24].

Beck depression inventory (BDI-II)

The Beck Depression Inventory Second Edition (BDI-II) is one of the most widely used self-report measures of depression in both research and clinical practice, with high validity and good psychometric properties [25]. The questionnaire consists of 21 items, and answers are rated on a four-point scale (0 = low, 3 = high). The total score ranges from 0 to 63. For persons who have been clinically investigated for depression, scores from 0–13 represent minimal depressive symptoms, scores of 14–19 indicate mild, scores of 20–28 indicate moderate, and scores of 29–63 indicate severe depressive symptoms [25]. Question number 16 evaluates sleep disturbances. Since sleep disturbances may be associated both with depression and stress reactivity, this variable was extracted, dichotomised and used in statistical analyses.

Swedish universities scales of personality (SSP)

The SSP is a thorough revision of the older Karolinska Scales of Personality (KSP). In contrast to many other personality inventories, SSP does not intend to measure "the entire personality", but has been developed to identify stable traits of psychological vulnerability and psychopathology. Psychological vulnerability is believed to predispose the individual to psychological problems [26]. The questionnaire comprises 91 items with a 4-point Likert response scale. The items are sorted into 13 subscales, each designed to measure one personality trait: (1) Somatic Trait anxiety, (2) Psychic Trait Anxiety, (3) Stress Susceptibility, (4) Lack of Assertiveness, (5) Impulsiveness, (6) Adventure Seeking, (7) Detachment, (8) Social Desirability, (9) Embitterment, (10) Trait Irritability, (11) Mistrust, (12) Verbal Trait Aggression, and (13) Physical Trait Aggression [27]. The SSP has been standardised in a large representative Swedish national sample, and the internal consistency with regard to Cronbach's alpha coefficient ranged from 0.59 to 0.84 in a normative sample [26]. The subscales are transformed into T scores according to the SSP computer algorithm. T scores (mean 50, SD 10) are standardised with regard to age and sex on the basis of a normal control group. Values of 10 points above or below 50 in each SSP scale indicate a difference from the standard population by 1.0 SD [27].

Psoriasis area and severity index (PASI)

Clinical assessment of PASI was conducted on 48 patients recruited during autumn 2009. The PASI scoring system is currently the best evaluated and the most widely used objective method to evaluate clinical severity of psoriasis [28]. The PASI combines the assessment of the area affected and the severity of lesions into a single score ranging from 0 (no disease) to 72 (severe disease). Severity has been categorised as follows: PASI < 7 = mild plaque psoriasis, PASI 7–12 = moderate plaque psoriasis, PASI > 12 = severe plaque psoriasis [29].

Statistical analysis

Independent samples t-tests, Chi-square tests and one-way ANOVA analyses were used for group comparisons when appropriate. Post hoc multiple comparisons were performed, using Tukey's test to identify pairwise significant differences. A logistic regression model was designed with SR as the dependent variable. All psychometric variables with a significant difference between SR and NSR in group comparisons were included and analysed in the model. The psychometric variables were first analysed separately, then adjusted for potential covariates, and finally with all psychometric variables and covariates included in the same model. Covariates used in the final model were age, gender, psoriasis impact on daily life, and age at debut of psoriasis. Age at debut was included since an association between this variable and psychological vulnerability has previously been found [30]. Other potential covariates that did not reach significance in the first adjustment were excluded from the final model, and they were: psychosocial variables sleep disturbances, alcohol consumption, PASI, pruritus and BMI. Two-tailed p-values < 0.05 were considered to be statistically significant. Statistical analyses were carried out using the Statistical Package for the Social Sciences, version 21.0 (SPSS™, Chicago, IL, USA).

The Ethics Committee of the Medical Faculty, University of Lund approved the study.

Results

Socio-demographic and clinical characteristics of the sample are given in Table 1.

Psychosocial interview

Most patients were satisfied with living conditions (93%), working conditions (98% of n = 90), private economy (89%) and also with relationships with mother (92% of n = 99), father (86% of n = 94), partner (91% of n = 77),

Table 1 Socio-demographic and clinical characteristics (N = 101)

Characteristics	
Gender, n (%)	
Male	56 (55)
Female	45 (45)
Age (years)	
Mean (SD), Mdn (range)	43.5 (13.8), 45 (18–65)
Age at onset of disease (years)	
Mean (SD), Mdn (range)	24.7 (14.5), 20 (0–61)
Duration of disease (years)	
Mean (SD), Mdn (range)	18.8 (12.7), 18 (1–56)
BMI	
Mean (SD), Mdn (range)	26.2 (4.5), 26.3 (17.6-38.5)
PASI (n = 48)	
Mean (SD), Mdn (range)	5.4 (4.3), 4.2 (0–21.7)
Mild psoriasis, n (%)	37 (77)
Moderate psoriasis, n (%)	8 (17)
Severe psoriasis, n (%)	3 (6)
Marital status, n (%)	
Single	18 (18)
Partner/cohabiting	35 (35)
Married	39 (38)
Divorced or widow/widower	9 (9)
Educational level, n (%)	
1-9 years	11 (11)
10-12 years	37 (37)
>12 years	53 (52)
Employment, n (%)	
Full time	66 (65)
Part time	13 (13)
Unemployed / retired	22 (22)
Tobacco consumption, n (%)	
Smokers	32 (32)
Nonsmokers	69 (68)
Alcohol consumption (gram/week)	
Mean (SD), Mdn (range)	45.9 (59.8), 30 (0–360)
Risk consumption:[a]	
Men, n (%)	3 (3)
Women, n (%)	2 (2)

BMI, Body Mass Index; PASI, Psoriasis Area and Severity Index.
[a]Alcohol risk consumption (standard drinks/week); men > 14, women > 9.

own children (100% of n = 66), friends (94%) and colleagues (98% of n = 80). Forty-nine patients (48%) reported that their psoriasis had a high impact on their daily life, and 27 patients (27%) reported that their psoriasis had a high impact on sexual relations.

Stress and exacerbation

Sixty-four patients (63%) were defined as "stress reactors" (SRs), 26 patients (26%) "non- stress reactors" (NSRs), seven patients (7%) answered "don't know" and four patients (4%) "sometimes". Statistically significant differences between SRs and NSRs were found regarding mean scores of state, and trait anxiety, BDI-II and five personality traits on the SSP scale, i.e. somatic trait anxiety, psychic trait anxiety, stress susceptibility, lack of assertiveness and mistrust. Results are presented in Table 2 together with descriptive mean scores for the total sample and all four groups of subjective stress-reactivity. No statistically significant differences between SRs and NSRs were found regarding all socio-demographic and clinical variables shown in Table 1, psychosocial variables, psoriasis-related distress or sleep disturbances.

In multivariate logistic regression analysis, the psychometric variables tested were all significant explanatory variables for SR when analysed as single variables. When these analyses were controlled for potential covariates, all psychometric variables remained significant, except SSP-mistrust. When analysing all psychometric variables with covariates in the same model, SSP-stress susceptibility was the only significant explanatory variable for SR. Due to multi-collinearity between the psychometric variables, the other psychometric variables did not remain significant. Odds-ratios (95% CI) and p-values are presented in Table 3.

SSP-stress susceptibility

Scores of SSP-stress susceptibility were positively correlated with scores of state and trait anxiety (r = 0.61 and r = 0.73 respectively, $p < 0.0001$), scores of BDI-II (r = 0.61, $p < 0.0001$), SSP-somatic trait anxiety (r = 0.60, $p < 0.0001$), SSP-psychic trait anxiety (r = 0.75, $p < 0.0001$), SSP-lack of assertiveness (r = 0.47, $p < 0.0001$) and SSP-mistrust (r = 0.50, $p < 0.0001$). No significant correlation or mean differences were found between SSP-stress susceptibility and of the socio-demographic and clinical variables shown in Table 1, psychosocial variables or sleep disturbances.

Stress and onset of psoriasis

Fifty patients (49%) reported an experience of disease onset during a stressful life situation. Thirty-seven patients (37%) did not, and 14 patients (14%) answered "don't know". Patients with onset related to stress had significantly higher mean age at onset compared with those who answered "no" (29.2 years vs 21.8 years, $p = 0.040$) and those who answered "don't know" (15.9 years, $p = 0.005$). Compared with those who answered "no", patients with onset related to stress had significantly higher mean scores of state anxiety (40.1 vs. 34.1, $p = 0.045$), trait anxiety (38.9 vs. 32.2, $p = 0.023$), BDI-II (10.0 vs. 5.8, $p = 0.043$) and SSP-psychic trait anxiety

Table 2 Results from the psychometric scales *Mean scores from the total sample, for the different groups of subjective stress reactivity and group comparisons of SRs vs. NSRs*

	Total Mean (SD) (N = 101)	"Yes" (SR) Mean (SD) (n = 64)	"No" (NSR) Mean (SD) (n = 26)	"Don't know" Mean (SD) (n = 7)	"Sometimes" Mean (SD) (n = 4)	SR vs. NSR Significance of difference, p
STAI						
State anxiety	38.0 (12.2)	40.5 (12.5)	29.9 (8.0)	44.0 (10.1)	40.8 (10.9)	<0.0001
Trait anxiety	36.5 (11.9)	38.3 (12.1)	28.0 (6.4)	43.1 (13.3)	35.0 (12.0)	<0.0001
BDI-II Depression	8.4 (8.1)	10.0 (8.5)	3.4 (3.6)	13.1 (10.4)	7.0 (4.1)	<0.0001
SSP						
Somatic Trait Anxiety	51.2 (10.8)	53.2 (10.4)	45.1 (9.8)	58.1 (10.8)	47.1 (4.9)	0.001
Psychic Trait Anxiety	47.5 (9.9)	49.2 (10.6)	42.1 (6.3)	53.3 (6.7)	46.6 (12.6)	<0.0001
Stress Susceptibility	50.7 (10.9)	53.5 (10.9)	42.1 (7.7)	55.4 (7.1)	53.9 (7.8)	<0.0001
Lack of Assertiveness	47.0 (9.9)	48.9 (10.6)	42.1 (6.1)	49.9 (10.8)	43.5 (4.5)	<0.0001
Impulsiveness	50.8 (9.9)	51.3 (10.0)	50.0 (10.9)	52.3 (6.7)	46.6 (9.1)	n.s.
Adventure seeking	49.7 (9.3)	49.5 (9.9)	49.5 (8.5)	51.6 (8.6)	52.4 (8.5)	n.s.
Detachment	47.0 (10.2)	47.2 (10.3)	44.6 (9.6)	53.5 (7.7)	47.5 (15.7)	n.s
Social Desirability	51.2 (9.7)	51.6 (10.5)	51.5 (9.9)	47.4 (7.6)	49.5 (5.4)	n.s
Embitterment	50.6 (10.1)	51.9 (10.0)	47.7 (8.3)	51.9 (8.2)	45.3 (2.6)	n.s.
Trait Irritability	49.3 (10.4)	49.9 (11.2)	46.3 (9.1)	55.0 (9.4)	48.7 (2.0)	n.s.
Mistrust	48.9 (11.6)	49.8 (11.7)	43.7 (10.6)	59.1 (8.2)	50.3 (6.1)	0.024
Verbal Trait Aggression	49.5 (10.7)	48.9 (11.1)	50.3 (10.4)	53.5 (10.7)	48.2 (7.9)	n.s.
Physical Trait Aggression	48.0 (10.2)	47.8 (9.6)	48.2 (11.0)	54.2 (12.7)	39.3 (5.9)	n.s.

SR: stress reactors; NSR: non-stress reactors; STAI: State- and Trait anxiety Inventory; BDI-II: Beck Depression Inventory-II; SSP: Swedish Universities Scales of Personality.

(49.3 vs. 43.9 $p = 0.016$). No statistically significant differences between the three groups were found regarding the other socio-demographic and clinical variables shown in Table 1, other SSP-traits, psychosocial variables, psoriasis-related distress or sleep disturbances.

Discussion

In our study, more than half of the patients reported stress as a causative agent for exacerbation of their psoriasis. Subjective stress reactivity (SR) was associated with both higher scores of depression, anxiety, and also five personality traits on the SSP scale, i.e. stress-susceptibility, somatic anxiety, psychic anxiety, lack of assertiveness and mistrust. SSP-stress susceptibility showed the strongest association with SR in multivariate regression analysis and seems to be the most relevant personality trait in this study.

Individuals with high scores of SSP-stress susceptibility more often state that they "get tired and hurried too easily", "can not handle being interrupted when working

Table 3 Results from the logistic regression analyses with "stress reactor" as dependent variable *(N =90)*

Psychometric variables	Analysed as single variables OR (95% CI)	p	Analysed as single variables with covariates[a] OR (95% CI)	p	All psychometric variables with covariates[a] in the same model OR (95% CI)	p
STAI Trait anxiety	1.14 (1.06 – 1.22)	<0.0001	1.14 (1.06 – 1.23)	<0.0001	1.10 (0.97 – 1.24)	0.136
BDI-II Depression	1.20 (1.07 – 1.34)	0.001	1.22 (1.08 – 1.38)	0.002	1.11 (0.92 – 1.35)	0.269
SSP Somatic trait anxiety	1.08 (1.03 – 1.14)	0.002	1.08 (1.02 – 1.14)	0.005	1.05 (0.96 – 1.14)	0.322
Psychic trait anxiety	1.09 (1.03 – 1.16)	0.004	1.09 (1.02 – 1.16)	0.007	0.85 (0.71 – 1.02)	0.083
Stress susceptibility	1.14 (1.07 – 1.23)	<0.0001	1.15 (1.07 – 1.24)	<0.0001	1.13 (1.02 – 1.24)	0.018
Lack of assertiveness	1.09 (1.03 – 1.15)	0.005	1.09 (1.02 – 1.16)	0.008	1.08 (0.98 – 1.19)	0.104
Mistrust	1.06 (1.01 – 1.11)	0.028	1.05 (0.99 – 1.10)	0.061	0.98 (0.91 – 1.06)	0.657

STAI: Spielberger State- and Trait anxiety Inventory, BDI-II: Beck Depression Inventory-II, SSP: Swedish Universities Scales of Personality.
[a]Covariates: age, gender, psoriasis impact on daily life, age at debut of psoriasis.

with something", "in order to get something done have to spend more energy than most others do", "have difficulties to concentrate on what I'm doing if the environment is distracting", "easily feel pressure when told to speed up work", "feel insecure when facing new tasks", "think I have less energy than most people I know" [27]. SSP-stress susceptibility showed medium to high correlations with scores of anxiety, depression, SSP-somatic- and -psychic anxiety, SSP-lack of assertiveness and SSP-mistrust. Hence, these individuals are likely to experience and encounter more stress in their daily life compared with less psychologically vulnerable individuals, which in turn may increase stress- related immune dysregulation [31].

To the best of our knowledge, this study is one of the few to thoroughly investigate psychological traits in relation to subjective stress-reactivity in patients with psoriasis. Some previous researchers have examined this subject [7-9,13,14,23], however with different methodology and never with the SSP-scale or, to our knowledge, with any other validated personality scale.

In a large Nordic psoriasis study by Zachariae et al., [8] 66% of the patients reported a subjective stress reactivity, as compared with 63% in our study. Their results suggested an indirect association between stress-reactivity and psychological vulnerability, since stress reactivity was significantly associated with more frequent use of tranquillisers, anti-depressants and tobacco, as compared with non-stress reactors.

In a study by O'Leary et al. [13] 61% of the sample reported a strong belief in stress/psychological attributes as a causal factor in their psoriasis. Consistent with our results, this belief was significantly associated with poorer levels of psychological well-being, in terms of higher levels of anxiety, depression and also with more perceived stress. Perceived stress was measured by a questionnaire and may correspond to some of the questions measuring SSP-stress susceptibility this study [13]. In accordance with our study and the O'Leary study, Fortune et al. [23] found that patients with psoriasis and a strong belief in an emotional cause of their psoriasis were more likely to experience pathological worry than those who believed the cause to be physical.

Gupta et al. [9] showed that approximately 50% of 127 patients with psoriasis reported high stress-reactivity (≥7 on a 10-point scale). High stress reactors were more likely to report difficulties with the assertion of anger. Interestingly, in our study, traits of verbal and physical aggressiveness were the only personality traits where SRs showed lower mean scores than NSRs. This may indicate that the ability to express anger is a resource in coping with stress. Furthermore, Gupta et al. [9] found that high stress reactors more often had a tendency to rely upon the approval of others. This is similar to our findings of higher scores of SSP-lack of assertiveness in patients

with stress reactivity. Submissiveness and wanting approval of others is likely to create more daily stress, since social support and a sense of coherence are important factors in stress management [32,33]. In a longitudinal stydy, Kupfer and colleagues [34] found that patients with a low sense of coherence experienced their first psoriasis relapse 3.5 months after completion of treatment, whereas patients with a high sense of coherence experienced their first relapse after 10 months.

In a study of 50 patients with psoriasis, Devrimci-Ozguven et al. [14] did not find any significant differences between stress reactors and non-stress reactors regarding psychological morbidity in terms of Beck Depression Inventory and Spielberger state and trait anxiety scores. Due to a relatively small sample size, their results may be interpreted with some caution.

Patients defined as "non-stress reactors" (NSRs) in our study reported lower scores of both state and trait anxiety compared with a normative sample. Furthermore, they showed lower scores of SSP-somatic trait anxiety, SSP-psychic trait anxiety, SSP-stress-susceptibility, SSP-lack of assertiveness and SSP-mistrust. NSRs thus seem to be psychologically stable individuals, and may probably tolerate and overcome the effects of stressors in many situations. In clinical practice, it is always important to be attentive to psychological morbidity of the patients; however, these results indicate that clinicians may be less concerned about psychological morbidity in patients who do not associate their disease with stress.

Previous researchers have found stress reactivity to be associated with younger age, more psoriasis-related distress [9], greater disease severity and poorer disease-related quality of life [8], compared with non-stress reactors. However, in our study we found no significant differences between SRs and NSRs regarding disease severity, psoriasis related distress or any of the other clinical or socio-demographic variables shown in Table 1.

Onset and stress

Nearly 50% of the patients in our study experienced that onset of their psoriasis was related to a particular stressful period or situation in life. Our results differ slightly from Zachariae's study [8], where 35% of the subjects reported that the onset of their psoriasis occurred during a time of worry and stress. Due to the potential risk of retrospective recall bias, these results should be interpreted with caution. However, it is interesting that also patients with an experienced association between onset and stress reported significantly higher scores of both depression and traits of anxiety, compared with those without this association.

Subjective reporting and retrospective studies will always involve some degree of scientific uncertainty regarding the potential influence of recall and cognitive bias. Despite the lack of strong aetiological evidence for the association between psychological distress and psoriasis, a substantial portion of the patients in this, and previous studies [8-13], perceived psychological distress to be a causative factor in the manifestation of their disease. Patients with a chronic condition are likely to construct their own personal perceptions and ideas about their disease, in an attempt to better deal with it [35]. The beliefs that patients have about the causes of symptoms or diseases can have a profound effect on clinical management, compliance with treatment and prognosis [36]. The use of a single question for stress reactivity would provide a simple method in clinical practice to identify potentially psychologically vulnerable individuals. Results from this and previous studies [7-9,13,23] suggest important opportunities for clinicians to identify those patients who might benefit from a deeper psychological exploration.

PASI scores were estimated in the latter half of our study sample (48%), which is a limitation. However, all patients were interviewed during the same time of year i.e. early autumn, which might implicate relatively similar levels of disease severity in the entire sample. The great majority (77%) of the 48 patients scored had PASI scores representing mild disease; hence this variable was not used in the logistic regression analysis, which may be a limitation. However, PASI has often not been significantly associated with psychological morbidity in previous studies [37-39].

The methodological strengths of this study are the high participation rate and that all patients were interviewed by the same researcher. All patients were consecutively recruited from the same clinic, and only eight of 109 patients declined participation. Moreover, the total study sample showed a homogeneous personality profile and was not more anxious or depressed than the general population [24,25]. Thus, it may be assumed that the patients in this study represent a psychiatrically normal sample in further analyses of stress reactivity and interpretation of results.

Conclusions

According to our results, patients who perceive stress as a causal factor for exacerbation of their disease seem to have a more vulnerable psychological constitution. This finding suggests important opportunities for clinicians to identify patients who might benefit from additional psychological exploration and support.

Competing interests
The authors declare that they have no competing interests.

Authors' contributions
CR participated in the design of the study, met each patient and carried out the psychocoial interviews, acquisition, analysis and interpretation of data, performed the statistical analysis and drafted the manuscript. KS participated

in the design of the study, analysis and interpretation of data and have been involved in drafting the manuscript. ÅS participated in the design of the study, analysis and interpretation of data and have been involved in drafting the manuscript. All authors read and approved the final manuscript.

Authors' information
KS is a senior psychiatrist with many years of experience within the field of psychosomatics, both in clinical practice and research.

Acknowledgements
We are grateful to statistician Per-Erik Isberg, University of Lund, for his statistical guidance and valuable comments on the manuscript.

Author details
[1]Department of Dermatology and Venereology, University of Lund, Hudkliniken, Skåne University Hospital, Jan Waldenströmsg. 16, Malmö 205 02, Sweden. [2]Psychiatric consultant at the Department of Dermatology and Venereology, Hudkliniken, Skåne University Hospital, Jan Waldenströmsg. 16, Malmö 205 02, Sweden.

References
1. Nestle FO, Kaplan DH, Barker J. Psoriasis. N Engl J Med. 2009;361:496–509.
2. Griffiths CE, Barker JN. Pathogenesis and clinical features of psoriasis. Lancet. 2007;370:263–71.
3. Lofvendahl S, Theander E, Svensson A, Carlsson KS, Englund M, Petersson IF. Validity of diagnostic codes and prevalence of physician-diagnosed psoriasis and psoriatic arthritis in southern Sweden–a population-based register study. PLoS One. 2014;9, e98024.
4. Gaston L, Lassonde M, Bernier-Buzzanga J, Hodgins S, Crombez JC. Psoriasis and stress: A prospective study. J Am Acad Dermatol. 1987;17:82–6.
5. Hunter HJ, Griffiths CE, Kleyn CE. Does psychosocial stress play a role in the exacerbation of psoriasis? Br J Dermatol. 2013;169:965–74.
6. Berg M, Svensson M, Brandberg M, Nordlind K. Psoriasis and stress: A prospective study. J Eur Acad Dermatol Venereol. 2008;22:670–4.
7. Verhoeven EW, Kraaimaat FW, de Jong EM, Schalkwijk J, van de Kerkhof PC, Evers AW. Individual differences in the effect of daily stressors on psoriasis: A prospective study. Br J Dermatol. 2009;161:295–9.
8. Zachariae R, Zachariae H, Blomqvist K, Davidsson S, Molin L, Mørk C, et al. Self-reported stress reactivity and psoriasis-related stress of nordic psoriasis sufferers. J Eur Acad Dermatol Venereol. 2004;18:27–36.
9. Gupta MA, Gupta AK, Kirkby S, Schork NJ, Gorr SK, Ellis CN, et al. A psychocutaneous profile of psoriasis patients who are stress reactors. A study of 127 patients. Gen Hosp Psychiatry. 1989;11:166–73.
10. Nevitt GJ, Hutchinson PE. Psoriasis in the community: Prevalence, severity and patients' beliefs and attitudes towards the disease. Br J Dermatol. 1996;135:533–7.
11. Al'Abadie MS, Kent GG, Gawkrodger DJ. The relationship between stress and the onset and exacerbation of psoriasis and other skin conditions. Br J Dermatol. 1994;130:199–203.
12. Fortune DG, Richards HL, Main CJ, Griffiths CE. What patients with psoriasis believe about their condition. J Am Acad Dermatol. 1998;39:196–201.
13. O'Leary CJ, Creamer D, Higgins E, Weinman J. Perceived stress, stress attributions and psychological distress in psoriasis. J Psychosom Res. 2004;57:465–71.
14. Devrimci-Ozguven H, Kundakci TN, Kumbasar H, Boyvat A. The depression, anxiety, life satisfaction and affective expression levels in psoriasis patients. J Eur Acad Dermatol Venereol. 2000;14:267–71.
15. Manolache L, Petrescu-Seceleanu D, Benea V. Life events involvement in psoriasis onset/recurrence. Int J Dermatol. 2010;49:636–41.
16. Fortune DG, Richards HL, Kirby B, McElhone K, Markham T, Rogers S, et al. Psychological distress impairs clearance of psoriasis in patients treated with photochemotherapy. Arch Dermatol. 2003;139:752–6.
17. Fortune DG, Richards HL, Kirby B, Bowcock S, Main CJ, Griffiths CE. A cognitive-behavioural symptom management programme as an adjunct in psoriasis therapy. Br J Dermatol. 2002;146:458–65.
18. Fordham B, Griffiths CE, Bundy C. A pilot study examining mindfulness-based cognitive therapy in psoriasis. Psychol Health Med. 2015;20:121–7.
19. Vollrath M. Personality and stress. Scand J Psychol. 2001;42:335–47.

20. Selye H. Stress without distress. New York: JB Lippincott; 1974.

21. Brosschot JF, Gerin W, Thayer JF. The perseverative cognition hypothesis: A review of worry, prolonged stress-related physiological activation, and health. J Psychosom Res. 2006;60:113–24.

22. Watson D, Clark LA. Negative affectivity: The disposition to experience aversive emotional states. Psychol Bull. 1984;96:465–90.

23. Fortune D, Richards H, Main C, Griffiths C. Pathological worrying, illness perceptions and disease severity in patients with psoriasis. Br J Health Psychol. 2000;5:71–82.

24. Spielberger C, editor. Manual for the state-trait anxiety inventory, STAI (form-Y). Palo Alto, CA: Consulting Psychologists Press Inc; 1983.

25. Beck A, Steer R. Garbin. Psychometric Properties of the Beck Depression Inventory, 2nd edn. Manual. Swedish version. San Antonio, TX, U.S.A.: Psykologiförlaget AB under license from Harcourt Assessment Inc.; 1996.

26. Gustavsson JP, Bergman H, Edman G, Ekselius L, von Knorring L, Linder J. Swedish universities scales of personality (SSP): Construction, internal consistency and normative data. Acta Psychiatr Scand. 2000;102:217–25.

27. Gustavsson J, Bergman H, Edman G, Ekselius L, von Knorring L, Linder JM. Swedish universities Scales of Personality (SSP) Manual. Version 2.1. Uppsala: Karolinska Institutet, Stockholm and Uppsala University; 2000.

28. Naldi L, Svensson A, Zenoni D, Diepgen T, Elsner P, Grob JJ, et al. Comparators, study duration, outcome measures and sponsorship in therapeutic trials of psoriasis: Update of the EDEN psoriasis survey 2001–2006. Br J Dermatol. 2010;162:384–9.

29. Schmitt J, Wozel G. The psoriasis area and severity index is the adequate criterion to define severity in chronic plaque-type psoriasis. Dermatology. 2005;210:194–9.

30. Remrod C, Sjostrom K, Svensson A. Psychological differences between early- and late-onset psoriasis: A study of personality traits, anxiety and depression in psoriasis. Br J Dermatol. 2013;169:344–50.

31. Segerstrom SC, Miller GE. Psychological stress and the human immune system: A meta-analytic study of 30 years of inquiry. Psychol Bull. 2004;130:601–30.

32. Antonovsky H, Sagy S. The development of a sense of coherence and its impact on responses to stress situations. J Soc Psychol. 1986;126:213–25.

33. Antonovsky A. The structure and properties of the sense of coherence scale. Soc Sci Med. 1993;36:725–33.

34. Kupfer J, Niemeier V, Brosig B, Pauli-Pott U, Karpinski G, Küster W, et al. Sense of coherence among psoriatics as a predictor of symptom-free time following dermatological inpatient therapy. Dermatol Psychosom. 2003;4:200–6.

35. Petrie KJ, Jago LA, Devcich DA. The role of illness perceptions in patients with medical conditions. Curr Opin Psychiatry. 2007;20:163–7.

36. Sensky T. Causal attributions in physical illness. J Psychosom Res. 1997;43:565–73.

37. Rieder E, Tausk F. Psoriasis, a model of dermatologic psychosomatic disease: psychiatric implications and treatments. Int J Dermatol. 2012;5:12–26.

38. Magin PJ, Pond CD, Smith WT, Watson AB, Goode SM. Correlation and agreement of self-assessed and objective skin disease severity in a cross-sectional study of patients with acne, psoriasis, and atopic eczema. Int J Dermatol. 2011;50:1486–90.

39. Sampogna F, Sera F, Abeni D. IDI Multipurpose Psoriasis Research on Vital Experiences (IMPROVE) Investigators. Measures of clinical severity, quality of life, and psychological distress in patients with psoriasis: a cluster analysis. J Invest Dermatol. 2004;122:602–7.

10

Prevalence, incidence and predictive factors for hand eczema in young adults – a follow-up study

Arne Johannisson[1*], Ann Pontén[2,3] and Åke Svensson[4,5]

Abstract

Background: Hand eczema is common in the general population and affects women twice as often as men. It is also the most frequent occupational skin disease. The economic consequences are considerable for society and for the affected individuals.

Methods: To investigate the prevalence and incidence of hand eczema and to evaluate risk factors for development of hand eczema in young adults. Subjects and methods; This is a prospective follow-up study of 2,403 young adults, 16 – 19 years old in 1995 and aged 29 – 32 years, 13 years later, in 2008. They completed a postal questionnaire that included questions regarding one-year prevalence of hand eczema, childhood eczema, asthma, rhino-conjunctivitis and factors considered to affect hand eczema such as hand-washing, washing and cleaning, cooking, taking care of small children and usage of moisturisers. These factors were evaluated with the multinominal logistic regression analysis.

Results: The one-year prevalence of hand eczema was 15.8% (females 20.3% and males 10.0%, p < 0.001). The incidence was 11.6 cases per 1000 person-years (females 14.3 and males 5.2, p < 0.001). Childhood eczema was the most important risk factor for hand eczema. The odds ratios were 13.17 when having hand eczema 1995 and 2008 compared to 5.17 in 2008 (p < 0.001). A high frequency of hand washing was important in predicting hand eczema only when having 1-year prevalence 2008, OR 1.02 (p = 0.038).

Conclusions: After 13 years an increased 1-year prevalence of hand eczema was found. The significant risk factors for hand eczema changed over time from endogenous to exogenous factors.

Keywords: Hand eczema, Childhood eczema, Prevalence, Incidence, Cohort, Gender, Skin care, Hand-wash

Background

Hand eczema is common in the general population. In a recent review of studies in the general population from mostly European countries, the 1-year prevalence rates ranged from 6.5% to 17.5% [1]. Hand eczema is 1.5 – 2 times more common in females compared with males [2,3]. Swedish estimates of 1-year prevalence of hand eczema in different age-groups have varied from 6.5% to 11.8% [4-6]. Among Swedish 20–29 year-olds, the 1-year prevalence of hand eczema was reported to range from 7.5% to 10.8% [3,4]. Furthermore, hand eczema is the most common occupational skin disease [7].

Occupation-related hand eczema has many negative consequences. The economic costs are considerable for affected individuals and for society [8,9]. Hand eczema has been shown to have an unfavourable long-term prognosis [10] and to impair quality of life [11]. These consequences could be reduced by identifying and preventing risk factors.

Several exogenous risk factors for hand eczema have been reported: occupational exposure, use of detergents and wet work at home [4,12-14]. The identification and evaluation of risk factors for the development and persistence of hand eczema are important especially among young adults. During this period of life, type of occupation, household work and childcare are factors that are important to study because they might be related to the development of hand eczema. Taken together, these circumstances justify follow-up studies in early adulthood.

The aim of the present study was to investigate the prevalence and cumulative incidence of hand eczema

* Correspondence: arne.johannisson@med.lu.se
[1]Department of Health Sciences, Lund University, Box 157, 221 00 Lund, Sweden
Full list of author information is available at the end of the article

and to evaluate factors that can influence the development and recurrence of hand eczema in young adults.

Methods

Study group

This is the 13 year prospective follow-up study of a cohort of pupils in upper secondary school, 16–19 years old at the baseline assessment, and consequently they were 29–32 years old at follow-up. In 1995, 2,572 pupils in the four secondary schools in Växjö completed a self-administered questionnaire regarding hand eczema, the response rate was 98.6%. Växjö is a town in southern Sweden with approximately 70,000 inhabitants [15,16]. In 1995, 74% of 16 – 19 years-olds attended secondary school in the study area, which was consistent with the overall attendance rate in Sweden. The 13-year follow-up of this cohort was performed in 2008. At both occasions the questionnaire was mailed in springtime. Swedish personal identification numbers were used to get updated addresses from the Swedish Population Address Register (SPAR). Addresses were found for 2,403 of the original 2,572 participants (Figure 1); 169 were unreachable: 106 had personal identification numbers not matching the SPAR register, 35 had emigrated, 21 had moved without providing a forwarding address, five were deceased, and two were not traceable for reasons of secrecy.

Questionnaire

In 1995 the questionnaire was based on the Toulihampi questionnaire [17]. The questionnaire in 2008 was based on the Nordic Occupational Skin Questionnaire 2002 (NOSQ-2002), [18]. The questions regarding hand eczema were almost the same in the two questionnaires and the answer alternatives were exactly the same. Some additional questions constructed by the investigators were included in the 2008 questionnaire (See Additional file 1).

Topics surveyed by the questionnaire were: hand eczema, childhood eczema, asthma and rhino-conjunctivitis, household size and family structure, occupation and everyday activities, hand washing and skin care.

Distribution of the questionnaire

A self-administered postal questionnaire and a pre-paid return envelope were distributed in late May 2008. A postcard was sent at the beginning of June as a first reminder. At the end of August, a second reminder was sent which included a copy of the questionnaire, a pencil and a pre-paid return envelope. Finally, a postcard was sent in the middle of September as a third and final reminder.

Data analysis and statistics

One-year prevalence of hand eczema was estimated from reported hand eczema at present or having had hand eczema some time during the last 12 months (See Additional file 1). The question regarding the 1-year prevalence was previously validated [19,20]. The question on point prevalence was validated, and sensitivity (73%) and specificity (99%) were calculated [15]. To estimate the true 1-year prevalence for this cohort, a calculation of the 1-year prevalence in relation to sensitivity and specificity was made by using the formula: $P = (P * + (\text{specificity}-1))/(\text{sensitivity} + (\text{specificity}-1))$. P is the estimated true 1-year prevalence in the population and $P*$ is the 1-year prevalence in the sample [5,15,21].

The cumulative incidence was calculated on the individuals reporting having 1-year prevalence or ever having had hand eczema 2008 minus those who had 1-year prevalence or ever had had hand eczema in 1995. The cumulative incidence is presented as the percentage of new cases of hand eczema in the cohort. Incidence rate is presented as new cases per 1000 person-years, i. e. the cumulative incidence/13 years × 1000.

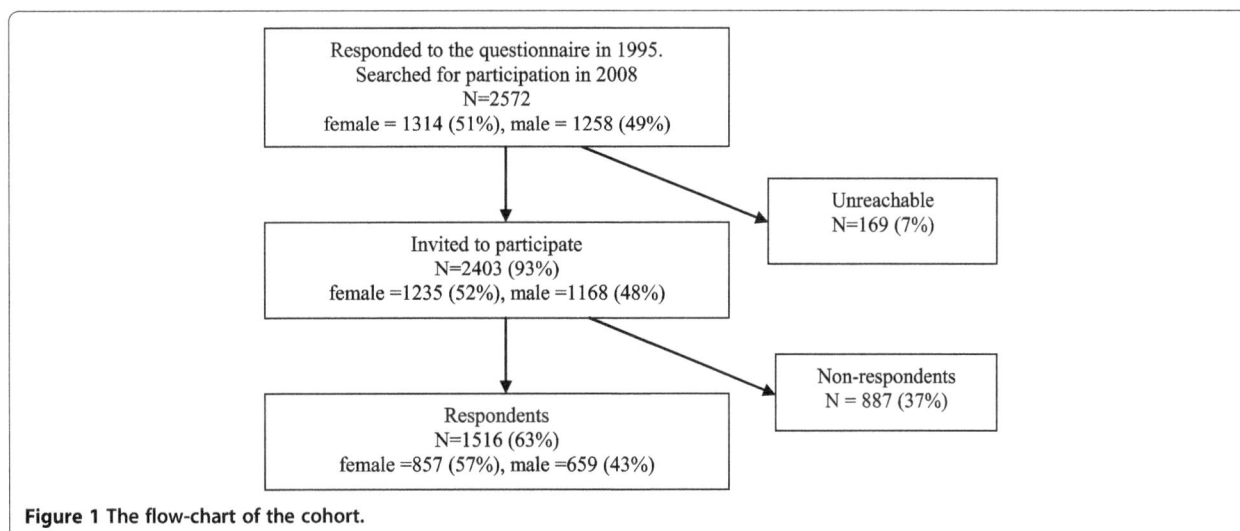

Figure 1 The flow-chart of the cohort.

Four groups were constructed with the intention to analyse risk factors and the development of hand eczema over time. The groups were constructed as follows: those who reported having a 1-year-prevalence in 1995 and in 2008 are in group HX9508, those who reported having a 1-year-prevalence in 1995 but not in 2008 are in group HX95, those who reported having a 1-year-prevalence in 2008 but not in 1995 are in group HX08, and those who reported that they never had hand eczema are in group NoHX.

The reliability over time of self-reported childhood eczema in 1995 and then reporting the same in 2008 was determined by calculating positive predictive value (PPV); i.e. the percentage positive agreement in 2008 among the yes-respondents from 1995. The negative predictive value (NPV); i.e. the agreement of no-answers in 1995 and 2008 was also calculated.

Potential exogenous risk factors for developing hand eczema such as household size, time required for household work, frequency of hand washing, skin protective habits, working hours outside home and leisure activities were investigated by dividing the cohort into two groups. The respondents who had 1-year prevalence of hand eczema 2008, i.e. the merged groups HX9508 and HX08, denominated the HX group, and the group that reported never having had hand eczema, the NoHX group. Furthermore, hand eczema was also studied in the two hand eczema groups separately regarding these factors.

Regarding occupation, the respondents were asked not only to tell their profession, but also to give information about work tasks.

The groups HX9508, HX95 and HX08 were compared to the group NoHX using a multinominal logistic regression model. The endogenous factors childhood eczema, asthma and rhino-conjunctivitis as reported in 2008 were used. The response choices in this calculation were Yes/No. Exogenous factors such as hand-washing (times a day), usage of moisturisers (dichotomised Daily/Some time each week, some time each month, never), cooking, cleaning/washing laundry, and taking care of children 0–4 years of age (hours a day) were investigated.

Categorical data were presented as numbers and/or proportions in groups; quantitative data were presented by mean, median and quartiles. Nominal data were tested with the Chi-squared test. When the number of expected values was insufficient, Fisher's exact test was used. When comparing groups over time, McNemar's test was used. Ordinal and interval data were tested with Kruskal-Wallis H test and Mann–Whitney U-test in independent group comparisons. In the multinominal logistic regression analysis odds-ratios, 95% confidence intervals and p-values were given for all the covariates. If data was missing for any covariate, the individual was not included in the analysis. A p-value <0.05 was considered significant

in all calculations. All statistical analyses were performed with SPSS 20.0 for Windows.

Ethics

The study was approved by the The Regional Ethical Review Board in Lund, (application no 156/2008).

Results

The flow-chart of the cohort is shown in Figure 1. Out of the 2,403 participants from the original cohort who received a questionnaire in the mail, 1,516 responded to the questionnaire, which was a response rate of 63%; 56% of the respondents were females. Significantly more females than males answered the questionnaire, 69.4% of the reachable original female cohort and 56.4% of the males (p < 0.001). However, in 2008 there were no significant differences between the respondents and non-respondents in reporting 1-year prevalence of hand eczema in 1995 (p = 0.677). No significant differences were found within the genders in reported hand eczema in 1995 (females, p = 0.490; males, p = 0.297).

In the first dispatch, 899 (37%) responded, the first postcard reminder yielded 158 (10%) responses. On the second reminder 437 (32%) responded. With the final postcard reminder, 22 (2%) responded, which left 887 non-respondents.

One-year prevalence of hand eczema

The 1-year prevalence of hand eczema in 2008 was 15.8%, Figure 2; females reported hand eczema twice as often as males, 20.3% versus 10.0%, (p < 0.001). The estimated true 1-year prevalence for this cohort was: (0.158 + (0.99 − 1)) / (0.73 + (0.99 − 1)) = 20.6%, 26.8% for females and 12.5% for males.The 1516 participants were allocated to any of the four groups as previously defined; HX9508 (83/1516, 5.5%, 7.2% females and 3.2% males), HX95 (71/1516, 4.7%; 5.6% females and 3.5% males), HX08 (157/1516, 10.4%; 13.1% females and 6.8% males) and NoHX (1016/1516, 67.0%; 61.4% females and 74.4% males). One hundred and sixty respondents (10.6%) reported that they had had hand eczema at some time, but not in 1995 nor in 2008, 29 individuals, 1.9%, did not answer the question. The higher proportion of females compared with males in the hand eczema groups compared with the NoHX group was significant (p < 0.001).

Incidence of hand eczema

In 1995 in total 13.3% (202/1516) reported they had or had had hand eczema, 139 females, (16.2%) and 63 males (9.6%), p < 0.001. In 2008 an additional 198 individuals reported themselves having or having had hand eczema. Thus the cumulative incidence over the 13 years was 15.1% (198/1314), for the females 18.6% and for the males 10.7%, p < 0.001. The incidence rate was estimated

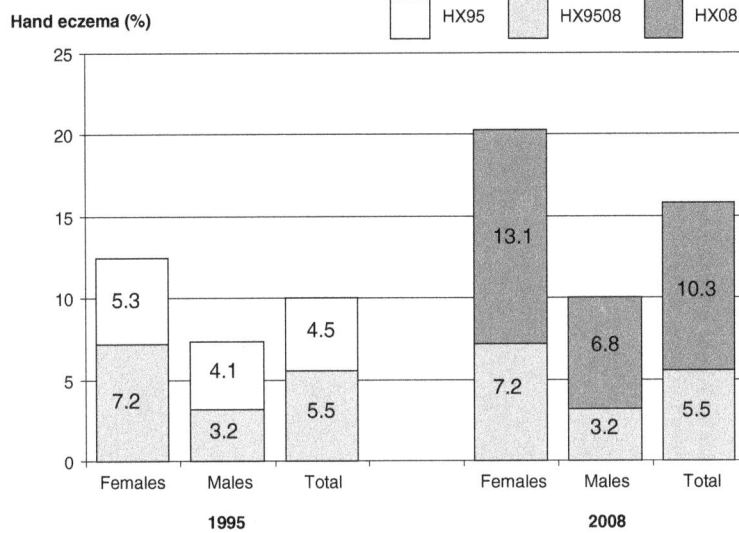

Figure 2 The proportions reporting hand eczema in 1995 but not 2008 (HX95), both 1995 and 2008 (HX9508), and only 2008 (HX08).

as 11.6 cases per 1000 person-years, 14.3 for females and 5.2 for males (p < 0.001).

Hand eczema versus childhood eczema, asthma, rhino-conjunctivitis and gender

Childhood eczema was reported by 400/1516 (26.4%) of the participants. The proportions of having had childhood eczema, asthma and rhino-conjunctivitis in the four groups in total and by gender for 2008 are shown in Table 1. The proportions of the individuals reporting only childhood eczema; i.e. not in combination with asthma and/or rhino-conjunctivitis (146/1516, 9.6%), were found to be: HX9508, 73.9%; HX95, 41.7%, HX08, 45.5% and NoHX, 17.3% (p < 0.001). Only having had asthma was reported by 22/1516 (1.5%); within the groups: 1, 1, 0 and 20 individuals respectively, (p = 0.366). Only having had rhino-conjunctivitis was reported by 201/1516 (13.3%). Within the groups 4, 7, 11 and 179 individuals, respectively (p = 0.124).

Self-reported childhood eczema in 2008 compared to 1995

The question about childhood eczema was answered by 1323 of the 1516 respondents (87.3%) in 2008. In 1995, 297/1323 individuals (22.4%) reported childhood eczema, and 239 of these gave the same answer in 2008. This gives the positive predictive value (PPV) of 80.5% (239/297). The negative predictive value (NPV), i.e. reporting not having had childhood eczema in 1995 as well as in 2008, was 76.7% (610/795). When comparing genders, the PPV for females was 82.3% and the NPV was 77.0%. The PPV for males was 75.6% and the NPV was 76.5%. There were significant differences within three of the four groups between PPV and NPV; HX9508 group: PPV = 90.6% and NPV = 35.0% (p = 0.016); HX95 group: PPV = 76.7% and NPV = 60.7% (p = 0.611); HX08 group: PPV = 94.0% and NPV = 55.3% (p < 0.001); NoHX group: PPV = 73.8% and NPV = 77.6% (p < 0.001).

Hand eczema and exogenous factors

The results regarding potential exogenous risk factors for developing hand eczema are shown in Table 2. The individuals in the HX group reported a significantly higher frequency of hand washing compared to the NoHX group, mean 15.4 versus 11.7 times per day (p < 0.001). The females in the HX group had a significantly higher number of daily hand washing compared to the females in the NoHX-group, 17.4 versus 14.5 times per day (p < 0.001).

Concerning skin care, daily use of moisturisers was reported by 60.5% in the HX group (females 67.6% males 41.5%), and by 30.6% in the NoHX group (females 47.4% and males 12.7%). The differences were significant between the two groups and between the genders within the groups (p < 0.001). Regardless of hand eczema, females used moisturisers significantly more often than males; 52.9% female versus 16.2% male daily users (p < 0.001), However, having hand eczema raised the reported usage of moisturizers by a factor 1.4 for females and 3.3 for males.

The exogenous factors were analysed between all four groups, in total as well as between genders (HX9508, HX95, HX08 and NoHX) and within genders in all groups, Table 3. In total as well as within females, the HX08 group had a significantly higher frequency of hand washing at home and at work than the NoHX group (p < 0.001). Regarding time spent at ordinary work; the HX08 group worked significantly less than the NoHX group (p = 0.001). The HX08 group spent significantly more time cooking, cleaning and doing laundry than the

Table 1 Prevalence of self-reported childhood eczema and/or asthma and/or rhino-conjunctivitis in 2008 with respect to 1-year prevalence of hand eczema and gender in the groups HX9508 (1-year prevalence of hand eczema 1995 and 2008), HX95 (1-year prevalence of hand eczema only 1995), HX08 (1-year prevalence of hand eczema only 2008) and NoHX (never having had hand eczema)

The 2008 questionnaire	Group HX9508			Group HX95			Group HX08			Group NoHX		
	Females n (%)	Males n (%)	Total n (%)	Females n (%)	Males n (%)	Total n (%)	Females n (%)	Males n (%)	Total n (%)	Females n (%)	Males n (%)	Total n (%)
"Did you have eczema in your childhood?" (n = 1325, 100%)												
"No" (n = 792, 59.8%)	10 (16.1) **a>**	3 (14.3)	13 (15.7)	19 (39.6)	6 (27.3)	25 (35.7)	38 (33.9)	14 (31.1)	52 (33.1)	349 (66.5)	353 (72.0)	702 (69.2)
"Yes" (n = 400, 30.2%)	48 (77.4) **a>**	15 (71.4) **a>**	63 (75.9) **b>**	22 (45.8) **a>**	14 (63.6) **a>**	36 (51.4) **b>**	63 (56.3) **a>**	23 (51.1) **a>**	86 (54.8) **b>**	140 (26.7) **a<, c>**	75 (15.3) **a<**	215 (21.2) **b<**
"I do not know" (n = 133, 10.0%)	4 (6.5)	3 (14.3)	7 (8.4)	7 (14.6)	2 (9.1)	9 (12.9)	11 (9.8)	8 (17.8)	19 (12.1)	36 (6.9)	62 (12.7)	98 (6.6)
"Have you ever had asthma?" (n = 1326)												
"No" (n = 1082, 81.6%)	37 (59.7)	15 (71.4)	52 (62.7)	38 (79.2)	19 (86.4)	57 (81.4)	84 (75.0)	35 (77.8)	119 (75.8)	433 (82.3)	421 (85.9)	854 (84.0)
"Yes" (n = 217, 16.4%)	23 (37.1)	6 (28.6)	29 (34.9) **b>**	8 (16.7)	2 (9.1)	10 (14.3) **b<**	23 (20.5)	10 (22.2)	33 (21.0) **b>**	84 (16.0)	61 (12.4)	145 (14.3) **b<**
"I do not know" (n = 27, 2.0%)	2 (3.2)	0	2 (2.4)	2 (4.2)	1 (4.5)	3 (4.3)	5 (4.5)	0	5 (3.2)	9 (1.7)	8 (1.6)	17 (1.7)
"Have you ever had allergic symptoms from your nose or eyes?" (n = 1306)												
"No" (n = 664, 50.8%)	20 (32.3)	5 (25.0)	25 (30.5)	26 (54.2)	11 (52.4)	37 (53.6)	41 (36.9)	16 (36.4)	57 (36.3)	280 (54.2)	265 (54.9)	545 (54.5)
"Yes" (n = 582, 44.6%)	40 (64.5) **a>**	15 (75.0) **a>**	55 (67.1) **b>**	21 (43.8) **a<**	10 (47.6) **a<**	31 (44.9) **b<**	63 (56.8) **a<**	24 (54.5) **a<**	87 (55.4) **b>**	211 (40.8) **a<**	198 (41.0) **a<**	409 (40.9) **b<**
"I do not know" (n = 60, 4.6%)	2 (3.2)	0	2 (2.4)	1 (2.1)	0	1 (1.5)	7 (6.3)	4 (9.1)	13 (8.3)	26 (5.0)	20 (4.1)	46 (4.6)

Significant differences ($p < 0.05$) between groups, totals and/or genders are **marked with bold letters**. **a**: significant differences within females or within males in different groups. **b**: significant difference between totals. **c**: significant difference between females and males in a group. < or >: the group or the gender has significantly lower or significantly higher frequency than the compared group. Chi-squared test.

Table 2 Comparisons of exogenous factors between the group with a 1-year prevalence of hand eczema in 2008 (Group HX), and the group reporting never having had hand eczema (Group NoHX)

| | Group HX | | | Group NoHX | | |
| | Mean, Median, (Q1 – Q3) | | | Mean, Median, (Q1 – Q3) | | |
	Females	Males	Total	Females	Males	Total
Number of persons in the household, yourself included (n = 1254)	3.0, 3, (2 – 4) **a>**, **c>**	2.5, 2, (2 – 3)	2.8, 3, (2 – 4) **b>**	2.7, 3, (2 – 4) **c>**	2.4, 2, (1 – 3)	2.6, 2, (2 – 4)
Number of children below 4 years of age (n = 1191)	0.8, 1, (0 – 1) **c>**	0.5, 0, (0 – 1)	0.7, 1, (0 – 1)	0.7, 0, (0 – 1) **c>**	0.6, 0, (0 – 1)	0.6, 0, (0 – 1)
Hours a day taking care of children 0 – 4 y (n = 1165)	5.3, 3, (0 – 8) **c>**	1.6, 0, (0 – 3)	4.3, 1, (0 – 6) **b>**	5.1, 0, (0 – 6) **c>**	2.0, 0, (0 – 3)	3.6, 0, (0 – 5)
Hours a day cooking (n = 1245)	1.3, 1, (1 – 1.5) **c>**	1.2, 1, (1 – 1)	1.2, 1, (1 – 1) **b>**	1.3, 1, (1 – 1.5) **c>**	1.0, 1, (0.5 – 1)	1.1, 1, (1 – 1)
Hours a day cleaning/making laundry (n = 1236)	1.3, 1, (1 – 2) **a>**, **c>**	0.7, 1, (0.3 – 1)	1.2, 1, (1 – 1) **b>**	1.1, 1, (1 – 1) **c>**	0.7, 1, (0.2 – 1)	0.9, 1, (0.5 – 1)
Number of times a day washing hands at home (n = 1241)	8.8, 7, (5 – 10) **a>**, **c>**	4.4, 3.5, (3 – 5)	7.6, 6, (4 – 10) **b>**	7.2, 5, (4 – 10) **c>**	4.4, 4, (3 – 5)	5.9, 5, (3 – 7)
Number of times a day washing hands at work (n = 1193)	9.2, 6, (4 – 10) **a>**, **c>**	6.2, 3.5, (3 – 8) **a>**	8.3, 5, (3 – 10) **b>**	7.5, 5, (3 – 10) **c>**	4.5, 3, (2 – 5)	6.0, 4, (3 – 6)
Number of times a day washing hands, at home and at work (n = 1189)	17.4, 13.3, (10–20)**a>**, **c>**	10.6, 8 (5.8 – 14)	15.4, 12, (8 –17.8) **b>**	14.5, 11, (8 – 15) **c>**	8.8, 7 (5 – 10)	11.7, 9, (6 – 14)
If smoking; number of cigarettes a day (n = 112)	9.6, 8, (3.5 – 15)	7.3, 5, (2 – 15)	9.3, 8,(3.3 – 15)	6.5, 5, (2 – 10)	7.6, 5.5, (2 – 11.5)	7.1, 5, (2 – 10)
If using protective gloves at work: hours a day using them (n = 398)	2.8, 2, (1 – 3) **c<**	3.5, 3, (1.5 – 5.5)	2.9, 2, (1 – 4)	2.3, 2, (1 – 3)	3.8, 2, (1 – 6)	3.1, 2, (1 – 4)
Number of working hours at ordinary work (n = 1212)	35.6, 40, (30 – 40) **c<**	41.7, 40, (40 – 45)	37.3, 40, (34 – 40) **b<**	36.7, 40, (34 – 40)	41.9, 40, (40 – 45)	39.2, 40, (38 – 40)
Number of working hours at additional work (n = 107)	4.7, 3, (2 – 7.3)	11.2, 12.5(1.5 –20)	6.1, 3.5, (2 – 8)	10.4, 5, (2 – 12)	9.0, 6, (3 – 10)	9.6, 5, (3 – 10)
Number of working hours at ordinary and additional work (n = 101)	39.8, 41, (30 – 48) **c<**	51.0, 56,(41–59)	42.0, 42.5,(31-51)	44.3, 43 (39 – 50)	50.6, 50, (44 – 55)	47.9, 46, (41 – 53)
Hours a week gardening (during summer season). (n = 1201)	2.3, 1, (0 – 3)	2.5, 1, (0 – 3)	2.4, 1, (0 – 3)	2.5, 1, (0 – 3)	2.7, 1, (0 – 3)	2.6, 1, (0 – 3)
Hours a week repairing cars/engines (n = 1168)	0.2, 0, (0 – 0) **c<**	2.9, 0, (0 – 1)	1.0, 0, (0 – 0)	0.1, 0, (0 – 0)	1.5, 0, (0 – 1)	0.8, 0, (0 – 0)
Hours a week doing building work, restoration (n = 1179)	2.4, 0, (0 – 1) **c<**	3.6, 1, (0 – 3)	2.7, 0, (0 – 2)	2.4, 0, (0 – 1) **c<**	5.1, 1, (0 – 4.75)	3.8, 0, (0 – 2)
Hours a week doing sports/athletics (n = 1184)	4.4, 2, (1 – 4)	3.3, 2, (1 – 4)	4.1, 2, (1 – 4)	4.0, 2, (1 – 5)	4.2, 2, (1 – 4)	4.1, 2, (1 – 4)
Hours a week doing hobbies (n = 979)	4.3, 2, (0 – 5) **c<**	4.6, 2, (0 – 4.5)	4.4, 2, (0 – 5)	3.4, 2, (0 – 4.5)	5.2, 2, (0 – 5)	4.3, 2, (0 – 5)

Significant differences (p < 0.05) between groups, totals and/or genders are **marked with bold letters**. **a**: significant differences within females or within males in different groups, **b**: significant difference between totals, **c**: significant difference between females and males in a group, < or >: the group or the gender has significantly lower or significantly higher frequency than the compared group. Mann-Whitney U test.

Table 3 Comparisons of exogenous factors between the group HX9508, i.e. having had hand eczema 1995 and 2008, the group HX95, i.e. having had 1-year prevalence of hand eczema 1995 and 2008, the group HX08, i.e. having eczema only 2008 and the group NoHX, i.e. the group reporting never having had hand eczema

	HX9508 Mean (Q1-Q3)			HX95 Mean (Q1-Q3)			HX08 Mean (Q1-Q3)			NoHX Mean (Q1-Q3)		
	Females	Males	Total	Females	Males	Total	Females	Males	Total	Females	Males	Total
Number of persons in the household, yourself included (n = 1324)	2.9 (2-4)	2.5 (1-3)	2.8 (2-4)	2.9 (2-4)	2.6 (2-4)	2.8 (2-4)	3.0 (2-4) a>, ◇	2.4 (2-3)	2.9 (2-4) b>	2.7 (2-4) a<, c<	2.4 (1-3)	2.6 (2-4) b<
Number of children below 4 years of age (n = 1259)	0.8 (0-1)	0.7 (0-1)	0.7 (0-1)	0.6 (0-1)	0.5 (0-1)	0.6 (0-1)	0.8 (0-1) a>	0.5 (0-1)	0.7 (0-1)	0.7 (0-1) a<	0.6 (0-1)	0.6 (0-1)
Hours a day taking care of children 0 – 4 years of age (n = 1234)	4.9 (0-8) a<	1.9 (0-3)	4.2 (0-6)	5.8 (0-8) a>	1.0 (0-1.5)	4.3 (0-5)	5.5 (0-8) a>	1.5 (0-2)	4.4 (0-6.3)	5.1 (0-6) a>	2.0 (0-3)	3.6 (0-5)
Hours a day cooking (n = 1314)	1.2 (1-1.3)	1.2 (1-1)	1.2 (1-1)	1.3 (1-2) ◇	0.9 (0.5-1)	1.2 (1-1)	1.3 (1-2) ◇	1.2 (0.8-1)	1.3 (1-1.3) b>	1.3 (1-1.5) ◇	1.0 (0.5-1)	1.1 (1-1) b<
Hours a day cleaning/ making laundry (n = 1304)	1.3 (1-1.6) ◇	0.8 (0.3-1)	1.2 (1-1) b>	1.1 (1-1) ◇	0.7 (0.4-1)	1.0 (1-1)	1.3 (1-2) a>, ◇	0.7 (0.4-1)	1.2 (1-1) b>	1.1 (1-1) a<, ◇	0.7 (0.2-1)	0.9 (0.5-1) b<
Number of times a day washing hands at home (n = 1309)	7.8 (4-10) ◇	3.8 (2-5)	6.8 (3-10)	6.3 (5-8) a<, ◇	5.0 (3-5.3)	5.9 (4-8) b<	9.3 (5-10) a>, ◇	4.7 (3-5)	8.0 (4-10) b>	7.2 (4-10) a<, ◇	4.4 (3-5)	5.9 (3-7) b<
Number of times a day washing hands at work (n = 1260)	8.3 (4-10) ◇	5.2 (2.5-4)	7.4 (3 –10) b>	7.6 (3.5-11) ◇	4.3 (3-4)	6.5 (3-8)	9.7 (4-10) a>, ◇	6.6 (3-10) a>	8.7 (3-10) b>	7.5 (3-10) a> c<	4.5 (2-5) a<	6.0 (3-6) b<
Number of times a day washing hands, at home and at work (n = 1255)	14.9 (9-17) ◇	9.0 (5-11.5)	13.3 (7-16)	14.0 (9-19.5) ◇	9.3 (6.8-10)	12.4 (8-16) b<	18.7 (10-21.5) a>, ◇	11.3 (6-15) a>	16.5 (8-20) b<	14.5 (8-16) a> c<	8.8 (5-10) a>	11.7 (6-14) b<
If smoking, number of cigarettes a day (n = 112)	7.5 (5.8,7.8)	3.5 (2-5)	6.7 (2.9,7.3) b<	8.1 (5-11.8)	1 (1.0)	7.7 (4.5– 10.5)	10.9 (6-15) a>	15 (1.0)	11.1 (7-15) b>	6.5 (2-10) a<	7.6 (2-11.5)	7.1 (2-10) b>
If using protective gloves at work: hours a day using them (n = 398)	2.8 (13-.5)	3.9 (2-5.8)	3.1 (1.5-4.5) b>	1.6 (1-2)	2.4 (0.5-4.5)	1.8 (1 – 2.8) b<	2.8 (1-3)	3.2 (1.5-5.5)	2.9 (1-3.3)	2.3 (1-3) c<	3.8 (1-6)	3.1 (1-4)
Number of working hours at ordinary work (n = 1279)	38.3 (35 – 40.5) a>	41.7 (40-44)	39.2 (38-42) b>	35.5 (32-40) c<	44.7 (40-50)	38.5 (36 – 45)	34.1 (30-40) a<, c<	41.8 (40-45)	36.3 (30-40) b<	36.7 (32-40) a>, c<	41.9 (40-45)	39.2 (38-40) b>
Number of working hours at ordinary and additional work (n = 107)	42.7 (32-49)	57.0 (57.0)	44.1 (33-51.8)	33.5 (29-38)	49.5 (45-54.5)	44.2 (35.8,51.5)	37.7 (29.3,47.3)	49.5 (39-59)	40.7 (30.5,51.8)	44.3 (38.5,49.5) c<	50.6 (44-55)	47.9 (41-53)
Hours a week gardening (n = 1270)	2.1 (0-3)	1.9 (0.3.5)	2.1 (0-3)	3.5 (0-3)	1.4 (0-2)	2.8 (0 – 2.5)	2.4 (0-2.3)	2.8 (0-3)	2.5 (0-2.5)	2.5 (0-3)	2.7 (0-3)	2.6 (0-3)
Hours a week repairing cars/engines (n = 1236)	0.2 (0-0)<	3.6 (0-1)	1.0 (0 -0)	0.1 (0-0) c<	0.5 (0-1)	0.2 (0-0)	0.3 (0-0) c<	2.6 (0-1)	1.0 (0-0)	0.1 (0-0) c<	1.5 (0-1)	0.8 (0-0)
Hours a week doing building work, restoration (n = 1245)	1.7 (0-2) c<	4.2 (0.6-5)	2.3 (0-2)	1.1 (0-1.5)	3.1 (0-3.5)	1.7 (0-2)	2.8 (0-1)	3.3 (0-2)	2.9 (0-1.5)	2.4 (0-1) c<	5.1 (0-4.8)	3.8 (0-2)
Hours a week doing sports (n = 1251)	4.2 (1-4)	2.7 (1-3.7)	3.8 (1-4)	2.5 (1-4)	2.7 (1-3.3)	2.6 (1-4)	4.5 (1-4.8)	3.6 (0.5-4)	4.2 (1-4)	4.0 (1-5)	4.2 (1-4)	4.1 (1-4)
Hours a week doing hobbies (n = 1035)	4.7 (2-5)	3.4 (0-6)	4.4 (2-5)	3.2 (0-4.8)	1.8 (0-3)	2.7 (0-4)	4.0 (0-4)	5.0 (0-4)	4.3 (0-4)	3.4 (0-4.5) c<	5.2 (0-5)	4.3 (0-5)

Significant differences (p < 0.05) between groups, totals and/or genders are **marked with bold letters**. **a**: significant differences within females or within males in different groups; **b**: significant difference between totals, **c**: significant difference between females and males in a group, < or >: the group or the gender has significantly lower or significantly higher frequency than the compared group/groups. Kruskal-Wallis Test and Mann-Whitney U test.

NoHX group. The HX08 group smoked significantly more cigarettes than those in the HX9508 and NoHX groups (p = 0.023 and 0.012 respectively).

Among the respondents 487/1323 (36.8%) used moisturisers daily. The HX9508 group used moisturisers significantly more than the other groups, 71.1%, followed by the HX08 group, 54.8%, the HX95group, 45.7% and the NoHX group, 30.6%, (p < 0.001). Among females 52.7% (n = 746), used moisturisers every day; 79% in the HX9508 group, 61.3% in the HX08 group, 56.2% in the HX95 group and 47.4% in the NoHX group (p < 0.001). Among males 16.3% used moisturisers daily: 47.6% in the HX9508 group, 38.6% in the HX08 group, 22.7% in the HX95 group and 12.7% in the NoHX group (p < 0.001). Males *with* hand eczema used moisturisers as often as women *without* hand eczema.

Factors predicting hand eczema

The analysis of endogenous and exogenous factors was performed with multinominal logistic regression. The results are shown in Table 4. Having had childhood eczema was the most significant predictor for 1-year prevalence of hand eczema 2008 with odds ratios of 13.17 in the group HX9508 and 5.17 in the group HX08 compared to the group NoHX. The frequency of daily hand washing was significantly associated with the 1-year prevalence of hand eczema only in the HX08 group. The daily usage of moisturisers was significantly associated with 1-year prevalence of hand eczema in the groups HX9508 and HX08. High odds ratios, 1.40, for predicting 1-year prevalence of hand eczema was found for female gender in the group HX9508. In the group HX08 the higher odds ratio for females was 1.19. However, none of these differences were significant.

Discussion

In this study comprising 1,516 young adults, the 1-year prevalence of hand eczema was more than 15%. One third of these individuals also had 1-year prevalence at the baseline 1995. The 1-year prevalence, and not the point prevalence, was used in all calculations because it better reflects the persistency, the relapsing course and the seasonal variations of the disease [2,19]. The increase in the one-year prevalence between the two occasions is in accordance with previous large Swedish cross-sectional studies with respect to the age groups [3-5,22].

The estimated incidence of hand eczema in our study was 11.6 cases per 1000 person-years, 14.3 among females and 5.2 among males. Our figures are in the upper amplitude compared to an earlier population based study from Sweden, which showed between 11.4 and 3.7 cases/1000 person-years among 20–29 year-old females and males, respectively [23]. One explanation could be that our study is prospective, and underreporting is to

be expected in retrospective questionnaire studies [24]. Based on 7 European hand eczema studies performed among 16–77 years-olds, the median incidence rate of hand eczema was 9.6 cases/1000 person-years (range 4.6–11.4) among women and 4.0 cases/1000 person-years (range 1.4–7.4) among men [1], which is also slightly lower than our current findings, probably due to age-differences. To the best of our knowledge there are no comparable studies of the cumulative incidence in this age group. The cumulative incidence of hand eczema in our study across 13 years was 15.1% (18.6% for females and 10.7% for males). This can be considered to be a high proportion [15]. When using a questionnaire for estimating the true occurrence of a disease it is important to know the sensitivity and specificity of the question used. The question on 1-year prevalence of hand eczema underestimates the occurrence. [25]. However, regarding childhood eczema the occurrence has been found to be overestimated especially if the true prevalence is low [5,19]. Based on prevalence as well as incidence, the occurrence of hand eczema is approximately twice as common among females compared to men, which is similar to other population-based studies [1,26,27].

The advantage of a longitudinal cohort study compared with a cross-sectional study is that it enables the estimation of both cumulative incidence and incidence rate. Another advantage of performing a follow-up study is the possibility to compare the development of hand eczema over time in relation to different risk factors.

The four groups (HX9508, HX95, HX08 and NoHX) were used to investigate the relationship between childhood eczema and the incidence of hand eczema. The assumption was that a smaller proportion of individuals who had hand eczema in 2008 but not in 1995 reported childhood eczema. However, there were no significant differences between the three hand eczema groups concerning childhood eczema. Furthermore, it was found that a higher proportion of individuals who had hand eczema at both occasions reported childhood eczema.

Thus, in this cohort childhood eczema was the most important predicting factor regardless of the debut of hand eczema. In 2008, around 30% of our sample reported childhood eczema (females 36%, males 20%). In a large population-based Swedish study performed from 2002–2003, among 21–30 years-olds, childhood eczema was reported by 30.1% of females and 20.8% of males, [4,28,29]. The corresponding figures in the 31–40 year-olds were 21.8% and 16.2% [30]. Thus, in our study, the prevalence of childhood eczema was higher. Similar to other studies, the relationship between having had hand eczema and reporting childhood eczema was highly significant [31]. The agreement in self-reports of childhood eczema at the two occasions was high. This high reliability over time in

Table 4 Endogenous and exogenous factors associated with hand eczema analysed with logistic multinominal regression method, Group NoHX: never having had hand eczema, Group HX9508: having hand eczema 1995 as well as 2008, Group HX95: having had hand eczema only 1995 and Group HX08: having hand eczema only 2008

Group	Group HX9508 vs Group NoHX (N = 852)		Group HX95 vs Group NoHX (N = 836)		Group HX08 vs Group NoHX (N = 895)	
	Odds-ratio	95% CI for OR (p-value)	Odds-ratio	95% CI for OR (p-value)	Odds-ratio	95% CI for OR (p-value)
Having had childhood eczema	**13.17**	**6.74 – 25.72 (<0.001)**	**4.12**	**2.31 – 7.33 (<0.001)**	**5.17**	**3.33 – 8.03 (<0.001)**
Having had asthma	1.89	0.99 – 3.62 (0.54)	0.81	0.34 – 1.89 (0.619)	1.12	0.64 – 1.94 (0.699)
Having had rhino-conjunctivitis	1.64	0.86 – 3.10 (0.132)	0.98	0.53 – 1.81 (0.945)	1.51	0.95 – 2.40 (0.084)
Female gender	1.40	0.71 – 2.75 (0.334)	1.42	0.73 – 2.79 (0.304)	1.19	0.72 – 1.97 (0.500)
Number of times a day washing hands, at home and at work	0.99	0.97 – 1.02 (0.696)	1.00	0.97 – 1.03 (0.858)	**1.02**	**1.01 – 1.04 (0.038)**
Usage of moisturisers: daily vs less than daily	**5.17**	**2.82 – 9.51 (<0.001)**	1.49	0.81 – 2.73 (0.199)	**2.11**	**1.34 – 3.30 (0.001)**
Cooking:hours a day	1.00	0.69 – 1.43 (0.987)	1.00	0.66 – 1.51 (0.997)	1.10	0.87 – 1.37 (0.433)
Washing and cleaning: hours a day	1.19	0.81 – 1.77 (0.377)	0.81	0.48 – 1.39 (0.446)	1.23	0.94 – 1.60 (0.126)
Taking care of children < 4 years old: hours a day	1.01	0.97 – 1.06 (0.616)	1.02	0.98 – 1.07 (0.321)	0.99	0.96 – 1.03 (0.707)

Odds-ratios (OR) in predicting 1-year prevalence of hand eczema 2008 compared to the group NoHX, group HX9508 compared to group NoHX and group HX08 compared to group NoHX. Confidence intervals (CI), 95%, and p-values are given for all variables. **Significant OR, CI and p-values are in bold text.**

this age-group can be useful to know when hand eczema is diagnosed. However, the lower rate of reported childhood eczema in 2008 can be explained by recall bias as was found in a study comprising respondents aged 31 to 42 years [32]. For the individuals who reported only rhino-conjunctivitis, there was no significant association with one-year prevalence of hand eczema. Also, there was no association with asthma only, but there were very few respondents. Thus in our study no additional information concerning risk for hand eczema was obtained by asking about asthma or rhino-conjunctivitis. These results are in accordance with Meding et al. who showed that asthma and rhino-conjuntivitis in adults were only associated with hand eczema at an age below 30 years [23]; in another study, including adolescents, a marginally significant association with inhalant allergy was found [33].

Analyses of exogenous factors showed that the individuals with hand eczema only in 2008, reported a significantly higher frequency of hand washing compared to the individuals without hand eczema.

Females with hand eczema spent significantly more time doing household activities than men with hand eczema (Table 3). Hand washing was more frequent among females with hand eczema than females without hand eczema as well as compared with men with hand eczema. In the multinominal regression analyses hand washing in the group HX08 was the only significant exogenous risk factor associated with hand eczema. In the majority of hand eczema studies hand washing is found to be the most significant risk factor for developing hand eczema [34]. In our cohort, other exogenous risk factors such as cooking, washing and cleaning and taking care of young children did not have any significant association with hand eczema. Furthermore, female gender was not a significant risk factor. However, it is well known that females have hand eczema more often than men. This can be explained by the high exposure to water and other skin irritants. Experimental as well as epidemiological studies [14,35] have demonstrated that female skin is not more sensitive to irritants than male skin [35] which is in line with our findings.

An interesting finding was the high odds-ratio in daily use of moisturisers in the two groups with current 1-year prevalence of hand eczema (HX9508 and HX08). This pattern was not seen in the group having had hand eczema in 1995 (HX95).

When self-administrated questionnaires are used, it is important for the results to be adjusted based on sensitivity and specificity of validated questions. This is especially important in diseases that are common and affect the general health and well-being of individuals, such as hand eczema. The development of specific instruments like questionnaires implicates problems. In this case the questions regarding childhood and hand eczema were not validated in 1995 but 2,535 of the 2,572 pupils

(98.6%) were clinically examined, and the sensitivity of 73% and the specificity of 99% were found [15]. The question regarding the 1-year prevalence of hand eczema, which was used in the present study and in the first study, was previously validated [19]. Thus, the true one-year prevalence of hand eczema can be estimated from our data and is 20.6% for all; 26.8% among females and 12.5% among males.

The answers to the open questions on occupation as well as work tasks gave no further information regarding risk factors for developing or maintaining hand eczema. This circumstance seems to be a common problem in questionnaire studies [3]. In a study regarding occupational exposure to water as a risk factor for hand eczema, it was found that the title of an occupation gave misclassified results; exposure time and frequency of water use were more appropriate measures [36]. For result validity, it is important to have high response rates in general population studies [37-39]. The response rate in this study was almost two thirds of the individuals who received a questionnaire in the mail. Females were significantly more willing to participate than the males. There were, however, no significant differences within the female or the male groups regarding having had 1-year prevalence of hand eczema at the two occasions. The response rate was similar to the annual national public health questionnaire performed by Swedish National Institute of Public Health [40].

Conclusions

This study demonstrated that incidence of hand eczema in early adulthood tends to be associated with factors in everyday life such as frequent hand-washing. Regarding childhood eczema, the odds ratio for having hand eczema was twice as high in the HX9508 group compared to the group HX08, indicating a high vulnerability in this group. Furthermore, early onset of hand eczema seemed to be related to endogenous risk factors such as a history of childhood eczema. The higher frequency of hand eczema among women depended on exogenous factors.

Competing interests
The authors declare that they have no competing interests.

Authors' contributions
The authors together designed the study, analysed the data and wrote the manuscript. All authors read and approved the final manuscript.

Acknowledgments
This study was supported by grants from the Swedish Asthma and Allergy Research Foundation and the Finsen-Welander Foundation. We will also

express our gratitude to Steven Schmidt for valuable comments and for revising the English text.

Author details
[1]Department of Health Sciences, Lund University, Box 157, 221 00 Lund, Sweden. [2]Department of Occupational and Environmental Dermatology, Lund University, Malmö, Sweden. [3]Department of Occupational and Environmental Dermatology, Malmö University Hospital, Malmö, Sweden. [4]Department of Dermatology, Lund University, Malmö, Sweden. [5]Department of Dermatology, Malmö University Hospital, Malmö, Sweden.

References

1. Thyssen JP, Johansen JD, Linneberg A, Menné T: The epidemiology of hand eczema in the general population – prevalence and main findings. *Contact Dermatitis* 2010, **62**:75–87.
2. Meding B: Epidemiology of hand eczema in an industrial city. *Acta Derm Venereol* 1990, **153**(Suppl):1–43.
3. Montnemery P, Nihlen U, Lofdahl CG, Nyberg P, Svensson A: Prevalence of hand eczema in an adult Swedish population and the relationship to risk occupation and smoking. *Acta Derm Venereol* 2005, **85**:429–432.
4. Meding B, Jarvholm B: Hand eczema in Swedish adults – changes in prevalence between 1983 and 1996. *J Invest Dermatol* 2002, **118**:719–723.
5. Stenberg B, Meding B, Svensson A: Dermatology in public health - a model for surveillance of common skin diseases. *Scandinavian J Public Health* 2010, **38**:368–374.
6. Bingefors K, Lindberg M, Isacson D: Quality of life, use of topical medications and socio-economic data in hand eczema: a Swedish nationwide survey. *Acta Derm Venereol* 2011, **91**:452–458.
7. Flyvholm M, Bach B, Rose M, Frydendall Jepsen K: Self-reported hand eczema in a hospital population. *Contact Dermatitis* 2007, **57**:110–115.
8. Van der Meer EW, Boot CR, Jungbauer FH, van der Klink JJ, Rustemeyer T, Coenraads PJ, van der Gulden JW, Anema JR: Hands4U: a multifaceted strategy to implement guideline-based recommendations to prevent hand eczema in health care workers: design of a randomised control trial and (cost) effectiveness evaluation. *BMC Public Health* 2011, **11**:669.
9. Augustin M: Versorgungsforschung in der Dermatologie. *Hautarzt* 2011, **62**:168–169.
10. Meding B, Wrangsjö K, Järvholm B: Fifteen-year follow-up of hand eczema: persistence and consequences. *Br J Dermatol* 2005, **152**:975–980.
11. Moberg C, Alderling M, Meding B: Hand eczema and quality of life: a population-based study. *Br J Dermatol* 2009, **161**:397–403.
12. Dickel H, Kuss O, Schmidt A, Kretz J, Diepgen TL: Importance of irritant contact dermatitis in occupational skin disease. *Am J Clin Dermatol* 2002, **3**:283–289.
13. Nielsen NH, Linneberg A, Menne T, Madsen F, Frolund L, Dirksen A, Jorgensen T: The association between contact allergy and hand eczema in 2 cross-sectional surveys 8 years apart. The Copenhagen allergy study. *Contact Dermatitis* 2002, **47**:71–77.
14. Bryld LE, Hindsberger C, Kyvik KO, Agner T, Menne T: Risk factors influencing the development of hand eczema in a population-based twin sample. *Br J Dermatol* 2003, **149**:1214–1220.
15. Yngveson M, Svensson A, Isacsson A: Evaluation of a selfreported questionnaire on hand dermatosis in secondary school children. *Acta Derm Venereol* 1997, **77**:455–457.
16. Yngveson M, Svensson A, Isacsson A: Prevalence of self-reported hand dermatosis in upper secondary school pupils. *Acta Derm Venereol* 1998, **78**:371–4.
17. Susitaival P, Kanerva L, Hannuksela M, Jolanki R, Estlander T: *Touhilampi Questionnaire for Epidemiological Studies of Contact Dermatitis and Atopy*, People and Work. Research Report 10. Helsinki: Finnish Institute of Occupational Health; 1996.
18. Susitaival P, Flyvholm MA, Meding B, Kanerva L, Lindberg M, Svensson A, Olufsson JH: Nordic occupational skin questionnaire (NOSQ-2002): a new tool for surveying occupational skin diseases and exposure. *Contact Dermatitis* 2003, **49**:70–76.
19. Meding B, Barregård L: Validity of self-reports of hand eczema. *Contact Dermatitis* 2001, **45**:99–103.
20. Anveden I, Lidén C, Alderling M, Meding B: Self-reported skin exposure – validation of questions by observation. *Contact Dermatitis* 2006, **55**:186–91.
21. Ahlbom A, Norell S: *Introduction to Modern Epidemiology*. Chestnut Hill: Epidemiology Resources Inc.; 1990:25–6.
22. Meding B, Lidén C, Berglind N: Self-diagnosed dermatitis in adults. Results from a population survey in Stockholm. *Contact Dermatitis* 2001, **45**:341–345.
23. Meding B, Järvholm B: Incidence of hand eczema-a population-based retrospective study. *J Invest Dermatol* 2004, **122**:873–877.
24. Bregnhøj A, Søsted H, Menné T, Johansen Duus J: Validation of self-reporting of hand eczema among Danish hairdressing apprentices. *Contact Dermatitis* 2011, **65**:146–150.
25. Stenberg B, Lindberg M, Meding B, Svensson Å: Is the question "Have you had childhood eczema?" useful for assessing childhood atopic eczema in adult population surveys? *Contact Dermatitis* 2006, **54**:334–337.
26. Yngveson M, Svensson A, Johannisson A, Isacsson A: Hand dermatosis in upper secondary school pupils: 2-year comparison and follow-up. *Br J Dermatol* 2000, **142**:485–489.
27. Meding B: Differences between the sexes with regard to work-related skin disease. *Contact Dermatitis* 2000, **43**:65.
28. Rystedt I: Hand eczema and long-term prognosis in atopic dermatitis. *Acta Derm Venereol* 1985, **117**:1–59.
29. Nilsson E: Individual and environmental risk factors for hand eczema in hospital workers. *Acta Derm Venereol* 1986, **128**(Suppl):1–63.
30. Röhrl K, Stenberg B: Lifestyle factors and hand eczema in a Swedish adolescent population. *Contact Dermatitis* 2010, **62**:170–176.
31. Nyrén M, Lindberg M, Stenberg B, Svensson M, Svensson Å, Meding B: Influence of childhood atopic dermatitis on future worklife. *Scand J Work Environ Health* 2005, **31**:474–478.
32. Moberg C, Meding B, Stenberg B, Svensson A, Lindberg M: Remembering childhood atopic dermatitis as an adult: factors that influence recollection. *Br J Dermatol* 2006, **155**:557–560.
33. Mortz CG, Lauritsen JM, Bindslev-Jensen C, Andersen KE: Prevalence of atopic dermatitis, asthma, allergic rhinitis, and hand and contact dermatitis in adolescents. The Odense adolescence cohort study on atopic diseases and dermatitis. *Br J Dermatol* 2001, **144**:523–532.
34. Anveden I, Wrangsjö K, Järvholm B, Meding B: Self-reported skin exposure – a population-based study. *Contact Dermatitis* 2006, **54**:272–277.
35. Agner T: Noninvasive measuring methods for the investigation of irritant patch test reactions; a study of patients with hand eczema, atopic dermatitis and controls. *Acta Derm Venereol* 1992, **173**(Suppl):1–26.
36. Anveden Berglind I, Alderling M, Järvholm B, Lidén C, Meding B: Occupational skin exposure to water: a population-based study. *Br J Dermatol* 2009, **160**:616–621.
37. Edwards PJ, Roberts I, Clarke MJ, DiGuiseppi C, Wentz R, Kwan I, Cooper R, Felix LM, Pratap S: Methods to increase response to postal and electronic questionnaires (Review). *Cochrane Database Syst Rev* 2009(3):MR000008. doi:10.1002/14651858.MR000008.pub4.
38. Data quality for the 2006 survey of labour and income dynamics (SLID). http://www.statcan.gc.ca/pub/75f0002m/2008005/section5-eng.htm.
39. Tolonen H, Helakorpi S, Talala K, Helasoja V, Martelin T, Prättälä R: 25-year trends and socio-demographic differences in response rates: Finnish adult health behaviour survey. *Eur J Epidemiol* 2006, **21**:409–415.
40. Swedish National Institute of Public Health: http://www.fhi.se/Documents/Statistik-uppfoljning/Folkhalsoenkaten/vad_betyder_bortfallet100330.pdf.

11

High glycemic load diet, milk and ice cream consumption are related to acne vulgaris in Malaysian young adults: a case control study

Noor Hasnani Ismail[1], Zahara Abdul Manaf[1*] and Noor Zalmy Azizan[2]

Abstract

Background: The role of dietary factors in the pathophysiology of acne vulgaris is highly controversial. Hence, the aim of this study was to determine the association between dietary factors and acne vulgaris among Malaysian young adults.

Methods: A case–control study was conducted among 44 acne vulgaris patients and 44 controls aged 18 to 30 years from October 2010 to January 2011. Comprehensive acne severity scale (CASS) was used to determine acne severity. A questionnaire comprising items enquiring into the respondent's family history and dietary patterns was distributed. Subjects were asked to record their food intake on two weekdays and one day on a weekend in a three day food diary. Anthropometric measurements including body weight, height and body fat percentage were taken. Acne severity was assessed by a dermatologist.

Results: Cases had a significantly higher dietary glycemic load (175 ± 35) compared to controls (122 ± 28) ($p < 0.001$). The frequency of milk ($p < 0.01$) and ice-cream ($p < 0.01$) consumptions was significantly higher in cases compared to controls. Females in the case group had a higher daily energy intake compared to their counterparts in the control group, 1812 ± 331 and 1590 ± 148 kcal respectively ($p < 0.05$). No significant difference was found in other nutrient intakes, Body Mass Index, and body fat percentage between case and control groups ($p > 0.05$).

Conclusions: Glycemic load diet and frequencies of milk and ice cream intake were positively associated with acne vulgaris.

Keywords: Acne vulgaris, Diet, Glycemic index, Young adults, Dairy products

Background

Acne vulgaris affects up to 85% of adolescent population in the United Kingdom [1]. In Malaysia, the prevalence of facial acne vulgaris among teenagers was 67.5% [2]. The condition was more common among males (71.1%) compared to females (64.6%). Previous studies enquiring into the potential link between diet and acne vulgaris have shown controversial results. Historically, milk was found to be positively associated with acne flares [3] while in 1969, a study reported that there was no association between chocolate and acne vulgaris [4]. However, the crossover study by Fulton et al. [4] was methodologically flawed by comparing chocolate and sweet vegetable oil bars that had the same glycemic index (GI). In addition, the placebo bars had higher content of partially hydrogenated vegetable fat, which may contribute to inflammation due to the trans-fatty acids [5]. This is because, in prostaglandins production, competition between trans and essential fatty acids may lead to inflammation [6]. Later, in the early 70's, a cross sectional study reported that foods such as chocolate, milk, roasted peanuts or cola have no influence on acne vulgaris conditions [7].

Recently, there has been an increasing number of studies investigating the role of diet as one of the underlying causes of acne vulgaris. Several studies on the effects of ingesting certain dairy products [8-10], carbohydrates, glycemic index (GI) and high glycemic load (GL) diet [11-13] in exacerbating acne vulgaris have

* Correspondence: zaharamanaf@yahoo.com
[1]Dietetic Program, School of Healthcare Sciences, Faculty of Health Sciences, Universiti Kebangsaan Malaysia, Jalan Raja Muda Abdul Aziz, 50300 Kuala Lumpur, Malaysia
Full list of author information is available at the end of the article

been carried out to support the hypothesis that what is eaten may affect the skin. However, the findings of these studies are inconsistent. Retrospective and prospective epidemiological studies reported by Adebamowo et al. [8-10] in the United States of America are the first to provide direct clinical evidence on the association between milk/dairy consumption and acne.

Knowledge on how diet and acne vulgaris is related enables the identification and management of the condition and community education in preventing and improving the acne condition, besides the primary systemic and topical treatment. Therefore, this study was conducted to determine the relationship between dietary variables and acne vulgaris among young adults. Based on previous studies, we hypothesized that high glycemic load diet, milk and dairy products intake, Body Mass Index (BMI) as well as body fat percentage may be the risk factors of acne vulgaris.

Methods

Study design

This study was designed as a case–control study. Based on the formula [14], it was calculated that 35 subjects were required to provide 80% power at a significant level of 5%. Standard deviation and magnitude difference was obtained from a previous study on acne patients [11]. After an estimation of 20% drop outs, 44 acne vulgaris patients were recruited as participants in the case group and 44 participants as the control group. Ethical approval was obtained from the Universiti Kebangsaan Malaysia Research Ethics Committee and permission to conduct this study was granted by the Director of Hospital Kuala Lumpur. All participants were given an information sheet about the study and written informed consent was obtained from each respondent.

Study population

From October 2010 to January 2011, 44 people attending a tertiary hospital Dermatology Clinic in Kuala Lumpur for acne vulgaris treatment were enrolled as participants in the case group. The 44 controls were healthy individuals without acne vulgaris recruited among students and staff members of Universiti Kebangsaan Malaysia Kuala Lumpur Campus. Both the case and control groups were recruited through a convenience sampling method, and then matched by age, gender and ethnicity. People with acne vulgaris aged between 18 to 30 years and referred to dermatologists were included in this study. Patients with chronic diseases such as Systemic Lupus Erythematosus (SLE), diabetic mellitus and heart disease were excluded. Control group participants scored 0 (clear) or 1 (almost clear) for acne severity on the Comprehensive acne severity scale (CASS) [15] as assessed by a qualified dermatologist.

Measurements

Anthropometric measurements that included body weight, height and body fat percentage were conducted. Body weight was measured using a TANITA digital scale HD-306 (TANITA Corporation, Japan) and height using a SECA 208 body meter (SECA, German) to the nearest 0.1 kg and 0.1 cm respectively. During body weight measurement, participants were required to wear minimal clothing and stand on the centre of the scales with the weight distributed evenly on both feet. Height measurement was performed using the stretch stature method. Participants were asked to stand with the feet together and the heels, buttocks and upper part of the back touching the scale and the head positioned in the Frankfort's plane. BMI was calculated by dividing the weight (kg) over the square of height (m) and classified according to WHO 2004 classification [16]. Body fat percentage was measured using an Omron Karada Scan Fat Body Analyzer Scale HBF-356 (Omron, Japan).

Questionnaires

Data related to respondent's family history, perceptions and beliefs on food that affect acne vulgaris occurrence were obtained using a validated questionnaire with Cronbach-α value of 0.684. Meanwhile, the frequency of milk and dairy products intake were collected through face-to-face interviews using an adapted structured, validated questionnaire [17]. Dietary pattern was assessed using a three day food diary. Participants were asked to record their food intake on two weekdays and one day on a weekend. The three day food diary was attached together with a stamped envelope addressed to the researcher and participants were requested to return the diet record within a period of two weeks. Participants were contacted through phone calls and emails to clarify the information.

Diet analysis

Daily dietary GL were calculated from the three day food diaries as $\sum$(GI for food item x its carbohydrate content in grams (g)/100). The GI values were taken from the International Table of Glycemic Index and the Glycemic Load Values [18], International Table of Glycemic Index and the Glycemic Load Values: 2008 [19] and Table of Glycemic Index Value of Selected Malaysian Foods [20]. The GI was estimated by using similar food of known value, if the GI of a food type from Malaysia was not available. Nutrient intakes were calculated using Nutritionist Pro™ 2003 software. The Malaysian Food Composition Table (FCT) [21] was used as the nutrient database. However, since the Malaysian FCT did not contain values for vitamin E and selenium, the United States Department of Agriculture (USDA) A National Nutrient Database for Standard [22] and the Food and

Nutrient Database for Dietary Studies were used to estimate the intake of these nutrients.

Statistical analysis

Statistical analyses were conducted using the Statistical Package for the Social Sciences (SPSS) version 19.0. Shapiro-Wilk test was used to test data normality. Descriptive analysis was done in order to elicit the percentage, mean and standard deviation (SD) for quantitative data. Chi-Square test was used to compare milk and dairy products intake between the two groups. Continuous quantitative variables such as anthropometric measurements, glycemic load as well as dietary intake were compared by using unpaired t-test. Binary Logistic Regression was used to calculate adjusted odd ratio with the inclusion of confounding factors such as family history, frequency of milk and the intake of dairy products.

Results

Demographic data

A total of 94 subjects initially agreed to participate in this study; however 6 subjects were excluded as they did not return their three day diet records. Therefore, 88 subjects, comprising 44 cases and 44 controls aged 18 to 30 years were included in the final analysis of this study. The case group consisted of 29 females (69.5%) and 15 males (34.1%) (Table 1). The subjects included Malays (79.5%) and non-Malays (20.5%) for both groups. Both the case and control groups were mostly single or divorced (86.4%). Significantly more subjects in the control group (95.5%) obtained their education at the tertiary level compared to the case group (68.2%) (p < 0.05). In the case group, 56.8% were employed while 43.2% of them were students. In the control group, the majority (63.6%) were students, and the rest were employed (36.4%).

Family history of acne vulgaris

More case group participants were found to have a family history of acne vulgaris compared to controls, $\chi2$ (1, N = 88) = 20.566 (p < 0.001). Among the cases, 81.8% reported that they had a close relative, such as parents or siblings with acne vulgaris whereas the majority of control group participants had no family history of the disease (Table 1).

Anthropometric measurements

No statistically significant difference (p > 0.05) was found between the case and control groups in body weight, height and BMI for both sexes with the exception of body fat percentage in male participants (Table 2). Male in the case group had a higher body fat percentage (18.2 ± 5.0%) compared to the males in the control group (16.6 ± 5.6%) (p < 0.05).

Table 1 Sociodemographic profile and family history of case and control groups

Parameter	Cases (n = 44)		Controls (n = 44)		P value
	n	(%)	n	(%)	
Gender					
Male	15	(34.1)	15	(34.1)	1.000
Female	29	(65.9)	29	(65.9)	
Ethnicity					
Malay	35	(79.5)	35	(79.5)	1.000
Non Malay	9	(20.5)	9	(20.5)	
Marital status					
Single/Divorced	38	(86.4)	38	(86.4)	1.000
Married	6	(13.6)	6	(13.6)	
Educational level					
Upper Secondary School	14	(31.8)	2	(4.5)	0.002**
Pre-University/Higher education institute	30	(68.2)	42	(95.5)	
Occupation					
Students	19	(43.2)	28	(63.6)	0.054
Employed	25	(56.8)	16	(36.4)	
Income status (monthly), RM (USD)					
≤ RM 2000 (USD6666)	37	(84.1)	40	(90.9)	0.334
> RM 2000 (USD6666)	7	(15.9)	4	(9.1)	
Family history of acne vulgaris					
Yes	36	(81.8)	15	(34.1)	<0.001***
No	8	(18.2)	29	(65.9)	

Chi-Square test.

Glycemic load and dietary intake

Overall, the case group had a higher glycemic load (175 ± 35) than the controls (122 ± 28) (p < 0.001) (Table 3). Based on multivariate analysis and taking into account BMI and gender, glycemic load of diet was significantly associated with acne vulgaris occurrence (F(1,86) = 59.412, p < 0.001).

Female acne vulgaris patients had a higher mean of daily energy intake (1812 ± 331) compared to their counterparts in the control group (1590 ± 148 kcal) (p < 0.05) (Table 4). However, no significant differences were found in other nutrients intake between the case and control groups (p > 0.05).

There were no significant differences between case and control participants in energy intake, carbohydrates, fat, protein, vitamin A, vitamin E, fiber, zinc and selenium at the 25th, 50th and 75th percentile (Table 5). Conversely, there was a significant difference in glycemic load at the 50th and 75th percentiles between cases and controls (p < 0.05). At the 75th percentile, glycemic load value of more than 175 increased the risk of occurrence of acne vulgaris by 21 fold. In addition, there was an

Table 2 Comparison of mean (±SD) of body weight, height, BMI and body fat percentage between case and control groups according to gender

	Male (n = 30)			Female (n = 58)		
	Cases (n = 15)	Controls (n = 15)	p value	Cases (n = 29)	Controls (n = 29)	p value
	Mean ± SD	Mean ± SD		Mean ± SD	Mean ± SD	
Body weight (kg)	61.7 ± 13.2	64.4 ± 10.0	0.15	61.7 ± 18.3	55.9 ±11.1	0.53
Height (cm)	169.0 ± 8.1	173.9 ± 6.5	0.48	157.9 ± 5.4	156.9 ± 5.0	0.08
BMI(kg/m^2)	21.8 ± 4.5	21.3 ± 3.1	0.19	24.8 ± 7.2	22.7 ± 4.1	0.72
Body fat (%)	18.2 ± 5.0*	16.6 ± 5.6	0.03	31.2 ± 6.9	29.6 ± 4.7	0.42

* Significant difference using Independent t-test ($p < 0.05$).

increase of OR with an increase in the percentile of the dietary glycemic load (25th percentile, OR = 0.05; 50th percentile, OR = 15.75; 75th percentile, OR = 21.00). This showed that the higher the glycemic load, the higher was the risk of acne vulgaris occurrence.

However, after adjusting for confounding variables including family history of acne vulgaris as well as frequency of milk and ice cream consumption using the binary logistic regression analysis, we found that the risk of acne vulgaris remains statistically significant only for the glycemic load value of ≥ 175 with increased odds of having acne vulgaris 25 times higher (Table 6).

Milk and dairy products, chocolates and nuts intake
Higher frequency of milk and ice cream intake were positively associated with acne vulgaris occurrence (Table 7). Consumption of milk ≥ once a week increased the risk of acne vulgaris occurrence by 4 times (OR = 3.99, 95% CI = 1.39 - 11.43). Consumption of ice cream ≥ once a week also increased the risk of having acne by 4 times compared to those who did not take ice cream (OR = 4.47, 95% CI = 2.44 - 19.72). The majority of cases (86.4%) drank milk more frequently (≥once a week) compared to 61.4% of the control subjects (p < 0.01). In addition, more cases (56.8%) also consumed a higher frequency of ice cream, (≥once a week) than their counterparts in the control group (22.7%) (p < 0.01). However, no significant differences were found in terms of frequencies of yoghurt, cheese, chocolate and nuts intake (p > 0.05).

Discussion
This study suggested that glycemic load has a significant positive relationship with acne vulgaris occurrence after considering factors like BMI and gender. The risk of

Table 3 Dietary glycemic load comparisons between case and control groups

	Case (n = 44)	Control (n = 44)
	Mean ± SD	Mean ± SD
Glycemic load (GL)	175 ± 35***	122 ± 28

***Significant difference using Independent t-test, ($p < 0.001$).

acne vulgaris decreased with the decreasing percentile of glycemic load, with a significant association noted at the 50th and 75th percentile. The association remained significant after adjustment for other confounding factors. Among the western population, high glycemic load diet was reported as a significant contributor to high acne vulgaris prevalence [23]. The result of this study provides further support to a randomized controlled trial study among male acne patients aged between 15 – 25 years which demonstrated that low glycemic load diet was effective in improving acne vulgaris symptoms [12]. Another study found improvements in biochemical parameters associated with acne vulgaris due to a high-protein, low glycemic-load diet intervention [24]. A study also reported that a low glycemic load diet known as the South Beach Diet was effective to ameliorate the acne conditions of 86.7% of 2995 acne vulgaris respondents in a three months period and reduced the use of conventional systemic as well as topical treatments [25]. In contrast to our study, these studies [12,24,25] found that the effect of the low glycemic load diet was lost when the data was statistically adjusted for changes in BMI.

The underlying mechanism of dietary effect on acne vulgaris formation might be the role of insulin-like growth factor-1 (IGF-1) in facilitating cell proliferation involved in acne vulgaris pathogenesis [26]. Acute hyperinsulinemia due to consumption of high glycemic load diet would cause an increase in IGF-1/insulin-like growth factor binding protein-3 (IGFBP-3) ratio, thus enhancing the effects of IGF-1 [23]. Hyperinsulinemia resulting from high glycemic load diet would also increase circulating androgens and decrease sex hormone binding protein, leading to increased sebum synthesis, which was crucial in acne development.

This study found that frequency of milk and ice cream intake was positively associated with acne vulgaris occurrence. The result is in accordance to a cross-sectional study in South Korea which reported that milk and dairy products intake was associated with acne vulgaris development [27]. They reported that the intake of milk and dairy products was higher among acne vulgaris subjects

Table 4 Gender based comparison of mean (±SD) of energy intake, percentage of macronutrients contribution to energy and micronutrients intake between case and control groups

Energy and nutrients intake	Case (n = 44)		Control (n = 44)	
	Male (n = 15)	Female (n = 29)	Male (n = 15)	Female (n = 29)
	Mean ± SD	Mean ± SD	Mean ± SD	Mean ± SD
Energy (Kcal)	2056 ± 210	1812 ± 331 *	2011 ± 224	1590 ± 148
Percentage of macronutrients contribution to energy Carbohydrate (%)	50.5 ± 3.6	51.8 ± 6.6	51.7 ± 4.7	53.1 ± 4.3
Fat (%)	33.3 ± 4.1	33.3 ± 5.5	33.7 ± 4.0	31.9 ± 3.9
Protein (%)	16.2 ± 3.5	14.9 ± 3.0	15.1 ± 2.2	15.0 ± 1.7
Micronutrients Vitamin A (RE)	1259.7 ± 432.4	1514.6 ± 503.4	1462.4 ± 515.8	1398.3 ± 470.1
Vitamin E (mg)	5.9 ± 2.6	5.7 ± 3.5	5.6 ± 2.3	4.1 ± 1.9
Fiber (g)	7.6 ± 4.0	6.2 ± 3.2	7.4 ± 3.9	5.3 ± 1.8
Zinc (mg)	6.7 ± 2.3	4.7 ± 2.2	6.3 ± 3.2	4.8 ± 1.8
Selenium (μg)	49.6 ± 34.8	30.7 ± 12.7	27.7 ± 9.9	35.8 ± 17.2

*Significant difference using Independent t-test (p < 0.05).

compared to non-acne subjects [27]. Our data also confirmed epidemiological studies performed in the United States [8-10]. Women, who consumed two or more servings of skimmed milk everyday, were 22% more likely to suffer from severe acne and 44% more likely to develop cystic or nodular acne than those who consumed only one glass of skimmed milk a day [8]. Endocrine factors involved in acne may be affected by milk consumption because milk is an insulinotropic nutrient and has a high insulinemic index [28] which would increase serum insulin and IGF-1 levels [29-32]. Milk produced persistently by pregnant cows contains substantial amounts of steroids and androgen-precursors, which have been suggested to play another role in acne pathogenesis [33,34]. Moreover, another group has proposed a hypothesis for the diet-induced impact of insulin/IGF-1 signaling in acne, as both high glycemic load and dairy proteins increase the serum levels of insulin and IGF-1, important

promoters of sebaceous glands and sebaceous lipogenesis [35,36]. In contrast to our study, a positive association between acne with cheese intake was found [8]. The difference may be partly attributed to lower frequency of cheese intake among subjects in this study.

This study confirmed earlier findings that acne vulgaris patients were more likely to have family history of acne vulgaris compared to the control group. In Jordan [37], it was reported that 69.3% of acne vulgaris patients had family history of acne vulgaris while in the United Kingdom, a study involving 458 pairs of monozygotic and 1099 dizygotic female twins [38] found that genetic factors attributed to 81% of acne vulgaris variant and only 19% involved environmental factors. A higher prevalence of acne vulgaris was also found among students with parents having a history of acne vulgaris [39].

Our study has found that acne vulgaris was neither related to BMI nor body fat percentage. This provides

Table 5 Glycemic loads of diet, macronutrients and micronutrients intake in percentiles and crude ORs

Parameter	Percentiles					
	25th	OR (95% CI)	50th	OR (95% CI)	75th	OR (95% CI)
Glycemic load	120	0.05 (0.007 – 0.308)	145	15.75** (1.773 – 139.935)	175	21.00** (2.390 – 184.515)
Energy (kcal)	1497	4.08 (1.161 – 13.904)	1782	6.43 (1.662 – 24.860)	2100	1.15 (0.319 – 4.167)
Carbohydrate (g)	197.5	4.67 (1.299 – 16.761)	226.9	8.53 (2.159 – 33.727)	271.3	1.24 (0.340 – 4.558)
Fat (g)	53.1	12.14 (2.655 – 55.537)	62.3	6.80 (1.537 – 30.077)	80.9	8.19 (1.839 – 36.424)
Protein (g)	56.7	4.08 (1.108 – 15.020)	65.0	11.56 (2.822 – 47.356)	83.7	2.83 (0.770 – 10.430)
Vitamin A (RE)	943.4	3.852 (1.086 – 13.661)	1246.7	0.93 (0.282 – 3.062)	1762.2	1.31 (0.393 – 4.388)
Vitamin E (mg)	3.1	4.06 (1.115 – 14.804)	4.5	6.50 (1.603 – 26.360)	6.3	1.35 (0.360 – 5.036)
Fiber (g)	3.6	2.53 (0.750 – 8.522)	5.0	2.14 (0.621 – 7.370)	8.0	1.75 (0.537 – 5.701)
Zinc (mg)	3.6	2.528 (0.750 – 8.522)	4.8	2.528 (0.750 – 8.522)	6.5	1.46 (0.436 – 4.880)
Selenium (μg)	21.1	1.733 (0.525 – 5.723)	28.4	0.45 (0.128 – 1.585)	45.0	2.57 (0.753 – 8.784)

** Significant difference, p < 0.01.

Table 6 Binary logistic regression model for glycemic load

Parameter	Crude OR	(95% CI)	Adjusted OR†	(95% CI)
Glycemic load				
<145/≥145	15.75**	(1.773 – 139.935)	1.94	(0.460 – 8.180)
≥175/<175	21.00**	(2.390 – 184.515)	24.96**	(2.285– 272.722)

†Adjusted OR for family history, level of education, frequencies of milk and ice cream consumption.
** Significant difference, $p < 0.01$.

further support to a study which discovered no correlation between BMI and leptin levels secreted by adipose tissue with the presence of acne vulgaris or its degree of severity [40]. A retrospective cohort in Turkey [10] also found no significant difference in serum leptin levels between cases and controls. Other studies among female twins [38] and female acne patients [41,42] also found no significant correlation between BMI and acne vulgaris severity among female acne vulgaris patients.

Our study found that yoghurt consumption was not correlated with acne vulgaris occurrence and is consistent with the findings by several studies [8-10]. When added to milk during fermentation process, probiotic bacteria (specifically Lactobacilli) utilize IGF-1 and lowered IGF-1 level in fermented milk by fourfold compared to skim milk [43]. It was hypothesized that increased intestinal permeability occurred in acne vulgaris patients, thus enhancing IGF-1 absorption in the gut [44]. Hence, milk consumption would cause an increased IGF-1 absorption rather than fermented milk products, which have lower levels of IGF-1. This might explain the association of milk with acne vulgaris occurrence in contrast to fermented dairy products such as

yoghurt. However, it is proposed that the most important mechanism of milk signalling is the postprandial fast upregulation of insulin secretion and the long-lasting increase in serum IGF-1 levels [35,36]. Recently, lactoferrin-enriched fermented milk was discovered to be effective in decreasing triglycerides in skin surface lipids, resulting in improvement of acne vulgaris symptoms through reduction in sebum production [45].

In contrast to common food beliefs, the present study found no statistically significant association between chocolate and nuts with acne vulgaris occurrences. Chocolate [25] and nuts [23] are commonly believed to cause or aggravate acne condition but previous studies regarding the effects of chocolate and nuts on acne vulgaris condition were inconsistent. An experiment on the effects of milk chocolate bars consumption in subjects with acne vulgaris found no exacerbation in their condition [46]. Subsequently, it was reported that acne lesion counts as well as composition and synthesis of sebum were also not affected after consumption of chocolates bar containing 10 times higher than normal cocoa solids [4]. Another case series study also concluded that chocolate and roasted nuts did not aggravate acne vulgaris condition [7]. Contrary to our findings, a cross sectional study among Koreans involving 783 acne vulgaris patients and 502 controls showed that consumption of nuts among cases were significantly higher than acne-free subjects [27].Thus, there is a clear need to conduct a randomized clinical trial to have a better understanding of the association between these food items with acne occurrence.

A few limitations of the study should be mentioned. Firstly, due to the nature of the study design used, this study was only able to determine the association, but

Table 7 Comparison of milk and dairy products, chocolate and nuts intake frequencies between cases and controls

Milk and dairy products	Frequencies	Cases(n = 44) n (%)	Controls(n = 44) n (%)	p value	Odds Ratio (OR)	95% Confidence Interval
Milk	≥Once a week	38** (86.4)	27 (61.4)	0.008	3.988	(1.391 - 11.434)
	0 - < Once a week	6 (13.6)	17 (38.6)			
Yoghurt	≥Once a week	10 (22.7)	8 (18.2)	0.597	1.324	(0.467 – 3.749)
	0 - < Once a week	34 (77.3)	36 (81.8)			
Cheese	≥Once a week	10 (22.7)	4 (9.1)	0.080	2.941	(0.846 – 10.229)
	0 - < Once a week	34 (77.3)	40 (90.9)			
Ice cream	≥Once a week	25** (56.8)	10 (22.7)	0.001	4.474	(1.777 – 11.266)
	0 - < Once a week	19 (43.2)	34 (77.3)			
Chocolate	≥Once a week	9 (20.5)	6 (13.6)	0.395	1.629	(0.526 – 5.044)
	0 - < Once a week	35 (79.5)	38 (86.4)			
Nuts	≥ Once a week	9 (20.5)	5 (11.4)	0.244	2.066	(0.613 – 6.558)
	0- < Once a week	35 (79.5)	39 (88.6)			

** Significant difference using Chi-Square test, $p < 0.01$.

not the cause and effect of diet on acne vulgaris. The severity of acne vulgaris condition should also be taken into account through acne lesion counts on patients in order to relate specific types of food and the frequency of their consumption. Furthermore, a retrospective food frequency questionnaire would be the most appropriate tool to determine the association between dietary intake such as dairy products and acne development. Repeated 3 day food records would have been a better method to calculate glycemic load and determine its association with acne. However, a 3 day food record was used in this study to measure the glycemic load due to the limited study duration. Additionally, this study did not measure the amount of consumed dairy protein, which may be the most important determinant for the acne-promoting effects of milk. Other confounding factors such as stress, inadequate sleep, smoking, alcohol consumption and facial hygiene care should also been taken into account in future studies. Despite these limitations, the findings from our study have provided further support to the existing evidence for the role of diet in acne vulgaris occurrence.

Conclusions

In conclusion, dietary factors particularly high glycemic load diets as well as higher frequency of milk and ice cream intake were positively associated with acne vulgaris development. Findings from this study further support the hypothesis that dietary factors play a fundamental role in acne vulgaris occurrences. Randomized clinical trials are needed to confirm the role of food items such as peanuts, chocolate and dietary fat in acne occurrence.

Competing interest
The authors declare that they have no competing interests.

Authors' contributions
NHI managed the literature searches, data collection and statistical analysis, and wrote the first draft of the manuscript. ZAM designed the study, developed the protocol, undertook the data interpretation and improved the manuscript. NZA was involved in assessing acne severity, development and improvement of the protocol, and improvement of the manuscript. All authors contributed to and have approved the final manuscript.

Acknowledgements
We are grateful to all the participants involved in this study. We would also like to thank the staff members of Department of Dermatology, Hospital Kuala Lumpur and others for facilitating the study.

Author details
[1]Dietetic Program, School of Healthcare Sciences, Faculty of Health Sciences, Universiti Kebangsaan Malaysia, Jalan Raja Muda Abdul Aziz, 50300 Kuala Lumpur, Malaysia. [2]Department of Dermatology, Hospital Kuala Lumpur, 50300 Kuala Lumpur, Malaysia.

References
1. Shaw L, Kennedy C: The treatment of acne. Paediatr Child Health 2007, 17(10):385–389.
2. Hanisah A, Khairani O, Shamsul AS: Prevalence of acne and its impact on the quality of life in school-aged adolescents in Malaysia. J Primary Health Care 2009, 1(1):20–25.
3. Robinson HM: The acne problem. South Med J 1949, 42:1050–1060.
4. Fulton JE, Plewig G, Kligman AM: Effect of chocolate on acne vulgaris. JAMA 1969, 210(11):2071–2074.
5. Treloar V: Diet and acne redux. Arch Dermatol 2003, 139:941–943.
6. Calder PC: Dietary modification of inflammation with lipids. Proc Nutr Soc 2002, 61(3):345–358.
7. Anderson PC: Foods as the cause of acne. Am Fam Physician 1971, 3(3):102.
8. Adebamowo CA, Spiegelman D, Danby FW, Frazier AL, Willett WC, Holmes MD: High school dietary dairy intake and teenage acne. J Am Acad Dermatol 2005, 52(2):207–214.
9. Adebamowo CA, Spiegelman D, Berkey CS, Danby W, Rockett HH, Colditz GA, Willet WC, Homes MD: Milk consumption and acne in adolescent girls. Dermatol Online J 2006, 12(4):1.
10. Adebamowo CA, Spiegelman D, Berkey CS, Danby W, Rockett HH, Colditz GA, Willet WC, Homes MD: Milk consumption and acne in teenaged boys. J Am Acad Dermatol 2008, 58(5):787–793.
11. Kaymak Y, Adisen E, Ilter N, Bideci A, Gurler D, Celik B: Dietary glycemic index and glucose, insulin, insulin-like growth factor-I, insulin-like growth factor binding protein 3, and leptin levels in patients with acne. J Am Acad Dermatol 2007, 57(5):819–823.
12. Smith RN, Mann NJ, Braue A, Makelainen H, Varigos GA: A low-glycemic-load diet improves symptoms in acne vulgaris patients: a randomized controlled trial. Am J Clin Nutr 2007, 86(1):107–115.
13. Smith R, Varigos G, Braue A, Mann NJ: The effect of a low glycemic load diet on acne vulgaris and the fatty acid composition of skin surface triglycerides. J Dermatol Sci 2008, 50(1):41–52.
14. Lehr R: Sixteen s squared over d squared: a relation for crude sample size estimates. Stat Med 1992, 11:1099–1102.
15. Tan JK, Tang J, Fung K, Gupta AK, Thomas DR, Sapra S, Lynde C, Poulin Y, Gulliver W, Sebaldt RJ: Development and validation of a comprehensive acne severity scale. J Cutan Med Surg 2007, 11(6):211–216.
16. WHO: Appropriate body-mass index for Asian populations and its implications for policy and intervention strategies. Lancet 2004, 363:157–163.
17. Kalkwarf HJ, Khoury JC, Lanphear BP: Milk intake during childhood and adolescence, adult bone density, and osteoporotic fractures in US women. Am J Clin Nutr 2003, 77(1):257–265.
18. Foster-Powell K, Holt SHA, Brand-Miller JC: International Table of Glycemic Index and Glycemic Load Values. Am J Clin Nutr 2002, 76:5–56.
19. Atkinson FS, Foster-Powell K, Brand-Miller JC: International Table of Glycemic Index and Glycemic Load Values: 2008. Diabetes Care 2008, 31:2281–2283.
20. Nik Shanita S, Nik Mazlan M: Chapter 4 Carbohydrates. In Recommended Nutrient Intakes for Malaysia. National Coordinating Committee on Food and Nutrition (NCCFN). A report of the Technical Working Group on Nutritional Guidelines. Edited by Mohd Ismail N, Khor GL, Tee ES. Putrajaya: Ministry of Health Malaysia; 2005:42–51.
21. Tee ES, Mohd Ismail N, Mohd Nasir A, Khatijah I: Nutrient composition of Malaysian foods. Kuala Lumpur: Inst. Medical Res; 1997.
22. United State Department for Agriculture. http://www.ars.usda.gov.
23. Cordain L, Lindeberg S, Hurtado M, Hill K, Eaton SB, Brand-Miller J: Acne vulgaris: a disease of Western civilization. Arch Dermatol 2002, 138(12):1584–1590.
24. Smith R, Mann N, Braue A, Makelainen H, Varigos G: The effect of a high-protein, low glycemic–load diet versus a conventional, high glycemic–load diet on biochemical parameters associated with acne vulgaris: A randomized, investigator-masked, controlled trial. J Am Acad Dermatol 2007, 57(2):247–256.
25. Rouhani P, Berman B, Rouhani G: Acne improves with a popular, low glycemic diet from South Beach. J Am Acad Dermatol 2009, 60(suppl):706.
26. Cordain L: Implications for the Role of Diet in Acne. Semin Cutan Med Surg 2005, 24(2):84–91.
27. Jung JY, Yoon MY, Min SU, Hong JS, Choi YS, Suh DH: The influence of dietary patterns on acne vulgaris in Koreans. Eur J Dermatol 2010, 20:768–772.

28. Hoyt G, Hickey MS, Cordain L: **Dissociation of the glycaemic and insulinaemic responses to whole and skimmed milk.** *Br J Nutr* 2005, **93**:175–177.

29. Hoppe C, Mølgaard C, Vaag A, Barkholt V, Michaelsen KF: **High intakes of milk, but not meat, increase s-insulin and insulin resistance in 8-year-old boys.** *Eur J Clin Nutr* 2005, **59**:393–398.

30. Rich-Edwards JW, Ganmaa D, Pollak MN, Nakamoto EK, Kleinman K, Tserendolgor U, Willet WC, Frazier AL: **Milk consumption and the prepubertal somatotropic axis.** *Nutr J* 2007, **6**:28.

31. Norat T, Dossus L, Rinaldi S, Overvad K, Grønbaek H, Tjønneland A, Olsen A, Clavel-Chapelon F, Boutron-Ruault MC, Boeing H, Lahmann PH, Linseisen J, Nagel G, Trichopoulou A, Trichopoulos D, Kalapothaki V, Sieri S, Palli D, Panico S, Tumino R, Sacerdote C, Bueno-de-Mesquita HB, Peeters PHM, van Gils CH, Agudo A, Amiano P, Ardanoz E, Martinez C, Quirós R, Tormo MJ, *et al*: **Diet, serum insulin-like growth factor-I and IGF-binding protein-3 in European women.** *Eur J Clin Nutr* 2007, **6**:91–98.

32. Crowe FL, Key TJ, Allen NE, Appleby PN, Roddam A, Overvad K, Grønbaek H, Tjønneland A, Halkjær J, Dossus L, Boeing H, Kröger J, Trichopoulou A, Dilis V, Trichopoulos D, Boutron-Ruault MC, De Lauzon B, Clavel-Chapelon F, Palli D, Berrino F, Panico S, Tumino R, Sacerdote C, Bas Bueno-de-Mesquita H, Vrieling A, van Gils CH, Peeters PHM, Gram IT, Skeie G, Lund E, *et al*: **The association between diet and serum concentrations of IGF-I, IGFBP-1, IGFBP-2, and IGFBP-3 in the European Prospective Investigation into Cancer and Nutrition.** *Canc Epidemiol Biomarkers Prev* 2009, **18**:1333–1340.

33. Danby FW: **Nutrition and acne.** *Clin Dermatol* 2010, **28**:598–604.

34. Danby FW: **Acne: Diet and acneigenesis.** *Indian Dermatol Online J* 2011, **2**:2–5.

35. Melnik BC: **Evidence for acne-promoting effects of milk and other insulinotropic dairy products.** *Nestle Nutr Workshop Ser Pediatr Program* 2011, **67**:131–145.

36. Melnik BC, John SM, Schmitz G: **Over-stimulation of insulin/IGF-1 signaling by Western diet may promote diseases of civilization: lessons learnt from Laron syndrome.** *Nutr Metab (Lond)* 2011, **8**:41.

37. El-Akawi Z, Abdel-Latif NA, Abdul-Razzak K, Al-Aboosi M: **Factors believed by Jordanian acne patients to affect their acne condition.** *East Mediterr Health J* 2006, **12**(6):840–846.

38. Bataille V, Snieder H, MacGregor A, Sasieni P, Spector T: **The influence of genetics and environmental factors in the pathogenesis of acne: a twin study of acne in women.** *J Invest Dermatol* 2002, **119**(6):1317–1322.

39. Rigopoulos D, Gregoriou S, Ifandi A, Efstathiou G, Georgala S: **Coping with acne: beliefs and perceptions in a sample of secondary school Greek pupils.** *J Eur Acad Dermatol Venereol* 2007, **21**(6):806–810.

40. Hunter N, Shaker O: **Diet and body mass index, do they have a role in acne vulgaris? A study using serum leptin and serum Insulin like growth factor-1.** *Egypt J Derm Androl* 2009, **9**(2):73–80.

41. Cibula D, Hill M, Fanta M, Sindelka G, Zivny J: **Does obesity diminish the positive effect of oral contraceptive treatment on hyperandrogenism in women with polycystic ovarian syndrome?** *Hum Reprod* 2001, **16**(5):940.

42. Borgia F, Cannavò S, Guarneri F, Cannavò SP, Vaccaro M, Guarneri B: **Correlation between endocrinological parameters and acne severity in adult women.** *Acta Derm Venereol* 2004, **84**(3):201–204.

43. Kang S, Kim J, Imm J, Oh S, Kim S: **The effects of dairy processes and storage on insulin-like growth factor-I (IGF-I) content in milk and in model IGF-I-fortified dairy products.** *J Dairy Sci* 2006, **89**(2):402–409.

44. Bowe WP, Logan AC: **Acne vulgaris, probiotics and the gut-brain-skin axis-back to the future?** *Gut Pathogens* 2011, **3**(1):1–11.

45. Kim J, Ko Y, Park YK, Kim NI, Ha WK, Cho Y: **Dietary effect of lactoferrin-enriched fermented milk on skin surface lipid and clinical improvement of acne vulgaris.** *Nutrition* 2010, **26**(9):902–909.

46. Grant J, Anderson P: **Chocolate as a cause of acne: a dissenting view.** *Mo Med* 1965, **62**:459.

12

Topical treatment with fresh human milk versus emollient on atopic eczema spots in young children: a small, randomized, split body, controlled, blinded pilot study

Teresa Løvold Berents[1,2]*, Jørgen Rønnevig[1,2], Elisabeth Søyland[3], Peter Gaustad[1,4], Gro Nylander[5] and Beate Fossum Løland[5]

Abstract

Background: Public health nurses report on effects of fresh human milk as treatment for conjunctivitis, rhinitis and atopic eczema (AE), the latter being highly prevalent in early childhood. Emollients and topical corticosteroids are first line treatment of AE. As many caregivers have steroid phobia, alternative treatment options for mild AE are of interest. The aim of this small pilot study was to assess the potential effects and risks of applying fresh human milk locally on eczema spots in children with AE.

Methods: This was a split body, controlled, randomized and physician blinded pilot study, of children with AE with two similar contralateral eczema spots having a mother breastfeeding the child or a sibling. Fresh expressed milk and emollient was applied on the intervention spot and emollient alone on the control area, three times a day for four weeks. The severity and area of the eczema spots was evaluated weekly, and samples from milk and the spots were analysed weekly with respect to bacterial colonisation.

Results: Of nine patients included, six completed the study. Mean age at inclusion was 18.5 months. The spots examined were localized on the arms, legs or cheeks. The spots were similar in severity, but differed in area. In one patient the eczema ceased after inclusion. In four patients both control and intervention areas increased during the intervention. The relative change in eczema area compared to baseline showed less increase in the intervention spots in two patients, whereas the opposite was observed in three. In four children *Staphylococcus aureus* was found in their eczema once or more. In three of the 28 human milk samples, *Staphylococcus aureus*, *alfa haemolytic streptococci* or *coagulase negative staphylococci* were detected. *Staphylococcus aureus* was found once both in human milk and in the eczema spots, no clinical signs of infection were however observed. No secondary infection due to milk application was detected.

Conclusion: In this small pilot study, no effect was found on eczema spots treated with topical application of fresh human milk. (ClinicalTrials.gov Identifier, NCT02381028).

Keywords: Atopic eczema, Children, Human milk, Emollient, Topical treatment, Pilot study

* Correspondence: t.l.berents@medisin.uio.no
[1]Institute of Clinical Medicine, University of Oslo, Oslo, Norway
[2]Department of Dermatology, Oslo University Hospital, Oslo, Norway
Full list of author information is available at the end of the article

Background

Atopic eczema (AE) is a common, chronic, pruritic, relapsing skin disease which affects up to 20% of children in the Nordic European countries [1]. AE is strongly associated with other atopic disorders, such as allergic rhinitis and asthma [2]. The pathogenesis is interplay between barrier dysfunction, genetic, immunological, environmental factors and colonization by *Staphylococcus aureus* (*S. aureus*) [3].

The treatment algorithm in AE is based on treating the barrier defect, the inflammation, the infection and the pruritus [4]. First line treatment is treating the barrier defect with optimal skin care by the use of emollients and baths. If a clinical infection is present in the eczema, local antiseptics may be utilized; for severe cases systemic antibiotics are needed. The inflammation is treated with topical steroid creams. Topical steroids have been shown to be a well-tolerated treatment, but in spite of this many caregivers have steroid phobia, mainly because of the potential side effects [5]. A treatment option in chronic eczema is topical calcineurin inhibitors; these are however not to be used in children under two years of age [4]. Alternatives without side effects for young children are therefore of interest.

Human milk may represent a source with potential treatment properties. Knowledge of the immunological qualities of mammalian milk can be traced back to 1892, when Paul Ehrlich demonstrated that newborn mice were protected against the toxic effects of phytotoxins if they were fed milk from an immunized mouse [6]. Today, numerous studies have contributed to our present knowledge of the short- and long-term effects of human milk in the breastfed child [7]. Mammalian milk is species specific. Human milk contains specialized immune components, including factors with anti-microbial and anti-inflammatory properties [8], which theoretically could be responsible for an effect on eczema spots when applied topically.

In Norway, public health nurses report several cases where parents have had positive experiences with topic applications of expressed human milk in eyes of children with conjunctivitis and on eczema spots in children with AE. We have not been able to find any studies investigating such treatment in children with AE. However, local use of expressed human milk has been studied for diaper dermatitis, rhinitis and conjunctivitis [9,10].

The aim of this small pilot study was to assess the potential positive and/or negative effects of topical use of expressed, fresh human milk on eczema spots in young children with AE by evaluating the eczema areas. A secondary aim was to evaluate any bacterial transmission from human milk to the eczema spots, causing infection in the child. Finally the mothers' compliance to the treatment was of interest.

Methods

Trial design

This was a split body controlled, randomized and physician blinded study of expressed human milk and emollients on contralateral eczema spots in children, the trial was registered at ClinicalTrials.gov Identifier, NCT02381028.

Inclusion criteria were children with AE according to Hanifin and Rajkas criteria [11] with a mother breastfeeding the child or a sibling. The eczema spots in the treatment and control areas were to be similar in features and extent as well as being localized on contralateral parts of the body. Children were excluded if the severity of the eczema spots indicated need for treatment with antibiotics and/or steroids.

The study was approved by the Regional Committee for Medical and Health Research Ethics - South East Norway. Mothers of participating children were informed verbally and in writing, and signed an informed consent prior to commencing the study.

Recruitment

Study patients were recruited through advertisement posters from three different well baby clinics in Oslo, Norway, in the period 2008–2011. Mothers interested in the study contacted the study team. The consultations mainly took place at the hospital; a few were carried out in the child's home. The mothers were able to contact the examining physician if they experienced any problems with the treatment.

Intervention

The study intervention was local application of fresh human milk on the study area. By hand milking, the mothers were to squeeze out and throw away the first few droplets of milk, and then squeeze the next droplets directly from the nipple to the eczema spot. The number of milk droplets depended on the size of the eczema area; the mothers were instructed to cover the whole eczema spot with milk. After absorption of the milk droplets, both treatment and control areas were treated with moisturizing cream (Apobase creme®, Actavis Norway AS). The cream contains: Aqua, Paraffinum Liquidum, Petrolatum, Cetearyl Alcohol, Ceteareth-20, Ceteareth-12, Sodium Gluconate, Caprylyl Glycol, Phenoxyethanol, with a total lipid content of 30 percent. Both intervention and control areas were treated with this regimen three times a day for four weeks.

Randomization and blinding

The same physician examined all the children, and was blinded as to which areas were the control or intervention sites. At inclusion the physician diagnosed the AE according to Hanifin and Rajkas criteria [11]. The two contra-lateral eczema spots to be randomized were elected; i.e. flexural aspect of elbow, flexural aspect of knees or cheeks. Another

Flow Diagram

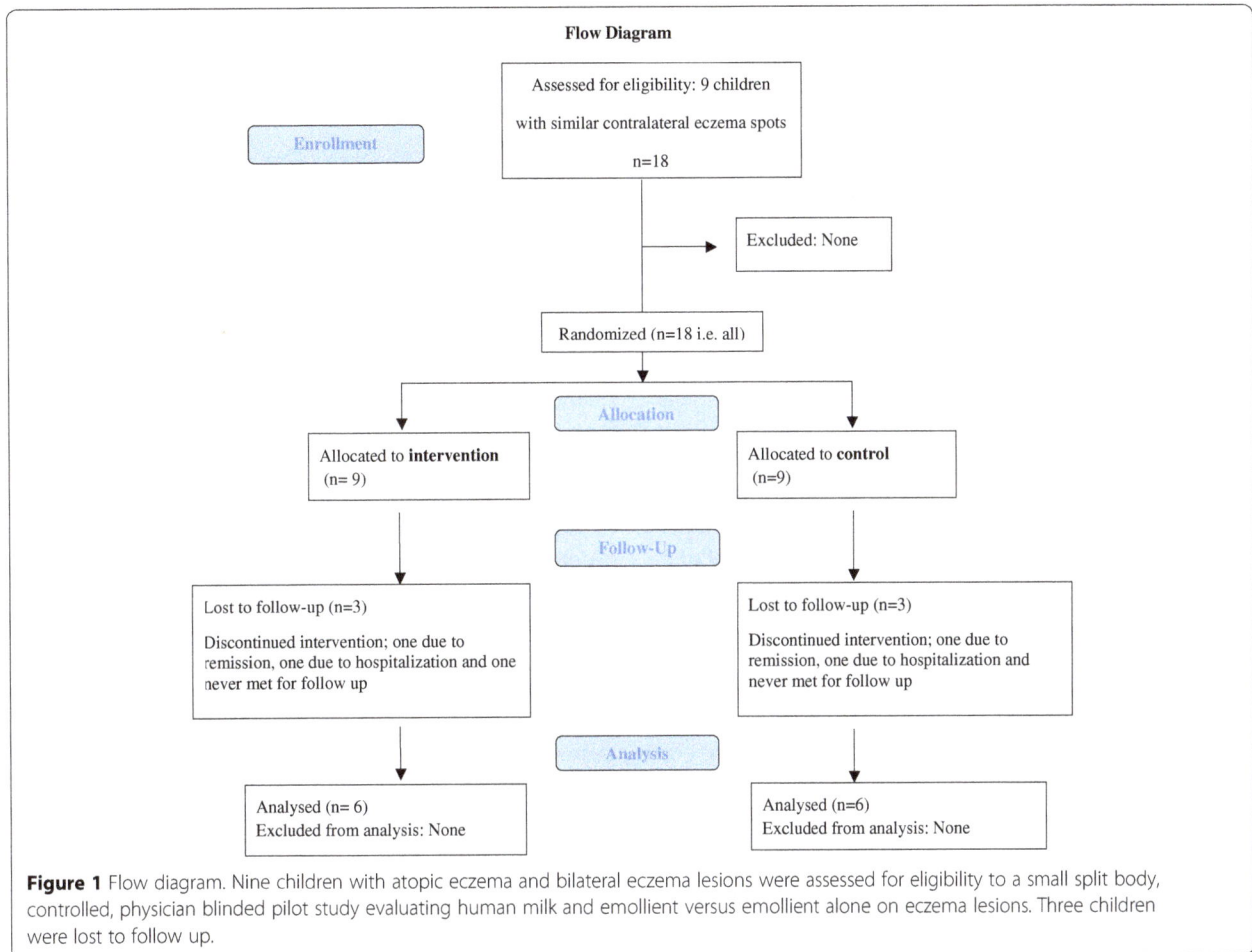

Figure 1 Flow diagram. Nine children with atopic eczema and bilateral eczema lesions were assessed for eligibility to a small split body, controlled, physician blinded pilot study evaluating human milk and emollient versus emollient alone on eczema lesions. Three children were lost to follow up.

physician, who did not see the child, was responsible for the randomization. The child was given a randomization number and the mothers were then informed on which side to apply the fresh expressed human milk and emollient, and on which side to apply emollient alone.

Follow-up

After inclusion, the children were examined once weekly for four consecutive weeks. The overall severity of AE was evaluated by the use of SCORAD, which defines mild disease as score <25, moderate disease between 25–50 and severe disease as scores >50 [12]. The severity of the study and control areas were evaluated by scoring the erythema, lichenification, excoriation and pruritus on a scale from 0 to 3, where 0 is none and 3 is severe. Study and control areas were measured using Visitrak™ (Smith & Nephew), a portable device used to measure the area of wounds [13]. A transparent folio is placed over the area and the borders are outlined, whereafter a computer determines the area measured in cm². In the present study this device was used to follow the development of the extent of the eczema spots.

At each visit, samples for bacterial cultures were taken at eczema spots and from breastmilk, using Amies Agar Gel with Charcoal™, Copan Venturi Transystem® (Copan, Brescia, Italy). Sampling from eczema spots was done by carefully rubbing the cotton swab over the eczema spot. Sampling of breastmilk was done from milk expressed by hand milking. The specimens were cultivated on blood agar plates and selective media for *S. aureus* and for gram-negative rods.

Outcome

The primary outcome was to register proportional change in the area of the eczema spot from baseline, as measured by Visitrak™. The secondary outcome was to assess transmission of bacteria from mother's milk to eczema spots in the child. The mother's compliance was also evaluated.

Statistical methods

Descriptive statistics were performed. The areas of the intervention and control sites for each child were not identical; therefore differences were calculated as percentages: Changes in the areas of the control and intervention sites each week were calculated as change in proportion of area related to baseline area.

Results
Study population
Nine children, four male, were recruited for the study through advertisement posters from three different well baby clinics in Oslo, Norway in the period 2008–2011. Three of these nine children were lost to follow-up consultations; one experienced remission from AE, the second suffered from severe AE and was hospitalized, the third never met for follow up (Figure 1). Two children were treated with mothers' milk produced for a younger sibling. The mean age of the children was 18.5 months (min, max; 4, 32). At inclusion mean SCORAD was 35 (min, max; 22, 45) and at the end of the study mean SCORAD was 34 (min, max; 18, 52). The spots examined were localized on the arms or legs in five of the children and on the cheeks in one. The spots were similar in severity, however the extent differed some.

Changes in measured area of eczema
The weekly change in the control and intervention eczema area related to baseline eczema area is illustrated in Figure 2. At the end of the study, child number one and seven displayed less area involvement in the area treated with human milk compared to the emollient treated area. In child number two, five and nine the emollient treated area showed at study end less involvement than the area treated with human milk. The eczema spots in child number eight disappeared after inclusion.

Most of the children showed an improvement of their general eczema, except for child five, who showed a slight increase. Child seven differs from the other children: this child experienced a worsening of the total eczema, having mild atopic eczema at inclusion, and severe atopic eczema at week four.

Changes in presence of bacterial species
Four of the children had positive *S. aureus* cultures in their eczema once or more (Table 1). However, only in four of twelve occasions this coincided with clinical signs of infection. Gram-negative rods were found in child number one at one visit. *S. aureus, alfa haemolytic streptococci* or *coagulase-negative staphylococci* were detected in three of the 28 human milk samples. Only on one occasion the same bacteria (*S. aureus*) were detected in both the eczema lesions and the human milk (child number five), and signs of clinical infection were present (Table 1). The intervention areas differed some from the control areas, as *S. aureus* was found in intervention area but not in the control area on four occasions in three different children (Table 1).

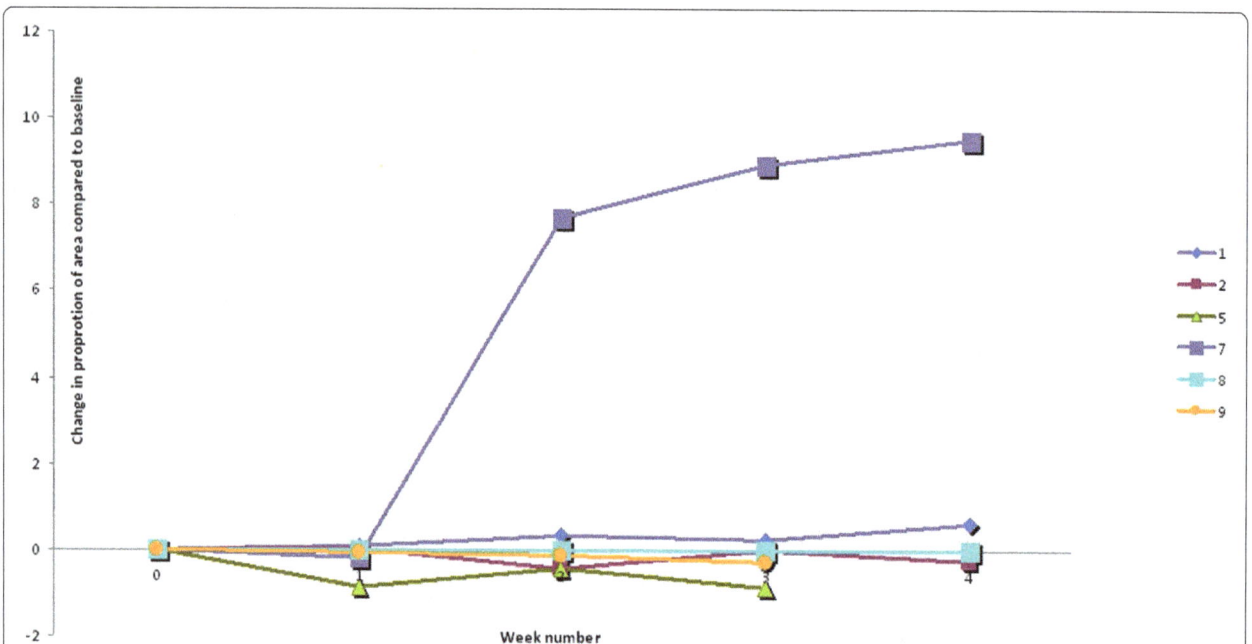

Figure 2 Change in eczema area. This figure illustrates the weekly difference between control and intervention sites based on the area change from baseline in six children with atopic eczema included in a split body, controlled, physician blinded pilot study evaluating human milk and emollient versus emollient alone on eczema lesions. Each line represents one child. The difference is calculated as: control area week 1, 2, 3 or 4 divided by control area at week 0 minus intervention area week 1, 2, 3 or 4 divided by intervention area at week 0. Lines above zero represent improvement of the intervention area, and lines below zero represent the relative increase of the eczema areas of the intervention sites.

Table 1 Bacteria in eczema spots and human milk

Child	Week	Clinical infected	Study area	Control area	Human milk
1	0	No	No growth	No growth	Skin flora[1]
	1	No	No growth	No growth	Missing
	2	No	No growth	Skin flora	Missing
	3	No	Gram negative rods	Gram negative rods	Skin flora
	4	No	Skin flora	No growth	Skin flora
2	0	No	Skin flora	Skin flora	Skin flora
	1	No	Skin flora	Skin flora	Skin flora
	2	No	Skin flora	Skin flora	Skin flora
	3	No	Skin flora	Skin flora	Skin flora
	4	No	No growth	No growth	Skin flora
5	0	No	*S. aureus* (rich)	*S. aureus* (mod.[2])	Skin flora
	1	No	*S. aureus* (rich)	*S. aureus* (rich)	*S. aureus* (some col.[3])
	2	Yes	*S. aureus* (mod.)	*S. aureus* (sparse)	Skin flora
	3	No	*S. aureus* (rich)	*S. aureus* (rich)	Skin flora
	4	Yes	*S. aureus* (mod.)	Skin flora	Skin flora
7	0	No	Skin flora	Skin flora	Skin flora
	1	Yes	Skin flora	Skin flora	CNS[4]
	2	No	*S. aureus* (some col.)	Skin flora	Skin flora
	3	No	Skin flora	Skin flora	Skin flora
	4	No	*S. aureus* (some col.)	Skin flora	Skin flora
8	0	No	Missing	Missing	Missing
	1	No	Skin flora	Skin flora	Skin flora
	2	No	Skin flora	Skin flora	Skin flora
	3	No	*S. aureus* (some col.)	Skin flora	Skin flora
	4	No	Skin flora	Skin flora	Skin flora
9	0	No	*S. aureus* (some col.)	*S. aureus* (sparse)	Skin flora
	1	Yes	*S. aureus* (mod.)	*S. aureus* (rich)	*AHST*[5]
	2	No	*S. aureus* (sparse)	*S. aureus* (mod.)	No growth
	3	Yes	*S. aureus* (mod.)	*S. aureus* (some col.)	Skin flora

[1]Skin flora: non-pathogen bacteria belonging to the skin flora [2] mod.: moderate, [3]col. colonies, [4]CNS: coagulase negative staphylococci, [5]AHST alfa haemolytic streptococci.
Bacterial presence in samples taken from eczema spots and human milk weekly, and the presence of clinically judged infection in control and intervention sites of six children with atopic eczema included in a split body, controlled, physician blinded pilot study evaluating human milk and emollient versus emollient alone on eczema lesions.

Compliance

The mothers experienced the application of human milk as an uncomplicated treatment option.

Discussion

In this small, split body controlled randomized pilot study of human milk and emollient applied topically on eczema spots in six children, no effect was found on eczema spots treated with the topical application of fresh human milk. In two of five children with persistent eczema lesions during the study, there was less involvement of the human milk treated area compared to the emollient area at study end compared to baseline. However, the opposite was found in three children.

There are few studies looking at the effect of human milk on eczema. One study of children with diaper dermatitis examined the effect of applying human milk after each breastfeeding or hydrocortisone 1% ointment twice a day, detecting after one week an effect of human milk comparable to that of hydrocortisone [9]. The application frequency was higher than in our study, but we still believe that an application rate of three times a day would be enough to show an effect of human milk, after four weeks of treatment.

There are many theoretical indications of how human milk can be effective on eczema lesions. One aspect of atopic disease is the type 2 helper T cell (Th2) dysbalance with production of interleukin- 4 (IL-4), IL-5, and IL-13 in the acute phase. In the chronic phase there is a Th1/Th0 dominance with production of interferon-γ, IL-2, IL-5 and granulocyte-macrophage colony-stimulating factor [2]. Of interest, therefore, are findings from an animal model, where the effect of human colostrum used locally on an acute inflammatory process was shown to be as potent as oral indomethacin and superior to oral dexamethasone at suppressing polymorphonuclear leukocyte influx [14,15]. In humans, the milk contains, among a wide variety of biologically active hormones, glucocorticoids. These are transferred from plasma to the milk in levels fairly highly correlated (in the .6-.7 range) [16].

Milk samples from healthy donors have revealed bacteria in 10–23% of the samples [17]. In the present study, bacteria were found in three of 28 samples; 11%. In one child only (child number five), S. aureus was found once in both the eczema spot and in the milk. Clinically, however, the eczema was not infected, and this child had S. aureus on both eczema lesions at every visit. This suggests that no iatrogenic infections due to application of fresh mothers milk occurred. Surprisingly, S. aureus was found in the intervention area but not in the control area on four occasions in three different children. One speculation might be that the preservative (eg. phenoxyethanol) in the emollient had some antimicrobial effect when applied alone.

Human milk contains several different substances that act against bacteria, virus and fungi, such as Secretory IgA and Secretory IgM [18], lactoferrin, lysozyme, oligosaccharides, Toll-like receptors and fatty acids [8]. In a study evaluating the inhibition in vitro of human colostrum against bacterial cultures from eye swabs of neonates with neonatal conjunctivitis, the inhibitory activity was ≥ 50% against S. aureus and coliform bacteria, demonstrating an antimicrobial effect also in vitro [19]. A consistent inhibitory effect of human milk was found against Neisseria gonorrhea in children with conjunctivitis. A significant but less pronounced effect was also found against Moraxella catarrhalis [10]. This strengthens the evidence for an antimicrobial effect of human milk also when used topically. When comparing different methods for preventing omphalitis in newborns, an application frequency of topical human milk twice a day demonstrated a shorter separation time of the umbilical stump compared to the use of antiseptics [20]. In the study of Ibhanesebhor [19], the mean duration of inhibition of human milk against S. aureus was three hours. Considering the huge amount of different biologically active components and cells in human milk, there might be a variety of candidates for explaining the positive effects described above.

The children participating in the present study were recruited through advertisement posters in well baby clinics, and responding mothers were presumably highly motivated and inclined to trust alternative/new treatment methods. We cannot rule out that the mothers co-treated the intervention sites with for instance steroid cream, but the instructions with respect to treatment of the intervention and control site were clear, and the results do not indicate performance bias.

Conclusions

The results of this small randomized, controlled pilot study of six children with AE does not support an effect of topical applied human milk. Treatment with fresh expressed human milk seems safe and easy for mothers to carry out.

Competing interests

The authors declare that they have no competing interests.

Authors' contributions

TLB, BFL, JR, ES and GN were all involved in the design of the study, drafting the protocol, analysing results and writing the paper. TLB provided methodological considerations and carried out the clinical part. PG was involved in analysing the bacteria cultures and in writing the paper. All authors read and approved the final manuscript.

Acknowledgements

We thank the children and their parents for cooperation in this study. The study team gratefully acknowledge Dr. PhD. Kristin Bergersen, Institute of Clinical Medicine, University of Oslo and Department of Dermatology, Oslo University Hospital, Oslo, Norway, for her important contribution to the initial study design. The team also acknowledge preliminary analyses provided by Mari Vårdal, Department of Biostatistics, Epidemiology and Health Economy, Oslo University Hospital, Oslo, Norway.

Author details

[1]Institute of Clinical Medicine, University of Oslo, Oslo, Norway. [2]Department of Dermatology, Oslo University Hospital, Oslo, Norway. [3]Department of Research, Education and Innovation, Oslo University Hospital, Oslo, Norway. [4]Department of Microbiology, Oslo University Hospital, Oslo, Norway. [5]Norwegian National Advisory Unit on Breastfeeding, Womens and Children´s Division, Oslo University Hospital, Oslo, Norway.

References

1. Odhiambo JA, Williams HC, Clayton TO, Robertson CF, Asher MI. Global variations in prevalence of eczema symptoms in children from ISAAC phase three. J Allergy Clin Immunol. 2009;124(6):1251–58 e1223.
2. Bieber T. Atopic dermatitis. N Engl J Med. 2008;358(14):1483–94.
3. Leyden JJ, Marples RR, Kligman AM. Staphylococcus aureus in the lesions of atopic dermatitis. British J Dermatol. 1974;90(5):525–30.
4. Eichenfield LF, Tom WL, Berger TG, Krol A, Paller AS, Schwarzenberger K, et al. Guidelines of care for the management of atopic dermatitis: section 2. Management and treatment of atopic dermatitis with topical therapies. J Am Acad Dermatol. 2014;71(1):116–32.
5. Kojima R, Fujiwara T, Matsuda A, Narita M, Matsubara O, Nonoyama S, et al. Factors associated with steroid phobia in caregivers of children with atopic dermatitis. Pediat Dermatol. 2013;30(1):29–35.
6. Ehrlich P. Über Immunität durch Vererbung und Säugung. Zeitschrift für Hygiene und Infectionkrankheiten. 1892;12:183–203.
7. Hornell A, Lagstrom H, Lande B, Thorsdottir I. Breastfeeding, introduction of other foods and effects on health: a systematic literature review for the 5th Nordic Nutrition Recommendations. Food Nutrition Res. 2013;57:20823.

8. Hosea Blewett HJ, Cicalo MC, Holland CD, Field CJ. The immunological components of human milk. Adv Food Nutr Res. 2008;54:45–80.

9. Farahani LA, Ghobadzadeh M, Yousefi P. Comparison of the Effect of Human Milk and Topical Hydrocortisone 1% on Diaper Dermatitis. Pediat Dermatol. 2013;30(6):725–9.

10. Baynham JT, Moorman MA, Donnellan C, Cevallos V, Keenan JD. Antibacterial effect of human milk for common causes of paediatric conjunctivitis. Br J Ophthalmol. 2013;97(3):377–9.

11. Hanifin JM, Rajka G. Diagnostic features of atopic dermatitis. Acta Derm Venereol (Stockholm). 1980;92:44–7.

12. European Task Force on Atopic Dermatitis. Severity scoring of atopic dermatitis: the SCORAD index. Consensus Report of the European Task Force on Atopic Dermatitis. Dermatology. 1993;186(1):23–31.

13. Sugama J, Matsui Y, Sanada H, Konya C, Okuwa M, Kitagawa A. A study of the efficiency and convenience of an advanced portable wound measurement system (VISITRAK). J Clin Nurs. 2007;16(7):1265–9.

14. Buescher ES. Anti-inflammatory characteristics of human milk: how, where, why. Adv Exp Med Biol. 2001;501:207–22.

15. Murphey DK, Buescher ES. Human colostrum has anti-inflammatory activity in a rat subcutaneous air pouch model of inflammation. Pediatr Res. 1993;34(2):208–12.

16. Grey KR, Davis EP, Sandman CA, Glynn LM. Human milk cortisol is associated with infant temperament. Psychoneuroendocrinology. 2013;38(7):1178–85.

17. Lindemann PC, Foshaugen I, Lindemann R. Characteristics of breast milk and serology of women donating breast milk to a milk bank. Arch Dis Child Fetal Neonatal Ed. 2004;89(5):F440–1.

18. Brandtzaeg P. The mucosal immune system and its integration with the mammary glands. J Pediatr. 2010;156(2 Suppl):S8–15.

19. Ibhanesebhor SE, Otobo ES. In vitro activity of human milk against the causative organisms of ophthalmia neonatorum in Benin City. Nigeria J Trop Pediatr. 1996;42(6):327–9.

20. Vural G, Kisa S. Umbilical cord care: a pilot study comparing topical human milk, povidone-iodine, and dry care. J Obstet Gynecol Neonatal Nurs. 2006;35(1):123–8.

Comparison of publication trends in dermatology among Japan, South Korea and Mainland China

Huibin Man[1†], Shujun Xin[2†], Weiping Bi[1], Chengzhi Lv[2], Theodora M Mauro[3,4], Peter M Elias[3,4] and Mao-Qiang Man[2,3,4*]

Abstract

Background: We previously showed that the number of publications in dermatology is increasing year by year, and positively correlates with improved economic conditions in mainland China, a still developing Asian country. However, the characteristics of publications in dermatology departments in more developed Asian countries such as Japan and South Korea are unknown.

Methods: In the present study, publications from 2003 through 2012 in dermatology in Japan, South Korea and mainland China were characterized. All data were obtained from www.pubmed.com.

Results: Dermatology departments in Japan published 4,094 papers, while mainland China and South Korea published 1528 and 1,758 articles, respectively. 48% of articles from dermatology in Japan were original research and 36% were case reports; The number of publications in Japan remained stable over time, but the overall impact factors per paper increased linearly over the last 10 year period ($p < 0.05$). In mainland China, 67% of articles from dermatology were original research, while 19% were case reports; The number of publications and their impact factors per paper increased markedly. In South Korea, 65% of articles from dermatology were original research and 20% were case reports. The impact factors per paper remained unchanged, despite of the fact that the number of publications increased over the last 10 year period ($r^2 = 0.6820$, $p = 0.0032$). Only mainland China showed a positive correlation of the number of publications with gross domestic product per capita during this study period.

Conclusions: These results suggest that the total number of publications in dermatology correlates with economic conditions only in developing country, but not in more developed countries in Asia. The extent of economic development could determine both the publication quantity and quality.

Keywords: Publication, Dermatology, Gross domestic product, China, Japan, South Korea

Background

The total number of publications is considered as a key indicator of scientific productivity and is often used to evaluate the success of research [1-3]. The total number of publications tends to increase yearly in medical field. For instance, number of publications in otolaryngology research increased by over 80% from the year 1995 to 2000 [4]. The number of publications also increased in the dermatology field year by year [5,6]. There are many determinants, such as gross domestic product (GDP), number of medical school, number of dermatologists, language skills as well as population size that influence the quantity and quality of publications [1,7,8]. Funding, which is closely associated with economic conditions, is a key factor that impacts scientific productivity [9,10]. Although the number of publications strongly correlates with GDP [1,6], GDP does not always influence scientific productivity in certain nations. For example, from 2001 to 2010, the number of publications in anesthesia journals from the United States declined from 412 to 361, despite the fact that NIH funding for anesthesia research increased [11] and the GDP per capita increased from \$35,912 to \$46,612 during that period. Similarly, the number of publications from dermatology in Finland decreased slightly

---

* Correspondence: mqman@hotmail.com
†Equal contributors
[2]The Center for Skin Physiology Research, Dalian Skin Disease Hospital, Liaoning 116021, P.R. China
[3]Dermatology Service, Veterans Affairs Medical Center, San Francisco, CA, USA
Full list of author information is available at the end of the article

from 1989 to 2008 [8], although GDP per capita increased from \$23,527 to \$51,186. We have reported that the number of publications in dermatology from mainland China, a developing country, markedly increased over the last 10 years, strongly correlating with GDP per capita. These results suggest that the correlation between the number of publications and GDP varies from country to country, and that the number of publications could remain relative stable, or even decline in well-developed countries, despite increases in GDP and/or overall funding for research. In the present study, we compared the characteristics of publications over ten year period in dermatology in mainland China, South Korea and Japan which represent developing, developed and well-developed countries, respectively, in Asia.

Methods

For publication searches, the internet address, http://www.ncbi.nlm.nih.gov/pubmed, was used to search articles in English from January 1, 2003 to December 31, 2012. The terms used to search each type of articles were listed in Table 1. Online Epub (ahead online electronically, but not yet printed) articles and papers published by authors not from each respective country were excluded. If publications were collaborated among countries, these papers were considered from all collaborating countries as long as the country names were listed in authors' affiliations. Meeting abstracts, announcements or papers without author list were not included. Papers identified as case report with review were considered as review articles. Since English is thought to be the universal scientific language [4], only papers published in English were included. Since China was used for the search term for publications from dermatology in mainland China, articles from dermatology inTaiwan, Hongkong and Macau were excluded from the search results. Because the number of published papers is usually proportional to data for gross domestic product per capita (GDPPC), GDPPC from 2002 to 2011 (since usually prior year fund supports current year production) also were obtained from

http://data.worldbank.org/indicator/NY.GDP.PCAP.CD. (Obtained on April 5, 2013).

There were some limitations in this study. For example, if either respective nation's name and/or dermatology were not listed as the authors' affiliations in papers, they would not be disclosed by the search terms in the present study.

Statistics

GraphPad Prism 4 software (San Diego, CA, USA) was used for all statistical analyses. Two-tailed nonparametric correlation and linear regression were used to determine significance.

Results

The number of annual publications increased linearly in Mainland China and South Korea, but not in Japan from 2003 to 2012

Dermatology in Japan published 4094 articles in 395 journals at an average of 10.37 articles per journal; 48% of papers were original research and 36% were case report (Table 2). Dermatology in mainland China published 1528 articles in 306 journals at an average of 4.99 articles per journal; 67% of papers were original research and 19% were case report (Table 2). A total of 1758 articles from dermatology in South Korea were published in 167 journals with an average of 10.53 articles per journal; 65% of papers were original research and 20% were case report (Table 2).

More than 50% of papers from South Korea and Japan were published in their favored10 journals (Table 3). Only 37% of articles from dermatology in mainland China were published in their favored 10 journals. In Japan, 23.55% of papers were published in Japanese journals, the Journal of Dermatology and the Journal of Dermatological Science. Likewise, the largest portion (30%) of articles from dermatology in South Korea was published in the Annals of Dermatology and the Journal of Korean Medical Science, both of which are Korean journals. In contrast, 9.2% of articles from dermatology in mainland China were published in the Chinese-owned journals, the Chinese Medical Journal and the Journal of Huazhong University of Science and Technology [Medical Sciences]. During this period, the Journal of Investigative Dermatology, the number one journal in dermatology field, published 209 articles from Japan, 34 from mainland China and 35 from South Korea.

The number of publications both in mainland China and South Korea rose linearly over the last 10 years, while the number of annual publications in Japan was similar during that period (Figure 1). Linear regression analysis showed that slopes for Japan, mainland China and South Korea were 1.05515, 29.67 and 24.93, respectively. Taken together with values of Y intercept for each

Table 1 Search terms used in the study

Types of articles searched	Search terms
All types of articles	Dermatology, Japan or China or Korea
Review	Review, Dermatology, Japan or China or Korea
Case report	Case report, Dermatology, Japan or China or Korea
Clinical trial	Clinical trial , dermatology, Japan or China or Korea
Meta-analysis and letter	Meta-analysis, letter, Dermatology, Japan or China or Korea
Randomized controlled trial	Randomized controlled trial, dermatology, Japan or China or Korea

Table 2 Characteristics of overall publications in each country over the last 10 years

Country	Number of publications (% of total publications)						
	Original research	Case report	Review	Clinical trial	Randomized controlled trial	Letter	Total
Japan	1978 (49.31%)	1468 (35.86%)	440 (10.75%)	143 (3.49%)	47 (1.15%)	18 (0.44%)	4094 (100%)
South Korea	1142 (64.96%)	351 (19.97%)	71 (4.04%)	129 (7.34%)	64 (3.64%)	1 (0.06%)	1758 (100%)
Mainland China	1022 (66.88%)	290 (18.98%)	90 (5.89%)	81 (5.3%)	18 (2.42%)	8 (0.52%)	1528 (100%)

country (1519 for Japan, -49880 for South Korea, and –59420 for mainland China), it was predicted that by middle of 2016 the number of publications in dermatology in mainland China would be comparable to that in Japan and the number of publications in dermatology in South Korea could catch Japan by early 2017.

Changes in the quality of publications from 2003 to 2012

Journal impact factors are often used to measure the quality of published research although only a small portion (25-30%) of publications in a journal can largely determine the impact factor for that journal [12-15]. We used the journals' impact factors to determine changes in the quality of publications in Japan and South Korea between 2003 and 2012. Since the average impact factors rose steadily from 2002 to 2011 in a developing country, mainland China [6], we next assessed whether the quality of publications in South Korea and Japan also improved over the last 10 years. For better comparison, data of impact factor per paper in dermatology in mainland China over this period were also added. As seen in Figure 2a, over the whole 10 year period the average impact factor per paper in Japan and mainland China increased significantly, while in South Korea the average impact factors per paper did not change significantly. It is worth noting that the average impact factor per paper

in both South Korea and Japan had tended to decline in the last 3 years. Since product quality can correlate negatively with quantity, we next correlated the average impact factor per paper with the number of papers. Indeed, the average impact factor per paper correlated negatively but weakly with the number of publications both in Japan and South Korea (Figure 2b). In contrast, in mainland China the average impact factor per paper correlated positively with the number of publications. These results suggest that remarkable improvement in publication quality occurs in developing country and publication quantity could trades for its quality in some countries.

The impact of economic conditions on publications between 2003 and 2012

Previous study showed that the number of publication correlated strongly with GDPPC in mainland China, a developing country in Asia [6]. We next determined whether GDPPC also influenced the quantity and quality of publications in South Korea and Japan, two developed countries in Asia. As seen in Figure 3a, GDPPCs in both Japan and South Korea increased linearly from 2002 to 2011. In contrast to the finding in developing country, mainland China [6], the number of publications did not correlate with the GDPPC in either Japan or South Korea

Table 3 Leading journals for each country from 2003 to 2012

Japan			South Korea			Mainland China		
Journals	Number of papers	% of total papers	Journals	Number of papers	% of total papers	Journals	Number of papers	% of total papers
J Dermatol.	695	16.98	Ann Dermatol	463	26.34	Chin Med J (Engl).	82	5.37
J Dermatol Sci.	269	6.57	Dermatol Surg.	131	7.47	Int J Dermatol.	82	5.37
Br J Dermatol	233	5.69	J Dermatol.	121	6.90	Clin Exp Dermatol	79	5.17
J Invest Dermatol	209	5.11	Int J Dermatol	74	4.22	Arch Dermatol Res.	60	3.93
Clin Exp Dermatol.	174	4.25	Br J Dermatol.	72	4.10	Br J Dermatol.	60	3.93
Eur J Dermatol.	148	3.62	J Korean Med Sci.	66	3.75	J Huazhong Univ Sci Technolog Med Sci.	59	3.86
Dermatology.	142	3.47	Clin Exp Dermatol	65	3.71	J Eur Acad Dermatol Venereol.	43	2.81
Int J Dermatol.	126	3.08	Exp Dermatol	46	2.62	Mycopathologia.	40	2.62
Arch Dermatol Res	109	2.66	J Am Acad Dermatol.	45	2.57	J Invest Dermatol.	34	2.23
J Am Acad Dermatol.	107	2.61	J Dermatol Sci.	39	2.22	Eur J Dermatol.	33	2.16
Total	2212	54.03	Total	1122	63.83	Total	572	37.43

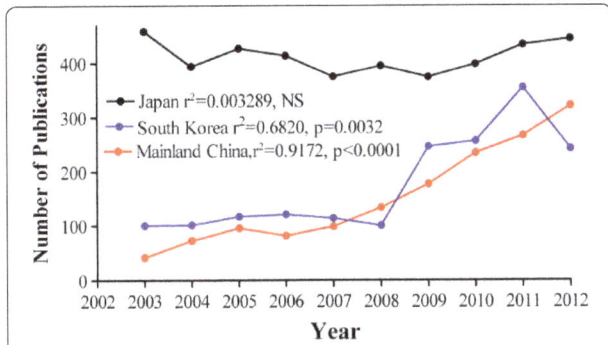

Figure 1 Changes in the number of publications from 2003 to 2012. Publication data were collected as described in materials and methods section. Linear regression was used to analyze the significance. Part of data (2003–2011) for mainland China was reported earlier [6].

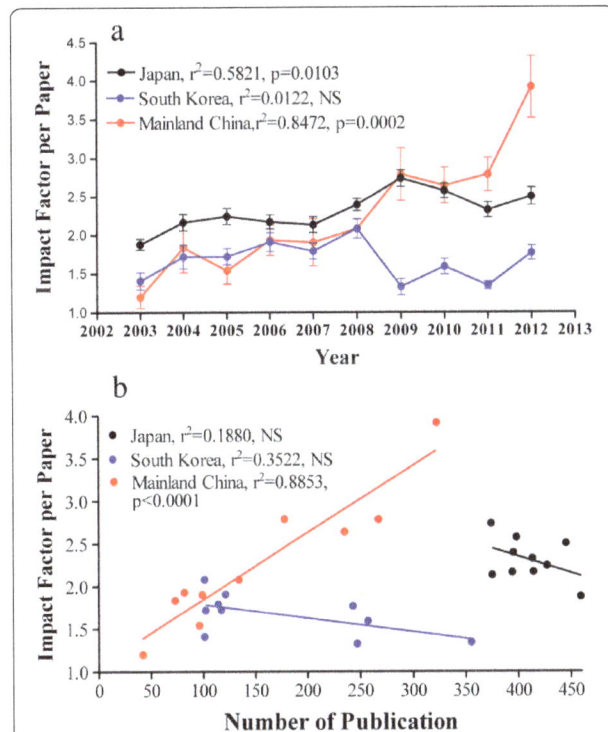

Figure 2 The changes of average impact factor per paper and their relationship to number of publications. Publication data were collected as described in materials and methods section. The impact factor per paper was calculated by dividing total impact factor by total number of published papers in each year. Linear regression was used to analyze the significant changes of impact factor per paper over the study period (Figure 2**a**). For correlation of impact factor per paper with the number of publication, Two-tailed Pearson test was used to determine significance (Figure 2**b**). Part of data (2003–2011) for mainland China in 3a was reported earlier [6].

(Figure 3b). The increased in GDPPC without increasing the number of publications could reflect an improvement in the quality of publications, as measured by impact factor per paper. Hence, we next correlated the average impact factor per paper with GDPPC. As seen in Figure 3c, the average impact factor per paper correlated positively and strongly with GDPPC in mainland China, weakly in Japan, but not in South Korea. The results indicate that economic conditions significantly impact both the quantity and quality of publications in dermatology in developing country, not developed countries in Asia.

To further reveal the impact of economic conditions on the number of publications in dermatology, changes in number of publication per GDPPC over the last 10 years were analyzed. The results showed that the number of publication per GDPPC in mainland China slightly increased over the last 10 years and was higher than that in Japan and South Korea (Figure 3d). A significant increase in the number of publication per GDPPC was observed in South Korea over this period. However, the number of publication per GDPPC in Japan declined significantly. These results demonstrate that mainland China, a developing country, yields higher number of publication per GDPPC in dermatology and further confirm that the impact of GDPPC on publications varies with nations.

Discussion

In the present study, we compared the publication trends in dermatology in developing, developed and well-developed countries in Asia. Dermatology in Japan, the well-developed country, published papers more than the total of mainland China and South Korea over the last 10 years. It is reported that the number of publications in dermatology has been increasing yearly in both developing and developed countries [6,16] and the increase in the number of publications is associated with improvement of economic conditions [1,6,17]. In contrast, the present study revealed that the number of publications in dermatology in Japan remained unchanged from 2003 to 2012 despite the linearly increase of GDPPC. This result is consistent with the observation in other developed countries such as Sweden and Norway where the number of publications in dermatology was relatively stable from 1989 to 2008 [8]. But overall the number of publications in mainland China and South Korea increased over the last 10 years. These data suggest that well-developed countries can reach maximum research productivity in dermatology and GDPPC may no longer be the key determinant that influences the number of publications. In contrast to the number of publications, the impact factor per paper in Japan increased from 2003 to 2012. Although GDPPC did not correlated with the number of publications at all, the quality of publications was likely associated with GDPPC. Coupling with the findings that the number of publications slightly and reversely

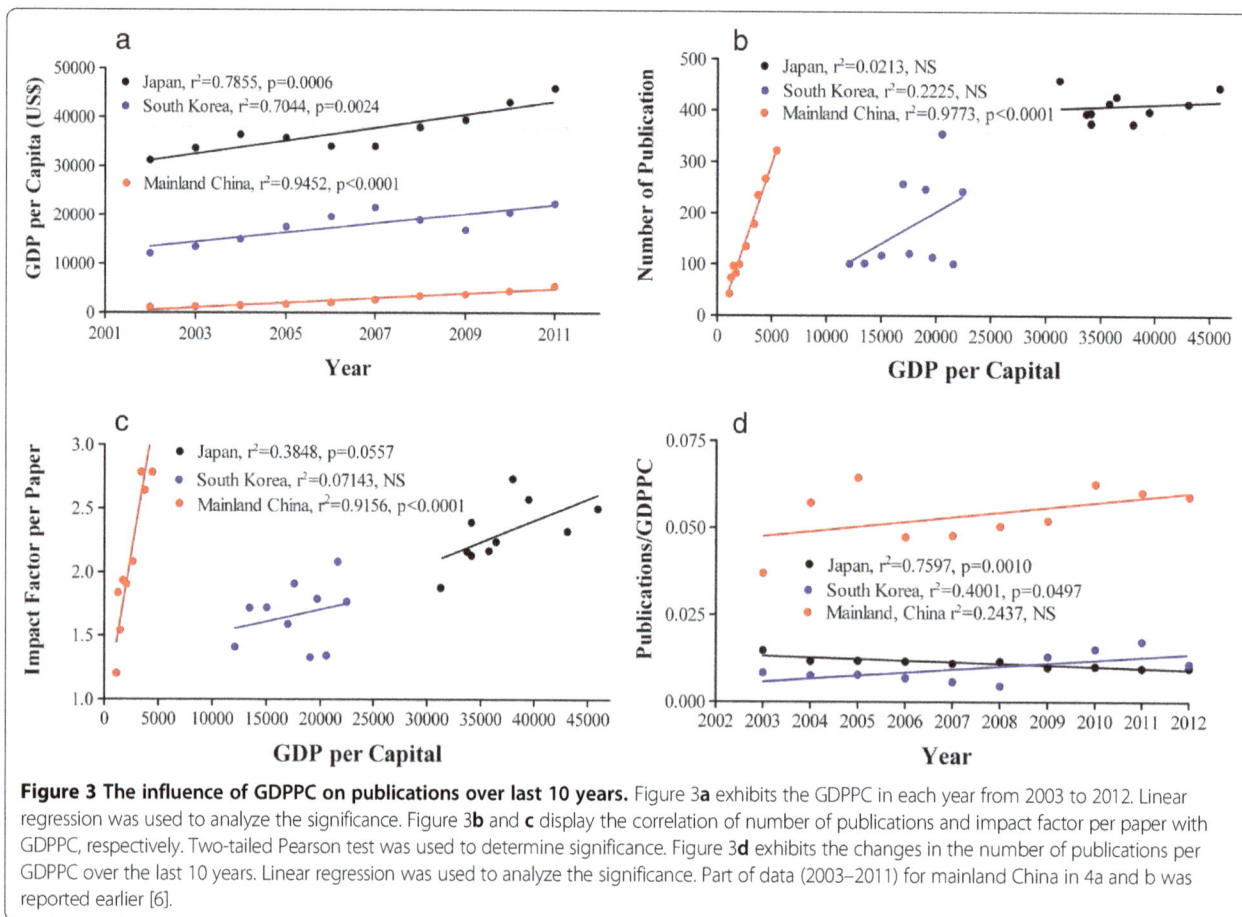

Figure 3 The influence of GDPPC on publications over last 10 years. Figure 3**a** exhibits the GDPPC in each year from 2003 to 2012. Linear regression was used to analyze the significance. Figure 3**b** and **c** display the correlation of number of publications and impact factor per paper with GDPPC, respectively. Two-tailed Pearson test was used to determine significance. Figure 3**d** exhibits the changes in the number of publications per GDPPC over the last 10 years. Linear regression was used to analyze the significance. Part of data (2003–2011) for mainland China in 4a and b was reported earlier [6].

correlated with impact factor per paper, it suggests that dermatology researchers in Japan sacrifice publication quantity for quality. Therefore, the impact of GDPPC on dermatology research in Japan reflected in linearly increase of impact factor per paper from 2003 to 2012. Another potential factor refraining Japan from increasing the number of publications could be the stable population. It has been reported that the number of publications correlates with population [1]. The change in population was negligible in Japan from 2002 to 2011 (from 127445000 in 2002 to 127817277 in 2011, 0.29% increase; data were from http://data.worldbank.org/indicator/SP.POP.TOTL.). Thus, the changes of article number were marginal over the last 10 years. Regarding the decreased number of publications per GDPPC from 2003 to 2012, it could result from improved publication quality. Nevertheless, the present study indicates that the quality of publications in Japan improved from 2003 to 2012 although the quantity remains unchanged.

South Korea is a developed country in Asia. The number of publications dramatically increased in the last 10 years. There was a big increase in the number of publications in 2009 when a significant drop in impact factor per paper occurred. These changes could represent an

example of trade-off between quantity and quality. The sudden increase of publication in 2009 could be also ascribed to the sharp addition of papers (over 40%) published in Annals of Dermatology, which was first indexed in PubMed in 2009. The overall increase of publications over the last 10 years could be attributed to both improved economic condition and increased population (from 47622000 in 2002 to 49779000 in 2011, 4.53% increase). GDPPC did not correlate with either the quantity or the quality of publications over the last 10 years in South Korea.

Both the quantity and the quality of publications in dermatology in mainland China were remarkably improved over the last 10 years. In addition to economic condition, manpower, language skills and promotion requirement [6], incentive award programs could also motivate researchers to publish more papers, especially in the journals with higher impact factor. Some institutions offer as much as 10,000 yuan RMB (about US$1,500) per impact factor for those papers published in high impact journals. Additionally, some institutions in mainland China use impact factors to determine the employment and promotion. Thus, incentive award programs and professional career requirement would definitely stimulate scientific research productivity, including dermatology research, in mainland China. In contrast to developed countries in Asia, GDPPC strongly correlate with both the quantity and the quality of publications in dermatology in mainland China.

Notably dermatology in both South Korea and Japan published significant portion of their papers in their top 10 favored journals. This is in agreement with those finding in mainland China [6]. However, the average number of papers per journal was much lower in mainland China (4.9 papers/journal) than in South Korea (10.53 papers/journal) and Japan (10.37 papers/journal). This may reflect that mainland China has a larger number of dermatologists and the broader range of research interests than South Korea and Japan.

In the present study, there are some limitations for using impact factor as a tool measuring the publication quality. First of all, although the impact factor usually represents the quality of a journal, approximately only 25% of papers largely determine the impact factor for a journal [12-15]. This means that not all papers published in journals with higher impact factor have higher impact. It is not uncommon that articles published in journals with lower impact factor have higher citations. Secondly, sometimes where to publish papers depends on the authors' preference. Likewise, the acceptance of a manuscript could mainly rely on editor and reviewers' preferences. For example, the present study revealed that authors in dermatology in South Korea prefer to publish their papers in the Annals of Dermatology and authors in dermatology in Japan prefer to publish their papers in the Journal of Dermatology. Finally, there are many factors such as the number of papers published by the journal, study field and type of articles that could affect journal impact factor [18]. Thus, impact factor may not truly reflect the impact or quality of every paper and extra caution should be taken when average impact factor per paper are compared between countries.

Conclusions

The present study shows that the publication characteristics in dermatology over the last 10 years vary among developing, developed and well-developed country in Asia. The results also suggest that the quality of dermatology research could reversely correlate with quantity.

Competing interests
All authors declare that they have no competing interests.

Authors' contributions
MH, XS, BW and LC collected and organized data from pubmed website; MMQ made figures and write draft; MTM and EPM helped design and critically reviewed manuscript. All authors read and approved the final manuscript.

Acknowledgement
This work was partially supported by grants (AR19089, PEM; AR051930, TM) from the National Institutes of Health.

Author details
[1]Wendeng Central Hospital, Shandong, P.R. China. [2]The Center for Skin Physiology Research, Dalian Skin Disease Hospital, Liaoning 116021, P.R. China. [3]Dermatology Service, Veterans Affairs Medical Center, San Francisco, CA, USA. [4]Department of Dermatology, University of California, 4150 Clement Street, San Francisco, CA 94121, USA.

References
1. Tasli L, Kacar N, Aydemir EH: Scientific productivity of OECD countries in dermatology journals within the last 10-year period. *Intl J Dermatol* 2012, **51**:665–671.
2. Lewison G: Gastroenterology research in the United Kingdom: funding sources and impact. *Gut* 1998, **43**:288–293.
3. Belinchon I, Ramos JM, Sanchez-Yus E, Betlloch I: Dermatological scientific production from European Union authors (1987–2000). *Scientometrics* 2004, **61**:271–281.
4. Cimmino MA, Maio T, Ugolini D, Borasi F, Mela GS: Trends in otolaryngology research during the period 1995–2000: a bibliometric approach. *Otolaryngol Head Neck Surg* 2005, **132**:295–302.
5. Jemec GB, Nybaek H: A bibliometric study of dermatology in central Europe 1991–2002. *Int J Dermatol* 2006, **45**:922–926.
6. Xin SJ, Mauro JA, Mauro TM, Elias PM, Man MQ: 10 year publication trends in dermatology in Mainland China. *Int J Dermatol* 2013. doi: 10.1111/ijd.12272.
7. Brambrink AM, Ehrler D, Dick WF: Publications on paediatric anaesthesia: a quantitative analysis of publication activity and international recognition. *Br J Anaesth* 2000, **85**:556–562.
8. Gjersvik P, Nylenna M, Jemec GB, Haraldstad AM: Dermatologic research in the Nordic countries 1989–2008–a bibliometric study. *Int J Dermatol* 2010, **49**:1276–1281.
9. Bovier PA, Guillain H, Perneger TV: Productivity of medical research in Switzerland. *J Investig Med* 2001, **49**:77–84.
10. Schwinn DA, Balser JR: Anesthesiology physician scientists in academic medicine: a wake-up call. *Anesthesiology* 2006, **104**:170–178.
11. Pagel PS, Hudetz JA: Recent trends in publication of basic science and clinical research by United States investigators in anesthesia journals. *BMC Anesthesiol* 2012, **12**:5.
12. Not-so-deep impact. *Nature* 2005, **435**:1003–1004. doi:10.1038/4351003b
13. Dissecting our impact factor. *Nat Mater* 2011, **10**:645. doi:10.1038/nmat3114
14. Saha S, Saint S, Christakis DA: Impact factor: a valid measure of journal quality? *J Med Libr Assoc* 2003, **91**:42–46.
15. Rezaei-Ghaleh N, Azizi F: The impact factor-based quality assessment of biomedical research institutes in Iran: effect of impact factor normalization by subject. *Arch Iran Med* 2007, **10**:182–189.
16. Mimouni D, Pavlovsky L, Akerman L, David M, Mimouni FB: Trends in dermatology publications over the past 15 years. *Am J Clin Dermatol* 2010, **11**:55–58.
17. Rahman M, Fukui T: Biomedical research productivity: factors across the countries. *Int J Technol Assess Health Care* 2003, **19**:249–252.
18. Amin M, Mabe MA: Impact factors: use and abuse. *Medicina (B Aires)* 2003, **63**:347–354.

Single application of 4% dimeticone liquid gel versus two applications of 1% permethrin creme rinse for treatment of head louse infestation: a randomised controlled trial

Ian F Burgess[*], Elizabeth R Brunton and Nazma A Burgess

Abstract

Background: A previous study indicated that a single application of 4% dimeticone liquid gel was effective in treating head louse infestation. This study was designed to confirm this in comparison with two applications of 1% permethrin.

Methods: We have performed a single centre parallel group, randomised, controlled, open label, community based trial, with domiciliary visits, in Cambridgeshire, UK. Treatments were allocated through sealed instructions derived from a computer generated list. We enrolled 90 children and adults with confirmed head louse infestation analysed by intention to treat (80 per-protocol after 4 drop outs and 6 non-compliant). The comparison was between 4% dimeticone liquid gel applied once for 15 minutes and 1% permethrin creme rinse applied for 10 minutes, repeated after 7 days as per manufacturer's directions. Evaluated by elimination of louse infestation after completion of treatment application regimen.

Results: Intention to treat comparison of a single dimeticone liquid gel treatment with two of permethrin gave success for 30/43 (69.8%) of the dimeticone liquid gel group and 7/47 (14.9%) of the permethrin creme rinse group (OR 13.19, 95% CI 4.69 to 37.07) ($p < 0.001$). Per protocol results were similar with 27/35 (77.1%) success for dimeticone versus 7/45 (15.6%) for permethrin. Analyses by household gave essentially similar outcomes.

Conclusions: The study showed one 15 minute application of 4% dimeticone liquid gel was superior to two applications of 1% permethrin creme rinse ($p < 0.001$). The low efficacy of permethrin suggests it should be withdrawn.

Keywords: Dimeticone, Head lice, Insecticides, Pediculosis, Permethrin, Physical mode of action, Treatment regimen

Background

In Europe control of head louse infestation is now mainly achieved by use of physically acting preparations [1]. The majority of these are based on the polydimethysiloxane, known as dimeticone. This compound exists in a variety of forms from the volatile hexamethyldisiloxane, with a viscosity of just 0.65 centistokes (cSt) through to high molecular weight gums with a viscosity of several million cSt. The level of polymerisation during manufacture results in a range of materials with such variable physical characteristics that selection of the right molecular weight and viscosity is potentially critical for gaining maximum effectiveness in this application.

The first dimeticone based product was Hedrin 4% lotion, approved as a medicine for sale in the UK in 2005, which used dimeticone of 100K cSt viscosity in a decamethylcyclopentasiloxane (cyclomethicone D5) volatile fluid vehicle. This product is also widely used in Europe, mostly as a class I medical device, and has been shown efficacious in several clinical field studies [2-4]. Since that time variant formulations have been developed

* Correspondence: ian@insectresearch.com
Medical Entomology Centre, Insect Research & Development Limited, 6 Quy Court, Colliers Lane, Stow-cum-Quy, Cambridge CB25 9AU, UK

in order to improve handling and application of the product and also the cosmetic characteristics.

The original 4% dimeticone lotion is applied for 8 hours or overnight on two occasions a week apart. Subsequent investigations both in the laboratory and in clinical trials have looked at shorter application times for this product and for the variants. One recently described study outcome found that no lice of any development stage were present following the first application of product in a two treatment regimen using a 15 minutes exposure time for a spray gel variant [5]. This report describes the first study investigating the efficacy of a single application regimen for Hedrin 4% dimeticone liquid gel, tested in a comparison trial against two applications of 1% permethrin creme rinse.

Methods

Participants

We recruited participants mostly through contact with families who had expressed a wish to be involved in research and advertising on local radio and in parish magazines. An information booklet was sent to each family and an appointment arranged for an investigator to visit. All household members were offered screening for head lice using a standard detection comb ("PDC", KSL Consulting, Denmark). The intensity of infestation was graded as heavy, medium, or light using criteria employed in previous studies [2-4].

We also used eligibility criteria from previous studies [2-4], excluding those with known sensitivity to treatment components or long terms scalp conditions other than lice, those treated for lice within 2 weeks previously, and who had used hair bleach, dyes, or permanent waves, or had been treated with trimethoprim containing preparations within the last month. Pregnancy, breast feeding, participation in another clinical study within 4 weeks or prior participation in the current study, were also grounds for exclusion. All eligible family members could be enrolled and on agreement were conducted through a standard informed consent and assent procedure. The practical lower age limit was 2 years although approval for the products was as young as 6 months. There was no upper age limit.

Demographic data were collected after consent was taken, including gender, age, hair characteristics, and appointments made for subsequent assessment and treatment visits. No payment was offered for participation. Ineligible household members with lice were offered standard of care treatment using 4% dimeticone liquid gel to minimise reinfestation of study participants.

Ethics

Ethical approval was granted by Central London Research Ethics Committee 2 (EudraCT 2011-000257-23).

The study was conducted in compliance with Good Clinical Practices, and conformity with the principles of the Declaration of Helsinki and of European Union Directive 2001/20/EC. All participants received study information at least 24 hours before enrolment and all stated that they understood the purpose and requirements of the investigation before giving consent. Parents or guardians gave written consent for children younger than 16 years and children also provided written assent, where able to do so, witnessed by the parent or guardian.

Treatments

The products used for this randomised controlled trial were different in both appearance and method of application so blinding at the time of treatment was not possible.

4% dimeticone liquid gel (Hedrin Once liquid gel, Thornton & Ross Ltd, Huddersfield, UK) contains 4% high molecular weight dimeticone, 1,6,10-dodecatrien-3-ol,3,7,11-trimethyl, PEG/PPG dimeticone co-polymer, and silica silylate. It was supplied in 150mL polyethylene bottles and applied systematically to dry hair over the whole scalp using the inbuilt dropper cap. In each case the investigators spread the fluid through the hair using their fingers to ensure thorough coverage. The product was applied once for 15 minutes and then washed out using shampoo and water.

1% permethrin creme rinse (Lyclear creme rinse, Omega Pharma UK, London, UK) contains 1% permethrin in a conditioner base with 20% isopropanol. It was supplied in 59mL HDPE bottles with a flip cap. It was applied liberally to shampoo washed and towel dried hair. Investigators ensured that all parts of the hair and scalp were thoroughly coated, which in most cases required more than one bottle. This product was applied for 10 minutes on two occasions 7 days apart followed by rinsing with water only.

In each case parent/guardians were advised of the time to wash the treatments off. Use of nit combs or other pediculicides during the course of the studies was not permitted.

Outcome measures

The primary outcome measure was elimination of infestation after completion of the treatment regimen. Following treatment on Day 0 we performed follow-ups on Days 1, 6, 9, and 14 by dry detection combing using the "PDC" comb to assess the efficacy of treatment. If any lice were found they were fixed in the case record and the development stage subsequently recorded.

Outcomes of treatment were classified as cure, reinfestation following cure, or treatment failure (with a sub-category for ovicidal failure). Because one of the treatments in this study used one application only we found it necessary to redraft the algorithm used in previous studies for determining outcome criteria.

Sample size

We anticipated that there was likely to be a disparity in efficacy between dimeticone liquid gel and permethrin creme rinse, based on previous data. Consequently, it was possible that, if different members of a family were randomly allocated different treatments, those receiving the more effective preparation could be reinfested from those receiving the less effective product. Although the protocol allowed for identification of reinfestation at a low level it could not address problems resulting from heavy reinfestation. Therefore a different randomisation model was employed in which all members of a household received the same treatment allocation, with randomisation by family rather than by individual.

An analysis of the variance of the cure rates in relation to household sizes was made using data from previous studies and from this we estimated that the number of participants required using the randomise-by-family approach was higher than the number required using the randomise-by-individual approach (assuming independence and ignoring dropout) by a factor of 1.46.

For a randomise-by-individual approach, assuming a confidence level of 95% and a power of 95%, and conservatively taking the expected cure rates to be 90% for dimeticone liquid gel and 50% for permethrin creme rinse, we estimated the required sample size as 29 participants per treatment. Under the same assumptions, the required number of participants per treatment under the randomise-by-family approach was 42, equivalent to an estimated 22 families per treatment.

Randomisation and blinding

The randomised treatment allocation sequence was derived using a free to access online computer generated list from http://www.randomization.com (seed 25270, 22nd June 2011). Allocation at the point of delivery was made from instruction sheets enclosed in opaque, sealed, sequentially numbered envelopes distributed to investigators in balanced blocks of eight. Participant families were allocated the next available numbered envelope held by the investigator. Investigators conducting follow up visits were separate from those involved in treatment and thus remained blind of treatment allocation.

Statistical analysis

We conducted analyses based on both the "intention-to-treat" (ITT) and the "per-protocol" (PP) populations. Differences between groups in baseline characteristics, safety, acceptability, and efficacy were tested using Fisher's exact test for yes/no variables and the Mann–Whitney U test for ranked variables. Where analyses showed important differences in baseline characteristics between the groups, chi-squared and rank tests stratified for these characteristics were conducted and 95% confidence limits presented for the difference between groups in the primary endpoint.

Results

Participants

Ninety participants from 44 households were enrolled between 1st July and 3rd November 2011, of whom four participants in two households later dropped out or were lost to follow up (Figure 1). A further six participants completed the study but were non-compliant, either combing out lice (five participants) or out of time on one assessment visit (one participant). Therefore the ITT population analysed was 90, but as a result of the protocol violations the per-protocol population was 80 across 40 households broken down as follows: dimeticone liquid gel = 35 participants from 20 households; permethrin creme rinse = 45 from 20 households.

Baseline characteristics were recorded for all participants at Day 0 of whom 73 (81.1%) were female and ranged from 2 to 45 years in age, mean age 11.7 years. The 44 households, varied in size from 2 to 9 occupants (mean 4.39). Numbers of participants per household were: 1 (17 households), 2 (16 households), 3 (6 households), 4 (3 households), 5 or 6 participants (1 household each). Of the 90 participants, the initial infestation was classified as "light" in 52, "moderate" in 17 and "heavy" in 21. There was no difference between treatments in this characteristic.

Consistent with the large proportion of females in the study, the proportion with hair "ears to shoulders" or "below shoulders" was very high (89.3% in the dimeticone group and 84.9% in the permethrin group). There were similarly high numbers of participants with "thick" hair (61.7% and 53.8% respectively). Both groups had approximately 37% of participants with "wavy" or "slightly curly" hair, which is a recently observed increased trend toward "wavy" hair compared with older studies. Only a small proportion of participants had hair that was dry (7.4%) or oily (8.1%).

Outcomes

The Day 1 analyses included all 90 participants; Day 6 analyses related to 89 participants following a drop out, with a subsequent drop out of 2 other participants from the same household so that 87 participants remained on Day 9. The Day 14 analyses included 86 participants due to one lost to follow up, with exclusion of a further 6 participants from the PP analyses for protocol violations.

For the intention to treat outcomes by individual, we conducted an endpoint analysis of rate of cure (or exceptionally cure followed by reinfestation as defined by

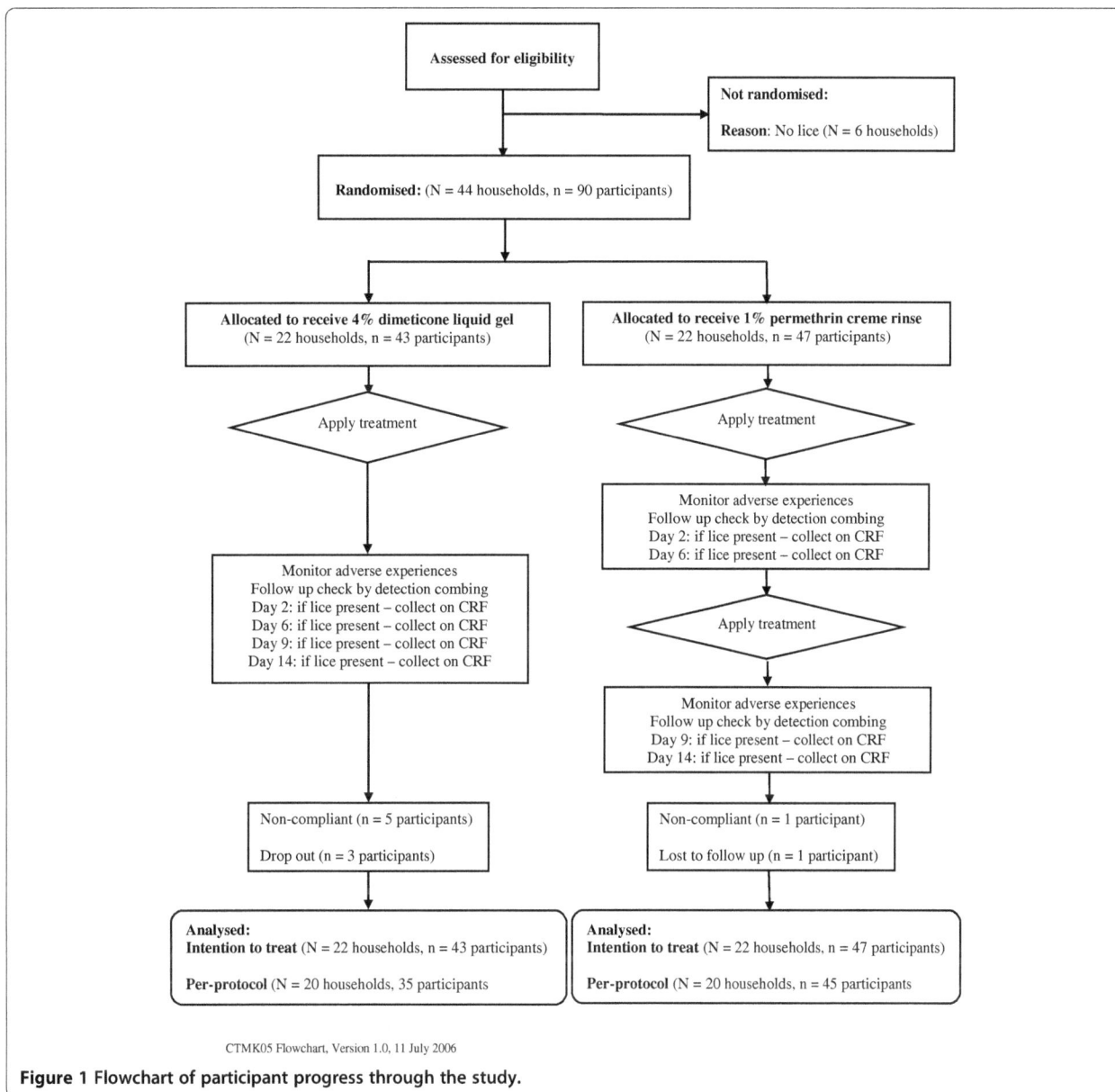

Figure 1 Flowchart of participant progress through the study.

algorithm) in the 90 participants in the ITT population. According to these criteria, success was achieved overall by 30/43 (69.8%) for dimeticone liquid gel group (26 cure, 4 reinfestation) and by 7/47 (14.9%) for the permethrin creme rinse group (6 cure, 1 reinfestation). The difference in rate of success between the dimeticone and permethrin groups was estimated as 54.9% (95% CI of 35% to 75%) (OR 13.19, 95% CI 4.69 to 37.07) which meant that there was a highly significant ($p < 0.001$) superiority of dimeticone liquid gel compared with permethrin creme rinse in the population tested. Dimeticone liquid gel not only showed a high ovicidal effect, as judged by not finding young nymphs following the single application of the product (32 participants),

but also a high proportion were entirely louse free throughout (the "cure" group of 26 participants) (Table 1). In contrast, nearly all participants in the permethrin group were found to have newly hatched nymphs at some point in the study, showing the product has a low capacity to inhibit eggs from hatching in addition to any impact on efficacy resulting from insecticide resistance (Table 2).

We obtained per-protocol outcomes by individual by elimination of protocol violators from the analysis to give PP success rates of 27/35 (77.1%) for the dimeticone liquid gel group (25 cure, 2 reinfestation) and 7/45 (15.6%) for the permethrin creme rinse group (6 cure, 1 reinfestation), giving an advantage of 61.6% (95% CI,

Table 1 Comparison of outcomes by participant – 4% dimeticone versus 1% permethrin

Outcome measurement	4% Dimeticone		1% Permethrin		P value
ITT analysis					
Number of households	22		22		
Number of participants	43		47		
Cure or cure followed by reinfestation	30	69.8%	7	14.9%	< 0.001
Relative success rate (95% CI)			4.68 (2.30 – 9.35)		
Cure	26	60.5%	6	12.8%	< 0.001
Inhibition of egg hatching	32	74.4%	6	12.8%	< 0.001
PP analysis					
Number of households	20		20		
Number of participants	35		45		
Cure or cure followed by reinfestation	27	77.1%	7	15.6%	< 0.001
Relative success rate (95% CI)			4.96 (2.45 – 10.03)		
Cure	26	71.4%	6	13.3%	< 0.001
Inhibition of egg hatching	30	85.7%	6	10.6%	< 0.001

40% to 80%) (OR 18.32, 95% CI 5.93 to 56.6) for the dimeticone treatment over permethrin, which was also highly significant (p < 0.001).

Using the same approach in the analysis of outcome by household, the advantage to dimeticone liquid gel

Table 2 Numbers of lice recovered – 4% dimeticone versus 1% permethrin

Endpoint	Lice collected			
	Day 1	Day 6	Day 9	Day 14
4% Dimeticone liquid gel				
Number of participants combed	43	42	40	40
Number of participants with lice	3	4	8	12
Total lice removed	3	27	24	45
Stage 1 nymphs removed	1	5	5	2
Stage 2 nymphs removed	2	18	8	10
Stage 3 nymphs removed	0	2	7	7
Adult males removed	0	0	2	9
Adult females removed	0	2	2	17
Participants louse free (%) ITT	**93.0%**	**90.5%**	**80.0%**	**70.0%**
Participants louse free (%) PP	**97.1%**	**94.3%**	**82.9%**	**77.1%**
1% Permethrin creme rinse				
Number of participants combed	47	47	47	46
Number of participants with lice	29	37	30	38
Total lice removed	359	741	259	375
Stage 1 nymphs removed	222	405	63	40
Stage 2 nymphs removed	18	204	46	51
Stage 3 nymphs removed	24	67	81	54
Adult males removed	23	17	27	91
Adult females removed	72	48	42	139
Participants louse free (%) ITT	**38.3%**	**21.3%**	**36.2%**	**17.4%**
Participants louse free (%) PP	**37.8%**	**20.0%**	**37.8%**	**17.7%**

was similar (p < 0.01 or p < 0.001) for all the outcomes, equivalent to a relative total success rate of 6.50 (95% confidence interval (CI) 1.66 to 25.5), or an odds ratio (OR) of 14.4 (95% CI 2.68 to 77.8), reflecting the difference of risk for a whole household compared with that for an individual.

All participants received the required number of treatments. Dimeticone liquid gel was given once, and the mean total product used was 63.91g (equivalent approximate cost = €6.20-€7.40). Permethrin creme rinse was given twice, and each treatment often involved two bottles and occasionally three. Over the two treatments combined, the mean number of bottles of creme rinse used per family member was 3.31, and the mean total product used, 141.58g (equivalent approximate cost = €8.30-€16.60), which was significantly (p < 0.001) more than for dimeticone.

Adverse events
Members of seven families experienced one or more adverse events, nine people treated with permethrin and eight with dimeticone. Only two people had an adverse event that was considered possibly related to treatment. One was a rash on the back of the neck following each treatment with permethrin creme rinse and the other, dry skin, following dimeticone liquid gel. There were no serious adverse events.

Discussion
It has long been considered that longer application times when using head louse treatment lotions are more effective than shorter applications. This was demonstrated *in vitro* using insecticide based products in which the formulation vehicle evaporates and concentrates the active material on the louse surface. The same approach

was initially taken with physically acting preparations such as 4% dimeticone lotion and preliminary results from a first small study did indicate that an 8 hour or overnight treatment was more effective than one of only 20 minutes [2]. However, in a later study we found that, contrary to expectation, reducing the application time for 4% dimeticone spray gel to 15 minutes not only increased the effectiveness but appeared to be wholly effective with a single application [5].

Although the majority action of 4% dimeticone lotion is derived from the dimeticone being deposited in the insect spiracular and tracheal systems, resulting in blocking of water excretion [6], it is necessary for it to be carried there by the solvent component of the product. If the solvent does not deliver sufficient dimeticone to the target site the activity may be reduced.

The perceived advantage of the 4% dimeticone gel over the original 4% lotion is that the gel seems to adhere to the lice more effectively and, in the spray form, is easier to direct and control ensuring all lice are killed and those eggs close to hatching are inhibited from doing so, as was demonstrated in our earlier study in which the product gave 100% efficacy after the first application in that two application trial [5]. In this study, most lice found by investigators during follow up assessments could be attributed to eggs that hatched after treatment, presumably because they had been missed as a result of inadequate spreading of the liquid gel using the dropper bottle. Some of the children had also been observed to present with hair dampened by sweat at the time of the treatment application, which may have acted as a barrier to the silicones forming a complete coating on some louse eggs, with the possible result that silicone was not able to reach the vulnerable surfaces of the eggs due to the presence of a water film. The four infestations in the ITT group without nymphs were all attributable to reinfestation from contacts either within the family or the local community.

This randomised controlled trial has clearly demonstrated a difference in overall activity between a physically acting preparation using a single application and two applications of an insecticide based product affected by insecticide resistance. Hitherto, the majority of claims that different products containing silicones, and other physically acting preparations, are effective with a single application have not been based on published clinical data but have been extrapolations either from *in vitro* data or else obtained in studies where the products were applied twice. This study has not only confirmed efficacy for a single application of Hedrin 4% dimeticone liquid gel, and demonstrated a difference in overall activity between a physically acting preparation and an insecticide based product affected by insecticide resistance, but has also demonstrated that extrapolations about treatment

outcomes may be misleading, in the absence of clinical confirmation.

This trial has also provided the first clear evidence that louse eggs do not all hatch within 7 days (Table 2). We and many other investigators in the past had assumed this hatching period primarily because previously we had no other experimental evidence upon which to base a conclusion. We found from our earlier double application study [5] that this does not necessarily constitute a significant problem for treatment because any lice hatching from eggs after a first treatment appear to be killed by a second treatment at 7 days. A treatment given at that time delivers more of the active material to any unhatched eggs, which further inhibits their chances of hatching. However, this information that eggs can take longer than one week to hatch emphasises the need for vigilance in confirming whether a treatment has been effective, by detection combing after completion of the treatment regimen, and also confirms the need for adequate application technique [7]. So, just because more than 90% of people appear louse free 2 days after a second treatment it does not mean that further checks are not necessary as some viable eggs may remain.

Although numerous lice were eliminated using the 1% permethrin creme rinse at each of the treatment applications, more than 60% of participants received no respite from infestation and, of those who appeared louse free one or two days after treatment, fewer than half were cured of their infestation, even though we used more than twice the supposedly adequate application dose on each participant. Why then did we choose 1% permethrin as the comparator product rather than some alternative preparation? The reason 1% permethrin was used in this study was to provide data in comparison with a known medicinal product for those territories where such data are required by decision makers before issuing approvals. On this basis the number of possible comparators is extremely limited because most products have a limited geographic distribution. The only other insecticide active used widely is 0.5% malathion but this was not selected because the range of formulations used in different territories are not comparable even within themselves (shampoos, alcohol based lotions with or without terpenoids added, and water based emulsions). Additionally, the one product still listed in the UK was not available at the time the study was conducted.

The outcome using permethrin mirrors closely the findings of a previous investigation comparing treatments using this product with and without combing [8], and also reflects the outcome found in other studies. Given the number of investigations in which permethrin and other insecticide products have delivered an unacceptably low efficacy [3,8-12], a review of the licensing of these preparations appears long overdue. It is understandable that sponsors may wish to use insecticide based products as comparators in clinical studies because they have a long history of use and are familiar to the decision makers within the various health services where the profile of new products needs to be raised. However, we have found that ethics review boards are increasingly reluctant to authorise their use in clinical investigations primarily because their efficacy is not much greater than using a placebo. Therefore, as long as these products retain a marketing authorisation, and the validity of this is not reviewed by the various competent authorities, consumers and prescribers will continue to use ineffective products. Consequently, now is probably the time for such a review to take place and for insecticide products to be removed from the market simply because so many treatments fail.

Conclusions

This study has shown that a single application of 4% dimeticone liquid gel is effective to eliminate head louse infestation and that the higher viscosity of this product allows this to be achieved using a treatment time of 15 minutes. However, as with all treatments, it is possible to miss some louse eggs during treatment, requiring post treatment vigilance for emerging nymphs more than 7 days after treatment.

Competing interests
IFB has been a consultant to Thornton & Ross Ltd, the sponsor of this study and manuscript, and to various other makers of pharmaceutical products, medical devices, and combs for treating infestations of head lice and their eggs. ERB and NAB declare no competing interests in this work.

Authors' contributions
IFB, ERB, NAB collectively conceived, designed, and carried out the investigation. IFB performed some analyses of the data and wrote the draft manuscript. ERB managed the documentation of the study. NAB collected data. All authors read and approved the final manuscript.

Acknowledgements
This study was sponsored by Thornton & Ross Ltd, Huddersfield, UK. The sponsor played no role in the study design, its execution, interpretation of the data, or the preparation of the manuscript. Statistical analyses were performed on behalf of the sponsor by Peter Lee of PN Lee Statistics and Computing Ltd, an independent statistical consultancy. Some treatments and assessments were performed by Audrey Pepperman, and assessments by Benedict Hall and Rebecca French. Product use and storage conditions for investigational product were monitored by Mark N Burgess. Dr Paul Silverston evaluated adverse events and acted as the medical contact throughout the course of the study. Katharine Coombs and Yvonne Cooper entered the data for statistical analysis and Dr. John Fry provided statistical assistance and review. The documents and conduct of Good Clinical Practice for this clinical trial were monitored by Janet Selby-Sievewright of Harrison Clinical Research Ltd.

References
1. Heukelbach J, Oliveira FA, Richter J, Häussinger D: **Dimeticone-based pediculicides: a physical approach to eradicate head lice.** *Open Dermatol J* 2010, **4**:77–81.
2. Burgess IF, Brown CM, Lee PN: **Treatment of head louse infestation with 4% dimeticone lotion: randomised controlled equivalence trial.** *BMJ* 2005, **330**:1423–1425.
3. Burgess IF, Lee PN, Matlock G: **Randomised, controlled, assessor blind trial comparing 4% dimeticone lotion with 0.5% malathion liquid for head louse infestation.** *PLoS ONE* 2007, **2**(11):e1127.
4. Kurt O, Balcioglu IC, Burgess IF, Limoncu ME, Girginkardesler N, Tabak T, Muslu H, Ermis O, Sahin MT, Bilac C, Kavur H, Ozbel Y: **Treatment of head lice with dimeticone 4% lotion: comparison of two formulations in a randomised controlled trial in rural Turkey.** *BMC Public Health* 2009, **9**:441.
5. Burgess IF, Burgess NA: **Dimeticone 4% liquid gel found to kill all lice and eggs with a single 15 minute application.** *BMC Res Notes* 2011, **4**:15.
6. Burgess IF: **The mode of action of dimeticone 4% lotion against head lice. Pediculus capitis.** *BMC Pharmacol* 2009, **9**:3.
7. Barker SC, Burgess I, Meinking TL, Mumcuoglu KY: **International guidelines for clinical trials with pediculicides.** *Int J Dermatol* 2012, **51**:853–858.
8. Meinking TL, Clineschmidt CM, Chen C, Kolber MA, Tipping RW, Furtek CI, Villar ME, Guzzo CA: **An observer-blinded study of 1% permethrin crème rinse with and without adjunctive combing in patients with head lice.** *J Pediatr* 2002, **141**:665–670.
9. Burgess IF, Lee PN, Brown CM: **Randomised, controlled, parallel group clinical trials to evaluate the efficacy of isopropyl myristate/cyclomethicone solution against head lice.** *Pharm J* 2008, **280**:371–375.
10. Burgess IF, Brunton ER, Burgess NA: **Clinical trial showing superiority of a coconut and anise spray over permethrin 0.43% lotion for head louse infestation, ISRCTN9646978.** *Eur J Pediatr* 2010, **169**:55–62.
11. Burgess IF, Burgess NA, Brunton ER: **Soya oil based shampoo superior to 0.5% permethrin lotion against head louse infestation: randomized clinical trial.** *Med Devices (Auckl)* 2011, **4**:35–42.
12. Burgess IF, Lee PN, Kay K, Jones R, Brunton ER: **1,2-octanediol, a novel surfactant, for treating head louse infestation: identification of activity, formulation, and randomised, controlled trials.** *PLoS ONE* 2012, **7**(4):e35419.

Association of variation in the *LAMA3* gene, encoding the alpha-chain of laminin 5, with atopic dermatitis in a German case–control cohort

Susanne Stemmler[1], Qumar Parwez[2], Elisabeth Petrasch-Parwez[3], Joerg T Epplen[1,4] and Sabine Hoffjan[1*]

Abstract

Background: Atopic dermatitis (AD) is a chronic inflammatory skin disorder caused by complex interaction of genetic and environmental factors. Besides mutations in the filaggrin gene, leading to impaired skin barrier function, variation in genes encoding additional skin proteins has been suggested to contribute to disease risk. Laminin 5, playing an important role in skin integrity, is composed of three subunits encoded by the *LAMA3*, *LAMB3* and *LAMC2* genes in which biallelic mutations cause epidermolysis bullosa junctionalis. We aimed at evaluating the role of variation in the *LAMA3*, *LAMB3* and *LAMC2* genes for AD pathogenesis.

Methods: 29 single nucleotide polymorphisms (SNPs) were genotyped in the three genes in a German AD case–control cohort comprising 470 unrelated AD patients and 320 non-atopic controls by means of restriction enzyme digestion. Allele, genotype and haplotype frequencies were compared between cases and controls using chi-square testing and the Haploview software.

Results: Several SNPs in the *LAMA3* gene showed significant association with AD in our cohort (p <0.01), while we did not detect association with variations in the *LAMB3* and *LAMC2* genes. Haplotype analysis additionally revealed several significantly associated haplotypes in the *LAMA3* gene. Due to extensive linkage disequilibrium, though, we were not able to further differentiate the specific disease causing variation(s) in this region.

Conclusions: We established the *LAMA3* gene as novel potential susceptibility gene for AD. Additional studies in independent cohorts are needed to replicate these results.

Keywords: Atopic dermatitis, Genetic factors, Laminin 5, *LAMA3*, Skin barrier function

Background

Atopic dermatitis (AD) is a chronic inflammatory skin disorder caused by complex interaction between genetic and environmental factors [1]. Besides dysregulated immune mechanisms that have long been suspected to play a major role for AD pathogenesis, the impact of an intact skin barrier in the protection against AD has gained increasing attention over the recent years [2]. In particular, the role of filaggrin, a major structural protein in the stratum corneum of the epidermis, has been extensively studied. Mutations in the *FLG* gene, located in the epidermal differentiation complex (EDC) on chromosome 1q21 [3], have consistently been associated with early-onset persistent AD [4]. It could be demonstrated that *FLG* mutations constitute the most significant known risk factor for AD development so far [5]. However, impaired skin barrier function has also been shown in AD patients without *FLG* mutations [6], suggesting that variation in genes encoding additional skin proteins may play a role in AD pathogenesis.

Laminin 5 is another protein that plays an important role for skin integrity [7]. It is comprised of three different subunits, built by the LAMA3 (alpha-3), LAMB3 (beta-3) and LAMC2 (gamma-2) polypeptide chains.

* Correspondence: sabine.hoffjan@rub.de
[1]Department of Human Genetics, Ruhr-University, Universitätsstrasse 150, 44801 Bochum, Germany
Full list of author information is available at the end of the article

Laminin 5 (also called laminin-332) is involved in connecting dermis and epidermis and induces adhesion, spreading and migration of human keratinocytes [8]. The three polypeptide chains are encoded by the *LAMA3*, *LAMB3* and *LAMC2* genes on chromosomes 18q11.2, 1q32.2 and 1q25.3, resp. [9]. Biallelic mutations in each of these three genes are known to cause epidermolysis bullosa junctionalis, a severe (type Herlitz) or less severe (type Non-Herlitz) skin disorder characterized by blisters and erosions of the skin [10]. Furthermore, laminin 5 synthesis is elevated during acute wound healing in healthy individuals [11].

Given the important role of mutations in skin barrier proteins in AD pathogenesis, we hypothesized that variation in one or more of the laminin 5 subunits may also confer risk for AD. Therefore we evaluated 29 single nucleotide polymorphisms (SNPs) in the three genes in a German AD case–control cohort and present first evidence that the *LAMA3* gene may be a novel susceptibility gene for AD.

Methods

Subjects

470 unrelated patients with AD with a mean age of 19 ± 15 years (median 11 years) were recruited by a consultant specialist for AD (Q.P., Gladbeck, Germany) as described before [12]. AD diagnosis was established based on the criteria by Hanifin and Rajka [13]. Since the risk remains very high for primarily asymptomatic children to develop an allergic disease during childhood or even adulthood [14,15], we chose to use non-allergic adults as a control group. Therefore, 320 individuals of at least 40 years (mean age 62 ± 11 years, median 63 years) that had neither self-reported allergies or allergic symptoms nor first degree relatives with allergic diseases were recruited in the same private practice as the patients. The controls further underwent clinical examination in order to exclude symptoms of AD, asthma or allergic rhinitis (see [12]). All participants were Germans of European ancestry and gave informed consent prior to enrolment. The Declaration of Helsinki protocols were followed and the study was approved by the Ethics Committee of the Ruhr-University Bochum.

Genotyping

DNA of AD patients and controls was extracted as described before [16]. We selected 29 SNPs in the three genes (17 in the *LAMA3* gene, 8 in *LAMB3*, and 4 in *LAMC2)* that represented the haplotype block structures according to HapMap [17]. Genotyping was performed by polymerase chain reaction (PCR) followed by restriction enzyme digestion. PCR was done in a total volume of 10 μl, containing 40 ng DNA, 200 mmol of each dNTP, 1.5-3 mmol $MgCl_2$, 5 pmol of each

primer, and 0.5 U Taq-DNA-polymerase (Genecraft, Münster, Germany) on the RoboCycler or Biometra *T* cycler (Stratagene, Heidelberg, Germany and Biometra GmbH, Göttingen, Germany, respectively). After two initial cycles at 6° C and 3°C above the annealing temperature, 28–32 cycles of 95°C (30 sec), annealing temperature (30 sec) and 72°C (30 sec) were run. PCR products were subsequently digested with the respective restriction enzyme, the fragments separated on 2.5%-3.5% agarose gels in 1xTBE buffer (30–60 min, 200 V) and visualized with ethidium bromide (0.5% [w/v]). Additional information about primer sequences, PCR conditions and restriction enzymes is summarized in Additional file 1.

Statistics

Genotype and allele frequencies were compared between AD patients and controls according to the χ2 method; the significance threshold was set at $p < 0.05$. We evaluated every SNP for deviations from Hardy-Weinberg equilibrium (HWE) using the deFinetti program [18]. The program Haploview 4.0 [19] was used to estimate haplotype frequencies and test for haplotypic association. We applied Bonferroni correction for multiple tests; however, since this approach has been controversially discussed for genetic case–control studies [20], especially if several tightly linked SNPs within one gene are analyzed as in the present study, we also present the uncorrected p-values and discuss them as hypothesis-generating.

Results

All 29 SNPs showed genotypic distributions according to HWE. Of the 17 SNPs chosen for the *LAMA3* gene, ten showed significant associations ($p < 0.01$ in the uncorrected analysis) with AD in the present cohort. The most significant results that also survived Bonferroni correction were obtained for rs8083184 and rs1711450, both located in the promoter region of *LAMA3* ($p = 0.0003$, $p_{corr} = 0.0087$, Table 1; full genotype data is presented in Additional file 2). A high degree of linkage disequilibrium (LD) was observed for the SNPs in the *LAMA3* gene region (Figure 1). Significant association extended into the 5′ region of *LAMA3*, including rs1613739 which is located in the neighbouring *ANKRD29* gene. Two other SNPs in *ANKRD29* (rs7238623 and rs8096061), however, did not show significant association results. Haplotype analyses revealed the existence of two haplo-blocks (Figure 1) with a common haplotype in block 1 that was highly significantly associated with AD (61.9% in cases *vs.* 51.1% in controls, $p = 2.94 \times 10^{-5}$, Table 2).

In the *LAMB3* gene, neither single SNP nor haplotype analyses revealed significant association with AD in the present cohort (Table 1; haplotype data not shown). In

Table 1 Allele frequencies of *LAMA3*, *LAMB3* and *LAMC2* polymorphisms in AD patients and controls

Gene	SNP	Location	Amino acid exchange	MAF in AD patients	MAF in controls	Uncorrected p-value	Corrected p-value*
LAMA3 18q11.2	rs7238623	5'UTR (*ANKRD29*)	-	0.107	0.083	0.123	n.s.
	rs8096061	5'UTR (*ANKRD29*)	-	0.036	0.044	0.441	n.s.
	rs1613739	5'UTR (*ANKRD29*)	-	0.143	0.200	**0.003**	0.087
	rs12960692	5'UTR	-	0.439	0.454	0.568	n.s.
	rs8083184	5'UTR	-	0.297	0.386	**0.0003**	**0.0087**
	rs1711450	5'UTR	-	0.319	0.410	**0.0003**	**0.0087**
	rs1711451	Intron 1	-	0.336	0.408	**0.005**	0.145
	rs4387667	Intron 2	-	0.336	0.408	**0.005**	0.145
	rs2337187	Intron 2	-	0.250	0.325	**0.001**	**0.029**
	rs1316950	Intron 2	-	0.331	0.407	**0.003**	0.087
	rs4044148	Intron 12	-	0.234	0.395	**0.007**	0.203
	rs1262340	Intron 44	-	0.143	0.196	**0.006**	0.174
	rs734731	Intron 55	-	0.079	0.104	0.096	n.s.
	rs1541836	Intron 59	-	0.086	0.106	0.195	n.s.
	rs1786310	Intron 62	-	0.076	0.103	**0.047**	**n.s.**
	rs1154232	Exon 65	Asn2815Lys	0.187	0.225	0.069	n.s.
	rs2288592	Intron 69	-	0.278	0.345	**0.005**	0.145
LAMB3 1q32.2	rs2566	3'UTR	-	0.283	0.271	0.611	n.s.
	rs2009292	Intron 18	-	0.323	0.336	0.617	n.s.
	rs3179860	Exon 18	Leu891Leu	0.161	0.144	0.375	n.s.
	rs12748250	Exon 17	Met852Leu	0.167	0.150	0.361	n.s.
	rs2072938	Intron 11	-	0.172	0.174	0.901	n.s.
	rs4844863	Intron 8	-	0.157	0.160	0.889	n.s.
	rs2236891	Intron 8	-	0.129	0.101	0.094	n.s.
	rs2236892	Intron 8	-	0.165	0.178	0.517	n.s.
LAMC2 1q25.3	rs483783	Intron 1	-	0.490	0.467	0.362	n.s.
	rs601508	Intron 1	-	0.476	0.440	0.158	n.s.
	rs2274980	Exon 3	Ser99Ser	0.166	0.173	0.723	n.s.
	rs11586699	Exon 3	Thr124Met	0.077	0.062	0.263	n.s.

*after Bonferroni correction for 29 SNPs; n.s.: not significant; bold: significant results.

LAMC2, no single SNP showed association with AD; however, haplotype analyses revealed the existence of a rare protective haplotype (4% in cases *vs.* 6.9% in controls, p = 0.01; Table 3).

Discussion

To our knowledge, this is the first report of an association of AD with variation in the *LAMA3* gene, encoding the alpha-chain of laminin 5. In a well-characterized German case–control cohort, we found significant association of both allelic and haplotypic frequencies in this gene with AD, suggesting that it may constitute a novel susceptibility gene for this frequent skin disease.

Of the 19 SNPs evaluated across the *LAMA3* gene, ten showed genotypic or allelic association with AD at p <

0.01 (uncorrected values). Due to the extensive LD evident at the *LAMA3* locus we were not able to further differentiate the specific disease causing variation(s) in this region. Significant association extended into the 5′ neighbouring gene *ANKRD29*, but additional SNPs in this gene did not show association with AD. The biological function of *ANKRD29*, encoding the ankyrin repeat domain-containing protein 29, is not yet known; however, for another protein of the same family, ANKRD17, a role in anti-bacterial innate immune pathways has been suggested [21]. For the gene located 3′ of *LAMA3* (*TTC39C*), encoding the tetratricopeptide repeat protein 39C, the biological function is not yet clear either, and since the most significant results for *LAMA3* were at the 5′ end of this large gene, we did not evaluate additional SNPs in the

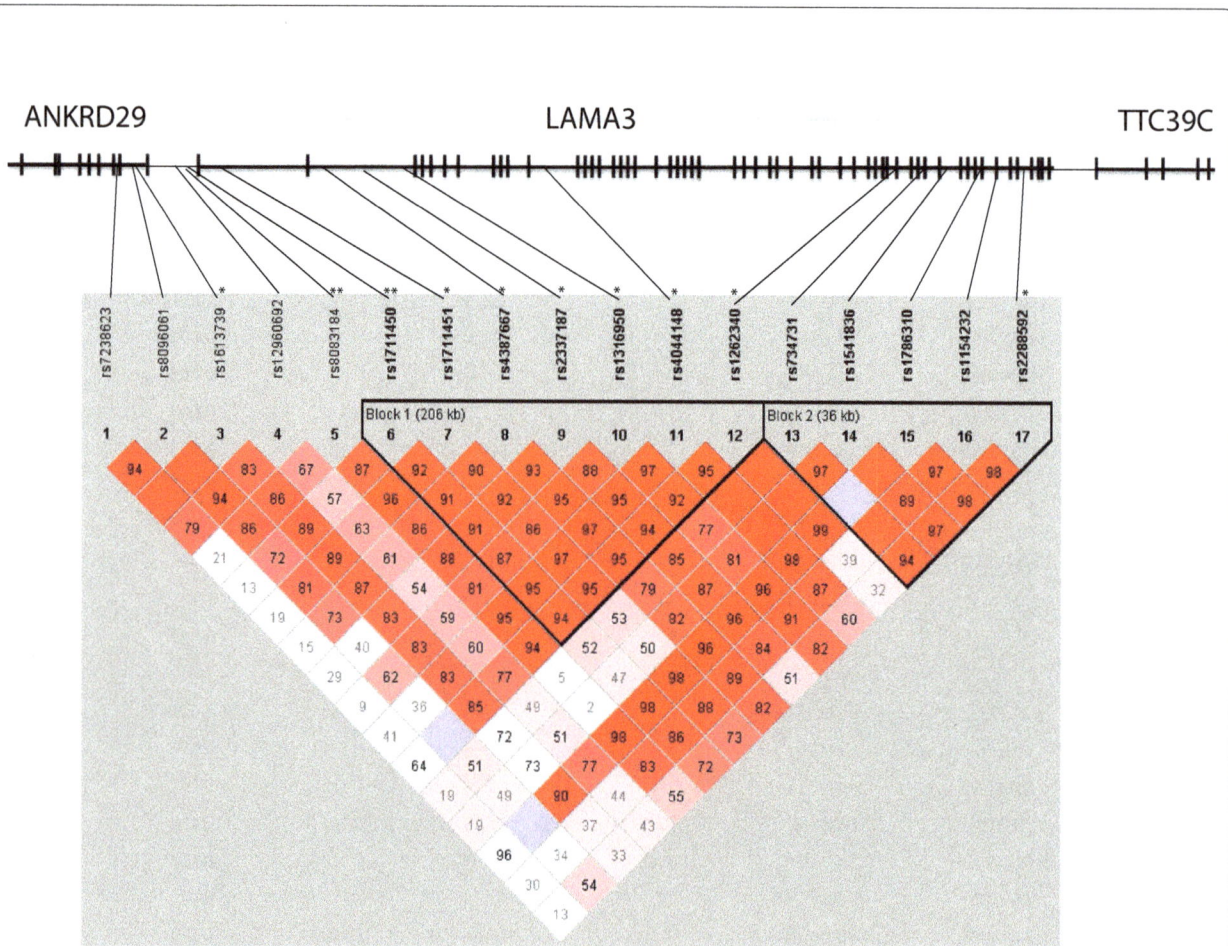

Figure 1 Haploblock structure of the *LAMA3* region as revealed by Haploview 4.0 [19]. *SNPs associated with AD at p < 0.01 (uncorrected values) **SNPs associated with AD at p < 0.001 (uncorrected values).

TTC39C gene. Taken together, even though we cannot exclude that the observed association with AD may be due to LD with a susceptibility variant in another gene in this region, our data highly points to *LAMA3* as susceptibility gene for AD in the 18q11.2 region. SNPs in the genes encoding the beta- and gamma-chains of laminin 5, on the other hand, did not show convincing evidence for association with AD in this analysis. However, haplotype analysis suggested the existence of a rare protective haplotype in *LAMC2*.

The main role of laminin 5 in normal tissues is the maintenance of epithelial-mesenchymal cohesion in tissues exposed to external forces, such as skin and stratified squamous mucosa [22]. Genetic variation in laminin 5 components may thus contribute to reduced skin integrity and barrier function, as has been observed for *FLG* mutations [5], even though the exact underlying mechanisms still have to be elucidated. In each of the three genes analysed here, rare null mutations are known to cause epidermolysis bullosa junctionalis, a severe autosomal recessive

skin disorder characterized by the development of blisters and skin erosions in response to minor injury or friction [10]. In contrast, we observed association of common variation in *LAMA3* with the common complex disorder AD. This phenomenon is in line with findings for the *SPINK5* gene, in which null mutations cause autosomal recessive Netherton syndrome while common variations have been associated with AD [23].

Our association results further contribute to the hypothesis that an intact skin barrier function plays a key part in AD pathogenesis. Additional to the established role of *FLG* mutations [24], associations with some other skin-related genes have been described recently. For example, mutations in the claudin-1 gene (*CLDN1*), encoding a major tight junction protein in the granular layer of the epidermis, were associated with AD in North American cohorts of both European and African American origin [25]. Further, polymorphisms near the *OVOL1* and *ACTL9* genes, both involved in epidermal proliferation and differentiation, showed genome-wide significant

Table 2 Frequencies and p-values of *LAMA3* haplotypes in AD patients and controls

Haplotype	Frequency in AD patients (n = 470)	Frequency in controls (n = 320)	p-value
Block 1			
1112122	0.619	0.511	**2.9×10^{-5}**
2221211	0.134	0.182	**0.0114**
2221212	0.086	0.088	0.8954
2222222	0.060	0.070	0.4447
1212122	0.023	0.019	0.607
1122222	0.022	0.016	0.4152
2221222	0.016	0.021	0.4906
2112122	0.012	0.025	0.0465
Block 2			
12121	0.718	0.650	**0.0043**
12112	0.113	0.110	0.8506
12212	0.074	0.106	**0.0305**
21122	0.079	0.093	0.3379
12122	0.007	0.022	**0.0083**

Bold: significant results.

association with AD in a large meta-analysis of GWAS data, including 5,606 AD patients and 20,565 controls [26]. In a study cohort comprising AD patients from Germany, Poland and the Czech Republic, a 24-bp deletion in the gene encoding small proline-rich protein 3 (*SPRR3*), located within the EDC, was significantly associated with disease risk [27]. On the other hand, a deletion of the cornified envelope 3B and 3C genes within in the EDC was not associated with AD in a European cohort [28]. All of these results still await replication in independent cohorts. Altogether, though, evidence is accumulating that additional genes involved in epidermal differentiation and stability may be important for AD pathogenesis.

We are conscious of the fact that the cohort sizes of the present study are comparatively small so that the

statistical power is only moderate. Furthermore, only for two SNPs in *LAMA3* results remained significant after strict Bonferroni correction for multiple testing, leaving open the risk for false-positive results. However, the Bonferroni correction has been controversially discussed for genetic case–control studies [20], especially if several tightly linked SNPs within one gene are analyzed, as was the case in the present study. Therefore, we regard the results as hypothesis-generating and strongly encourage replication in additional cohorts.

Conclusions

We presented initial evidence for association of *LAMA3* variation with AD, suggesting that variation in this gene may contribute to skin fragility and impaired barrier function underlying AD pathogenesis. Additional studies in independent populations as well as functional analyses of the associated variations appear warranted to replicate or extend these findings, since the genetic risk factors for AD might be increasingly included into prognostic and therapeutic strategies in the future. In more detail, an integrated approach including genotypic and phenotypic information as well as genetic and biological biomarkers has been proposed for example to identify patients who are prone to develop persistent AD and/ or additional asthma and start early intervention [29]. Further, therapeutic strategies targeting the skin barrier function are already under way [30]. Thus, elucidating the complex genetic background of AD is essential for paving the way towards a more individualized therapy in the future.

Abbreviations
AD: Atopic dermatitis; EDC: Epidermal differentiation complex; HWE: Hardy-Weinberg equilibrium; LD: Linkage disequilibrium; SNP: Single nucleotide polymorphism.

Competing interests
The authors declare that they have no competing interests.

Authors' contributions
SS was in charge of study design and statistical analysis and drafted the manuscript. QP and EPP were involved in patient recruitment and helped to draft the manuscript. JTE and SH conceived of the study, participated in its design and coordination and helped to draft the manuscript. All authors read and approved the final manuscript.

Acknowledgments
We thank Maike Kallenbach, Natascha Wirkus, Monika Harazin and Katharina Batzke for technical assistance and the patients for their cooperation in this study.

Table 3 Frequencies and p-values of *LAMC2* haplotypes in AD patients and controls

Haplotype	Frequency in AD patients (n = 470)	Frequency in controls (n = 320)	p-value
1221	0.356	0.341	0.5252
2121	0.347	0.343	0.8557
2111	0.099	0.086	0.3998
1222	0.068	0.053	0.2136
1121	0.040	0.069	**0.0102**
1111	0.037	0.058	0.0493
2211	0.022	0.016	0.4027
2221	0.015	0.014	0.8668

Bold: significant results.

Author details

[1]Department of Human Genetics, Ruhr-University, Universitätsstrasse 150, 44801 Bochum, Germany. [2]Private medical practice, Gladbeck, Germany. [3]Department of Neuroanatomy and Molecular Brain Research, Ruhr-University Bochum, Bochum, Germany. [4]Faculty of Health, Witten/Herdecke University, Witten, Germany.

References

1. Holloway JW, Yang IA, Holgate ST: **Genetics of allergic disease.** *J Allergy Clin Immunol* 2010, **125**:S81–S94.
2. Boguniewicz M, Leung DY: **Atopic dermatitis: a disease of altered skin barrier and immune dysregulation.** *Immunol Rev* 2011, **242**:233–246.
3. Kypriotou M, Huber M, Hohl D: **The human epidermal differentiation complex: cornified envelope precursors, S100 proteins and the 'fused genes' family.** *Exp Dermatol* 2012, **21**:643–649.
4. Irvine AD, McLean WH, Leung DY: **Filaggrin mutations associated with skin and allergic diseases.** *N Engl J Med* 2011, **365**:1315–1327.
5. McAleer MA, Irvine AD: **The multifunctional role of filaggrin in allergic skin disease.** *J Allergy Clin Immunol* 2013, **131**:280–291.
6. Jakasa I, Koster ES, Calkoen F, McLean WH, Campbell LE, Bos JD, Verberk MM, Kezic S: **Skin barrier function in healthy subjects and patients with atopic dermatitis in relation to filaggrin loss-of-function mutations.** *J Invest Dermatol* 2011, **131**:540–542.
7. Nishiyama T, Amano S, Tsunenaga M, Kadoya K, Takeda A, Adachi E, Burgeson RE: **The importance of laminin 5 in the dermal-epidermal basement membrane.** *J Dermatol Sci* 2000, **24**(Suppl 1):S51–S59.
8. Schneider H, Muhle C, Pacho F: **Biological function of laminin-5 and pathogenic impact of its deficiency.** *Eur J Cell Biol* 2007, **86**:701–717.
9. Akutsu N, Amano S, Nishiyama T: **Quantitative analysis of laminin 5 gene expression in human keratinocytes.** *Exp Dermatol* 2005, **14**:329–335.
10. Kiritsi D, Has C, Bruckner-Tuderman L: **Laminin 332 in junctional epidermolysis bullosa.** *Cell Adh Migr* 2013, **7**:135–141.
11. Amano S, Akutsu N, Ogura Y, Nishiyama T: **Increase of laminin 5 synthesis in human keratinocytes by acute wound fluid, inflammatory cytokines and growth factors, and lysophospholipids.** *Br J Dermatol* 2004, **151**:961–970.
12. Macaluso F, Nothnagel M, Parwez Q, Petrasch-Parwez E, Bechara FG, Epplen JT, Hoffjan S: **Polymorphisms in NACHT-LRR (NLR) genes in atopic dermatitis.** *Exp Dermatol* 2007, **16**:692–698.
13. Hanifin JM, Rajka G: **Diagnostic features of atopic dermatitis.** *Acta Derm Venereol* 1980, **92**:44–47.
14. Bel EH: **Clinical phenotypes of asthma.** *Curr Opin Pulm Med* 2004, **10**:44–50.
15. De Marco R, Locatelli F, Cerveri I, Bugiani M, Marinoni A, Giammanco G: **Incidence and remission of asthma: a retrospective study on the natural history of asthma in Italy.** *J Allergy Clin Immunol* 2002, **110**:228–235.
16. Miller SA, Dykes DD, Polesky HF: **A simple salting out procedure for extracting DNA from human nucleated cells.** *Nucleic Acids Res* 1988, **16**:1215.
17. International HapMap Consortium: **The International HapMap Project.** *Nature* 2003, **426**:789–796.
18. DeFinetti test for Hardy-Weinberg equilibrium. http://ihg.gsf.de/cgi-bin/hw/hwa1.pl.
19. Barrett JC: **Haploview: Visualization and analysis of SNP genotype data.** *Cold Spring Harb Protoc* 2009:pdb ip71.
20. Boehringer S, Epplen JT, Krawczak M: **Genetic association studies of bronchial asthma-a need for Bonferroni correction?** *Hum Genet* 2000, **107**:197.
21. Menning M, Kufer TA: **A role for the Ankyrin repeat containing protein Ankrd17 in Nod1- and Nod2-mediated inflammatory responses.** *FEBS Lett* 2013, **587**:2137–2142.
22. Rousselle P, Beck K: **Laminin 332 processing impacts cellular behavior.** *Cell Adh Migr* 2013, **7**:122–134.
23. Norgett EE, Kelsell DP: **SPINK5: both rare and common skin disease.** *Trends Mol Med* 2002, **8**:7.
24. McLean WH, Irvine AD: **Heritable filaggrin disorders: the paradigm of atopic dermatitis.** *J Invest Dermatol* 2012, **132**:E20–E21.
25. De Benedetto A, Rafaels NM, McGirt LY, Ivanov AI, Georas SN, Cheadle C, Berger AE, Zhang K, Vidyasagar S, Yoshida T, Boguniewicz M, Hata T, Schneider LC, Hanifin JM, Gallo RL, Novak N, Weidinger S, Beaty TH, Leung DY, Barnes KC, Beck LA: **Tight junction defects in patients with atopic dermatitis.** *J Allergy Clin Immunol* 2010, **127**:773–786.
26. Paternoster L, Standl M, Chen CM, Ramasamy A, Bonnelykke K, Duijts L, Ferreira MA, Alves AC, Thyssen JP, Albrecht E, Baurecht H, Feenstra B, Sleiman PM, Hysi P, Warrington NM, Curjuric I, Myhre R, Curtin JA, Groen-Blokhuis MM, Kerkhof M, Sääf A, Franke A, Ellinghaus D, Fölster-Holst R, Dermitzakis E, Montgomery SB, Prokisch H, Heim K, Hartikainen AL, Pouta A, et al: **Meta-analysis of genome-wide association studies identifies three new risk loci for atopic dermatitis.** *Nat Genet* 2012, **44**:187–192.
27. Marenholz I, Rivera VA, Esparza-Gordillo J, Bauerfeind A, Lee-Kirsch MA, Ciechanowicz A, Kurek M, Piskackova T, Macek M, Lee YA: **Association screening in the Epidermal Differentiation Complex (EDC) identifies an SPRR3 repeat number variant as a risk factor for eczema.** *J Invest Dermatol* 2011, **131**:1644–1649.
28. Bergboer JG, Zeeuwen PL, Irvine AD, Weidinger S, Giardina E, Novelli G, Den Heijer M, Rodriguez E, Illig T, Riveira-Munoz E, Campbell LE, Tyson J, Dannhauser EN, O'Regan GM, Galli E, Klopp N, Koppelman GH, Novak N, Estivill X, McLean WH, Postma DS, Armour JA, Schalkwijk J: **Deletion of Late Cornified Envelope 3B and 3C genes is not associated with atopic dermatitis.** *J Invest Dermatol* 2010, **130**:2057–2061.
29. Bieber T, Cork M, Reitamo S: **Atopic dermatitis: a candidate for disease-modifying strategy.** *Allergy* 2012, **67**:969–975.
30. Heimall J, Spergel JM: **Filaggrin mutations and atopy: consequences for future therapeutics.** *Expert Rev Clin Immunol* 2012, **8**:189–197.

16

Treatment and referral patterns for psoriasis in United Kingdom primary care: a retrospective cohort study

Javaria Mona Khalid[1], Gary Globe[2], Kathleen M Fox[3*], Dina Chau[2], Andrew Maguire[1] and Chio-Fang Chiou[4]

Abstract

Background: In the UK, referrals to specialists are initiated by general practitioners (GPs). Study objectives were to estimate the incidence of diagnosed psoriasis in the UK and identify factors associated with GP referrals to dermatologists.

Methods: Newly diagnosed patients with psoriasis were identified in The Health Improvement Network (THIN) database between 01 July 2007-31 Oct 2009. Incidence of diagnosed psoriasis was calculated using the number of new psoriasis patients in 2008 and the mid-year total patient count for THIN in 2008. A nested case–control design and conditional logistic regression were used to identify factors associated with referral.

Results: Incidence rate of diagnosed adult psoriasis in 2008 was 28/10,000 person-years. Referral rate to dermatologists was 18.1 (17.3-18.9) per 100 person-years. In the referred cohort (N=1,950), 61% were referred within 30 days of diagnosis and their median time to referral was 0 days from diagnosis. For those referred after 30 days (39%, median time to referral: 5.6 months), an increase in the number of GP visits prior to referral increased the likelihood of referral (OR=1.87 95% CI:1.73-2.01). A prescription of topical agents such as vitamin D3 analogues 30 days before referral increased the likelihood of being referred (OR=4.67 95% CI: 2.78-7.84), as did corticosteroids (OR=2.45 95% CI: 1.45-4.07) and tar products (OR=1.95 95% CI: 1.02-3.75).

Conclusions: Estimates of the incidence of diagnosed adult psoriasis, referral rates to dermatologists, and characteristics of referred patients may assist in understanding the burden on the UK healthcare system and managing this population in primary and secondary care.

Keywords: Primary care, General practice, Psoriasis, Referral patterns, UK

Background

Psoriasis is a serious chronic inflammatory skin disease with varying degrees of severity and disability. The most common type, accounting for 90% of all cases, is plaque psoriasis [1]. In the United Kingdom (UK), the prevalence of psoriasis has been reported to be between 0.24% - 1.5%, [2,3]. Higher mortality rates have been reported for severe psoriasis (patients with history of systemic therapy) in the UK [4] and hospital admission rate for patients with a primary diagnosis of psoriasis has been reported to be 2.9 per 10,000 population per year [2]. Psoriasis causes physical impairment, pain, and psychological stress, including impairment in social settings and workplace, and poor health-related quality of life [5-9].

In the UK, the National Institute for Health and Clinical Excellence (NICE) and the British Association of Dermatologists (BAD) treatment guidelines for psoriasis [10,11] recommend starting with prescription topical drugs including corticosteroids, coal tar, dithranol, retinoids (e.g. tazarotene), and vitamin D3 analogues (calcipotriol, calciotriol, tacalcitol) for mild to moderate psoriasis, and progressing to more potent therapies (phototherapy, systemic drugs including methotrexate, ciclosporin, acitretin, and hydroxycarbamide) for greater severity of psoriasis. Anti-tumor necrosis factor agents (e.g. etanercept, adalimumab, infliximab) are indicated in the UK for the treatment of severe plaque psoriasis

* Correspondence: kathyfox@gforcecable.com
[3]Strategic Healthcare Solutions, LLC, PO Box 543, Monkton, MD 21111, USA
Full list of author information is available at the end of the article

among patients who do not respond, or are intolerant to or contraindicated for standard systemic therapy [10-12]. At the time of this analysis, the British National Formulary (BNF) restricted the prescribing of systemic biologic drugs acting on the immune system to specialists.

To comprehensively understand psoriasis patients in the UK, the treatment patterns and characteristics of patients treated in primary care before they are referred to dermatologists needs to be elucidated. A previous study reported the number of prescriptions received by patients undergoing therapy [3]. However, data on psoriasis treatment patterns in primary care, especially for patients who are referred to specialist care, is lacking. Additionally, the most current estimates for the incidence of psoriasis in the UK utilized data for patients diagnosed about 15 years ago, in 1996–1997 [13]. It is important to understand the proportion and characteristics of patients who are currently being referred for specialist care to determine an updated disease burden on the UK health system. The objectives of the present study are to estimate the incidence of diagnosed psoriasis and describe the clinical characteristics and treatment patterns for incident psoriasis patients being referred to specialist (dermatologist) care.

Methods

A retrospective cohort study using The Health Improvement Network (THIN) data to identify patients with a new diagnosis between 1 July 2007 and 31 October 2009 was conducted. The THIN database contains anonymized medical records from 1500 GPs in over 427 primary care practices covering over 5% of the UK population (>7.6 million patients), which is broadly representative of the non-institutionalized UK population [14,15]. Approximately 98% of the UK population is registered with a GP. Diagnoses are recorded using the READ diagnostic code scheme and prescriptions are recorded using codes from the UK Prescription Pricing Authority [16]. THIN is the only UK primary care database that has complete mortality reporting indicated as the acceptable mortality reporting date [17] to ensure the completeness and accuracy of the enumeration of the total population during the study period. THIN data have been previously validated for the study of psoriasis in a population-based setting [18]. The study was reviewed and approved by the Cegedim Strategic Data Medical Research Scientific Review Committee (SRC) (Reference no. 10–035).

Study population

The study population was comprised of patients in THIN with a diagnosis of psoriasis and who were currently managed by their general practitioner (GP). Newly diagnosed psoriasis patients aged ≥18 years were identified by the first psoriasis Read Code (diagnosis code) in the medical records after 1 July 2007. The index date was defined as

the date of first psoriasis diagnosis. Patients were required to be registered with the GP practice for at least one day in the follow-up period (minimum follow-up). Twelve months of computerized records for each patient were required before the first diagnosis of psoriasis to ensure that true incident cases were identified. Patients were excluded if their diagnosis date was earlier than the practice's acceptable mortality reporting date to increase accuracy of the denominator in the incidence calculations. Follow-up was defined as the time from index date until the earliest of the following: 1) end of study period (i.e. 31 October 2009), 2) date patient left the practice, or 3) date of patient's death.

Study measures

Primary outcomes included incidence of diagnosed psoriasis in 2008, and the proportion, characteristics, and treatment patterns of patients referred to specialist (dermatologist) care between 1 July 2007 and 31 October 2009. Incidence of diagnosed psoriasis was defined as the number of new cases of psoriasis in 2008 with a denominator of the mid-year (June) patient count for THIN in 2008. For the incidence person-time calculation, prevalent cases of psoriasis were subtracted from the denominator, and age- and sex-specific rates were calculated from which a UK standardized rate was estimated for 2008.

Patient characterization of the incident cohort referred to dermatologist care included age at diagnosis, gender, body mass index (BMI), select comorbid conditions prior to index date (including hypertension, cardiovascular disease, chronic obstructive pulmonary disease, hyperlipidemia, diabetes mellitus, heart failure, renal insufficiency, cancer, psoriatic arthritis, liver disease, eczema, rheumatoid arthritis, other auto-immune conditions), social class, number of GP visits, and current psoriasis therapy. Psoriasis-related therapies included prescriptions at the index date (or within 30 days after the diagnosis) as well as therapies received during follow-up before a referral to a dermatologist. Social class was represented by the Townsend deprivation index, a census-based index of material deprivation [19].

For identifying factors associated with referral from the GP to dermatologists, a nested case–control design was used. Patients with psoriasis who were not referred to a dermatologist during follow-up were designated as controls. Patients referred to a dermatologist were matched to four controls by GP practice. Matched (by GP practice only) controls were assigned the date of referral of their matched case (referred patients) to investigate potential determinants of referral to a dermatologist.

Statistical analysis

Referral rates to dermatologists were expressed using survival analysis techniques which accounted for varying

Table 1 Characteristics of incident psoriasis patients at diagnosis, n = 10,832

Characteristics	Males (n = 5281)	Females (n = 5551)	All (n = 10,832)
Age, years (mean, SD)	48.5 (17.1)*	49.4 (18.3)	49.0 (17.8)
Body mass index, kg/m^2 (mean, SD)	27.4 (5.3)	27.6 (6.4)	27.5 (5.9)
Comorbidities at index, %			
Hypertension	24.1	24.6	24.3
Cardiovascular disease	10.7	7.7	9.1
Chronic obstructive pulmonary disease	7.0	7.2	7.1
Diabetes mellitus	7.5	6.8	7.1
Heart failure	1.2	0.8	1.0
Cancer	4.3	6.3	5.3
Rheumatoid arthritis	4.4	6.3	5.4
Psoriatic arthritis	2.3	2.6	2.4
Eczema	29.0	34.1	31.6
Other autoimmune diseases†	5.5	11.4	8.5
Liver disease	0.04	0.2	0.1
Dyslipidemia	9.4	8.1	8.7
Number of comorbid conditions, %			
0	43.7	37.4	40.5
1	31.9	33.0	32.5
2 or more	24.4	29.6	27.1
Townsend deprivation quintile, %			
1	23.9	22.6	23.3
2	20.7	20.4	20.6
3	21.0	21.2	21.1
4	16.9	17.6	17.3
5	13.0	13.4	13.2
Psoriasis-related therapies at index, %			
Vitamin D3 analogues	45.5*	34.7	39.9
Retinoids	0.04	0.07	0.06
Tar & tar combination products	12.0	15.9	14.0
Anthracin & combination products	0.6	0.5	0.6
Salicylic acid	0.8	0.8	0.8
Corticosteroids	34.9	43.6	39.4
Phototherapy	0	0.04	0.02
Non-biologic systemic therapy	0.6	0.8	0.7
Any psoriasis-related medication at index, %	80.6	80.1	80.4

†includes ankylosing spondylitis, Crohn's disease, irritable bowel syndrome, metabolic syndrome, ulcerative colitis.
*P<0.05.

lengths of follow-up. Patients that were not referred were censored at the end of their follow-up. Kaplan-Meier survival method was used to calculate the time to referral. Conditional logistic regression was used to calculate adjusted odds ratios (OR) to identify factors associated with referral. The multivariate model was adjusted for age, gender, and variables that were significantly different between groups in an initial bivariate analysis.

Results

A total of 10,832 patients who were newly diagnosed with psoriasis between 1 July 2007 and 31 October 2009 and met the study inclusion and exclusion criteria were identified. Psoriasis was diagnosed around the age of 49 years for men and women (Table 1). BMI was not significantly different between males and females and its distribution was similar to the general UK population (28 kg/m^2) [20]. Eczema, present in 31% of newly diagnosed psoriasis patients, was the most commonly reported comorbid condition followed by hypertension (24%). Approximately 40% of patients did not have any of the selected comorbid conditions. The distribution of social class (Townsend deprivation quintiles) was similar to the social class distribution of the general population in THIN. At index date, approximately 80% of newly diagnosed psoriasis patients received topical pharmacological therapy for the treatment of psoriasis. Approximately, 24% of patients started therapy with a combination of vitamin D3 analogues, corticosteroids, and tar or tar combination products, with a total of 40% using vitamin D3 analogues, 39% using corticosteroids, and 14% using tar or tar combination products at index. All other therapies for psoriasis were used by < 1% of patients at index.

Incidence of diagnosed psoriasis

The standardized incidence rate of diagnosed adult psoriasis in 2008 was 28 (95% CI: 28–29) per 10,000 person-years. The incidence rate was highest for 60–69 year olds at 34 (95% CI: 31–36) per 10,000 person-years. Incidence did not vary by sex (Table 2).

Referrals to dermatologists

A total of 1,950 (18%) patients within the incident cohort had a referral to a dermatologist. The referral rate was 18.1 (95% CI: 17.3-18.9) per 100 person-years. Amongst those that were referred, 49% were male and median age at diagnosis was 49 (interquartile range: 35–62) years. The distribution of time to referral showed a clustering of patients who were referred very shortly after diagnosis (within 30 days of diagnosis). For patients referred after 30 days of diagnosis, the distribution of time to referral ranged from 31 days to 2.3 years with no clear clustering so these patients were grouped together as referral >30 days after diagnosis. Approximately 61% of referred patients (n = 1,183) were referred to a dermatologist within 30 days of diagnosis (immediately referred) and 39% were referred after 30 days post-diagnosis and were managed in primary care up to their referral date (Figure 1).

The median time to referral for patients referred within the first month was the day of diagnosis (day 0, interquartile range: 0–6 days). Demographic characteristics, including age (mean [SD]: 49.2 years [17.5] vs. 48.8 [17.9]), gender (46.8% vs. 48.8% men), BMI (28.1 kg/m^2 [6.4] vs. 27.6 [6.0]), and number of psoriasis-related prescriptions at index (0.6 [0.9] vs. 0.4 [0.7]) were similar between cases that were immediately referred and their matched controls that were not referred to a dermatologist. Mean number of GP visits in the year prior to referral was 2.0 [1.5] for immediately referred patients compared to 1.8 [1.4] for patients not referred to a dermatologist (p<0.05). Mean number of comorbid conditions was 1.2 [1.3] for immediately referred patients compared to 1.1 [1.2] for patients not referred (p<0.05). For those who were referred immediately, a greater number of GP visits prior to a dermatologist referral significantly increased the likelihood of referral (OR = 1.14, 95% CI: 1.08-1.20) compared to controls, after adjusting for age, gender, number of comorbid conditions, psoriatic arthritis diagnosis, and psoriasis-related prescription at index (Table 3). A prescription at index of tar products also increased the likelihood of being referred immediately (OR = 2.00, 95% CI: 1.45-2.76), as did vitamin D3 analogue (OR = 1.84, 95% CI: 1.50-2.25) and corticosteroid (OR = 1.56, 95% CI: 1.26-1.92) prescriptions compared to controls (Table 3).

For patients who were referred to a dermatologist > 30 days after diagnosis (later referred patients), demographic characteristics, including age (48.5 years [19.0] vs. 49.2 [17.8]), gender (51.1% vs. 50.3% men), BMI (28.1 kg/m^2 [6.2] vs. 27.6 [6.0]), and the number of comorbid conditions (1.3 [1.3] vs. 1.2 [1.3]) in the year period were similar between cases (later referred patients) and controls. The median time to referral to a dermatologist was 5.6 (interquartile range: 2.8-11.5) months after the psoriasis

diagnosis. The mean number of GP visits in the year prior to referral was 3.0 [2.0] for later referred patients compared to 1.4 [1.3] for patients not referred to a dermatologist (p<0.05); the mean number of psoriasis-related prescriptions at index was 0.6 [1.0] for later referred patients and 0.1 [0.5] for controls (p>0.05). Overall, later-referred patients made 5.34 visits to the GP before they were referred to a dermatologist. Of those GP visits, 2.73 visits were psoriasis-related.

After adjusting for age, gender, number of comorbid conditions, psoriatic arthritis diagnosis, and psoriasis-related prescription, a greater number of GP visits prior to referral increased the likelihood of later referral (OR = 1.87, 95% CI: 1.73-2.01) compared to controls (Table 3). A prescription for vitamin D3 analogues within 30 days before referral also increased the likelihood of being later referred (OR = 4.67, 95% CI: 2.78-7.84), as did corticosteroids (OR = 2.43) and tar products (OR = 1.95) compared to controls.

Discussion

Approximately 28 patients per 10,000 person-years were newly diagnosed with psoriasis in the UK. Among patients who were diagnosed in primary care, the referral rate to dermatology was 18 per 100 person-years, with most patients who were referred being referred immediately after a diagnosis is made. Having a greater number of GP visits in the year prior to referral, a prescription for vitamin D3 analogues, corticosteroids or tar products increased the likelihood of being referred to the dermatologist.

Previous population-based UK studies have reported psoriasis incidence to be lower as 14 per 10,000 person-years [13,21]. One possible explanation of the higher incidence estimate of diagnosed psoriasis in the present study is that previous studies were conducted prior to the introduction of the Quality Outcomes Framework (QOF) guidelines [22], which have improved the completeness of diagnostic recording in UK primary care since payment is performance-related under QOF. An increased awareness of psoriasis and new treatment options may also be a reason for the higher incidence of diagnosed psoriasis in recent years. The bimodal distribution of incidence of diagnosed psoriasis with rates peaking in the 30–39 and 60–69 year age groups in this study was also reported in a previous study of the UK population [13].

In the present study, approximately 18% of newly diagnosed psoriasis patients were referred to dermatologists. In the UK, the first point of contact with health professionals is the GP. The GP may decide to manage psoriasis patients in primary care, especially when the disease is mild, or refer patients to dermatologists in secondary care if the psoriasis is more severe. According to guidelines and the BNF, most systemic therapies including biologics can only be prescribed by a specialist [10-12].

Table 2 Incidence rates of diagnosed psoriasis for 2008 by age and sex per 100 person-years

Age group, years	Incidence rate per 100 person-years (95% CI)	
	Males	Females
18-29	0.25 (0.23-0.28)	0.35 (0.32-0.38)
30-39	0.29 (0.26-0.32)	0.32 (0.28-0.35)
40-49	0.22 (0.20-0.25)	0.22 (0.20-0.24)
50-59	0.32 (0.30-0.36)	0.31 (0.28-0.34)
60-69	0.37 (0.33-0.40)	0.31 (0.28-0.35)
70-79	0.29 (0.25-0.33)	0.29 (0.25-0.32)
80 and older	0.18 (0.14-0.23)	0.16 (0.13-0.19)

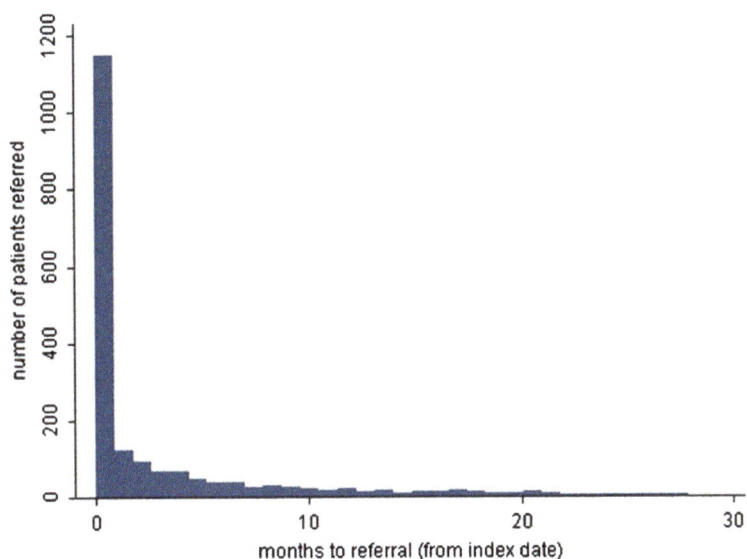

Figure 1 Distribution of time to referral to secondary care dermatology specialist (n = 1,950).

Recent evidence indicates that 25% to 44% of psoriasis patients are moderate to severe and would likely benefit from specialist attention [23-25]. However, the present study found that only 18% of patients were referred, suggesting under-utilization of specialist services. The referral rate of 18% is higher than the previously reported figure of 0.7% in 2003 using data from the Doctor's Information Network, a smaller primary care database in the UK [21]. The higher rate of referral in the present study may also be explained, in part, by the recent availability (since 2003) of biologics in secondary care and biologics can only be prescribed by a specialist in the UK.

Most patients in the present study were referred immediately after the psoriasis diagnosis. One possible reason is these patients may present with severe psoriasis at

Table 3 Risk of referral from conditional logistic regression for patients referred to a dermatologist

Variable	Immediately referred at diagnosis Adjusted† Odds ratio (95% CI)	Referred >30 days after diagnosis Adjusted† Odds ratio (95% CI)
Age	1.00 (0.98-1.00)	0.99 (0.98-1.00)
Males	1.07 (0.92-1.23)	0.87 (0.71-1.07)
Number of comorbidities in prior year	1.01 (0.94-1.08)	0.96 (0.87-1.06)
Number of GP visits in prior year	1.14 (1.08-1.20)*	1.87 (1.73-2.01)*
Psoriatic arthritis at index	1.16 (0.62-2.19)	1.15 (0.61-2.16)
No psoriasis-related prescription at index	Reference	NA
Corticosteroid prescription at index	1.56 (1.26-1.92)*	NA
Vitamin D3 analogue prescription at index	1.84 (1.50-2.25)*	NA
Tar & tar combination prescription at index	2.00 (1.45-2.76)*	NA
Non-biologic systemic therapy at index	0.30 (0.11-0.88)*	NA
No psoriasis-related prescription in 30 days prior to referral	NA	Reference
Corticosteroid prescription in 30 days prior to referral	NA	2.43 (1.45-4.07)*
Vitamin D3 analogue prescription in 30 days prior to referral	NA	4.67 (2.78-7.84)*
Tar & tar combination prescription in 30 days prior to referral	NA	1.95 (1.02-3.75)*
Non-biologic systemic therapy in 30 days prior to referral	NA	0.20 (0.05-0.90)*
Number of psoriasis-related prescriptions in 30 days prior to referral	NA	0.85 (0.31-1.17)

†Adjusted for age, gender, number of comorbidities, psoriatic arthritis diagnosis, and psoriasis-related prescriptions at index; NA not applicable.
*P<0.05.

the time of diagnosis, necessitating immediate referral to a dermatologist.

A greater number of GP visits in the year prior to referral, a prescription for vitamin D3 analogues, corticosteroids or tar products were all significantly associated with an increased likelihood of referral to a dermatologist amongst patients referred immediately or later. The factors associated with referral may help in understanding which patients need specialist care so that in the future, patients may be identified and referred earlier and, where appropriate, receive systemic therapies (biologic and non-biologic) to control their psoriasis. With the association between vitamin D3 analogues, corticosteroids and tar products and referral to a dermatologist, it appears that GPs are following the UK NICE and BAD guidelines [10,11] for step therapy of starting with prescription topical drugs since corticosteroids and vitamin D3 analogues were most frequently prescribed at index. Also, a greater proportion of referred patients received topical therapies within 30 days prior to referral than at index. Age, gender, BMI, concomitant psoriatic arthritis, and number of co-morbid conditions were found to not be associated with an increased likelihood of referral to a dermatologist.

One of the strengths of this study is that THIN is one of the few primary care databases validated to study psoriasis [18]. Furthermore, as a population-based database was used, the results from this study are broadly representative of the UK population in terms of age and gender. The study data are presented for a recent time period, after the introduction of incentivized guidelines on completeness of coding in primary care and represent estimates from a period where GPs may be coding more accurately.

The study does have some limitations. It was not possible to directly discern severity of the psoriasis amongst the patient population since medical Read codes do not consistently indicate severity of the condition. It is possible that patients with mild psoriasis may not have come to medical attention in which case diagnoses by GPs may underestimate the incidence of psoriasis. The clinical characteristics and treatment patterns described in this study are those that are prescribed in primary care by GPs and the treatment patterns for systemic therapy are not included in primary care data. Other factors such as psoriasis severity, patient understanding of the disease, and patient desire for improvement, may be associated with GP referrals to dermatologists; however, data for these factors were not recorded or available in the THIN database.

Conclusion

In conclusion, the current estimates of the magnitude of the diagnosed psoriasis population and referral rates to dermatologists may assist in understanding the burden on the UK healthcare system and allow for decision-making and planning for managing this chronic disease population in primary and secondary care.

Consent

The THIN database contains only anonymized and de-identified clinical data and no direct patient contact occurred in this retrospective study. As such, this study was exempt from obtaining patient consent.

Abbreviations
BAD: British association of dermatologists; BMI: Body mass index; BNF: British national formulary; GP: General practitioners; NICE: National institute for health and clinical excellence; OR: Odds ratio; QOF: Quality outcomes framework; THIN: The health improvement network; UK: United Kingdom.

Competing interests
Drs. Khalid, Fox, and Maguire received research funds from Amgen, Inc. Drs. Globe and Chau are employed by Amgen, Inc. and are stockholders. Dr. Chiou was employed by Amgen, Inc. at the time of this research.

Authors' contributions
JMK oversaw the data acquisition, conducted the data analysis and interpretation, performed the statistical testing, provided critical review and revision of the article, and approved of the final version of the article. GG contributed significantly to the study concept and study design, provided data interpretation, provided critical review and revision of the article, and approved of the final version of the article. KMF contributed significantly to the study concept and study design, provided data interpretation, drafted the article, provided critical revision of the article, and approved of the final version of the article. DC contributed to the data interpretation, provided funding for the study, provided critical review and revision of the article, and approved of the final version of the article. AM contributed significantly to the study concept and study design, provided data interpretation, provided critical review and revision of the article, and approved of the final version of the article. CC contributed significantly to the study concept and study design, provided data interpretation, provided critical review and revision of the article, and approved of the final version of the article. All authors read and approved the final manuscript.

Funding support
This study was supported by Amgen, Inc. The funder did not have involvement in the study design, data collection, data analysis, manuscript preparation or publication decision except through the authors who are employees of Amgen, Inc. (GG, DC).

Author details
[1]United Biosource Corporation, London, UK. [2]Amgen Inc., Thousand Oaks, CA, USA. [3]Strategic Healthcare Solutions, LLC, PO Box 543, Monkton, MD 21111, USA. [4]Janssen Global Services, Companies of Johnson & Johnson, New Jersey, USA.

References
1. Greaves MW, Weinstein GD: Treatment of psoriasis. N Engl J Med 1995, 332:581–588.
2. Conway P, Currie CJ: Descriptive epidemiology of hospitalisation for psoriasis. Curr Med Res Opin 2008, 24:3487–3491.
3. Gelfand JM, Weinstein R, Porter SB, Neimann AL, Berlin JA, Margolis DJ: Prevalence and treatment of psoriasis in the United Kingdom: a population-based study. Arch Dermatol 2005, 141:1537–1541.
4. Gelfand JM, Troxel AB, Lewis JD, et al: The risk of mortality in patients with psoriasis: results from a population-based study. Arch Dermatol 2007, 143:1493–1499.
5. Horn EJ, Fox KM, Patel V, et al: Association of patient-reported psoriasis severity with income and employment. J Am Acad Dermatol 2007, 57:963–971.

6. Rapp SR, Feldman SR, Exum ML, Fleischer AB Jr, Reboussin DM: **Psoriasis causes as much disability as other major medical diseases.** *J Am Acad Dermatol* 1999, **41**:401–407.

7. Duque MI, Yosipovitch G, Chan YH, Smith R, Levy P: **Itch, pain, and burning sensation are common symptoms in mild to moderate chronic venous insufficiency with an impact on quality of life.** *J Am Acad Dermatol* 2005, **53**:504–508.

8. Husted JA, Tom BD, Schentag CT, Farewell VT, Gladman DD: **Occurrence and correlates of fatigue in psoriatic arthritis.** *Ann Rheum Dis* 2009, **68**:1553–1558.

9. Chan B, Hales B, Shear N, *et al*: **Work-related lost productivity and its economic impact on Canadian patients with moderate to severe psoriasis.** *J Cutan Med Surg* 2009, **13**:192–197.

10. National Health Services: *Psoriasis.* www.nhs.uk/Conditions/Psoriasis/Pages/NICE.aspx.

11. Smith CH, Anstey AV, Barker JN, *et al*: **British association of dermatologists' guidelines for biologic interventions for psoriasis 2009.** *Br J Dermatol* 2009, **161**:987–1019.

12. British National Formulary: *Edition 59.* www.bnf.org.

13. Huerta C, Rivero E, Rodriguez LA: **Incidence and risk factors for psoriasis in the general population.** *Arch Dermatol* 2007, **143**:1559–1565.

14. *The THIN database.* www.ucl.ac.uk/pcph/research-groups-themes/THIN-pub/databases/pros-cons.

15. Lewis JD, Schinnar R, Bilker WB, Wang X, Strom BL: **Validation studies of the health improvement network (THIN) database for pharmacoepidemiology research.** *Pharmacoepidemiol Drug Saf* 2007, **16**:393–401.

16. Chisholm J: **The Read clinical classification.** *Br Med J* 1990, **300**:1467.

17. Maguire A, Blak BT, Thompson M: **The importance of defining periods of complete mortality reporting for research using automated data from primary care.** *Pharmacoepidemiol Drug Saf* 2009, **18**:76–83.

18. Seminara NM, Abuabara K, Shin DB, *et al*: **Validity of the health improvement network (THIN) for the study of psoriasis.** *Br J Dermatol* 2011, **164**:602–609.

19. Townsend Deprivation Index: www.geog.soton.ac.uk/gen-refer/go3_142_c15p19819999snsw.html.

20. Edwards P, Robert I: **Population adiposity and climate change.** *Int J Epidemiol* 2009, **38**:1137–1140.

21. Gillard SE, Finlay AY: **Current management of psoriasis in the United Kingdom: patterns of prescribing and resource use in primary care.** *Int J Clin Pract* 2005, **59**:1260–1267.

22. *Quality Outcomes Framework.* www.qof.ic.nhs.uk.

23. British Association of Dermatologists: *Treatment for moderate or severe psoriasis.* www.bad.org.uk/site/866/default.aspx.

24. Langan SM, Seminara NM, Shin DB, *et al*: **Prevalence of metabolic syndrome in patients with psoriasis: a population-based study in the United Kingdom.** *J Invest Dermatol* 2011. doi:10.1038/jid.2011.365.

25. Griffiths CE, Clark CM, Chalmers RJ, Li Wan Po A, Williams HC: **A systematic review of treatments for severe psoriasis.** *Health Technol Assess* 2000, **4**(1):1–25.

17

Topical application of RTA 408 lotion activates Nrf2 in human skin and is well-tolerated by healthy human volunteers

Scott A. Reisman[*], Angela R. Goldsberry, Chun-Yue I. Lee, Megan L. O'Grady, Joel W. Proksch, Keith W. Ward and Colin J. Meyer

Abstract

Background: Topical application of the synthetic triterpenoid RTA 408 to rodents elicits a potent dermal cytoprotective phenotype through activation of the transcription factor Nrf2. Therefore, studies were conducted to investigate if such cytoprotective properties translate to human dermal cells, and a topical lotion formulation was developed and evaluated clinically.

Methods: *In vitro*, RTA 408 (3–1000 nM) was incubated with primary human keratinocytes for 16 h. *Ex vivo*, RTA 408 (0.03, 0.3, or 3 %) was applied to healthy human skin explants twice daily for 3 days. A Phase 1 healthy volunteer clinical study with RTA 408 Lotion (NCT02029716) consisted of 3 sequential parts. In Part A, RTA 408 Lotion (0.5 %, 1 %, and 3 %) and lotion vehicle were applied to individual 4-cm^2 sites twice daily for 14 days. In Parts B and C, separate groups of subjects had 3 % RTA 408 Lotion applied twice daily to a 100-cm^2 site for 14 days or a 500-cm^2 site for 28 days.

Results: RTA 408 was well-tolerated in both *in vitro* and *ex vivo* settings up to the highest concentrations tested. Further, RTA 408 significantly and dose-dependently induced a variety of Nrf2 target genes. Clinically, RTA 408 Lotion was also well-tolerated up to the highest concentration, largest surface area, and longest duration tested. Moreover, significant increases in expression of the prototypical Nrf2 target gene NQO1 were observed in skin biopsies, suggesting robust activation of the pharmacological target.

Conclusions: Overall, these data suggest RTA 408 Lotion is well-tolerated, activates Nrf2 in human skin, and appears suitable for continued clinical development.

Keywords: RTA 408 lotion, Nrf2, Radiation dermatitis, Cancer supportive care

Background

Nuclear factor erythroid 2-related factor 2 (Nrf2) is the principal transcription factor that regulates the expression of greater than 90 % of all antioxidative genes [1]. Activation of Nrf2 induces the expression of a battery of such genes, which results in a coordinated intrinsic cellular defense effort to switch to a phenotype that protects against oxidative and electrophilic insult, highlighted by increased antioxidative capacity, induction of glutathione (GSH) synthesis, increased energy production, and elimination of potentially harmful molecules [2, 3]. Activation of Nrf2 also imparts potent anti-inflammatory properties in cells through detoxification of reactive oxygen species

(ROS), which activate the pro-inflammatory transcription factor nuclear factor-kappa B (NF-κB) [4].

Semi-synthetic oleanane triterpenoids are among the most potent activators of Nrf2 identified to date; they bind to specific cysteine residues on Kelch-like ECH-associated protein 1 (Keap1), resulting in subsequent translocation of Nrf2 to the nucleus, where it binds to specific antioxidant response elements, facilitating induction of a multitude of cytoprotective genes [5–8]. Recently, a newly developed semi-synthetic oleanane triterpenoid denoted RTA 408 has been described as an activator of Nrf2 in rat skin [9]. Specifically, topical application of RTA 408 to rats at concentrations of 0.1, 1, or 3 % led to significant and dose-dependent induction of many Nrf2 target genes in the skin, including the prototypical Nrf2 targets NAD(P)H:quinone

* Correspondence: scott.reisman@reatapharma.com
Reata Pharmaceuticals, Inc., 2801 Gateway Dr. Ste 150, Irving, TX 75063, USA

oxidoreductase (Nqo1), sulfiredoxin 1 (Srxn1), and the rate-limiting enzyme subunits for the synthesis of GSH, namely glutamate-cysteine ligase, catalytic and modifier subunits (Gclc and Gclm, respectively). Further, immunohistochemical methods demonstrated that increased staining for Nqo1 protein and total GSH of structures in both the epidermis and dermis was consistent with full transdermal penetration of RTA 408 [9].

The ability to activate Nrf2 and produce cytoprotection was also observed in mice in a model of fractionated radiation-induced dermatitis [10]. Topical application of RTA 408 was highly effective at decreasing the severity of dermatitis in mice exposed to fractionated radiation, where doses as low as 0.01 % RTA 408 demonstrated significant improvements, and a dose of 1 % RTA 408 restored normal appearance of skin by the end of the 40-day treatment period, including substantial hair regrowth [10]. The remarkable improvement in skin attributable to topical treatment with RTA 408 was associated with significant increases in antioxidative Nrf2 target mRNA expression in skin. In contrast, the same skin samples had marked decreases in pro-inflammatory NF-κB target mRNA expression. Overall, these data support the development of RTA 408 as a new therapy for the prevention and treatment of radiation-induced dermatitis in cancer patients undergoing radiation therapy and other conditions associated with oxidative stress and inflammation.

Nevertheless, the translatability of the effects of RTA 408 to human cells has yet to be evaluated. Therefore, this study was performed to investigate the effects of RTA 408 on activation of Nrf2 after exposure of human primary keratinocytes *in vitro* and cultured human skin explants *ex vivo*. Positive results from these *in vitro* and *ex vivo* studies in human cells and tissues suggested the efficacy of topical RTA 408 observed in the mouse model of fractionated radiation-induced dermatitis could be translated to humans. Therefore, a clinically feasible lotion formulation of RTA 408 was developed for a Phase 1 clinical study to evaluate safety, pharmacokinetics (PK), and pharmacodynamics (PD) after topical application to healthy volunteers.

Methods

Culturing of primary human keratinocytes

Fresh human abdominal skin, obtained from a Caucasian donor undergoing an abdominoplasty (female aged 46 years old) was collected and maintained in a holding medium consisting of HEPES buffered DMEM containing antibiotics and antifungals. The epidermis was removed from the dermis after overnight incubation at 4 °C with dispase in the holding medium and then underwent trypsin digestion. The keratinocyte suspension was seeded on 3 T3 fibroblasts and rendered mitotically inactive by mitomycin

C treatment. Human keratinocyte monolayers were cultured for 6 days in DMEM (2 mM Ca^{2+}), with 10 % FCS, L-glutamine (2 mM), insulin (5 µg/mL), hydrocortisone (0.4 µg/mL), epidermal growth factor (EGF, 10 ng/mL), penicillin (100 IU/mL), and streptomycin (100 µg/mL), at 37 °C, in 95 % air/5 % CO_2 atmosphere, with 95 % relative humidity. After 6 days, the 3T3 feeder cells were removed from the human keratinocyte cultures by a trypsin/EDTA treatment. The next day, the human keratinocytes were removed by trypsinization. The human keratinocyte suspension was centrifuged, resuspended in fresh culture medium, and then strained through a series of filters. Cells ($1.5x10^5$/well) were then seeded into 96-well plates with 200 µL of EpiLife® medium and 60 µM calcium, antibiotics, and human keratinocyte growth supplement (HKGS) per well. Human tissue samples for the isolation of keratinocytes (described above) and skin explants (described below) were obtained in accordance with the Human Tissue Act of 2004 (England Wales and Northern Ireland) and collected with the appropriate donor consent.

Treatment and harvesting of primary human keratinocytes

RTA 408 (3, 30, 100, 300, 700, and 1000 nM), vehicle (DMSO, 0.1 % final concentration), or nothing (media control) was incubated with cells in two separate 96-well plates (1.5×10^5 cells per well) for 16 h. At the time of harvest, one plate utilized the MTT assay (Invitrogen, V13154) to examine cell viability, and one plate was processed for QuantiGene Plex 2.0 analysis (*i.e.*, mRNA expression of Nrf2 target genes), according to manufacturer's instructions and as previously reported [9, 11].

Culturing of human skin explants

Skin, obtained from a female reduction mammoplasty (48 year old donor), was collected and placed in a holding medium consisting of HEPES buffered DMEM containing antibiotics and antifungals. The fat was removed, and a 5-mm punch biopsy was used to cut 30 biopsies. Biopsies were cultured at the air-liquid interface with 5 mL of DMEM media (2 mM Ca^{2+}), 10 % FCS, L-glutamine (2 mM), insulin (5 µg/mL), hydrocortisone (0.4 µg/mL), EGF (10 ng/mL), penicillin (100 IU/mL), and streptomycin (100 µg/mL), at 37 °C, in a 95 % air/ 5 % CO_2 atmosphere, with 95 % relative humidity. The dermis of each culture was immersed in the media, while the epidermis was in contact with air.

Ex vivo treatment and harvesting of human skin explants

Skin cultures were split into 5 treatment groups. RTA 408 (0.03, 0.3, or 3 %), vehicle (sesame oil), or nothing (media control) was applied topically twice daily for 2 days and once on Day 3. Approximately 50 µL of RTA 408 or vehicle was applied to the entire surface of the skin cultures. Prior to each application, a visual inspection of the skin cultures confirmed there was no residual RTA 408 or vehicle from the previous administration. All skin cultures were harvested 8 h after the final administration on Day 3, with half of the replicates fixed for 24 h in phosphate-buffered formalin (pH 7.0–7.4), transferred to 70 % ethanol, then processed and paraffin-embedded, according to standard histological techniques. The remaining skin samples were snapped frozen.

Quantigene 2.0 Plex mRNA expression analysis

Messenger RNA (mRNA) was quantified using Quantigene Plex 2.0 technology according to manufacturer's protocol (Affymetrix, Inc., Santa Clara, CA) and as previously described [12]. Probe sets were designed against the human genome for analysis of Nrf2 target genes, and a modified version of Panel 11834 (Affymetrix) was used. Human primary keratinocyte data were normalized to the housekeeping gene PPIB. Human skin explant data were normalized to the average of housekeeping genes RPL13A and PPIB.

Immunohistochemical analysis of NQO1 protein in cultured human skin explants and biopsies

Levels of NQO1 protein in skin sections were determined by immunohistochemistry (IHC) using previously described methods [9]. NQO1 staining intensity of 5X magnification photomicrographs was quantified using ImageJ software v1.46 with the Densitometry 1 plug-in, both freely available from the National Institutes of Health (http://rsbweb.nih.gov/ij/index.html).

Healthy volunteer clinical study design

The clinical study (https://clinicaltrials.gov/ct2/show/NCT02029716) enrolled healthy adults (male and female) aged 18 to 65 years, with Fitzpatrick skin type I to IV, and a body mass index (BMI) between 18 and 32 kg/m^2. Demographic data are presented in Table 1. The study was conducted sequentially in 3 parts to assess the safety, tolerability, PD, and PK of RTA 408 Lotion applied topically twice daily (BID), at 8:00 a.m. and 8:00 p.m., for up to 28 days. For each application, the appropriate amount of lotion was applied to the skin and gently massaged for the appropriate time (Parts A and B: 10–15 s; Part C: 45 s). The areas of application were allowed to dry for 5 min, and then the entire area was covered with loose-fitting gauze to keep the lotion confined during normal activities.

Part A was a randomized, double-blind, placebo-controlled assessment of the safety, local skin tolerability, PD, and PK of 3 concentrations of RTA 408 Lotion (0.5 %, 1 %, and 3 %, w/w) compared to lotion vehicle (0 %) applied topically to 12 healthy subjects BID for 14 days to a small skin surface area on the lower back (4 cm^2 for each concentration). Part B was open-label and assessed the safety, tolerability, PD, and PK of the highest tolerated

dose of RTA 408 Lotion from Part A (i.e., 3 %) applied topically to 10 healthy subjects BID for 14 days to a larger skin surface area on the lower back (100 cm^2). During the dosing period in Parts A and B, subjects were confined to the study site for 15 days. Part C was open-label and assessed the safety, tolerability, PD, and PK of RTA 408 Lotion (3 %) concentration applied BID to an even larger skin surface area (500 cm^2) on the backs of 10 healthy subjects for 28 days. During the dosing period in Part C, subjects were confined to the study site for 29 days. Total daily doses of RTA 408 for Parts A, B, and C were approximately 1.8, 30, and 150 mg/day, respectively. The assessment of safety was based primarily on the incidence, intensity, and type of adverse events, Modified Draize Skin Irritation Assessments, clinical laboratory assessments (hematology, clinical chemistry, and urinalysis), physical examinations, 12-lead electrocardiograms (ECG), and vital signs.

Analysis of RTA 408 plasma concentrations in healthy volunteers following topical administration of RTA 408 lotion

Blood samples for PK analysis were collected for determination of plasma RTA 408 concentrations prior to dosing and 1, 2, 4, 12, and 24 h after the first topical application of RTA 408 Lotion on Days 1, 7, and 14 of Parts A, B, and C and also on Day 28 for Part C. A validated LC/MS/MS method with a lower limit of quantitation (LLOQ) of 0.074 ng/mL and an upper limit of quantitation (ULOQ) of 37.0 ng/mL was used for quantification of RTA 408 in plasma samples.

Analysis of NQO1 protein expression in healthy volunteer skin punch biopsies

Punch biopsies (3 mm) for evaluation of induction of NQO1 protein expression, the prototypical Nrf2 target gene, were collected the day following the final dose in each part of the study. A local injection of lidocaine HCl (1 %) was used for anesthesia. Biopsies were incubated in formalin at room temperature for 24 h and then transferred to 70 % ethanol. NQO1 IHC on the skin biopsies was performed as described above.

The protocol and informed consent documents were submitted to and approved by the duly constituted Western Institutional Review Board prior to initiation of the clinical study. The study was conducted in accordance with the Declaration of Helsinki and with all applicable laws and regulations of the locale and country where the study was conducted, and in compliance with Good Clinical Practice Guidelines.

Statistics

Nrf2 target gene data were analyzed with Sigmaplot 12.0 (Systat, Inc., San Jose, CA) by student's t-test or by one way-analysis of variance (ANOVA) followed by Duncan's Multiple Range post-hoc test with significance set at $p < 0.05$.

Table 1 Phase 1 Clinical trial healthy volunteer baseline characteristics

Demographic/characteristic category/statistic	Part A	Part B	Part C	Total
N	12	10	10	32
Age				
Mean	41.9	40.2	42.0	41.4
S.D.	10.1	9.7	8.4	9.2
Median	38.5	40.5	40.0	39.0
Minimum	29	23	33	23
Maximum	59	53	59	59
Gender (N)				
Female	1 (8.3 %)	1 (10.0 %)	2 (20.0 %)	4 (12.5 %)
Male	11 (91.7 %)	9 (90.0 %)	8 (80.0)	28 (87.5 %)
Ethnicity				
Hispanic or Latino	1 (8.3 %)	0 (0.0 %)	2 (20.0 %)	3 (9.4 %)
Not Hispanic or Latino	11 (91.7 %)	10 (100.0 %)	8 (80.0 %)	29 (90.6 %)
Race				
White	11 (91.7 %)	10 (100.0 %)	8 (80.0 %)	29 (90.6 %)
Asian	1 (8.3 %)	0 (0.0 %)	0 (0.0 %)	1 (3.1 %)
Other	0 (0.0 %)	0 (0.0 %)	2 (20.0 %)	2 (6.3 %)
Fitzpatrick Skin Type				
I (0–7)	0 (0.0 %)	1 (10.0 %)	0 (0.0 %)	1 (3.1 %)
II (8–16)	4 (33.3 %)	5 (50.0 %)	4 (40.0 %)	13 (40.6 %)
III (17–25)	8 (66.7 %)	4 (40.0 %)	6 (60.0 %)	18 (56.3 %)
IV (26–30)	0 (0.0 %)	0 (0.0 %)	0 (0.0 %)	0 (0.0 %)
Baseline BMI				
Mean	27.9	27.7	25.9	27.2
S.D.	2.7	3.2	3.2	3.1
Median	27.6	28.5	27.3	27.7
Minimum	22.6	21.8	21.0	21.0
Maximum	31.2	31.3	29.8	31.3

Results

RTA 408 induces Nrf2 target genes in primary human keratinocytes

The effects of RTA 408 (3–1000 nM) on the mRNA expression of Nrf2 target genes were evaluated in freshly isolated primary human keratinocytes. There were no differences in percent cell viability among the groups (Additional file 1: Figure S1), indicating that RTA 408 was well-tolerated over the concentration range tested. Further, RTA 408 significantly induced the mRNA expression of many cytoprotective Nrf2 target genes in a concentration-dependent manner (Fig. 1). Remarkably, for most of the genes evaluated [*i.e.*, NQO1, SRXN1, thioredoxin reductase (TXNRD1), GCLC, GCLM, glutathione reductase (GSR), xCT, heme oxygenase-1 (HO-1), aldo-keto reductase 1C1 (AKR1C1), and ferritin heavy chain 1 (FTH1)], significant induction was observed beginning towards the lower range of the concentrations tested (*i.e.*, 3 and/or 30 nM), and induction continued to increase dose-dependently up to the highest concentration tested (*i.e.*, 1000 nM). Though the levels of induction of superoxide dismutase 1 (SOD1), catalase, glutathione peroxidase 3 (GPX3), epoxide hydrolase-1 (EH-1), glutaredoxin (GLRX), peroxiredoxin 1 (PRDX1), and thioredoxin (TXN) are less than other Nrf2 target genes, it is still quite meaningful for this particular subset of antioxidant proteins. Further, the combined coordinated upregulation of the mRNA expression of these antioxidant enzymes would likely have a profound antioxidant and cytoprotective effect on the cells.

Topical application of RTA 408 induces Nrf2 target genes in human skin explants

The effects of topical application of RTA 408 (0.03, 0.3, or 3.0 %) were evaluated *ex vivo* in cultured human skin explants. RTA 408 was well-tolerated with skin maintaining

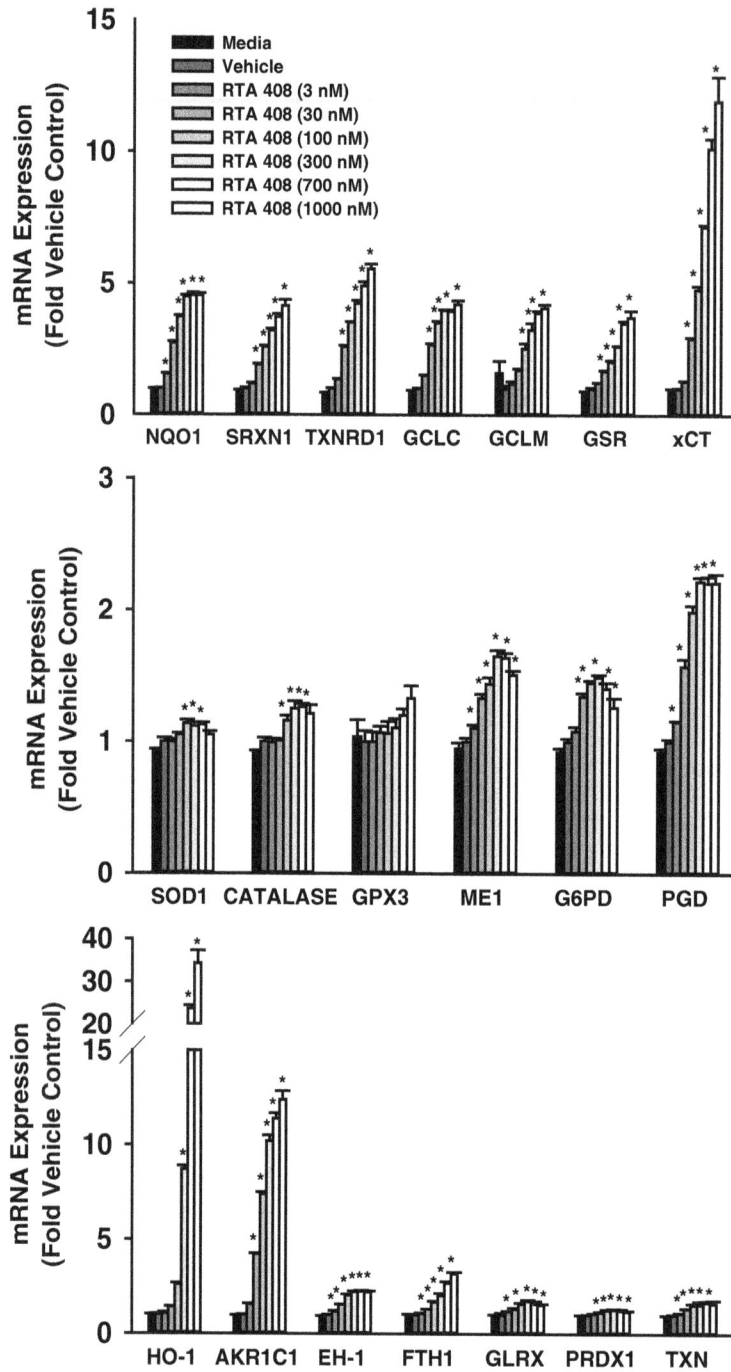

Fig. 1 Effect of RTA 408 on mRNA Expression of Nrf2 Target Genes in Primary Human Keratinocytes. Freshly isolated primary human keratinocytes were incubated with RTA 408 (3–1000 nM) or vehicle (DMSO, 0.1 % v/v) for 16 h and analyzed for mRNA expression of Nrf2 target genes. Data were normalized to the housekeeping gene PPIB and are presented as mean fold vehicle control ± standard error of the mean (S.E.M.). *$p < 0.05$ vs. vehicle control

normal appearance throughout the treatment period. Eight hours after the last dose, skin was harvested for determination of mRNA expression and NQO1 protein expression by IHC. Similar to the results in primary human keratinocytes, RTA 408 significantly and dose-dependently induced the

mRNA expression of a broad panel of Nrf2 target genes (Fig. 2). Very marked (>30-fold) induction of Nrf2 target genes such as NQO1, SRXN1, xCT, HO-1, and AKR1C1 was observed. The mRNA induction of the prototypical Nrf2 target gene NQO1 translated to significant and dose-dependent

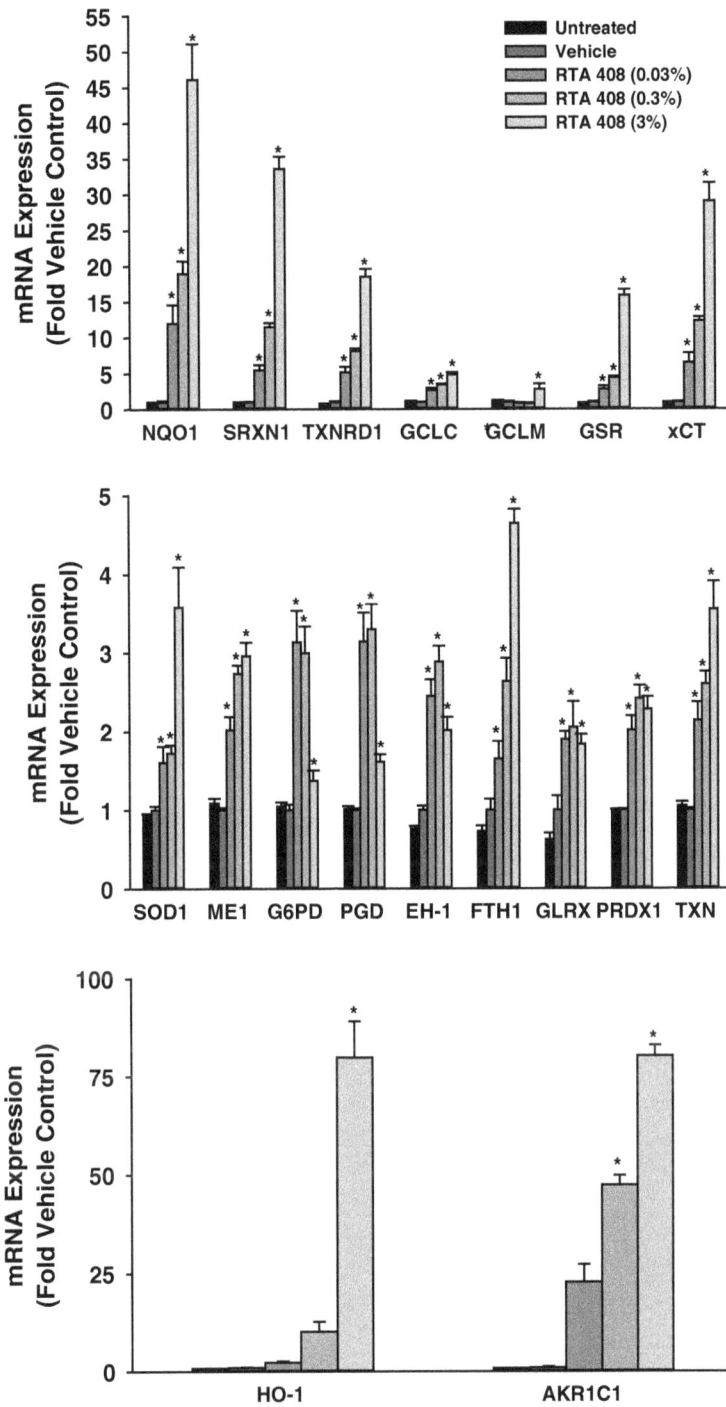

Fig. 2 Effect of RTA 408 on the mRNA Expression of Nrf2 Target Genes in Human Skin Explants. Human skin explants from a healthy donor were cultured. RTA 408 (0.03, 0.3, or 3 %) or vehicle (sesame oil) was applied topically up to twice daily for 3 days and skin was then processed and analyzed for mRNA expression of Nrf2 target genes. Data were normalized to the average of housekeeping genes RPL13A and PPIB and are presented as mean fold vehicle control ± S.E.M. *$p < 0.05$ vs. vehicle control

induction of NQO1 protein in the epidermis of the skin explants (Fig. 3). Statistically significant increases in most Nrf2 target genes at both the mRNA and protein levels were observed at the lowest concentration tested (*i.e.*, 0.03 %).

Topical application of RTA 408 lotion was well-tolerated and produced low systemic exposures in healthy volunteers

A Phase 1 study was completed to evaluate the safety, local PD, and systemic PK of RTA 408 following topical

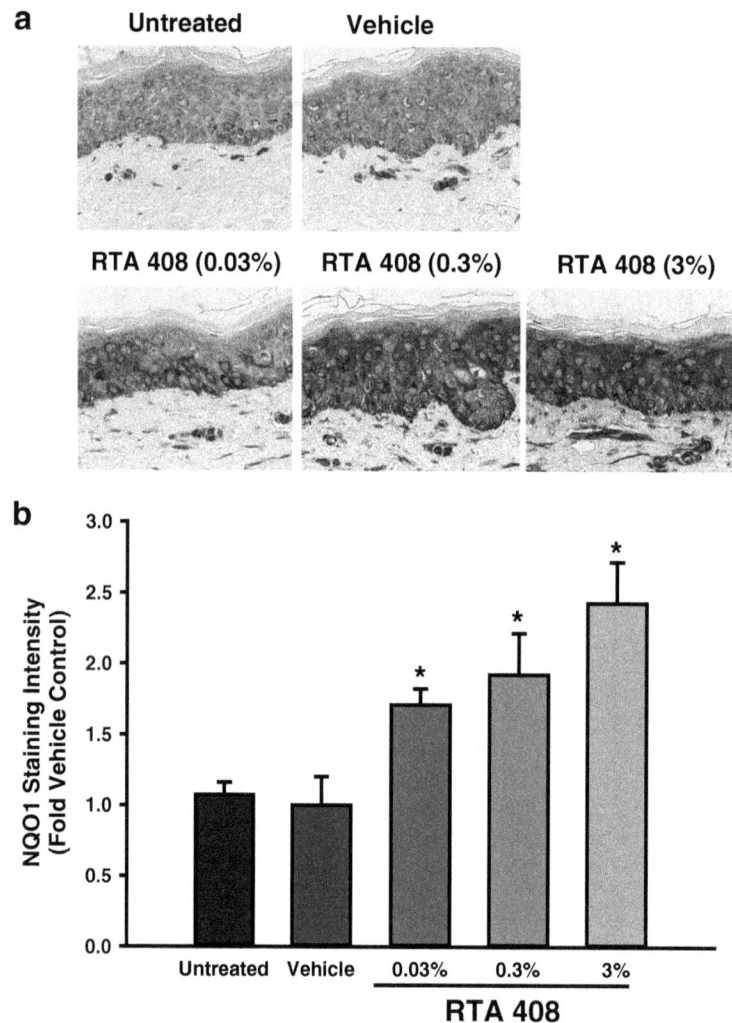

Fig. 3 Effect of RTA 408 on the Protein Expression of NQO1 in Human Skin Explants. Human skin explants from a healthy donor were cultured. RTA 408 (0.03, 0.3, or 3 %) or vehicle (sesame oil) was applied topically up to twice daily for 3 days and the skin was fixed in formalin. NQO1 protein was evaluated using standard immunohistochemical techniques. **a**. Representative photomicrographs (20X) are presented for each treatment group. **b**. Staining intensity was determined and presented as mean fold vehicle control ± S.E.M. *$p < 0.05$ vs. vehicle control

application of RTA 408 Lotion to healthy volunteers ($n = 32$). RTA 408 Lotion was well-tolerated, with only 1 (3.1 %) subject exhibiting mild application site erythema and pruritus (Table 2 and Additional file 2: Table S1). This subject was enrolled in Part C of the study, receiving 3 % RTA 408 Lotion twice daily for 28 days. This subject had a modified Draize Score of 1 (barely perceptible, faint to pink) on Days 5–9, which subsided on Day 10 with continued RTA 408 Lotion administration, and was not observed during the remainder of the study with continued dosing through Day 28. Modified Draize Scores for all other subjects on all other days were 0 (no erythema). There were no severe adverse effects, and no subjects discontinued treatment of RTA 408 Lotion. With the exception of one subject, all individual abnormal laboratory results

were considered to not be clinically significant. In Part C, one subject experienced an adverse event (not related to study drug) of increased alanine transaminase (ALT) levels (79 IU/L) on Day 7. As a result, study drug was stopped on Day 16; study drug was not restarted, but the subject completed the study. The subject also had elevated ALT (48 IU/L) on Day –1, which was recorded in the subject's medical history. The subject's ALT value at the end of the study (58 IU/L) was similar to the baseline value (48 IU/L), and the adverse event of increased alanine transaminase (ALT) levels was considered resolved and unrelated to study drug. Further, at no time during the study did this subject have measureable concentrations (<LLOQ of 0.074 ng/mL) of RTA 408 in plasma. Moreover, there were no clinically significant mean changes in vital signs or electrocardiogram (ECG) parameters

Table 2 Overview of adverse events

Category Preferred Term	Part A (N = 12) N (%)	Part B (N = 10) N (%)	Part C (N = 10) N (%)	Total (N = 32) N (%)
Subjects with Any Adverse Event	1 (8.3)	3 (30.0)	7 (70.0)	11 (34.4)
Subjects with Any Study Drug Related Adverse Event	0 (0.0)	0 (0.0)	1 (10.0)	1 (3.1)[a]
Subjects with Any Serious Adverse Event	0 (0.0)	0 (0.0)	0 (0.0)	0 (0.0)
Subjects with Any Study Drug Related Serious Adverse Event	0 (0.0)	0 (0.0)	0 (0.0)	0 (0.0)
Subjects with Any Adverse Event Leading to Discontinuation	0 (0.0)	0 (0.0)	0 (0.0)	0 (0.0)

[a]In total, 1 (3.1 %) subject, in Part C, had an RTA 408 Lotion-related adverse event, described as mild application site erythema and pruritus (Table 2). This subject had a modified Draize Score of 1 (barely perceptible, faint to pink) on Days 5–9, which subsided on Day 10, and was not observed during the remainder of the study. Scores for all other subjects on all other days were 0 (no erythema)

(heart rate and PR, RR, QRS, QT, QTc, and QTcF intervals) from baseline in any subject, and there were also no clinically significant drug-related abnormalities in clinical laboratory parameters. Overall, RTA 408 was well-tolerated at the doses and durations tested.

Topical administration of RTA 408 Lotion produced very low systemic exposures to RTA 408. The highest dose evaluated in the Phase 1 study was 3 % RTA 408 Lotion (or ~150 mg RTA 408) applied to a 500-cm^2 skin area (~2.6 % of total body surface area (BSA) based on the average total BSA of ~1.92 m^2 of volunteers in Part C) twice daily for 28 days, which produced plasma concentrations of RTA 408 near or below the LLOQ (0.074 ng/mL) for all healthy volunteers in the study, indicating that topical application of RTA 408 Lotion did not produce any meaningful systemic exposures. Only one healthy volunteer demonstrated measurable plasma RTA 408 concentrations; this subject was enrolled in the Part C cohort that received the highest dose evaluated, and had measurable plasma RTA 408 concentrations only on Day 28. The maximal plasma RTA 408 concentration quantifiable in this healthy volunteer was 0.0943 ng/mL, and the AUC$_{(0-24h)}$ was 0.0019 h*µg/mL. Overall, RTA 408 produced very low systemic exposures.

Topical application of RTA 408 lotion to healthy volunteers induced NQO1 protein in skin

Protein expression of NQO1, the prototypical Nrf2 target gene, was evaluated by IHC in skin biopsies collected from all subjects enrolled in each part of the study (Fig. 4). In Part A, RTA 408 Lotion tended to induce the protein expression of NQO1, but high variability precluded statistical significance. In Part A, the relatively small size of the treatment area (4-cm^2) may have contributed to the variability in NQO1 staining. However, statistically significant induction of NQO1 was observed in Parts B and C when RTA 408 Lotion was applied to larger surface areas (i.e., 100-cm^2 for Part B and 500-cm^2 for Part C).

Discussion

Similar to other semi-synthetic oleanane triterpenoids, RTA 408 is a potent activator of the cytoprotective and antioxidative transcription factor Nrf2 and a potent inhibitor of the pro-inflammatory transcription factor NF-κB [7]. Previous studies have demonstrated that topical dermal application of RTA 408 to rodents produces desirable dermal cytoprotective effects in both the naïve setting in rats and in a mouse model of dermatological injury produced by fractionated radiation exposure [10, 9]. Thus, the present series of nonclinical and clinical studies were conducted to evaluate the translatability of the cytoprotective effects in skin produced by RTA 408 to humans.

Because of their anatomical location within the epidermis, keratinocytes are constantly exposed to external stresses, including sunlight, radiation, and oxygen in air, all of which can contribute to production of excess ROS and ultimately, tissue injury [13]. Thus, human keratinocytes are an important cell type to investigate tolerability of RTA 408 and whether RTA 408 can elicit suitable pharmacologic activation of the Nrf2-mediated antioxidant response. Indeed, freshly isolated primary human keratinocytes demonstrated tolerability (i.e., lack of cytotoxicity) to RTA 408 (3–1000 nM), and RTA 408 produced dose-dependent induction of Nrf2 target genes over the entire concentration range. In addition, these in vitro keratinocyte data were consistent with a previous study demonstrating induction of NQO1 protein expression in keratinocytes after topical dermal application of RTA 408 to rat skin [9], suggesting that effects of RTA 408 previously observed in rodent skin may also be observed in human skin.

Full thickness human skin explants more closely mimic the in vivo setting and represent a practical model of intact skin that can be used to evaluate topical dermal application to human tissue ex vivo [14]. RTA 408 was well tolerated in human skin explants, and topical application of RTA 408 dose-dependently and significantly induced the mRNA expression of Nrf2 target

Part a:4 -cm² Dosing Site (14 Days)

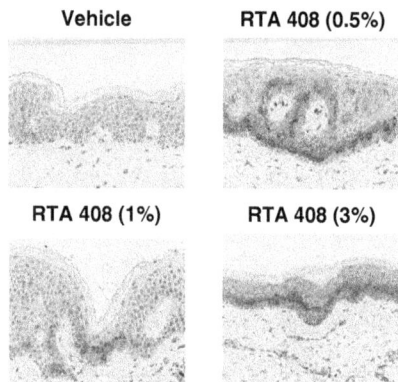

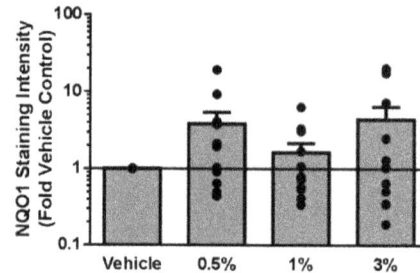

Part b:100 -cm² Dosing Site (14 Days)

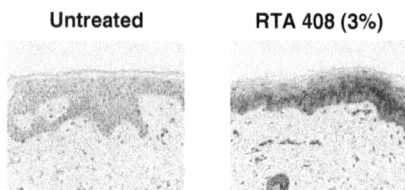

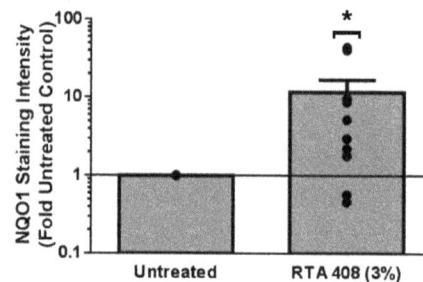

Part c:500 -cm² Dosing Site (28 Days)

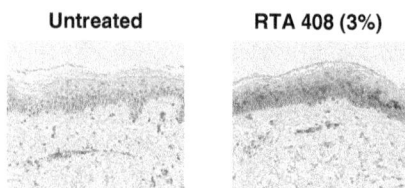

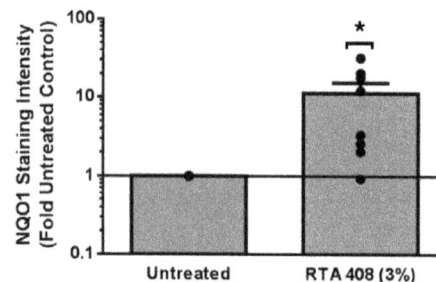

Fig. 4 Effect of RTA 408 Lotion on the Protein Expression of NQO1 in Human Skin Biopsies from Phase 1 Clinical Trial. Skin biopsies were collected from healthy volunteers one day after the final dose in Parts **a**, **b**, and **c** of the Phase 1 clinical trial. Part **a** evaluated 3 concentrations of RTA 408 Lotion (0.5, 1, and 3 %) compared to lotion vehicle applied topically to 12 healthy subjects BID for 14 days to a small skin surface area on the lower back (4 cm² for each concentration). Part **b** was open-label and assessed the RTA 408 Lotion (3 %) applied topically to 10 healthy subjects BID for 14 days to skin on the lower back (100 cm²). Part **c** was open-label and assessed the RTA 408 Lotion (3 %) applied topically to 10 healthy subjects BID for 28 days to skin on the lower back (500 cm²). Representative photomicrographs (20X) from each part are presented on the left with corresponding quantified staining intensities presented on the right. Dots represent individual data points for each subject. Bars present data as mean fold vehicle or untreated control ± S.E.M. *$p < 0.05$ vs. vehicle or untreated control

genes. Together, these data demonstrate that topical application of RTA 408 is well tolerated in a relevant nonclinical human skin model and produces robust Nrf2 activation.

Consistent with the nonclinical data, RTA 408 Lotion was very well tolerated, when applied topically to healthy human volunteers up to concentrations of 3 % to a 500-cm² area twice daily for 28 days. Notably, no systemic exposure was generally observed, suggesting that the pharmacological effects of RTA 408 were limited to locally treated skin sites. Finally, protein induction in skin biopsies of the prototypical Nrf2 target gene NQO1 was associated with administration of RTA 408 Lotion, indicating that local Nrf2 activation can be achieved in human skin.

The profound Nrf2 activation effects of RTA 408 in skin are consistent with, although more potent than, the activity previously observed with the polyphenol phytochemical and weak Nrf2 activator curcumin. Curcumin also activates Nrf2 and induces Nrf2 target genes when incubated with human primary keratinocytes or cultured skin biopsies, though less potently and efficaciously than RTA 408 (15). Curcumin was tested clinically in a recently completed trial investigating the effects of oral administration (6 g/day) to breast cancer patients undergoing radiation therapy (16). This high dose of curcumin only modestly reduced radiation dermatitis severity and moist desquamation, but overall, the data suggested that pharmacological activation of Nrf2 in skin may be a beneficial strategy for the prevention and treatment of radiation dermatitis (16). Therefore, a more potent activator of Nrf2, such as RTA 408, may provide the necessary level of cytoprotection to provide a meaningful clinical benefit.

Based in part on these results, RTA 408 Lotion has been advanced into clinical evaluation for the prevention and treatment of radiation dermatitis in cancer patients receiving radiotherapy (https://clinicaltrials.gov/ct2/show/NCT02142959). In such a radioprotection setting, one theoretical concern could be that such robust induction of the cytoprotective response may afford protection to cancer cells, as well as normal skin cells. However, available nonclinical data suggest that this will not be the case. A recent study evaluated the radioprotective effects of RTA 402, a potent Nrf2 activator and closely related analog to RTA 408, in normal epithelial cells and a panel of cancer cells exposed to ionizing radiation [15]. RTA 402 evoked significant Nrf2-dependent radioprotection in normal lung and breast epithelial cells, as well as lymphocytes, but provided no protection nor activated Nrf2 in any of the cancer cells evaluated. This suggests that RTA 402 and RTA 408 differentially affect Nrf2 in normal versus cancer cells. Similarly, RTA 408 increases survival and protects the rat gastrointestinal tract from a lethal dose of whole body irradiation [16], while also inhibiting growth of established xenografts with enhanced anti-cancer effects when coupled with radiation treatments [16]. Overall, these data suggest that RTA 408 will afford radioprotection to normal cells only and may enhance radiosensitivity to cancer cells; additional work to characterize these differential activities is ongoing.

Conclusions

Collectively, the present data demonstrate that topical application of RTA 408 Lotion is well-tolerated by healthy human volunteers, and RTA 408 Lotion produces an appropriate pharmacodynamic response of Nrf2 activation in skin that would be hypothesized to be cytoprotective under conditions of oxidative stress and inflammation. These safety data, coupled with the profound pharmacology observed in a clinically-relevant rodent model of radiation-induced skin injury [10], support the continued clinical development of topical RTA 408 Lotion.

Abbreviations

AKR1C1: Aldo-keto reductase 1C1; ALT: Alanine transaminase; ECG: Electrocardiogram; EH-1: Epoxide hydrolase-1; FTH1: Ferritin heavy chain 1; G6PD: Glucose-6-phosphate dehydrogenase; GCLC: Glutamate cysteine ligase, catalytic subunit; GCLM: Glutamate cysteine ligase, modifier subunit; GPX3: Glutathione peroxidase 3; GSH: Glutathione; GSR: Glutathione reductase; HO-1: Heme oxygenase-1; IHC: Immunohistochemistry; Keap1: Kelch-like ECH-associated protein 1; LLOQ: Lower limit of quantitation; ME1: Malic enzyme 1; NF-κB: Nuclear factor-kappa B; NQO1: NAD(P)H: quinone oxidoreductase 1; Nrf2: Nuclear factor erythroid 2-related factor 2; PD: Pharmacodynamics; PGD: 6-phosophoglucose dehydrogenase; PK: Pharmacokinetics; PRDX1: Peroxiredoxin; ROS: Reactive oxygen species; SOD1: Superoxide dismutase 1; SRXN1: Sulfiredoxin; TXN: Thioredoxin; TXNRD1: Thioredoxin reductase 1; ULOQ: Upper limit of quantitation; xCT: Cystine/glutamate transporter.

Competing interests

All authors are employed by and have a financial interest in Reata Pharmaceuticals, Inc.

Authors' contributions

SR was the primary author, aided in the design of nonclinical experiments, and conducted laboratory experiments and statistical analyses for the presented biochemical data. CL and JP designed the *in vitro* and *ex vivo* studies. CM, AG, JP, KW, and MO designed the protocol, performed statistical analyses, and interpreted data from the clinical study. All authors read and approved the final manuscript.

Acknowledgements

Human primary keratinocyte and human skin explant experiments were conducted by Epistem Ltd (Manchester, UK). Immunohistochemistry was conducted by HistoTox Labs, Inc. (Boulder, CO). LC-MS/MS experiments were performed by Abbvie, Inc. (North Chicago, IL).

References

1. Lisk C, McCord J, Bose S, Sullivan T, Loomis Z, Nozik-Grayck E, et al. Nrf2 activation: a potential strategy for the prevention of acute mountain sickness. Free Radic Biol Med. 2013;63:264–73. doi:10.1016/j.freeradbiomed.2013.05.024.
2. Ludtmann MH, Angelova PR, Zhang Y, Abramov AY, Dinkova-Kostova AT. Nrf2 affects the efficiency of mitochondrial fatty acid oxidation. Biochem J. 2014;457(3):415–24. doi:10.1042/BJ20130863.
3. Suzuki T, Motohashi H, Yamamoto M. Toward clinical application of the Keap1-Nrf2 pathway. Trends Pharmacol Sci. 2013;34(6):340–6. doi:10.1016/j.tips.2013.04.005.
4. Pedruzzi LM, Stockler-Pinto MB, Leite Jr M, Mafra D. Nrf2-keap1 system versus NF-kappaB: the good and the evil in chronic kidney disease? Biochimie. 2012;94(12):2461–6. doi:10.1016/j.biochi.2012.07.015.
5. Takaya K, Suzuki T, Motohashi H, Onodera K, Satomi S, Kensler TW, et al. Validation of the multiple sensor mechanism of the Keap1-Nrf2 system. Free Radic Biol Med. 2012;53(4):817–27. doi:10.1016/j.freeradbiomed.2012.06.023.
6. Sporn MB, Liby KT, Yore MM, Fu L, Lopchuk JM, Gribble GW. New synthetic triterpenoids: potent agents for prevention and treatment of tissue injury caused by inflammatory and oxidative stress. J Nat Prod. 2011;74(3):537–45. doi:10.1021/np100826q.
7. Liby KT, Sporn MB. Synthetic oleanane triterpenoids: multifunctional drugs with a broad range of applications for prevention and treatment of chronic disease. Pharmacol Rev. 2012;64(4):972–1003. doi:10.1124/pr.111.004846.
8. Cleasby A, Yon J, Day PJ, Richardson C, Tickle IJ, Williams PA, et al. Structure of the BTB domain of Keap1 and its interaction with the triterpenoid antagonist CDDO. PLoS One. 2014;9(6), e98896. doi:10.1371/journal.pone.0098896.
9. Reisman SA, Lee CY, Meyer CJ, Proksch JW, Ward KW. Topical application of the synthetic triterpenoid RTA 408 activates Nrf2 and induces cytoprotective genes in rat skin. Arch Dermatol Res. 2014;306(5):447–54. doi:10.1007/s00403-013-1433-7.

10. Reisman SA, Lee CY, Meyer CJ, Proksch JW, Sonis ST, Ward KW. Topical application of the synthetic triterpenoid RTA 408 protects mice from radiation-induced dermatitis. Radiat Res. 2014;181(5):512–20. doi:10.1667/RR13578.1.

11. Reisman SA, Ward KW, Klaassen CD, Meyer CJ. CDDO-9,11-dihydro-trifluoroethyl amide (CDDO-dhTFEA) induces hepatic cytoprotective genes and increases bile flow in rats. Xenobiotica. 2013;43(7):571–8. doi:10.3109/00498254.2012.750022.

12. Reisman SA, Yeager RL, Yamamoto M, Klaassen CD. Increased Nrf2 activation in livers from Keap1-knockdown mice increases expression of cytoprotective genes that detoxify electrophiles more than those that detoxify reactive oxygen species. Toxicol Sci. 2009;108(1):35–47. doi:10.1093/toxsci/kfn267.

13. Bito T, Nishigori C. Impact of reactive oxygen species on keratinocyte signaling pathways. J Dermatol Sci. 2012;68(1):3–8. doi:10.1016/j.jdermsci.2012.06.006.

14. Nakamura M, Rikimaru T, Yano T, Moore KG, Pula PJ, Schofield BH, et al. Full-thickness human skin explants for testing the toxicity of topically applied chemicals. J Invest Dermatol. 1990;95(3):325–32.

15. El-Ashmawy M, Delgado O, Cardentey A, Wright WE, Shay JW. CDDO-Me protects normal lung and breast epithelial cells but not cancer cells from radiation. PLoS One. 2014;9(12), e115600. doi:10.1371/journal.pone.0115600.

16. Alexeev V, Lash E, Aguillard A, Corsini L, Bitterman A, Ward K, et al. Radiation protection of the gastrointestinal tract and growth inhibition of prostate cancer xenografts by a single compound. Mol Cancer Ther. 2014;13(12):2968–77. doi:10.1158/1535-7163.MCT-14-0354.

Prevalence of head lice infestation and pediculicidal effect of permethrine shampoo in primary school girls in a low-income area in southeast of Iran

Moussa Soleimani-Ahmadi[1,2*], Seyed Aghil Jaberhashemi[3], Mehdi Zare[4] and Alireza Sanei-Dehkordi[2]

Abstract

Background: Head lice infestation is a common public health problem that is most prevalent in primary school children throughout the world, especially in developing countries including different parts of Iran. This study aimed to determine the prevalence and risk factors associated with head lice infestation and pediculicidal effect of 1% permethrin shampoo in primary schools girls of Bashagard County, one of the low socioeconomic areas in southeast of Iran.

Methods: In this interventional study six villages with similar demographical situations were selected and randomly assigned into intervention and control areas. In each area 150 girl students aged 7–12 years were selected randomly and screened for head lice infestation by visual scalp examination. In intervention area, treatment efficacy of 1% permethrin shampoo was evaluated via re-examination for infestation after one, two, and three weeks. Pre-tested structured questionnaire was used to collect data on socio-demographic and associated factors of head lice infestation.

Results: The prevalence of head lice infestation was 67.3%. There was significant association between head lice infestation and school grade, family size, parents' literacy, bathing facilities, frequency of hair washing, and use of shared articles ($p < 0.05$). The effectiveness of 1% permethrin shampoo for head lice treatment was 29.2, 68.9, and 90.3% after the first, second, and third weeks, respectively.

Conclusion: The head lice infestation is a health problem in primary school girls of Bashagard County. Improvement of socioeconomic status and providing appropriate educational programs about head lice risk factors and prevention can be effective for reduction of infestation in this area.

Keywords: Head lice infestation, Schoolchildren, Socio-demographic characteristics, Permethrin shampoo, Bashagard, Iran

Background

The human head louse, *Pediculus humanus capitis*, is an obligate ectoparasitic insect, which is readily transmitted by direct head-to-head contact, especially in crowded conditions [1]. Head lice infestation is a common health problem in children worldwide and a survey conducted in the south of Iran reported the prevalence to be 23.9% [2].

Although the biology of head lice is the same globally, the epidemiology depends on the society and cultural behaviour. Treatment options are dependent on the context and factors such as access to pediculicides and availability of educational interventions for adoption of a particular behaviours [3, 4]. For the treatment of head lice infestation two classes of insecticides are commonly used, organophosphates such as malathion and pyrethroids such as permethrin and phenothrin with pyrethroids being the most widely used ones due to their

* Correspondence: mussa.sahmadi@gmail.com; mussa.soleimai@yahoo.com
[1]Social Determinants in Health Promotion Research Center, Hormozgan University of Medical Sciences, Bandar Abbas, Iran
[2]Department of Medical Entomology and Vector Control, Faculty of Health, Hormozgan University of Medical Sciences, P.O. Box: 79145–3838, Bandar Abbas, Iran
Full list of author information is available at the end of the article

shorter contact time and less odor [5]. This is despite the fact that the efficacy of many of the insecticide products including permethrin has been now reduced because the head louse has acquired resistance to some of these chemicals [6, 7].

This study was conducted aiming to determine the prevalence and risk factors associated with head lice infestation and treatment efficacy of 1% permethrin shampoo in primary schools girls of Bashagard County, one of the low socioeconomic areas in the southeast of Iran.

Methods

Study design and data collection

This interventional community-based cross-sectional study was carried out in Bashagard County in the Hormozgan province, southeast of Iran. The county has an area of 16,000 km^2 and is located between latitudes 26°04′-26°58′ N and longitudes 57°23′-59°02′ E with an approximately 43,000 population in 2016.

Bashagard County has a warm climate with mean annual temperature of 27.8 °C ranging from 18.8 to 38 °C. The rainfall occurs through the January–October with a total annual average of 235.9 mm during 2015–2016. The annual averages of minimum and maximum relative humidity are respectively 16% in June and 38.2% in August. It is a low socioeconomic area with majority of the population living in houses made of cement and blocks and shelters made of palm tree branches (Fig. 1).

On the basis of available epidemiological data and unpublished data on the prevalence of head lice infestation in the Bashagard health center, six villages with similar topographical, epidemiological, and demographic characteristics were selected for conducting the study and assigned randomly into intervention and control areas

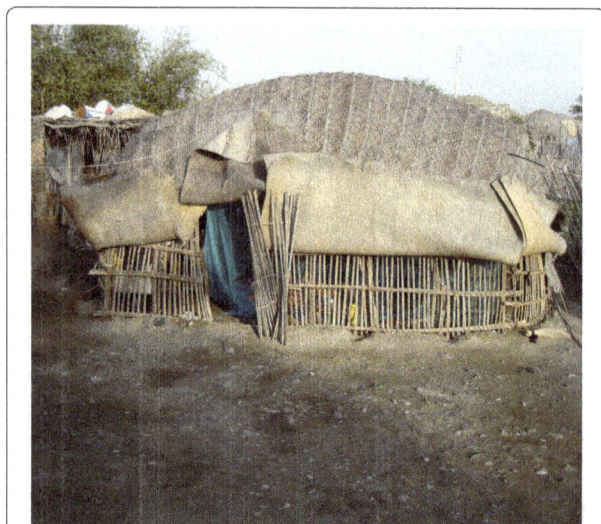

Fig. 1 Sheds made of palm leaves, a living place for people in Bashagard County, southeast of Iran

which received and did not received 1% permethrin shampoo, respectively. In each area 150 girl students aged 7–12 years were selected randomly. The study area is shown in Fig. 2.

A team including health workers of the study area and a medical entomologist inspected the hair and scalps of the students visually for eggs, nymphs, and adult lice.

The entire head was examined carefully and special attention was paid to the nape of the head and behind the ears, for a period of 5 min. Students whose hair had at least one of the developing stages of louse including egg, nymph, and adult was considered as head lice infested. In this regard the nits found less than about 1/4″ away from the scalp and eggs with a dark colour considered as viable. After the examination, each student was interviewed using a pre-tested structured questionnaire. The questionnaires were administered by trained field interviewers and supervised by the principal investigator. The questions included respondents' demographic characteristics, family size, parent's educational level and job, history of head lice infestation in family members, bathroom availability in the home, bathroom, and dwelling houses construction materials, electricity, and water supply.

In the intervention area, each student directly received three 60 ml bottles of 1% permethrin shampoo and through a face to face educational program students were advised to use shampoo at 7 day intervals and each time the shampoo should left on head for 10 min. The effectiveness of shampoo was evaluated via reexamination for head lice infestation after one, two, and three weeks and the therapeutic efficacy was calculated as the number of cured divided by the total number of initial infected cases.

Students were considered as infestation free if they did not have any of the developing stages of louse including egg, nymph, and adult. The therapeutic efficacy of permethrine shampoo was calculated as the number of cured cases divided by the total number of infested cases.

Statistical analysis

The data were analyzed using SPSS version 19. Descriptive statistics were used to show percentages, averages, and relative frequencies of the variables. Cross tabulation of variables and Chi-squared test were used to determine the statistical significance of differences of relative frequencies. The results were considered significant at 5% levels of significance ($p < 0.05$).

Ethical consideration

Students of study villages and their family were informed about the objectives and procedures of the investigation. The parents signed a consent form and the students

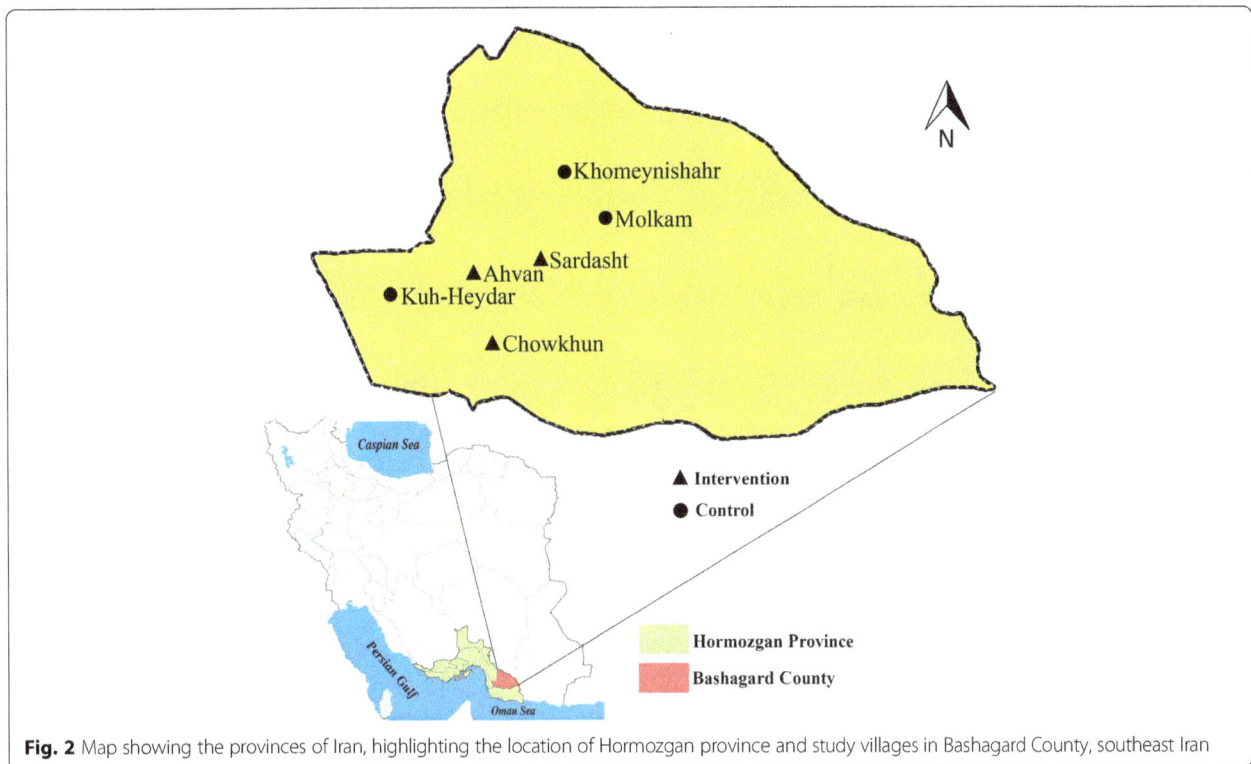

Fig. 2 Map showing the provinces of Iran, highlighting the location of Hormozgan province and study villages in Bashagard County, southeast Iran

were informed that their participation was purely voluntary and they were free to withdraw from the study at any time. In this study identification numbers were used instead of participant names and collected data were kept confidential.

Results

A total of 300 female students were interviewed. The ages of students ranged from 7 to 12 years with an average of 9.45 ± 1.15 years. The mean family size was 5.3 ± 2.1 people ranging from 2 to 12 people.

During this study, a total of 202 (67.3%) students were found to be infested with at least a single specimen of louse. Infestation rate was estimated 68.6% and 66% in the intervention and control groups, respectively. In 74 (36.6%) of the positive students, only louse eggs were found, whereas in 128 (63.4%) students, at least one of the live adult, nymph, and viable nit was observed.

The prevalence of head lice infestation was significantly higher in the highest grade students who aged 9 years ($p < 0.012$), and the lowest infestation rate was in 7 years age grade (Table 1).

In this study, the frequency of lice infestation was significantly higher (78.1%) among schoolchildren with no bathroom in their homes compared to those with bathroom in their homes (60.7%) ($p < 0.038$). Moreover, frequency of hair washing had significant relationship with infestation rate ($p < 0.021$). Students who regularly washed their hair three times or more per week had the

Table 1 Head lice infestation in female primary school girls by socio- demographic characteristics in Bashagard County, southeast Iran

Characteristics	Examinations (n)	infestations (%)	p-value[a]
School grade(age)			0.012
I(7)	50	50	
II(8)	52	57.7	
III(9)	43	81.4	
IV(10)	51	76.4	
V(11)	57	71.9	
VI(12)	47	68.1	
Bathroom within the house			0.038
Yes	186	60.7	
No	114	78.1	
Frequency of hair washing per week			0.021
1	211	72.9	
2	78	56.4	
≥ 3	11	27.2	
Sharing articles[b]			0.043
Yes	170	71.7	
No	130	60	

[a]Chi-square test
[b]combs, and scarves

least head lice infestation compared with the students who washed hairs once a week (Table 1).

As Table 1 indicates, the frequency of infestation is significantly higher among students who used shared articles such as combs and scarves (71.7%) compared with students who did not use shared articles (60%) (p = 0.043).

The study results also showed that head lice infestation rate was significantly related to the mothers' (p = 0.032) and fathers'(p = 0.021) educational levels and it was 82.4% and 81% in students with uneducated father and mother, respectively. Moreover, the students whose father and mother' educational level was higher than diploma had 6.7 and 14.3% infestation, respectively. Parents' job was not significantly associated with lice infestation (Table 2).

Analysis of another factors influencing head lice infestation showed that infestation rate was positively associated with family size of students (p = 0.0001). The prevalence of head lice infestation according to family demographic characteristics is demonstrated in Table 2.

Rates of head lice infestation detected at initial, 7, 14, and 21 days in intervention and control groups are reported in Table 3.

Table 2 Head lice infestation in primary school girls according to family demographic characteristics in Bashagard County, southeast Iran

Characteristics	Examinations (n)	Infestations (%)	p-value[a]
Father's education			0.021
Illiterate	159	82.4	
Primary	109	58.7	
Secondary	17	35.3	
High school / University	15	6.7	
Mother's education			0.032
Illiterate	137	81	
Primary	142	57	
Secondary	14	64.3	
High school / University	7	14.3	
Father's Job			0.89
Employee	259	67.6	
Self-employment	41	65.9	
Mother's Job			0.31
Employee	14	50	
Housewife	286	68.2	
Family size			0.0001
2–3	7	28.6	
4–5	92	52.1	
6–7	122	73.5	
≥ 8	79	79.7	

[a]Chi-square test

Table 3 Head lice infestation rate in intervention and control groups at initial, 7, 14, and 21 days during examinations

Examiation time	Intervention group		Control group		p-value[a]
	Examined (n)	Infested n(%)	Examined (n)	Infested n(%)	
Initial	150	103 (68.6)	150	99 (66.0)	0.622
7 days	148	73 (49.3)	149	98 (65.7)	0.003
14 days	150	32 (21.3)	150	96 (64.0)	0.0001
21 days	147	10 (6.8)	148	92 (62.1)	0.0001

[a]Chi-square test

In this study, the effectiveness of 1% permethrin shampoo was revealed to be 29.2%, 68.9%, and 90.3% at follow-up examinations after one, two and three weeks, respectively (Fig. 3).

Discussion

Infestation with head lice is a common health problem that is most prevalent in primary schools throughout the world, especially in developing countries including different regions of Iran [8, 9]. In this study the prevalence of head lice infestation was 67.3% in primary school girls which is higher than the mean of infestation rate which has been reported to be 8.8% in different parts of Iran [9]. High prevalence of head lice infestation in the study area can be attribute to factors such as low parents' educational level, use of shared personal hygiene items, large family size, poor health facilities, low frequency of bathing per week, lack of a school health educator, and low socioeconomic status. Obviously, many of these factors are due to the extreme poverty.

Results of the studies in primary schoolchildren from different parts of Iran show the infestation rate between 0.47% to 27.1% [9, 10] and the rate of lice infestation among school children in some Middle East and other regional countries ranges from 4.2 to 78% [11].

The variation of infestation rate may be due to several factors including personal hygiene, family size, economic condition and family income [9, 12].

In this study the highest rate of infestation was seen in 9-year-old students. This finding is similar to some studies in different parts of the world [8–10]. This can be explained by behavioral factors which make children at this age to have more direct physical contact with friend. Physical contacts, especially head-to-head contacts are the most important factors in transmission of head lice infestation [13].

In this study, there was a significant association between head lice infestation and the presence of bathroom in the home as well as the frequency of hair washing. This finding is supported by other studies in the northwest of Iran [9, 14]. Similarly, in studies conducted in Korea, Jordan, and Egypt, a strong association

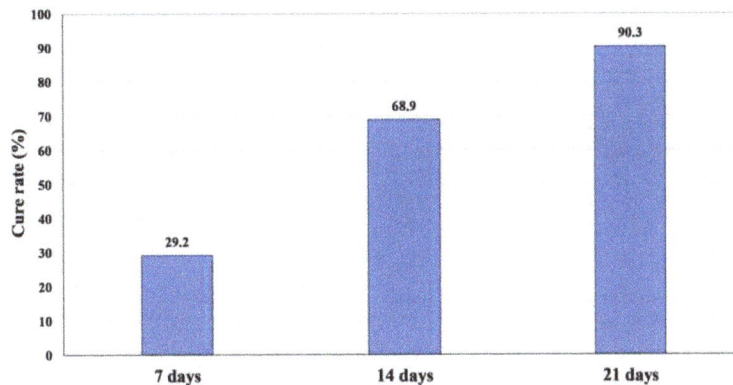

Fig. 3 Cure rates after 7,14,and 21 days of treatment with 1% permethrin shampoo in the intervention group in Bashagard County, southeast Iran

between head lice infestation and bathing facilities in the home was reported [15–17].

According to the results, use of shared articles such as combs, hair brushes, and scarves affects the head lice prevalence. Similar findings have been reported from Jordan, Egypt, Palestine, and Yemen [16, 18–20]. All the girls in this study were wearing scarves due to their Islam religion. Covering the head may facilitate the infestation because of creating a better and ideal scalp humidity and temperature for the head lice to thrive and multiply [21].

The results of this study also showed that the infestation was more common among students with low-educated parents. This finding is in agreement with results of previous studies which carried out in Iran, Egypt, Yemen, Palestine, and Turkey [9, 17, 19, 20, 22], which have shown that low educational levels of mothers and fathers increased the risk of infestation. The reason is that educated mothers and fathers have more information about head lice infestation and its prevention due to their awareness and social communication [23, 24]. Since educational intervention has been reported to be effective in increasing community involvement and reduction of prevalent insect-borne diseases in low socioeconomic areas such as Bashagard County [25], it is important to provide appropriate educational programs directed toward parents, teachers, and students to increase community awareness about head lice risk factors and prevention.

This study also showed a positive relationship between head lice infestation and family size.

This finding is in line with the results of other studies in different parts of Iran [16]. Similarly, in studies conducted in Korea, Jordan, Egypt, Yemen, Malaysia, and Turkey head lice infestation prevalence was more common among big size families [15–17, 19–21].

In an overcrowded home, close contact between family members facilitates the transmission of head lice. Moreover, having more children may lead to higher infestation

rates because parents pay less time per child to perform laundry and personal cleansing.

In this study, the effectiveness of 1% permethrin shampoo after the first, second, and third weeks were 29.2, 68.9, and 90.3%, respectively. A similar study in the south of Iran reported that 1% permethrin shampoo was effective as pediculicide product in schoolchildren with 64.1% and 89.7% cure rate after 6 and 14 days, respectively [26].

The dominant therapeutic effect of permethrin shampoo in our study can be attributed to effective face to face educational intervention and subsequent follow ups of infested cases.

Since the large insecticide selection pressure induced by conventional insecticides has led to the emergence and spread of resistance in many parts of the world [27, 28] which may lead to treatment failure, there is a need for regular monitoring of insecticide resistance in order to select suitable insecticides for successful control of head lice infestation.

Conclusion

Our study revealed that there is a high prevalence of head lice infestation among primary school girls in Bashagard County. Factors that may explain the high prevalence of head lice infestation in the studied girls may be attributed to low parents' educational level, shared use of personal hygiene items, large family size, poor health facilities, low frequency of bathing per week, lack of a school health educator, and low socioeconomic status. Moreover, since in this study 1% permethrin shampoo found to be suitable as a pediculicide for head lice infestation control in schoolchildren, regarding the socioeconomic status of Bashagard county population, free distribution of 1% permethrin shampoo and providing educational program for proper and regular use of the shampoo seems necessary for control of head lice infestation in primary school girls.

Acknowledgements

The authors would like to appreciate the collaboration received from Dr. Darakhshan, Head of Bashagard Health Center for providing facilities for implementation of this investigation. We especially thank Ms. F. Mirzadeh-Koshahi, Ms. F. Azimi, and Ms. M. Saadati, personnel of the Bashagard Health Center, for their cooperation in the field. We also thank Dr. Madani, for performing the statistical analyses. Finally, we are grateful to all school principals and the parents, teachers and students of the schools that participated in this study.

Funding

This study received financial support from Research and Technology Deputy of Hormozgan University of Medical Sciences (Project No.764).

Authors' contributions

MSA, SAJ, MZ, and ASD conceived and designed the study. MSA, and MZ drafted the manuscript. MSA and ASD participated in the data analysis. MSA and SAJ performed the data collection, and trained field researcher. All authors read and approved the final manuscript.

Ethics approval and consent to participate

The participation in the study was voluntary and the participants were free to withdraw from the study at any time. Students and their parents had received an adequate and understandable explanation about the intent of the study, the possible results, their meaning, and signed the informed consent form. In this study identification numbers were used instead of participant names and collected data were kept confidential. The study was approved by Hormozgan University of Medical Sciences ethical committee.

Competing interests

The authors declare that they have no competing interests.

Author details

[1]Social Determinants in Health Promotion Research Center, Hormozgan University of Medical Sciences, Bandar Abbas, Iran. [2]Department of Medical Entomology and Vector Control, Faculty of Health, Hormozgan University of Medical Sciences, P.O. Box: 79145–3838, Bandar Abbas, Iran. [3]Bashagard Health Center, Hormozgan University of Medical Sciences, Bashagard, Iran. [4]Department of Occupational Health Engineering, Faculty of Health, Hormozgan University of Medical Sciences, Bandar Abbas, Iran.

References

1. Service M. Medical entomology for students. New York: Cambridge University Press; 2012. p. 191–9.
2. Soleimani-Ahmadi M, Zare S, Hanafi-Bojd AA, Amir-Haydarsha M. The epidemiological aspect of pediculusis in primary school of Qeshm, south of Iran. J Med Sci. 2007;7:299–302.
3. Speare R, Harrington H, Canyon D, Massey PD. A systematic literature review of pediculosis due to head lice in the Pacific Island countries and territories: what country specific research on head lice is needed? BMC Dermatol. 2014;14:11.
4. Moshki M, Zamani-Alavijeh F, Mojadam M. Efficacy of peer education for adopting preventive behaviors against head lice infestation in female elementary school students: a randomised controlled trial. PLoS One. 2017;12:1.
5. Orion E, Marcos B, Davidovici B, Wolf R. Itch and scratch: scabies and pediculosis. Clin Dermatol. 2006;24:168–75.
6. Kristensen M, Knorr M, Rasmussen AM, Jespersen JB. Survey of permethrin and malathion resistance in human head lice populations from Denmark. J Med Entomol. 2006;43:533–8.

7. Rupes V, Moravec J, Chmela J, Ledvinka J, Zelenkova J. A resistance of head lice (Pediculus Capitis) to permethrin in Czech Republic. Cent Eur J Public Health. 1995;3:30–2.
8. Leung AK, Fong JH, Pinto-Rojas A. Pediculosis capitis. J Pediatr Health Care. 2005;19:369–73.
9. Moosazadeh M, Afshari M, Keianian H, Nezammahalleh A, Enayati AA. Prevalence of head lice infestation and its associated factors among primary school students in Iran: a systematic review and meta-analysis. Osong Public Health Res Perspect. 2015;6:346–56.
10. Kamiabi F, Nakhaei FH. Prevalence of pediculosis capitis and determination of risk factors in primary-school children in Kerman. East Mediterr Health J. 2005;11:988–92.
11. Hodjati MH, Mousavi N, Mousavi M. Head lice infestation in school children of a low socioeconomy area of Tabriz city. Iran African Journal of Biotechnology. 2008;7:2292–4.
12. Rukke BA, Birkemoe T, Soleng A, Lindstedt HH, Ottesen P. Head lice prevalence among households in Norway importance of spatial variables and individual and household characteristics. Parasitology. 2011;138:1296–304.
13. Toloza A, Vassena C, Gallardo A, Gonzalez-Audino P, Picollo MI. Epidemiology of pediculosis capitis in elementary schools of Buenos Aires. Argentina Parasitol Res. 2009;104:1295–8.
14. Tappeh KH, Chavshin A, Hajipirloo HM, Khashaveh S, Hanifian H, Bozorgomid A, et al. Pediculosis capitis among primary school children and related risk factors in Urmia, the Main City of West Azarbaijan. Iran J Arthropod Borne Dis. 2012;6:79–85.
15. Sim S, Lee WJ, Yu JR, Lee IY, Lee SH, Oh SY, et al. Risk factors associated with head louse infestation in Korea. Korean J Parasitol. 2011;49:95–8.
16. AlBashtawy M, Hasna F. Pediculosis capitis among primary-school children in Mafraq governorate. Jordan East Mediterr Health J. 2012;18:43–8.
17. Abd El Raheem TA, El Sherbiny NA, Elgameel A, El-Sayed GA, Moustafa N, Shahen S. Epidemiological comparative study of pediculosis capitis among primary school children in Fayoum and Minofiya governorates, Egypt. J Community Health. 2015;40:222–6.
18. Morsy TA, El-Ela RG, Mawla MY, Khalaf SA. The prevalence of lice infesting students of primary, preparatory and secondary schools in Cairo, Egypt. J Egypt Soc Parasitol. 2001;31:43–50.
19. Alzain B. Pediculosis capitis infestation in school children of a low socioeconomic area of the North Gaza Governorate. Turk J Med Sci. 2012; 42 Supp1:1286–91.
20. Al-Maktari MT. Head louse infestations in Yemen: prevalence and risk factors determination among primary schoolchildren, al-Mahweet governorate. Yemen J Egypt Soc Parasitol. 2008;38:741–8.
21. Bachok N, Nordin RB, Awang CW, Ibrahim NA, Naing L. Prevalence and associated factors of head lice infestation among primary schoolchildren in Kelantan, Malaysia. Southeast Asian J Trop Med Public Health. 2006;37:536–43.
22. Gulgun M, Balci E, Karaoglu A, Babacan O, Türker T. Pediculosis capitis: prevalence and its associated factors in primary school children living in rural and urban areas in Kayseri. Turkey Cent Eur J Public Health. 2013;21:104–8.
23. Vahabi A, Shemshad K, Sayyadi M, Biglarian A, Vahabi B, Sayyad S, et al. Prevalence and risk factors of Pediculus (humanus) capitis (Anoplura: Pediculidae), in primary schools in Sanandaj City, Kurdistan Province. Iran Trop Biomed. 2012; 29:207–11.
24. Davarpanah MA, Rasekhi Kazerouni A, Rahmati H, Neirami RN, Bakhtiary H, Sadeghi M. The prevalence of pediculus capitis among the middle schoolchildren in Fars Province, southern Iran. Caspian J Intern Med. 2013;4:607–10.
25. Soleimani-Ahmadi M, Vatandoost H, Zare M, Alizadeh A, Salehi M. Community knowledge and practices regarding malaria and long-lasting insecticidal nets during malaria elimination programme in an endemic area in Iran. Malar J. 2014;13:511.
26. Moemenbellah-Fard M, Nasiri Z, Azizi K, Fakoorziba M. Head lice treatment with two interventions: pediculosis capitis profile in female schoolchildren of a rural setting in the south of Iran. Annals of Tropical Medicine and Public Health. 2016;9:245–50.
27. Nasirian H, Ladonni H, Shayeghi M, Ahmadi MS. Iranian non-responding contact method German cockroach permethrin resistance strains resulting from field pressure pyrethroid spraying. Pak J Biol Sci. 2009;12:643–7.
28. Durand R, Bouvresse S, Berdjane Z, Izri A, Chosidow O, Clark JM. Insecticide resistance in head lice: clinical, parasitological and genetic aspects. Clin Microbiol Infect. 2012;18:338–44.

Enzymatic debridement for the treatment of severely burned upper extremities – early single center experiences

Tomke Cordts, Johannes Horter, Julian Vogelpohl, Thomas Kremer, Ulrich Kneser and Jochen-Frederick Hernekamp*

Abstract

Background: Severe burns of hands and arms are complex and challenging injuries. The Standard of care (SOC) – necrosectomy with skin grafting – is often associated with poor functional or aesthetic outcome. Enzymatic debridement (ED) is considered one promising alternative but, until recently, results proved to be highly variable.

Methods: Between 04/2014 and 04/2015, 16 patients with deep partial- to full-thickness burns of the upper extremities underwent enzymatic debridement (ED) in our Burn Center and were evaluated for extent of additional surgery, wound healing, pain management and functional parameters.

Results: Following ED, no further surgical intervention was required in 53.8 % of the study population. In patients who required surgical treatment, the the skin-grafted area could be reduced by 37.0 % when compared to initial assessment. Time from injury to ED was 24.4 h and patients were able to start physical therapy after 2.0 days but suffered from prolonged wound closure (28.0 days). Regionally administered anesthesia proved to be superior to pain medication alone as pain levels and consumed morphine-equivalent were lower. Post-demission follow-up showed good functional results and pain levels with low scores in two self-report questionnaires (DASH, PRWE-G) but 3 patients reported increased susceptibility to shear stress. Based on these early experiences, we developed a 3-step algorithm for consecutive patients allowing appropriate and individualized treatment selection.

Conclusions: We see a potential benefit for ED in the treatment of severely burned hands and forearms but further investigations and proper prospective, randomized controlled trials are needed to statistically support any outlined assumptions.

Keywords: Burn wound, Enzymatic debridement, Bromelain, Scarring, Skin grafting, Plexus catheter

Background

Burns are common injuries associated with substantial morbidity and mortality. Over 2000 cases have been treated in German Burn Centers in 2013 [1]. Estimates for the frequency of hand involvement vary between 30–60 and 80 % of newly admitted patients [2, 3]. Standard of care (SOC) for deep partial- and full-thickness burns is necrosectomy and skin grafting but, especially when conducted on hands and forearms, often associated with poor aesthetic and functional outcome [4].

Initial assessment of both burn extent and depth can prove to be difficult and inadequate. Additionally, burn wounds can progress and change over time, leading to an unanticipated need for surgery [5]. In combined partial- and full-thickness wounds, conventional surgical intervention may cause unnecessary tissue loss, since vital tissue might be unnecessarily removed. This can be detrimental for functional outcomes, especially when distal extremities with a thin soft tissue envelope are treated. Fingers and hands have a complex anatomy, sparse tissue coverage and present vessels, nerves and tendons confined on a very small space [4]. Since SOC might lead to unsatisfying outcomes in some patients, new therapeutic options are still required. Enzymatic

* Correspondence: jfhernekamp@bgu-ludwigshafen.de
Department of Hand, Plastic and Reconstructive Surgery – Burn Center, BG Trauma Center Ludwigshafen, Ludwig-Guttmann-Strasse 13, 67071 Ludwigshafen, Germany

debridement (ED) is considered one promising alternative and has therefore been extensively studied since the Second World War. But, until recently, results proved to be highly variable [6].

NexoBrid° (NXB) is an enzymatic debriding agent that was EMEA-approved in late 2012. Its active ingredient constitutes of a concentrate of proteolytic enzymes enriched in bromelain derived from the stem of the pineapple plant. It is indicated for enzymatic debridement in adults with deep partial- and full-thickness thermal burns [7]. Application is possible outside the operation theatre as long as sufficient analgesia is ensured during this otherwise painful debridement procedure.

Previous studies reported promising results. A large multi-center, randomized controlled clinical trial conducted on 182 patients between 2006 and 2009 postulated significant reductions in time from injury to complete debridement, need for surgery, autografting and area of burns excised when compared to SOC. In a subgroup of hand burns, additional benefit was seen as these patients exhibited earlier time to wound closure and better long-term results [8]. Similar findings had previously been reported in a retrospective data analysis of 69 hand burns [2]. Furthermore, the number of escharotomies could be reduced, since initial ED sufficiently decreased compartment or interstitial pressures. In both studies, no ED treated hand required escharotomy compared to about 10 % in SOC [2, 8]. However, although these results suggest a benefit of ED especially in hand burns, no prospective correlative studies have yet been conducted.

In April 2014, we started using NXB on qualifying burns of the upper extremities as a possible alternative to surgical necrosectomy and skin grafting. We hypothesized, that these patients would benefit from reduced need for surgery and absent morbidity often associated with SOC, e.g. functionally impairing tissue loss and subcutaneous tissue damage. We also evaluated the time to onset of physical therapy (PT), wound closure and early functional outcome. Additional emphasize was put on pain management accompanying ED when comparing local to regionally administered anesthetic measures.

With this article, we want to provide an overview of the problems, experiences and results gathered when using ED for deep burns of the hands and forearms.

Methods

Between 04/2014 and 04/2015, all patients admitted to our Burn Intensive Care Unit (BICU) showing deep partial- to full-thickness upper extremity burns were treated by ED on not more than 15 % TBSA within the first 48 h after admission. Fingers and hands were prioritized even when injuries were exceeding proximally or included additional body regions.

Upon arrival in the Burn Trauma Bay (BTB), standard admission protocol was performed which included complete undressing of the patient and initial debridement with opening of present blisters under antiseptic conditions. Standardized escharotomy by monopolar cautery was performed if injuries included circumferential burns. This was not regarded as exclusion criterion and ED was not performed as a replacement for surgical escharotomy. When wound bed was cleaned, a polihexanide gel was applied and sterile wound dressings were completed by multilayered greased gauzes, cotton and elastic bandages before admission to BICU. If burn depth on the upper extremities was categorized as potential deep partial- to full-thickness by the attending physician, dressings were opened and reassessed within 48 h (Fig. 1). If the patient qualified for ED, sufficient analgesia was ensured by either timely administration of p.o./i.v. pain medication or ultrasound-guided placement of brachial plexus nerve block by an anesthesiologist [9]. Additional pain medication was given if needed. Some patients received the application under anesthesia since severity of their total burn injuries had required intubation and ongoing sedation.

Wounds were covered in bandages rinsed in a 0.04 % polihexanide solution (Serasept™ 2, Serag-Wiessner, Naila, Germany) and soaked for 2 h before and after application of the actual debriding agent (Fig. 2). Preparation also included separation of the wound bed from intact skin by vaseline. Enzymatic reaction was then started by mixing the powder ingredient into the carrier gel, creating a golden viscous mass (Fig. 3) that was applied to the wound bed under sterile conditions (approx. 2 g/% TBSA). We then formed an occlusive dressing with two large plastic self-adhesing sheets (Fig. 4). Enzymatic debridement time was at least 4 h before dressings were opened and detritus was removed by sterile spatulas and rinsing in saline solution. The final step consisted of another 2 h soaking period before standardized greased gauze dressings were applied. In these first 16 cases, dressings were then changed every two days and reassessment was performed by an attending physician. To ensure proper and repeated wound bed evaluation, we abstained from using dermal substitutes or collagen matrices after the application of NXB.

In SOC, necrosectomy was conducted by Weck knife, Humby knife or Versajet™ (Smith & Nephew GmbH, Hamburg, Germany). We usually combined skin transplantation with spray application of fibrin sealant (ARTISS™, Baxter Deutschland GmbH, Unterschleißheim, Germany) to assure proper adhesion.

Throughout their stay on BICU, pain levels were monitored every hour, objectified by numeric rating scale (NRS) and patients received pain medication as required. Brachial plexus catheters were removed when analgesic

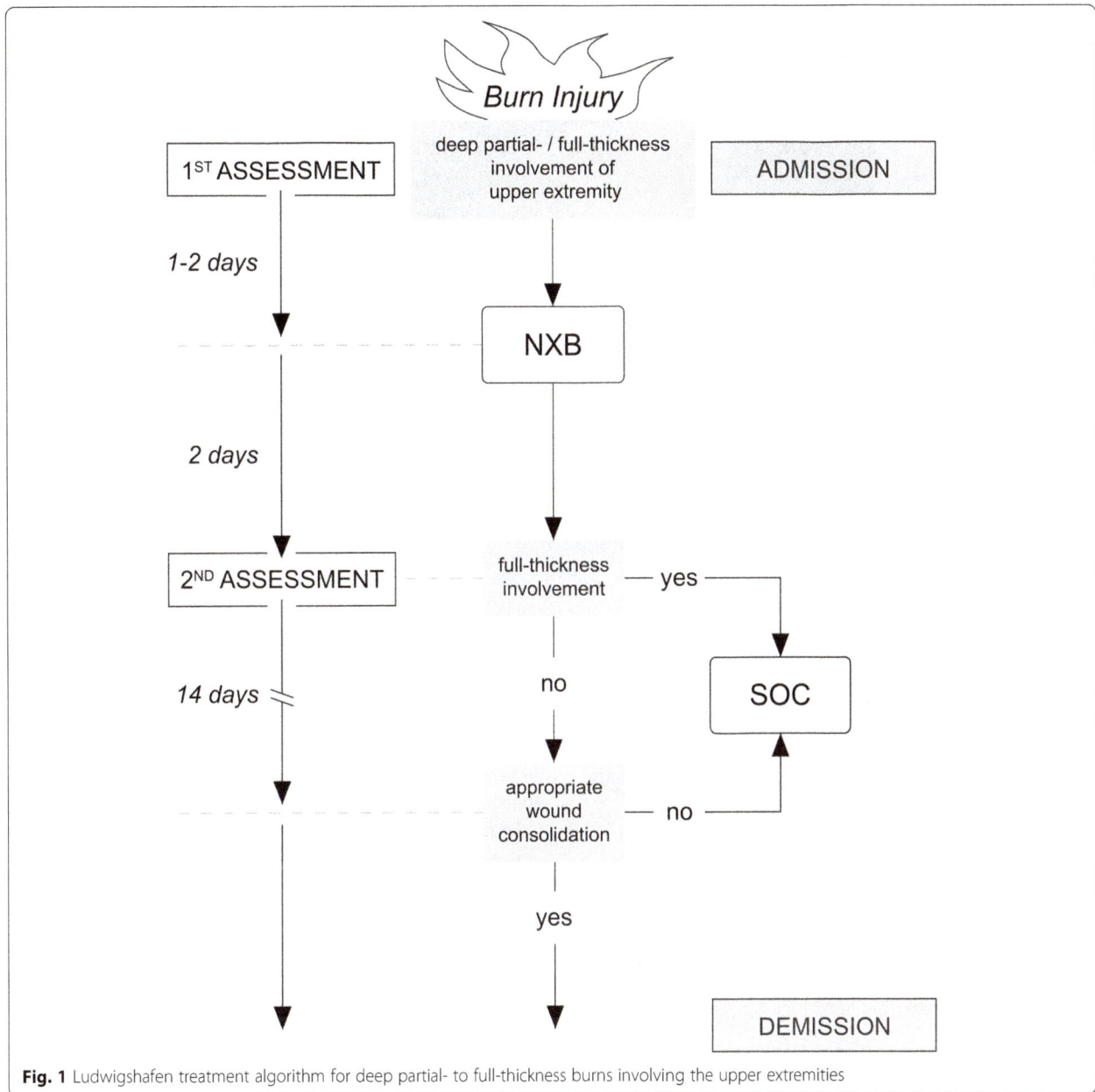

Fig. 1 Ludwigshafen treatment algorithm for deep partial- to full-thickness burns involving the upper extremities

effect decayed to insufficient levels or determined to be dispensable. Wound healing, signs of infection or other complications were assessed every two days by the attending physician when change of dressings took place. Following ED, physical therapy was started as soon as dressings would allow treatment by a professional therapist.

About 3 months after demission, patients were evaluated for remaining functional disabilities and pain levels using two German self-report questionnaires (Disabilities of the Shoulder, Arm and Hand – DASH; Patient-Related Wrist Evaluation Score – PRWE-G) as well as scar quality by a single physician (Vancouver Scar Scale – VSS).

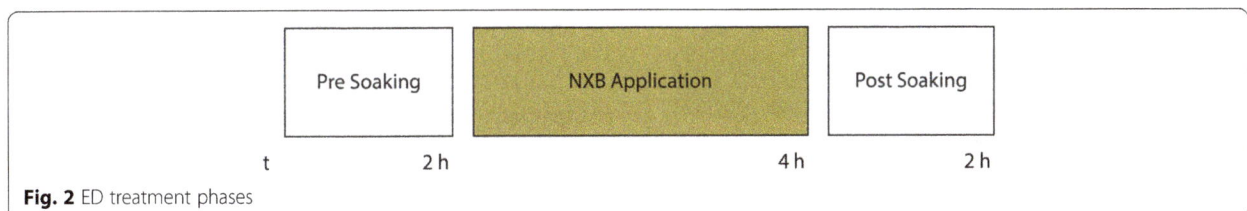

Fig. 2 ED treatment phases

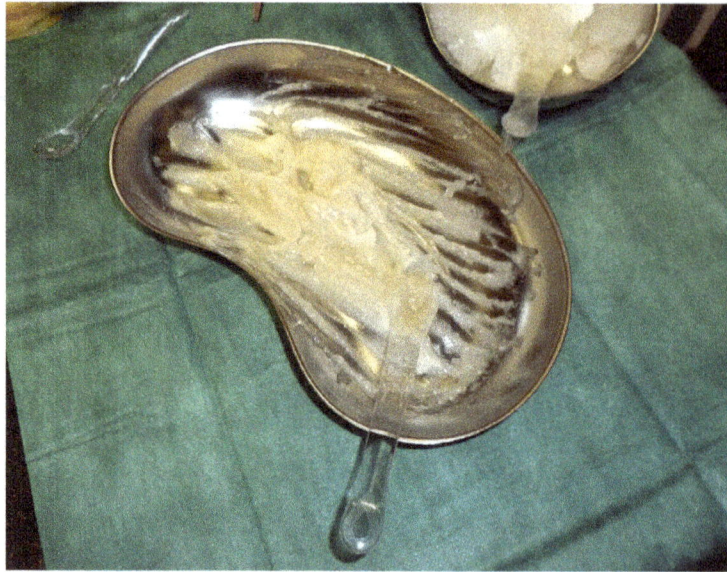

Fig. 3 Active NXB agent after mixing powder ingredient and carrier gel

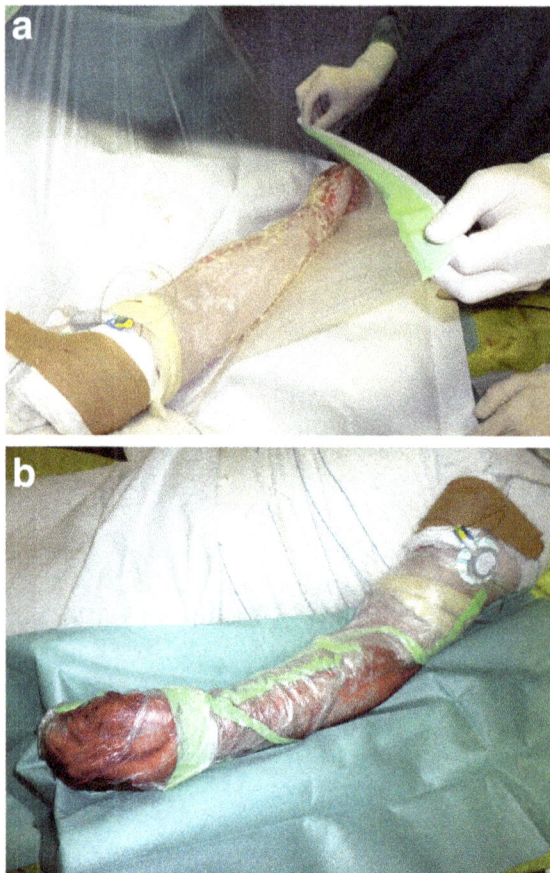

Fig. 4 NXB application phase. **a** Forming of occlusive dressing by self-adhesing sheets. Plexus catheter already in place. **b** Completed dressing and active enzymatic reaction as indicated by bleeding

Results

Sixteen patients (11 male, 5 female) with burns of 20.1 (2–66) % TBSA were included in the study. On the upper extremities, 7.3 (2–15) % TBSA were classified as deep partial- to full-thickness and treated by ED 24.4 (5–47) hours after injury (Table 1). NXB proved to be very effective in achieving a complete initial debridement for all cases.

Individual data sets are provided as supplemental file, see Additional file 1: Raw data.

Three patients deceased due to severity of accompanying injuries and therefore withdrew from follow-up. Out of the remaining 13, 7 patients completely avoided surgical intervention as necrosectomy by ED alone led to satisfactory wound healing. 6 required additional surgical debridement and skin grafting of 4.6 (0.5–12) % TBSA, equaling a 37.0 % reduction of transplanted skin area when compared to initial assessment. After ED patients were able to start PT after 2.0 (0–5) days but experienced prolonged wound closure with 28.0 (9–49) days on average.

Seven patients had been intubated on admission due to the severity of their injuries and were fully sedated during ED. According to the severity of the injury, patients underwent either p.o./i.v. pain medication (n = 3) or a brachial plexus nerve block was applied (n = 6). Regionally administered anesthesia proved to be superior to pain medication alone. Pain level, objectified by numeric rating scale (NRS), was 3.4 (1.1–5.2) in general analgesia and 2.9 (1.8–4.1) in plexus block group. This was accompanied by a 77.2 % reduction of morphine-equivalent consumed as general anesthesia group required 9.2 (0.0–17.2) mg/h and regional analgesia group required 2.1 (0.3–7.0) mg/h (Fig. 5).

Table 1 Patient injury and treatment characteristics

Characteristic	
Epidemiology	
Number of patients treated	16
Mean age (SD), years	47.8 ± 14.9
Males, no. (%)	11 (68.8 %)
Females, no. (%)	5 (31.2 %)
Drop outs, no. (%)	3 (18.8 %)
Injury and treatment	
Mean (SD) % TBSA	20.1 ± 18.1
Mean (SD) % TBSA treated by ED	7.3 ± 4.1
Patients requiring skin grafting after ED, no. (%)	6 (46.2 %)
Mean (SD) time to skin grafting after ED, days	16.3 ± 11.8
Mean (SD) % TBSA skin grafted after ED	4.6 ± 4.1

No wound infections or ED-related side effects were seen. No blood transfusions were necessary.

Eight of 16 patients (50.0 %) were available for follow-up examination regarding remaining pain levels and functional outcomes. Results were within the lowest quarter of the scoring range with 23/100 (0–45) points on DASH and 22/100 (1–46) points on PRWE-G. Overall scar quality was assessed as 6/14 (4–8) points on VSS. All follow-up examinations were conducted by the same physician. 3 patients (37.5 %) complained about increased skin susceptibility of ED treated areas. Reports consisted of persisting lesioning (Fig. 6), partly spontaneous but mostly induced by minimal sheer stress or otherwise negligible, everyday trauma.

Discussion

ED enabled patients to receive early initial debridement. With bedside application being practicable, patients would remain on ward and avoid cost-consuming surgical and anesthetic measures conducted in the OR. Also, in SOC, some days are usually allowed for wounds to completely demarcate the areas requiring necrosectomy and skin grafting, which further enhances time to debridement.

In our Burn Center, we were able to perform initial debridement 24.4 h after admission. ED phases itself will add up to at least 8 h of treatment (Fig. 2) and should therefore be started preferably in morning hours. Preceding plexus catheter placement further increases time by usually 1 or 2 h, rendering ED a long, laborsome procedure. We found this to be a limitation worth mentioning as ED requires a surgeon and nursing staff to be present at all times during the procedure.

ED reduced the % TBSA treated with surgical necrosectomy and skin grafting. Initial assessment of burn

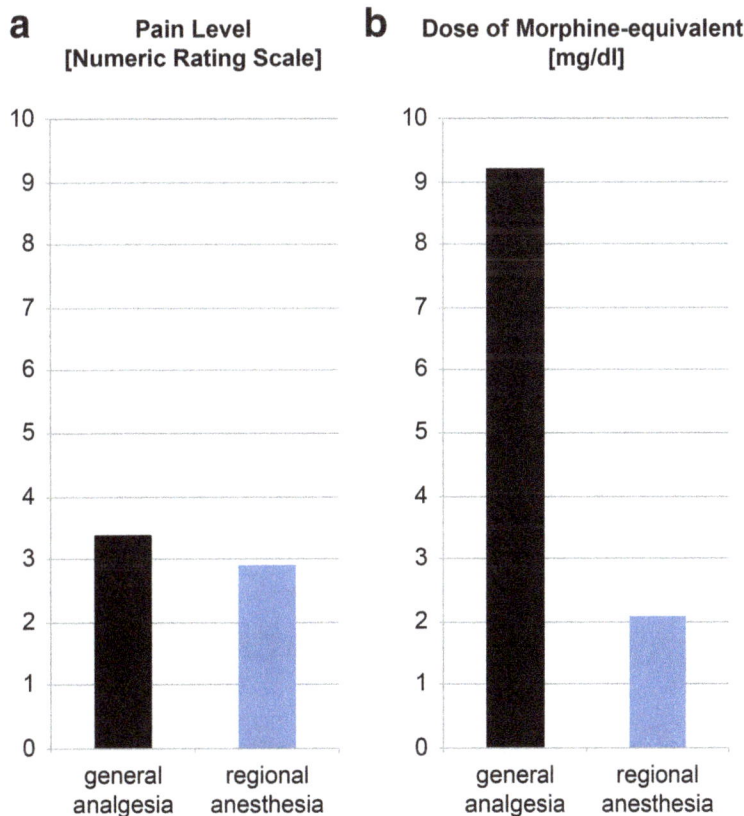

Fig. 5 Comparison of general analgesia and regional anesthesia during ED. **a** Lower NRS scores in plexus catheter group. **b** Higher morphine-equivalent dose in general analgesia

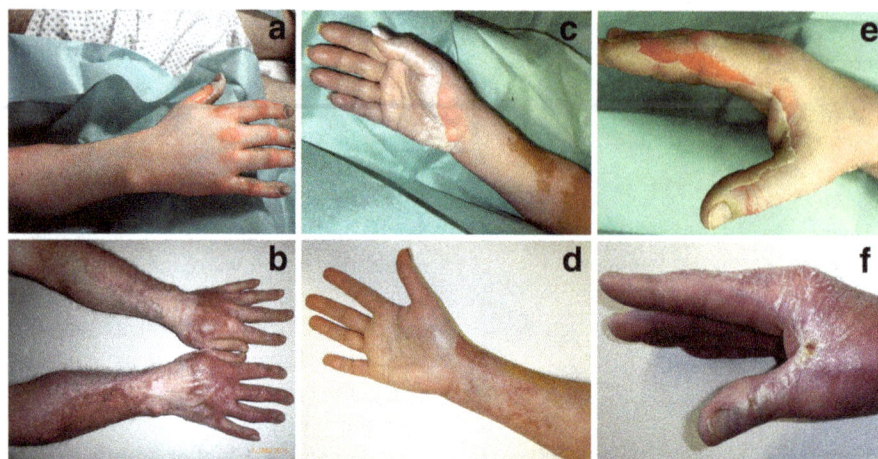

Fig. 6 Three representative patients before and after ED. **a** and **b** Closed wounds 23 weeks after treatment. Note the intense vascularization in originally full-thickness affected areas. **c** and **d** Good results 16.5 weeks after ED. **e** and **f** Unstable scars with possibly sheer stressed induced interdigital lesioning still present after 18 weeks

extent and depth is difficult and needs to be permanently scrutinized and reevaluated. Especially in the first days after injury, wounds can both progress or turn out to be overestimated by the admitting physician. The latter will result in unnecessary surgical interventions and morbidity, especially on delicate structures such as fingers and hands. In more than half of our collective initially classified as candidates for surgery, ED totally avoided necrosectomy and skin grafting. In the remaining patients, transplanted area was substantially smaller than initially anticipated, minimizing associated complications such as donor site morbidity, contractures and aesthetic disadvantages. Patients, however, exhibited prolonged wound healing and at least 14 days of close observation were allowed before additional debridement and skin grafting could be ruled out.

No differentiation was made between the treatment of deep partial- and full-thickness burns as NXB is approved for both. But experiences show that areas early identified as full-thickness often lacked any self-healing activity after ED. Furthermore, full-thickness wounds that successfully healed after ED were often observed with intense scar vascularization and discoloration as well as increased susceptibility to trauma (Fig. 6). Based on these findings, we changed our policy to earlier skin grafting of full-thickness areas after ED, actually combining SOC and ED (Fig. 1).

In these first 16 ED patients, no dermal substitutes or collagen matrices were used as application would have interfered with repeated wound assessment. However, products such as Matriderm™ (Dr. Suwelack Skin & Health Care AG, Billerbeck, Germany), Integra™ (Integra GmbH, Ratingen, Germany), Suprathel™(Polymedics Innovations GmbH, Denkendorf, Germany) and Biobrane™ (Smith & Nephew GmbH, Hamburg, Germany) are generally available and used in our Burn Center. Additional methods include allo- or xenografting and spray-on epidermal cells (Recell™, Avita Medical, Melbourn, United Kingdom). These products will presumably further facilitate burn wound consolidation but their exact effect on NXB treated areas is unknown and something we tend to elucidate in future investigations.

In our experience, ED does not necessarily require intubation and sedation, usually conducted in SOC. Pain is generally well tolerated by on ward anesthetic measures, with regionally administered analgesia being more effective when compared to p.o./i.v. medication alone. Ultrasound-guided placement of brachial plexus nerve blocks is safe and excludes morbidity possibly associated with intubation and sedation. These patients also exhibit decreased opioid doses essentially achieved by a continuously infused local anesthetic (mepivacaine or ropivacaine). Due to their additional anti-inflammatory properties, NSAIDs were given in both groups and were therefore not evaluated.

Grafted areas are immobilized for at least 5 days to ensure proper skin adhesion. This unfortunately excludes these regions from PT and subsequently leads to contractures, movement restrictions and often prolonged functional recovery. With ED, patients benefitted from early onset of PT measures, mostly on the first or

Table 2 Applied NXB exclusion criteria

NXB contraindications as listed by manufacturer (see [7])
Hypersensitivity to the active substance, to pineapples or papain or to any of the excipients
Additional exclusion criteria applied in our Burn Center
Pregnant and nursing women, Chemical or electrical burns, Age of burn injury >48 h

Enzymatic debridement for the treatment of severely burned upper extremities – early single center...

163

second day after admission. 3-month follow-up also yielded good functional outcomes and pain levels.

Conclusions

In conclusion, we see a potential benefit for ED in the treatment of deeply burned hands and arms but careful observation must be assured as full-thickness involvement might require treatment adjustments, possibly neglecting associated benefits. We found regional anesthesia by brachial plexus catheter being superior to pain medication alone but availability might be limited as placement usually requires a skilled anesthesiologist. Some patients complained of persistent lesioning and hypertrophic scarring which we attributed to our prolonged waiting for reepithelialization. Based on these findings, the following protocol is currently applied at our Burn Center (Fig. 1): All admitted patients with deep partial- to full-thickness burns of the upper extremities not meeting exclusion criteria (Table 2) will undergo ED within the first 48 h after trauma (1st Assessment), preferably accompanied by regional anesthesia via brachial plexus blockage. Two days later, during dressing changes, the patient is again evaluated for areas of demarcated full-thickness involvement (2nd Assessment), which would then be treated by additional necrosectomy and skin grafting. Absence of these would rule out SOC and allow wounds to consolidate for at least 2 more weeks before surgery is again taken into consideration.

We hereby report our experiences in using ED on 16 patients with deep partial- to full-thickness burns of the upper extremities. Although group size is small and obviously lacking appropriate controls, we feel that our observations will be of interest to any NXB using burn surgeon. Certain problems and obstacles had us adjust our initial treatment protocol but this current standard is solely based on expert opinion and clinical experience. Further investigations and prospective randomized controlled studies will be required to statistically support our conclusions.

Abbreviations

BICU, burn intensive care unit; BTB, burn trauma bay; DASH, disabilities of the arm, shoulder and hand; ED, enzymatic debridement; NXB, NexoBrid®; PRWE-G, patient-related wrist evaluation score, German; PT, physical therapy; SOC, standard of care; TBSA, total body surface area

Funding

No external funding was obtained. Study design, data collection, analysis and interpretation as well as writing of the manuscript was performed independent of any financial grants or affiliations with companies or other external institutions.

Authors' contributions

TC, TK, UK and JFH participated in the design of the study. Study coordination and statistical analysis was performed by TC with aid in data collection and patient recruitment by JH and JV. TC and JFH drafted the manuscript with senior revisions performed by TK und UK. All authors read and approved the final manuscript.

Competing interests

The authors whose names are listed immediately below certify that they have no current affiliations with or involvement in any organization or entity with any financial interest (such as honoraria; educational grants; participation in speakers' bureaus; membership, employment, consultancies, stock ownership, or other equity interest; and expert testimony or patent-licensing arrangements), or non-financial interest (such as personal or professional relationships, affiliations, knowledge or beliefs) in the subject matter or materials discussed in this manuscript. In 2013, Ulrich Kneser has had a one-time affiliation as consultant for Mediwound Germany.

References

1. German Burn Society. Excerpt from the 2013 Statistic for Adult Burn Centers. 2014.
2. Krieger Y, Bogdanov-Berezovsky A, Gurfinkel R, Silberstein E, Sagi A, Rosenberg L. Efficacy of enzymatic debridement of deeply burned hands. Burns. 2012;38:108–12.
3. Luce EA. The acute and subacute management of the burned hand. Clin Plast Surg. 2000;27:49–63.
4. van Zuijlen PP, Kreis RW, Vloemans AF, Groenevelt F, Mackie DP. The prognostic factors regarding long-term functional outcome of full-thickness hand burns. Burns. 1999;25:709–14.
5. Pham TN, Gibran NS, Heimbach DM. Evaluation of the burn wound. management decisions. In: Herndon D, editor. Total Burn Care. 3rd ed. London: Saunders Elsevier; 2007. p. 119–26.
6. Klasen HJ. A review on the nonoperative removal of necrotic tissue from burn wounds. Burns. 2000;26:207–22.
7. MediWound Germany GmbH. NexoBrid 2 G Powder and Gel for Gel Summary of Product Characteristics. 2014.
8. Rosenberg L, Krieger Y, Bogdanov-Berezovsky A, Silberstein E, Shoham Y, Singer AJ. A novel rapid and selective enzymatic debridement agent for burn wound management: a multi-center RCT. Burns. 2014;40:466–74.
9. Pfeiffer K, Weiss O, Krodel U, Hurtienne N, Kloss J, Heuser D. Ultrasound-guided perivascular axillary brachial plexus block. A simple, effective and efficient procedure. Anaesthesist. 2008;57:670–6.

20

Risk factors of keloids in Syrians

Abeer Shaheen[1*], Jamal Khaddam[1] and Fadi Kesh[2]

Abstract

Background: Keloid is a benign fibrous growth, which presents in scar tissue of predisposed individuals. It is a result of irregular wound healing, but the exact mechanism is unknown. However, several factors may play a role in keloid formation. To date, there are no studies of keloids in Syria, and limited studies on Caucasians, so we have investigated the risk factors of keloids in Syrians (Caucasians), and this is the main objective of this study.

Methods: Diagnosis of keloids was clinically made after an interview and physical examination. We did a histopathological study in case the physical examination was unclear.

The following information was taken for each patient; sex, Blood groups (ABO\Rh), cause of scarring, anatomical sites, age of onset, number of injured sites (single\multiple) and family history.

Results: We have studied the clinical characteristics of 259 patients with keloids,130 (50.2 %) females and 129 (49.8 %) males. There were 209 (80.7 %) patients with keloids in a single anatomical site compared to 50 (19.3 %) patients with 130 keloids in multiple anatomical sites, 253 (97.68 %) patients with keloids caused by a single cause for each patient compared to 6 (2.32 %) patients with keloids caused by two different causes for each patient.

Keloids could follow any form of skin injury, but burn was the most common (28.68 %). Also, keloids could develop at any anatomical sites, but upper limb (20 %) followed by sternum (19.17 %) was the most common. Over half of the patients developed keloids in the 11–30 age range. 19.3 % (50/259) of patients had family history, 76 % (38/50) of them had keloids located in the same anatomical sites of relative, also, 66 % (33\50) of them had keloids caused by the same cause.

The following information was found to be statistically significant; people with blood group A ($p = 0.01$) compared with other blood groups, spontaneous keloids in patients with blood group A ($p = 0.01$), acne in males ($p = 0.0008$) compared to females, acne in someone who has a previous acne keloid ($p = 0.0002$), burn in someone who has a previous burn keloid ($p = 0.029$), family history, especially for spontaneous ($p = 0.005$), presternal ($p = 0.039$) and shoulder ($p = 0.008$) keloids, people in second and third decades ($p = 0.02$) ($p = 0.01$) respectively.

Conclusion: Age of onset, sex, cause of scarring, blood groups, anatomical site, presence of family history and the number of site (multiple\single) were significant in keloid formation in Syrians.

Keywords: Keloids, Risk factors, Blood groups, Cause of scarring, Anatomical site, Single site, Multiple sites, Family history, Age of onset, Syrians

Background

Keloid is a benign fibrous growth, presents in scar tissue of predisposed individuals, extends beyond the borders of the original wound, doesn't usually regress spontaneously, and tends to recur after excision [1]. It is a result of irregular wound healing [2, 3], but the exact mechanism is unknown [1].

There is a clear genetic component given the correlation with family history, high occurrence in identical twins [4, 5], higher predisposition in Blacks, Hispanics and Asians, less frequently in Caucasians and rarity in albinos [1, 4, 6, 7]. Proposed inheritance patterns include autosomal recessive [1], autosomal dominant [1–3, 8, 9] with incomplete penetrance, and variable expression. Maybe the heredity of certain antigens like (HLA-B14, HLA-B21, HLA-Bw16, HLA-Bw35, HLA-DR5, HLA-DQw3, and blood group A) [1] is the underlying reason of genetic predisposition. Genetically susceptible individuals form keloids after wounding but not at every body

---

* Correspondence: dr.abeer.a.shaheen@gmail.com
[1]Department of dermatology, Tishreen University, Lattakia, Syria
Full list of author information is available at the end of the article

site, and not after all insults of skin [4], which suggest the effect of both anatomical site and form of skin injury in keloid formation. Although keloids can occur at any age, they are most likely to occur between the ages of 11 and 30 years, which demonstrates the importance of age in keloid formation [8]. Also, keloid growth may be stimulated by sexual hormones due to the higher incidence of keloid formation during puberty and pregnancy, and remarkable decrease after menopause [10].

To date, there are no studies of keloids in Syria, and limited studies on Caucasians, so we investigated the risk factors of keloids in Syrians (Caucasians), and this is the main objective of this study.

Methods

This study was conducted between March/2013 and August/2015 in the departments of dermatology, at Tishreen and Alassad Hospitals, Lattakia, Syria.

The diagnosis of keloids was clinically made after an interview and physical examination. We did a histopathologic study if the physical examination was unclear, especially for genitalia, buttock, palm and sole keloids, and for other uncertain scars.

Inclusion/exclusion criteria

All patients with keloids were included into this study, while patients with hypertrophic scare were excluded. Hypertrophic scars are defined as raised scars that remained within the boundaries of the original lesion, often regressing spontaneously after the initial injury and rarely recurring after surgical excision. In contrast, a keloid scar is defined as a dermal lesion that spreads beyond the margin of the original wound, continues to grow over time, does not regress spontaneously and commonly recurring after excision [4].

Data collection

The following information was taken for each patient: Sex (male/female), blood groups (ABO and Rh), cause of scarring or form of skin injury (which was divided into 7 causes:, burn, surgical wound, sharp wound or knife laceration and not surgical, trauma or laceration, acne, unknown (spontaneous) and other), the age of onset (which was divided into seven age groups: 0–10, 11–20, 21–30, 31–40, 41–50, 51–60 and >60), anatomical sites (face, neck, scalp, earlobe, pinna, upper limb, lower limb, shoulder, lower back, sternum, chest wall without sternum, abdominal wall, palm and sole, genitalia and buttock), the number of injured anatomical sites (single/multiple), family history, the anatomical site and the cause of relative when family history is positive.

Note: Multiple sites refer to keloids found in a multiple number of anatomical sites as opposed to multiple keloids found in the same anatomical site. Therefore, the presence of more than one scar in the same anatomical site was not considered to be multiple keloids. Also, a single site keloid refers to a keloid or a number of keloids found in only one anatomical site.

Control group

We have to compare some of our data (blood groups, sex and age groups) with similar society data, so we got the relative frequency of blood groups from National Blood Transfusion Center (NBTC) of Lattakia for 2015, and the relative frequency of sex and age groups from the Syrian Census Center (SCC) for 2011, which was the last data of SCC because of war conditions. We needed chi-square test to compare that data, so we created a miniature group containing 259 people reflecting society data (blood groups, sex and age groups). We considered it as a control group.

Statistical analysis

Microsoft Excel 2012 and Microsoft Word 2012 were used for tables and figures. Calculation for the chi-square test on http://www.quantpsy.org/chisq/chisq.htm was used for comparing data. A P-value of less than 0.05 was considered statistically significant.

Results

We studied the clinical characteristics of 259 patients with keloids,130 (50.2 %) females and 129 (49.8 %) males. There were 209 patients with keloids in single anatomical site compared to 50 patients with 130 keloids in multiple anatomical sites, and 253 patients with keloids caused by a single cause for each patient compared to 6 patients with keloids caused by two different causes for each patient. According to that, we had 259 patients with 339 keloids spread over 15 anatomical sites, and 265 causes of scarring as a final result to 7 different forms of skin injury (Table 1). The associations among the age of onset, sex, causes of scarring, blood groups, anatomical sites, presence of family history and number of injured anatomical sites (multiple/single) were analyzed in detail and were statistically evaluated.

Incidence of keloids was equal in females 130 (50.2 %) and males 129 (49.8 %), with statistical significance for developing keloids neither male nor female compared to control ($p = 0.79$) (Table 2). However, males who were older than forty had statistical significance for developing keloids compared to females in the same age ($p = 0.036$) (Table 1).

Keloids could follow any form of skin injury, but burn was the most common (76\265) (28.68 %), and trauma (20\265) (7.55 %) was the least (Table 1). Causes had almost coordinated distribution in males and females, but males had higher predisposition to develop acne keloids compared to females ($p = 0.0008$) (Table 1). Also, keloids

Table 1 Demographic details of patients with keloids

		Males	Females	Totals	Final total
Frequency of patients (%)		129 (49.8 %)	130 (50.2 %)	259 (100 %)	
Causes	Spontaneous	13	21	34 (12.83 %)	265 (100 %)
	Burn	34	42	76 (28.68 %)	
	Sharp wound	21	20	41 (15.47 %)	
	Surgical	33	32	65 (24.53 %)	
	Trauma	10	10	20 (7.55 %)	
	Acne	21*	5	26 (9.81 %)	
	Others (sting, varicella)	0	3	3 (1.13 %)	
Anatomical sites	Face	13	6	19 (5.6 %)	339 (100 %)
	Neck	14	9	23 (6.78 %)	
	Scalp	8	0	8 (2.36 %)	
	Ear lobe	0	9	9 (2.65 %)	
	Pinna	3	0	3 (0.885 %)	
	Upper limb	34	34	68 (20.06 %)	
	Lower limb	12	14	26 (7.67 %)	
	Shoulder	19	25	44 (12.98 %)	
	Lower back	9	6	15 (4.424 %)	
	Sternum	38	27	65 (19.17 %)	
	Chest wall	11	16	27 (7.96 %)	
	Abdominal wall	9	12	21 (6.19 %)	
	Palm and sole	1	2	3 (o.885 %)	
	Genital	2	2	4 (1.18 %)	
	Buttock	1	3	4 (1.18 %)	
Blood groups	A	62	53	115 (44.4 %)*	259 (100 %)
	B	17	18	35 (13.51 %)	
	AB	6	10	16 (6.2 %)	
	O	44	49	93 (35.9 %)	
	RH +	119	119	238 (91.9 %)	259 (100 %)
	RH−	10	11	21 (8.1 %)	
Age groups	A	18	29	47 (18.15 %)	259 (100 %)
	B	41	39	80 (30.89 %)	
	C	38	32	70 (27.03 %)	
	D	6	16	22 (8.5 %)	
	E	11	9	20 (7.72 %)	
	F	7	4	11 (4.25 %)	
	G	8	1	9 (3.47 %)	
Family history		29	21	50	
F.H in the same site		15	23	38	
F.H by the same cause		16	17	33	
Multiple sites		29	21	50 (19.3 %)	259 (100 %)
Single site		100	109	209 (80.7 %) S	

($*p < 0.05$)

Table 2 Comparison between blood groups, sex and age groups in both groups (patients versus controls)

Society data			Relative frequency of society data (%)	Control group	Frequency of patients	Relative frequency of patients (%)
Blood groups (ABO)	A		34	88	115*	44.4
	B		15.4	40	35	13.51
	AB		8.5	22	16	6.2
	O		42.1	109	93	35.9
Total			100	259	259	100
Blood groups	RH+		91.1	236	238	91.9
RH	RH−		8.9	23	21	8.1
Total			100	259	259	100
sex	Male		51	132	129	49.8
	Female		49	127	130	50.2
Total			100	259	159	100
Age groups Y	A	0–10	25.6	66	47*	18.15
	B	11–20	22.4	58	80*	30.89
	C	21–30	17.6	46	*70	27.03
	D	31–40	12.3	32	22	8.5
	E	41–50	9.3	24	20	7.72
	F	51–60	6.5	17	11	4.25
	G	60<	6.3	16	9	3.47
Total			100	259	259	100

(*$P < 0.05$)

could develop at any anatomical sites, but upper limb (68\339) (20 %) followed by sternum (65\339) (19.17 %) were the most common, while buttock, genitalia, palm and sole were the least. (Table 1). Distribution of causes of keloids according to anatomical sites are demonstrated at (Fig. 1) (Table 3).

Univariate analysis between each blood group in both groups (patients versus controls) found statistical significance for developing keloids in people with blood group A ($p = 0.01$) (Table 2) (Fig. 2), especially for spontaneous keloids ($P = 0.01$) (Table 4). However, the proportion of Rh + subjects wasn't significantly different between control (91.1 %) and patients (91.9 %) ($p = 0.7$) (Table 2).

Keloids occurred in patients, either in single or in multiple anatomical sites. 19.3 % (50/259) of patients had 130 keloids in multiple anatomical sites as opposed to 80.7 % (209/259), who had a keloid in a single site (Table 1). The upper limb was the most common site for patients with multiple site keloids (23\130) (17.7 %), and sternum was the most common one for patients with single site (51\209) (24.4 %) (Fig. 3). All causes tended to develop keloids in multiple sites, but burn was the most common (21\55) (38.2 %), while surgical wound was the most common one for patients with a single site (56\210) (26.67 %) (Table 5). There was statistical significance for developing both burn and acne keloids in multiple anatomical sites ($p = 0.029$) ($p = 0.0002$) respectively (Table 6). Also, keloids followed either single or multiple forms of skin injury. Only 2.32 % (6\259) of patients had keloids caused by two different causes for each patient, 5\6 of them had a surgical cause, and 5\6 of them had keloids in multiple sites.

Note: When we want to compare variables with causes or anatomical sites, we compare with number of patients (259) and not with number of causes (265) or number of sites (339)). As at (Table 5) (Table 6).

19.3 % (50/259) of patients had family history, 76 % (38/50) of them had keloids located in the same anatomical sites of relative. Also, 66 % (33\50) of them had

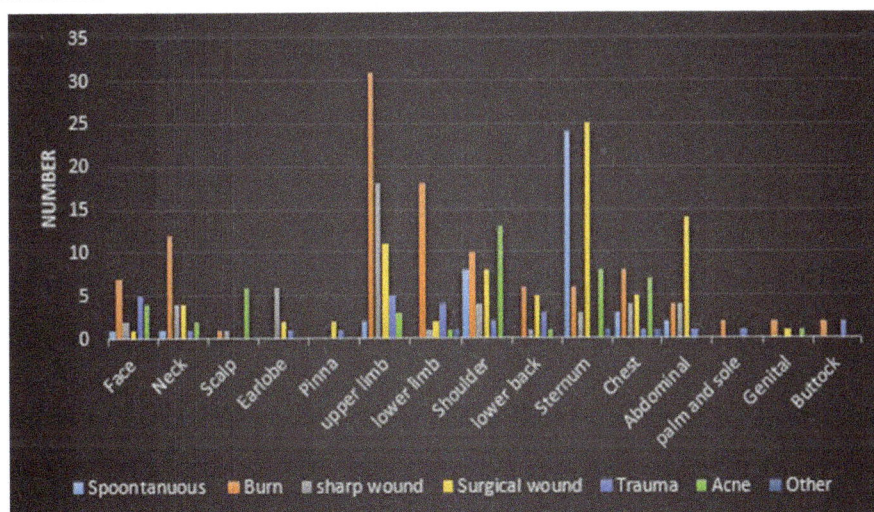

Fig. 1 Distribution of causes of scaring according to anatomical sites

Table 3 The most common causes of scarring according to anatomical sites, and the most common anatomical sites of keloids according to causes

Causes	The most common anatomical sites (%)	Anatomical sites	The most common causes (%)
Spontaneous	Sternum (58.54 %), shoulder (19.5 %)	Face	Burn (35 %)
Burn	Upper limb (28.44 %), lower limb (16.51 %)	Neck	Burn (50 %)
Sharp wound	Upper limb (37.5 %)	Scalp	Acne (75 %)
Surgical	Sternum (31.25 %), abdominal (17.5 %)	Ear lobe	Sharp wound (66.66 %)
Acne	Shoulder (28.26 %), sternum (17.4 %)	Pinna	Surgical (66.66 %)
Trauma	Face (18.52 %) upper limb (18.52 %)	Upper limb	Burn (44.29 %)
		Lower limb	Burn (66.66 %)
		Shoulder	Acne (28.88 %)
		Lower back	Burn (37.5 %)
		Sternum	Spontaneous (35.82 %) Surgical (37.13 %)
		Chest wall	Burn (27.59 %)
		Abdominal wall	Surgical (56 %)
		Palm and sole	Burn (66.66 %)
		Genital	Burn (50 %)
		Buttock	Trauma (50 %) Burn (50 %)

Table 4 The possible effect of blood group A on development of spontaneous keloids

Blood group (N)	Spontaneous keloids		Total
	Yes	No	
Blood group A	22	93	115
Blood groups B, AB, O	12	132	144
Total	34	255	259
P value (chi-square test)	0.01		

respectively (Fig. 5). We found statistical significance for heredity spontaneous, presternal and shoulder keloids ($p = 0.002$) ($p = 0.047$) ($p = 0.006$) respectively (Table 7).

Over half of the patients developed keloids in the 11–30 age range (Table 1) (Fig. 6).

Both age groups B and C (second and third decades) had statistical significance for developing keloids compared with control ($P = 0.02$) ($P = 0.01$) respectively, as opposed to age group A (first decade), that had statistical significance for not developing keloids compared with control ($p = 0.04$). (Table 2) (Fig. 6).

The distribution of causes and anatomical sites according to age groups were demonstrated at (Table 8) (Table 9) respectively. We have analyzed the relationship between each cause and each anatomical site according to 7 age groups. Then we selected the results that had statistical significance (Tables 10, 11, 12, 13 and 14).

This mean for each variable (each cause or each anatomical site) we have 7 independent tests. Therefore, because of multiple tests, we lowered the p value (to be less or equal 0.01) to reduce false positive.

In age group A (0-10Y), there was statistical significance for developing burn keloids ($p < 0.0001$), and for no developing spontaneous keloids ($p = 0.01$) (Table 10). Upper limb (26.98 %) followed by lower limb (19.05 %) were the most common anatomical sites for developing keloids in this age group.

keloids caused by the same cause (Table 1). Most of the causes and anatomical sites tended to be inherited, but in different proportions (Fig. 4) (Fig. 5). Patients with spontaneous and acne keloids had the highest percentage of family history (38.23 %) (30.77 %) respectively in contrast to patients with sharp wound keloids, who had the least percentage (9.76 %) (Fig. 4). Also, patients with shoulder and sternum keloids had the highest percentage of family history (34.1 %) (27.7 %)

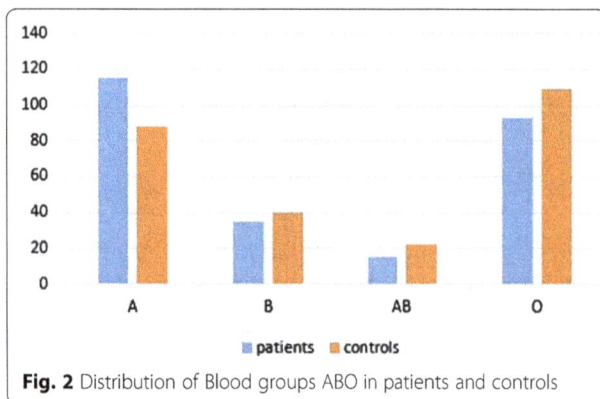

Fig. 2 Distribution of Blood groups ABO in patients and controls

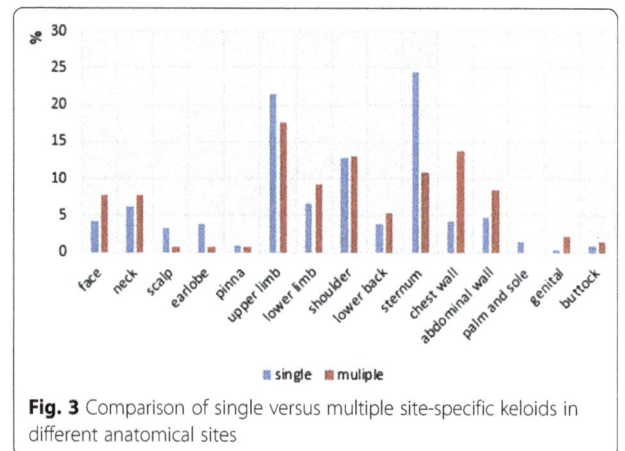

Fig. 3 Comparison of single versus multiple site-specific keloids in different anatomical sites

Table 5 Distribution of causes of scarring according to (single\multiple) sites

	Spontaneous	Burn	Acne	Trauma	Sharp wound	Surgical	other	Total	Number of patients
Single	29 (13.81 %)	55 (26.19 %)	14 (6.67 %)	15 (7.14 %)	38 (18.1 %)	56 (26.7 %)	3 (1.43 %)	210 (100 %)	209
Multiple	(5) 9.1%	21 (38.2 %)	12 (21.82 %)	5 (9.1 %)	3 (5.45 %)	9 (16.36 %)	0	55 (100 %)	50
Total	34	76	26	20	41	65	3	265	259

In age group B (11–20Y), causes had almost coordinated distribution. The shoulder (17.76 %) followed by sternum (15.88 %) were the most common sites for developing keloids in this age group. There was statistical significance for developing sharp wound, acne and earlobe keloids ($p = 0.002$) (0.008) ($p = 0.002$) respectively (Table 11).

In age group C (21–30Y), there was also a coordinated distribution of causes.

The upper limb (26.7 %) followed by sternum (16.7 %) were the most common sites. We found statistical significance for developing scalp keloids in this group ($p = 0.002$) (Table 12).

In age group D (31–40Y), causes had almost coordinated distribution considering the absence of acne keloids. The sternum (24.14 %) was the most common site for developing keloids in this age group without statistical significance.

In age groups E, F and G (41–70 Y), there was statistical significance for developing surgical keloids in these groups ($p = 0.00002$) ($p = 0.0002$) ($p = 0.003$) respectively (Table 13).

The sternum was the most common site for developing keloids in these groups (28.6 %) (53.8 %) (77.8 %) respectively with statistical significance for developing presternal keloids only in F and G groups ($p = 0.003$) ($p = 0.0002$) respectively (Table 14).

There were some pictures of keloids of our patients at Fig. 7.

Discussion

The exact mechanism of keloid formation is unknown, but several factors play a significant role in its formation. The genetic predisposition is the most important factor; other factors are the anatomical site, the form of skin injury, the age of onset and sex. In this study we have analyzed the associations among the age of onset, sex, the cause of scarring, blood groups, the anatomical site, presence of family history and the number of injured anatomical sites (multiple/single) to demonstrate some of the risk factors of keloids in Syrians (Caucasians).

Incidence of keloids was equal in females and males. That agree with most previous studies [5, 6, 11–13]. However, some studies found higher incidence of keloids in females [1, 4], while others found higher incidence in males [14].

Burn was the most common cause of keloid formation in our study (28.68 %), but laceration was the most common one in a Jamaican study [4]. We can explain this finding particularly because of war conditions in our country. The occurrence of acne keloids was higher in males compared to females ($p = 0.0008$), because only males have acne keloidalis nuchae. Also, the severity of acne is higher in them [15].

The most common anatomical site for developing keloids differs according to race, traditions and conditions of study's society, generally keloids tend to occur on highly mobile sites with high tension [16, 17]. In our study, upper limb (20 %) followed by sternum (19.17 %) were the most common sites for developing keloids, which was similar to a study of dark skin patients [11] (sternum 28.95 %, upper limb 15.8 % and head 16.7 %), and contrary to the Jamaican study [4] (ear 23 %), and Indian one [5] (sternum 33.6 %). On other hand, genitalia (1.18 %), buttock (1.18 %), palm and sole (0.9 %) were the rarest sites in our study, which agree with the previous studies [10, 14].

Table 6 Distribution of burn and acne keloids according to (single\multiple) sites

	Burn		Acne		Total
	Yes	No	Yes	No	
Single site	55	154	14	195	209
Multiple sites	21	29	12	38	50
Total	76	183	26	233	259
P value (chi-square test)	0.029		0.0002		

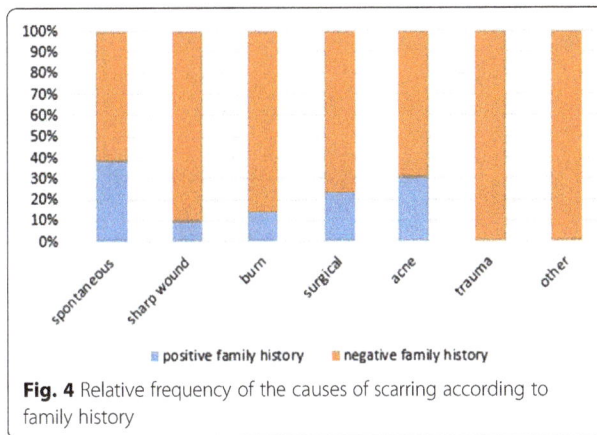

Fig. 4 Relative frequency of the causes of scarring according to family history

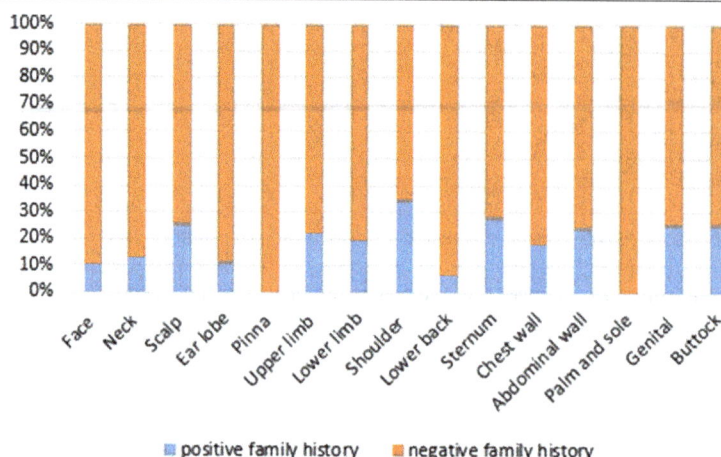

Fig. 5 Relative frequency of anatomical sites of keloids according to family history

People with blood group A have high probability to develop keloids compared with other blood groups ($p = 0.01$), that may be partly explained by the association between the effect of red cell antigens A (which present on the membrane surface of red blood cells and certain epithelial cells [11]) and other factors in these patients. Our findings agree with a previous study [5], and disagree with another one [11]. Spontaneous keloid is a rare condition, and it is controversial whether it is in fact spontaneous. The scar tissue may form after an insignificant inflammatory reaction or injury which the patient has no recollection of [18]. However, we found 13.4 % spontaneous keloids, which was similar to Togo study [11] (13.13 %), but lesser than an Iraqi one [13] (34 %). Also, we found statistical significance association between spontaneous keloids and blood group A ($p = 0.01$), which has not been previously reported. This result confirms the effect of red cell antigens A in development of keloids, as we discussed before.

Few studies discussed the development of keloids in single versus multiple anatomical sites [4, 19]. There were 19.3 % of patients who had keloids in multiple anatomical sites, while this percentage was 42 % in the Jamaican study [4]. All causes tended to develop keloids in multiple sites, but only burn and acne had statistical significance ($p = 0.029$) ($p = 0.0002$)

respectively, because both acne and burn could affect multiple sites more than other causes, which is more located. This means there was high probability to develop acne or burn keloids in another anatomical site in a patient who had a previous acne or burn keloid respectively. In our study, the upper limb was the most common anatomical site for developing keloids in patient with multiple sites (46 %), and sternum was the most common one in patients with a single site (26.84 %), while the earlobe was the most common site in both multiple (24 %) and single (48 %) sites in the Jamaican study [4]. Also, burn was the most common cause in patients with multiple sites (42 %), and surgical wound was the most common one in patients with a single site (26.8 %), while ear piercing was the most common cause in both sites in that study [4]. We didn't find any relationships between the development of keloids in multiple anatomical sites and the age of onset, the sex of patient or the presence of family history, while other studies [4, 19, 20] found statistically significant associations among these variables.

Table 7 Remarkable hereditary of spontaneous, sternum and shoulder keloids

Family history	Spontaneous		Sternum		Shoulder		Total
	Yes	No	Yes	No	Yes	No	
Positive	13	37	18	32	15	35	50
Negative	21	188	47	162	29	180	209
Total	34	225	65	194	44	215	259
P value (chi-square test)	0.002		0.047		0.006		

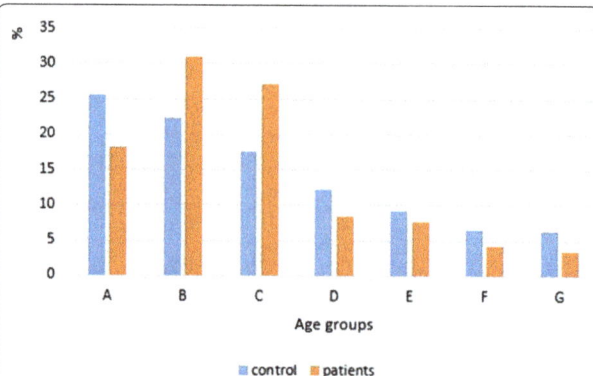

Fig. 6 Relative frequency of age groups in patients and control

Table 8 Distribution of causes of scarring according to age groups

Age groups	Causes							Total	Number of patients
	spontaneous	Burn	acne	trauma	Sharp wound	Surgical wound	others		
A	1	38	0	4	2	2	0	47	47
B	13	13	14	5	21	15	2	83	80
C	11	15	11	6	14	15	1	73	70
D	6	5	0	3	2	6	0	22	22
E	3	2	1	1	0	13	0	20	20
F	0	1	0	1	1	8	0	11	11
G	0	2	0	0	1	6	0	9	9
Total	34	76	26	20	41	65	3	265	259

Only (6/259) (2.32 %) of our patients had keloids caused by two different causes, compared to 15.9 % of patients in another study [11]. This result confirms the importance of the form of skin injury in keloid formation (not all insults lead to keloids even in the susceptible individuals [4]). (5\6) of these patients had surgical keloids, so we have to be careful when performing surgery for a patient who had a previous keloid. Only 5\259 (1.93 %) of patients had keloids caused by different causes, and distributed on multiple anatomical sites. This means there were only few people who have a high predisposition to develop keloids.

Most keloids occur sporadically, but some cases are familial, 19.3 % of our patients had family history,

Table 9 Distribution of anatomical sites of keloids according to age groups

Anatomical sites	Age groups							
	A	B	C	D	E	F	G	Total
Face	3	10	5	0	1	0	0	19
Neck	5	7	6	3	2	0	0	23
Scalp	0	2	6	0	0	0	0	8
Ear lobe	0	7	1	0	0	1	0	9
Pinna	1	2	0	0	0	0	0	3
Upper limb	17	14	24	5	5	1	2	68
Lower limb	12	6	2	2	4	0	0	26
Shoulder	5	19	13	4	1	2	0	44
Lower back	4	6	3	1	1	0	0	15
Sternum	4	17	15	7	8	7	7	65
Chest wall	5	8	8	3	2	1	0	27
Abdominal wall	2	7	5	3	3	1	0	21
Palm and sole	2	0	1	0	0	0	0	3
Genital	1	2	0	0	1	0	0	4
Buttock	2	0	1	1	0	0	0	4
Total	63	107	90	29	28	13	9	339
Number of patients	47	80	70	22	20	11	9	259

which was lower than previous studies [4, 14]. 76 % (38/50) of them had keloids located in the same anatomical sites of the relative. Also, 66 % (33\50) of them had keloids caused by the same cause. There was statistical significance for heredity spontaneous keloids ($p = 0.002$), which usually appears in the second decade (there was statistical significance for not developing spontaneous keloids in first decade ($p = 0.01$)) (Table 8), and for heredity presternal and shoulder keloids ($p = 0.047$), ($p = 0.006$) respectively. These results reflect the importance of the cause and anatomical site in heredity of keloid. Some recent studies confirmed the hereditary of spontaneous keloids [19, 21]. Other studies pointed to familial patterns of keloid distribution [9]. We didn't find any relationships between the family history and sex or the number of sites (single/multiple), while there were statistically significant associations between these variables in other studies [4, 19, 20].

Although keloids could occur at any age, they were rare in first decade (age group A) ($p = 0.04$), because people in this decade are not stimulated by sexual hormones (higher incidence of keloid formation during puberty) [10], most likely to occur in second and third decades (age groups B and C) ($P = 0.02$) ($P = 0.01$) respectively, and tend to decrease in older (Fig. 6), because younger people may have a higher frequency of trauma and their skin is more elastic than the skin of elderly people [22]. These findings agree with many studies [1, 4–6, 19, 20]. Burn was the most common

Table 10 Spontaneous and burn keloids in age group A compared with other age groups

Age group	Spontaneous		Burn		Total
	No	Yes	No	Yes	
A	46	1	9	38	47
B,C,D,E,F,G	179	33	174	38	212
Total	225	34	183	76	259
P value (chi-square test)	0.01		<0.0001		

Table 11 Acne, earlobe and sharp wound keloids in age group B compared with other age groups

Age group	Earlobe		sharp wound		Acne		Total
	No	Yes	No	Yes	No	Yes	
B	73	7	59	21	66	14	80
A,C,D,E,F,G	177	2	159	20	167	12	179
Total	250	9	218	41	233	26	259
P value (chi-square test)	0.002		0.002		0.008		

Table 13 Distribution of surgical keloids and other keloids (keloids caused by other causes) according to age groups G, F and G

Cause of keloid	Age group E		Age group F		Age group G		Total
	No	Yes	No	Yes	No	Yes	
Surgical keloid	52	13	57	8	59	6	65
Other keloids	187	7	191	3	191	3	194
Total	239	20	248	11	250	9	259
P value (chi-square test)	0.003		0.0002		0.00002		

cause for developing keloids in age group A compared with other groups ($p < 0.0001$), especially on upper and lower limbs. This is a logical result, because most of burn accidents exist in younger children especially on extremities. Occurrence of acne keloids was higher in age group B compared with other groups ($p = 0.008$), because the peak in prevalence and severity of acne occurs in second decade [23]. High frequency of sharp wound accidences and earlobe piercing in age group B explain the statistical significance for developing sharp wound ($p = 0.002$) and earlobe ($p = 0.002$) keloids in this age group. Also, development of scalp keloids was higher in age group C compared with other groups ($p = 0.002$), because most cases of acne keloidalis nuchae occur in persons aged 14–25 years [24] (acne keloidalis nuchae caused 75 % of scalp keloids in our study). We noted absence of acne keloids in age group D, because frequency of acne extremely decrease in this age [25, 26]. At last, development of surgical keloids was higher in age groups E, F and G compared with other groups ($p = 0.00002$) ($p = 0.0002$) ($p = 0.003$) respectively, especially on sternum. These results reflect an increase of open heart surgeries in older people, especially for males who were older than forty compared to females in the same age ($p = 0.036$).

Note: All patients with multiple site keloids had the same age group for each one.

We can explain this result; Patients with burn keloids were war or extensive burn victims, and patients with trauma and cut wound keloids were war or road accident victims. Patients with surgical keloids had extensive surgical wounds, or multiple surgical wounds which have occurred nearly in same time. As we know, acne keloids followed acne, which usually occur in specific age groups. It is surprising that all patients with multiple spontaneous keloid had the same age group for each one, that may reflect the predisposition for developing spontaneous keloid differs from one to another, or because we didn't follow up the patient, so we can't know if they will develop keloid later.

At last, we have demonstrated some of the risk factors of keloids:

- People with blood group A compared with other blood group.
- Spontaneous keloids in patients with blood group A.
- Acne in males compared to females.
- Acne in someone who has a previous acne keloid, because acne keloids tend to develop in multiple sites.
- Burn in someone who has a previous burn keloid, because burn keloids tend to develop in multiple sites.
- Family history, especially for developing spontaneous, presternal and shoulder keloids.
- People in second and third decades.

Conclusions

It is possible that several factors such as the age of onset, sex, the cause of scarring, blood groups, the anatomical site, the presence of family history and the number of injured sites (multiple/single) have an

Table 12 Scalp keloids in age group C compared with other age groups

Age group	Scalp keloids		Total
	No	Yes	
C	64	6	70
A,B,E,F,G	187	2	189
Total	251	8	259
P value (chi-square test)	0.002		

Table 14 Distribution of presternal keloids and other keloids (keloids in other anatomical sites) according to age groups G and F

Anatomical site of keloid	Age group F		Age group G		Total
	No	Yes	No	Yes	
Presternal keloid	58	7	58	7	65
Other keloids	190	4	192	2	194
Total	248	11	250	9	259
P value (chi-square test)	0.003		0.0002		

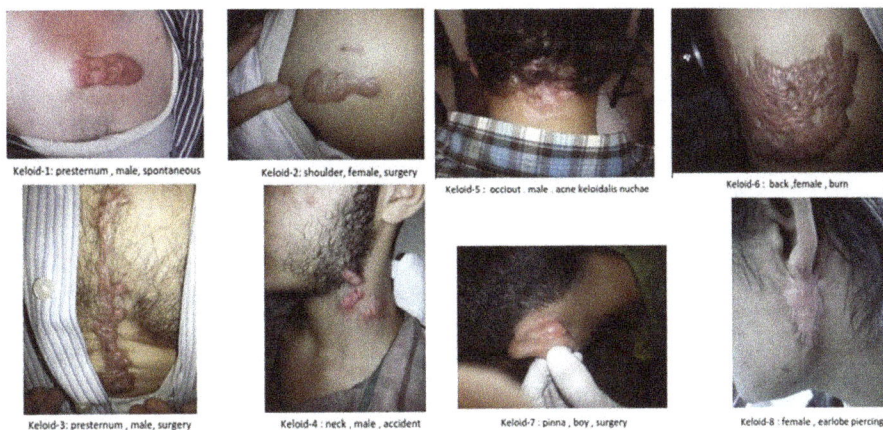

Fig. 7 Some keloids of our patients which located in different sites and caused by different forms of skin injury

important role in keloid formation and consequentially in predicting a keloid's behavior in response to treatment and prognosis. In this study we have demonstrated the significance of the previous factors in keloid formation in Syrian population. Therefore, we have to generalize these results, especially for dermatologists and surgeons. These observations could indicate a genetic basis in keloid formation, which justifies the need for genetic studies and more studies about families with keloids to define the type of heredity in our patients. (We noted that only females in two families (in three generations) had keloid formation. That suggests kind of sex-linked heredity, which has not been previously reported).

Abbreviations
NBTC: National blood transfusion center; SCC: Syrian census center

Acknowledgements
There is no one to acknowledge to.

Funding
There are no funding resources.

Authors' contributions
Dr. S carried out collecting data from the patients, analyzing it and drafting the manuscript. Dr. K and Dr. K helped in data collecting and reviewing the manuscript. All authors read and approved the final manuscript.

Competing interests
The authors declare that they have no competing interests.

Author details
[1]Department of dermatology, Tishreen University, Lattakia, Syria.
[2]Department of Plastic and Reconstructive Surgery, Tishreen University, Lattakia, Syria.

References
1. Burrows NP, Lovell CR. Rook textbook of dermatology. Eighth edition. volume 3. Chapter 45.54.
2. Nemeth AJ. Keloids and hypertrophic scars. J Dermatol Surg Oncol. 1993; 19(8):738–46.
3. Teofolia P, Barduagnia S, Ribuffob M, Campanellac A, De Pita'a O, Puddu P. Expression of Bcl-2, p53, c-jun and c-fos protooncogenes in keloids and hypertrophic scars. J Dermatol Sci. 1999;22(1):31–7.
4. Bayat A, Arscott G, Ollier WER, Mc Grouther DA, Ferguson MWJ. Keloid disease: clinical relevance of single versus multiple site scare. Br J Plast Surg. 2005;58(1):28–37.
5. Ramakrishnan K, Mathang FRCS, Thomas K, Pothan MS, Sundararajan Cheyyur R. Study of 1,000 patients with keloids in south India. J Am Soc Plastic Syrgeon. 1974;53(3):276–80.
6. Brian B, Bieley HC. Keloids. J Am Acad Dermatol. 1995;33(1):117–23.
7. Gao F-L, Jin R, Lu Z, Zhang Y-G. The contribution of melanocytes to pathological scar formation during wound healing. Int J Clin Exp Med. 2013; 6(7):609–13.
8. Chuma J, Chike O, Cole PD, Brissett AE. Keloids: Pathogenesis, Clinical Features, and Management. Semin Plast Surg. 2009;23(3):178–84.
9. Jason A Clark, Maria L Turner, Lillian Howard, Horia Stanescu, Robert Kleta and Jeffrey B Kopp. Description of familial keloids in five pedigrees: Evidence for autosomal dominant inheritance and phenotypic heterogeneity. *BMC Dermatology.* July 2009, DOI: 10.1186/1471-5945-9-8.
10. Gauglitz GG, Korting HC, Tatiana P, Thomas R, Jeschke MG. Hypertrophic Scarring and Keloids: Pathomechanisms and Current and Emerging Treatment Strategies. Mol Med. 2011;17:113–25. doi:10.2119/molmed.2009. 00153.
11. Abas Mouhari -Toure, Bayaki Saka, Koussak'e Kombat'e, Sefako Akakpo, Palakiyem Egbohou, Kissem Tchanga¨i-Walla, and Palokinam Pitche. Is There an Association between Keloids and Blood Groups? *International Scholarly Research Network ISRN Dermatology,* Volume 2012, Article ID 750908, 4 pages, doi:10.5402/2012/750908.
12. Kelly AP. Medical and surgical therapies for keloids. Dermatol Ther. 2004; 17(2):212–8.
13. Sharquie KE, Al-Dhalimi MA. Keloid in Iraqi Patients. A Clinicohistopathologic Study. Dermatol Surg. 2003;29(8):847–51.
14. Olaitan PB, Olabanji JK, Oladele AO, Oseni GA. Symptomatology of keloids in Africans. Sierra Leone J Biomed Res. 2013;5(1):29–33.
15. Lello J, Pearl A, Arroll B, Yallop J, Birchall NM. Prevalence of acne vulgaris in Auckland senior high school students. N Z Med J. 1995;108(1004):287–9.
16. Ogawa R, Okai K, Tokumura F, Mori K, Ohmori Y, Huang C, Hyakusoku H, Akaishi S. The relationship between skin stretching/contraction and pathologic scarring: The important role of mechanical forces in keloid generation. Int J Tissue Repair Regen. 2012;20(2):149–57.

17. Brissett AE, Sherris DA. Scar contractures, hypertrophic scars, and keloids. Facial Plast Surg. 2001;17(4):263–72.

18. Monarca C, Maruccia M, Palumbo F, Parisi P, Scuderi N. A Rare Case of Postauricular Spontaneous Keloid in an Elderly Patient. In vivo. 2012;26:173–6.

19. Park Tae H, Park Ji H, Tirgan Michael H, Halim Ahmad S, Chang Choong H. Clinical Implications of SingleVersus Multiple-Site Keloid Disorder: A Retrospective Study in an Asian population. Ann Plast Surg. 2015;74(2):248–51.

20. Wen-sheng L, Xiao-dong Z, Xiu-hua Y, Ian-fang Z. Clinical and epidemiological analysis of keloids in Chinese patients. Arch Dermatol Res. 2015;307(2):109–14.

21. Mandal A, Imran D, Rao GS. Spontaneous keloids in siblings. Ir Med J. 2004; 97(8):250–1.

22. Davies DM. Scars, hypertrophic scars and keloids. Br Med J. 1985;290:1056–8.

23. Burton JL, Cunliffe WJ, Stafford L, et al. The prevalence of acne vulgaris in adolescence. Br J Dermatol. 1971;85(2):119–26.

24. Perling LC, Homoky C, Pratt L, Sau P. Acne keloidalis is a form of primary scarring alopecia. Arch Dermatol. 2000;136(4):479–84.

25. Stathakis V, Kilkenny M, Marks R. Descriptive epidemiology of acne vulgaris in the community. Australas J Dermatol. 1997;38(3):115–23.

26. Collier CN, Harper JC, Cafardi JA, Cantrell WC, Wang W, Foster KW, Elewski BE. The prevalence of acne in adults 20 years and older. J Am Acad Dermatol. 2008;58(1):56–9. Epub 2007 Oct 22.

21

Skin cancer knowledge and attitudes in the region of Fez, Morocco: a cross-sectional study

Awatef kelati[1*], Hanane Baybay[1], Mariam Atassi[2], Samira Elfakir[2], Salim Gallouj[1], Mariame Meziane[1] and Fatima Zahra Mernissi[1]

Abstract

Background: The prevalence of skin cancers is constantly increasing in Morocco, and they have gradually become more aggressive due to a significant delay in the diagnosis. Our aim was to assess the levels of awareness and the influencing factors related to skin cancer knowledge in Morocco.

Methods: This cross-sectional study was carried out in Morocco through the medium of a validated questionnaire, which contained several items – demographics, skin cancer knowledge and attitudes towards skin cancer patients– during a period of 1 year (2014).

Results: Out of the 700 participants enrolled in the study, 17.9% had never heard of skin cancer, 32.5% had a low score of skin cancer knowledge, 66.7% had a moderate score, and only 0.85% had a high score of skin cancer knowledge. Further, 15.1% of the participants were under the assumption that this cancer is contagious. The sun was the most incriminated risk factor in skin cancer occurrence by 74.3% of the participants, and 57.9% of them believed that prevention is important through using various means of photoprotection. After univariate and multivariate analysis, the influencing factors related to the skin cancer knowledge in Morocco were: the socioeconomic status ($P = 0.003$, OR $= 7. 3$) and the educational level ($p < 0.001$, OR $= 20. 9$).

Conclusions: Due to the lack of knowledge or the underestimation of skin cancer in our study population, efforts are needed to promote skin cancer surveillance behaviors in Morocco.

Keywords: Cross-Sectional study, Skin cancer, Epidemiology, Knowledge, Attitudes, Morocco

Background

Skin cancer (SC) is the most common worldwide malignancy and it a preeminent global public health problem [1]. These SCs are divided into two main groups in Morocco: melanoma and non-melanoma SCs (NMSC), these last tumors are mainly basal cell carcinoma (BCC) and squamous cell carcinoma (SCC), and also cutaneous lymphomas, Sarcomas in addition to rare types such as adnexal tumors and Merkel cell carcinoma [2].

In Morocco, because of the absence of a national cancer registry, the exact number of incidence and mortality of SC is not available. However, according to regional records -Casablanca register of cancers (2004), Cancer registry of the National Institute of Oncology Sidi Mohamed Ben Abdellah, Rabat (2002–2007) and Rabat register of cancers (2009)- and a few publications, a change in the distribution of different SCs was noted; the prevalence of melanoma and lymphoma increased from 3,5% and 1,5% to 10,4% and 18,6% of skin malignancies in a period of 19 years; while the prevalence of the SCC and BCC decreased from 58% and 32% to 26,9% and 23,7% in the same period [2]; with a decrease in the proportion of skin carcinomas at the expense of Melanoma: 50.6% of carcinomas during the period 1992–2011 against 90% during the period 1971–1991.

* Correspondence: awatkelati@gmail.com
[1]Department of dermatology, University Hospital Hassan II, 202 Hay Mohamadi, Fez, Morocco
Full list of author information is available at the end of the article

There were also an increase in melanomas' aggressivity, in a study of 30 melanomas made in the region of Fez-Boulmane [3], Breslow index was more than 4 mm in 33%, 56 patients had metastasis and 2 patients died; while these numbers have almost doubled in a recent cohort of 70 cases of melanoma, carried out in the same region (unpublished data of the Moroccan Society of Dermatology), the Breslow at the moment of the diagnosis was > 4 mm in 50% of cases, with 4 cases of death.

Because of this increase, the costs attributable to the diagnostic delay and noneffective health care procedures are now an economic burden and they are a problem for health care services worldwide, for example, Medical costs to treat SCs in the USA are estimated at $3 billion annually [4].

However, the most important fact about SC is that it is mostly preventable with the health care promotion and the early detection endeavors. [5] When discovered early, the survival rate for individuals with melanoma is > 98%, as compared with 15% of those diagnosed with advanced disease. That's why health care providers should be promoting the establishment of appropriate strategies to ultimately improve the preventive provision of care for these cancers, by carrying out programs to evaluate the degree of awareness of populations with this problem and the benefit of the prevention of these risk factors especially sun exposure. Kyle and al. [5] reported that every dollar spent on sun safety educational initiatives saves the nation almost $4 in health care costs, in addition to a reduction in morbidity and mortality associated with SC.

In emerging Countries like Morocco, SC is not a public health priority, and it is usually underestimated. For this reason, before thinking about effective preventive measures, studies must be carried out to investigate SC knowledge in our populations.

The aim of the present study was to assess the level of awareness, and the influencing factors related to SC knowledge in Morocco, and to detect attitudes towards SC patients based on the degree of awareness of our population.

Methods
Study design
This was a cross-sectional study, spread over a period of 1 year between March 2014-March 2015 in the city of Fez in Morocco.

Participants
Participants aged more than 18 years old were randomly selected from different categories of the Moroccan population with different educational levels (ELs) and socioeconomic levels using a systematic sampling method: from the daily list of patients of other specialities' consultations and their accompanists in the Hospital Hassan II of Fez, Morocco.

Data collection
The data collection was based on filling a five-minute questionnaire by participants, in a "face to face" way with the investigator, in order to help them especially those with a low EL who can't read the questionnaire by themselves. Investigators were volunteers from the medical staff of the departments of dermatology and clinical epidemiology of the Hospital Hassan II of Fez.

The questionnaire consisted of 42 questions with several items: demographics, SC knowledge, attitudes towards SC patients, use of photoprotection measures, and the relationship with the doctor. The questions about SC knowledge were included in Table 1.

This questionnaire was validated in a multidisciplinary meeting, including experts in Dermatology, Clinical epidemiology, Scientific research and a psychiatrist.

Epidemiological and sociodemographic data of participants included: age, gender, highest level of education, health insurance status, profession and salary, medical records of participants and their phototype (filled by the investigator); then, participants were asked if they heard about SC and from who (health professional, relatives or media) and if they know someone who suffers from this disease and how he lived the experience; then, they completed questions regarding their knowledge about SC (risk factors especially sun exposure, clinical manifestations, location, contagiosity and treatment), in addition to SC eventually preventive measures (sunscreen use, shade seeking, and use of sun protective clothing).

Also, the questionnaire explored the participant's opinion of how must be the relationship between the physician and the patient, and how to announce the diagnosis (direct way or progressive way), and if the psychiatric care is obligatory for patients instead of, or accompanied by the family support.

Participants used a 3-point response scale (yes, no, I don't know or others) to indicate their response to the questions.

A score of SC knowledge level was established based on correct answers from 0 to 27: a low level of knowledge

Table 1 The questions about SC knowledge

Questions of SC knowledge
1) Have you ever/never heard of skin cancer?
2) Is it dangerous?
3) Could It kill
4) Clinical manifestations (multiples choices) (Table 3)
5) Alarming symptoms (multiples choices) (Table 3)
6) Skin cancer risk factors (multiples choices) (Table 3)
7) Its relationship with the phototype
8) Do you think that it appears in a pre-existing lesion?
9) Is mucosal involvement possible?
10) Do you know someone who has this skin cancer?
11) The reaction of the participant towards skin cancer patient
12) Relationship with the doctor: how should the doctor announce the diagnosis?

was described if the participant had less than 10 correct answers, a moderate level of knowledge if the participant had between 10 and 20 correct answers, and a high level of knowledge if the participant had more than 20 correct answers.

Socioeconomic level (SEL) was considered low if the monthly salary was less than 3000 DH (294.30 USD), moderate if it was between 2000DH (196.20 USD) and 7000DH (686.70 USD), and high if it was more than 7000 DH (686,70 USD).

Statistical analysis
A descriptive, univariate and multivariate analysis using the SPSS 20 software were performed.

In the descriptive analysis, quantitative variables were expressed by means ± standard deviation and qualitative variables by percentages. In the univariate analysis, the "Chi-square" test was used to compare percentages in order to determine the factors associated with the knowledge level. In the multivariate analysis, high and moderate levels of knowledge were grouped into one group of an appropriate level of SC knowledge, and a logistic binary regression was performed including variables for which the p value in the univariate analysis was less than 0.20, then a step down method was carried out. A p value less than 0.05 was considered statistically significant.

Results
We had included 700 subjects in this survey, the average age of participants was 33.6 years (SD = 13. 3 years). There was a female predominance (61.9%) and 64.1% of participants were in a moderate SEL (Table 2).

17.9% of the participants had never heard of SC, and 15.1% of them thought that it was contagious.

32,5% of the participants had a low score of SC knowledge level, 66.7% had a moderate score and only 0.85% had a high score of SC knowledge level (Table 3).

The sun was the factor the most incriminated in the pathogenesis of SC (74.3%) and 57.9% of the participants believed that it is important to use various means of photoprotection as sunscreens (34.2%), clothes (11%) or avoiding the exposition to the sun between 10 am and 16 pm (29%).

Regarding the relationship between the doctor and the patient, 58.4% of the participants thought that the doctor has to announce the diagnosis of cancer to the patient gradually, while 23.3% of the participants preferred the direct way, and 18.3% of them thought that the diagnosis must be hidden to the patient (Table 4).

In the univariate analysis, younger participants (<45 years) and subjects with a moderate or a high SEL ($p < 10–4$) and a high EL ($p < 0.001$) had an appropriate level of SC

Table 2 Descriptive analysis of epidemiological characteristics of participants

Epidemiological characteristics	N = 700	%
Age groups		
< 15 years old	5	0.7
15–45 years old	548	78.3
> 45 years old	147	21.1
Gender		
F	438	62.5
M	262	37.4
Phototype		
III	93	13.2
IV	489	69.8
V	118	16.8
Educational level		
Academic (university)	357	51
High school	164	23.4
Primary education	68	9.7
Illiterate	111	15.9
Socioeconomic level (SEL)		
Low SEL	167	23.8
High SEL	68	9.7
Moderate SEL	449	64.1

knowledge, and they emphasized the importance of the photoprotection and the psychiatric care for these patients.

Sources of information about SC varied according to the age ($P = 0. 03$) and the EL ($P = 0. 02$). Each category of the population had a different source of information; young persons with a moderate and a high EL used the internet, while television was the source of information of illiterates and aged persons.

Behaviors of the participants were influenced by their EL; the more the EL was increased, the more the participants preferred to stay away from SC patients or they remain indifferent to them because it could be contagious, and it was analphabets and the persons with a low EL who thought that they must support these patients even though it could be contagious ($p < 0.001$).

Men preferred the direct relationship between the doctor and the patient, especially the way to announce the diagnosis of cancer (38%), while women thought that the doctor must announce it gradually (60.5%) or not to announce it at all (20.3%) ($p = 0.02$) (Table 4).

After the multivariate analysis, the influencing factors related to SC knowledge in our Moroccan population were the SEL ($P = 0. 003$, OR = 7. 306, IC 95% = (1.9–27.5)), and the EL ($p < 0.001$, OR = 20.9, IC 95% = (10.5–41.6)) (Table 5).

Table 3 Descriptive analysis of the questionnaire items about skin cancer knowledge

Items	N = 700	%	Influencing factors	p value
Have you ever heard of skin cancer?				
Yes	486	69.7	None	
No	125	17.9		
I don't know	86	12.3		
Sources of Information			Age	0.03
Internet	350	50	Educational level	0.02
TV	290	41.4		
Patients and doctors	60	8.6		
Is it dangerous?			None	
Yes	384	54.8		
No	70	10		
I don't know	246	35.1		
It could kill				
Yes	304	44.3	None	
No	250	35.7		
I don't know	146	20		
Clinical manifestations			None	
Papules	234	54.3		
Nodules	126	30.1		
Tumors	174	41.5		
Ulcers	213	50.8		
Purulent bubbles	121	28.9		
Black patches	20	2.9		
Others	384	54.8		
Alarming symptoms			None	
Size increase	149	31.7		
Color change	143	30.4		
Resistance to usual treatment	118	25.2		
Pruritus	39	5.6		
Skin cancer risk factors			None	
Sun Exposure	344	74.3		
Genetic factors (Family history of skin cancer)	235	51.1		
Chemical products	230	49.8		
Irradiation	207	44.7		
Infection	171	37		
Smoking	121	26.5		
Relationship with the phototype (324/46.3%)			None	
Fair skin	300	42.8		
Dark skin	70	10		
Appears without pre existing lesion	142	20.2	None	

Table 3 Descriptive analysis of the questionnaire items about skin cancer knowledge *(Continued)*

Appears in pre existing lesion	331	47.2		
Mucosal involvement	312	44.5	None	
Treatments			None	
Surgery	174	24.8		
Chemotherapy	223	31.8		
Radiotherapy	194	27.7		
Total Score				
Low level of knowledge	228	32.5		
Moderate level of Knowledge	467	66.7	Socioeconomic level	<0.001
High level of knowledge	6	0.85	Educational level	<0.001

Discussion

SC is the most common malignancy [6–14]; and it increases dramatically, especially Melanoma [2], which has a faster growing incidence and a higher mortality rate than that of any other malignancy [15]. The underlying reasons for this increase were discussed in many studies that have confirmed the development of risk factors such as sun exposure; chronic and repeated in both BCC and SCC, while intense sun exposure and a history of sunburn was linked to melanoma [3]. Furthermore, a history of multiple moles (>50), atypical moles, light skin, red or blond hair, blue or green eyes, freckles, history of sunburn, or family history of melanoma are considered higher risks for developing melanoma [4], other risk factors especially for NMSC are an immunosuppression, human papilloma virus, chronic wounds and burns...

Compared with other cancer types, SC treatment costs are currently low because it can be primarily treated efficiently in an office-based setting. NMSC care cost stands in fifth place after prostate, lung, colon, and breast carcinomas. But, due to its considerable frequency, its final cost would be huge and depends on 2 factors: care settings and treatment modalities [2–16].

This present study is -to our knowledge- the first Moroccan, North African and among the first occidental studies interested in assessing the knowledge level, attitudes, and behaviors related to SC. Apart from three similar studies conducted on youths in Maryland [17] and in the USA [18], and the survey of Gordon R and al. that concluded to an overall low levels of knowledge about SCs especially melanoma [19, 20]. Other few studies interested only in the relationship between the sun, the photoprotection and SCs were performed [21–26], or conducted on minorities and targeted populations like golfers [6]. Similarly to these studies, the sun was the factor the most incriminated in the etiopathogenesis of skin cancer in our study (74.3%), and 57.9% of the

Table 4 Descriptive analysis of participants' responses about behaviors towards skin cancer patients and the relationship with the doctor

Items	N (%) = 700	Men N(%) 262 (37.4%)	Women N(%) 438(62.5%)	Influencing factors	p value
Relationship with skin cancer patients					
Do you know someone who has this skin cancer?				None	
Yes	139 (19.9)	55(21)	84 (19.2)		
No	561(80.1)	207(79)	354 (80.1)		
The reaction of the participant towards skin cancer patient				Educational level	<0.001
Remoteness (contagious)	90 (15.1)	34 (13)	56 (12.7)		
Indifferent	181 (30.4)	75 (28.6)	106 (24.2)		
Support	324 (54.5)	153 (58.4)	276 (63)		
The psychiatric care is obligatory for skin cancer patients				None	
Yes	358 (51.1)	122 (46.5)	233 (53.1)		
No	202 (29)	33 (12.6)	40 (9.1)		
I don't know	140 (20)	107 (40.8)	165 (37.6)		
Relationship with the doctor: how should the doctor announce the diagnosis?				Gender	0.02
Direct way	157 (23.3)	99 (38)	84 (19.1)		
Progressive way	393 (58.4)	147 (56.1)	265 (60.5)		
Hiding the diagnosis to the patient and inform just his family	123 (18.4)	16 (6.1%)	89 (20.3)		

participants believed that it is important for the SC prevention using various measures especially sunscreens.

We have found that 17.9% of participants, especially those with a low EL had never heard of SC, which is a real issue because this category not only underestimated this cancer and may have a poor sense of risk-reducing strategies for SC, but they would never come to see the doctor in the early stage of the disease, which explain why we still see historical tumors with bad prognosis and metastasis. Also, another possible factor of delay in our context is the frequent use of traditional medicine such as fire and plants.

Another common error in our population is the idea that SC is contagious, which was the participants' opinion in 15.1% of cases; and that it is due to germs (37%). This idea of contagious disease would not only influence the patient, but also his integrity in the society, which

will surely make the situation more complicated with a real impact on the patient's life quality.

What was surprising in our results was the fact that the more the EL increased, the more the participant preferred to stay away from SC patients or remain indifferent to them. While persons with a low EL thought that they must support these patients even though it could be contagious, this could be explained by the importance of the family and the religious links in our population, particularly in those with a low and moderate SEL who share a common home and a lifestyle.

From another perspective, 69.7% of our participants, especially younger patients with moderate or high SEL and EL had already heard of this type of cancer from different sources, such as SC patients, dermatologists and particularly the media (TV, internet..). This media tools may be an interesting way of sensitization that we can use as a strategy of SC prevention. According to our results, each category of the population may be educated using different media tools; for young educated persons the internet and the social media are the most effective way of giving information, while TV remains the best way of sensitization for illiterates and aged persons.

Regarding the way of announcing the diagnosis of cancer to the patient, Our results confirmed that it must vary according to the gender. This fact must be taken into account by the health care professionals in Morocco in order to decrease the disease burden, especially in women, but in the same time, we should be careful, because, it may lead the patient to neglect his disease if he did not know the gravity of it.

Table 5 Multivariate analysis showing the association between factors and SC knowledge score

Variables	P value	OR	CI 95%	
SEL				
Low SEL	0.000	4.232	2.550	7.023
Moderate and high SEL	0.003	7.306	1.936	27.567
Educationnal level				
Academic (university)	0.000	20.996	10.584	41.651
High school	0.000	3.332	1.834	6.052
Illiterates and primary education	0.038	2.136	1.041	4.382

Based on these results, we deduced that it's crucial to seek ways to correct the false ideas and the common errors regarding this special type of cancer in an attempt to prevent and to establish a SC surveillance and to facilitate its early detection.

Unfortunately, Guidelines regarding the SC screening are inconsistent and depend on the economic level of countries and natural factors (sunshine, climate, altitude), phototype and customs. However, several prominent national organizations recommended and emphasized sun-protective behaviors [27], education of health professionals, including nurses, in addition to improving strategies of SC and melanoma screening [28–32].

Ultimately, Despite all the barriers to SC prevention in Morocco, like financial issues, the lack of national guidelines, awareness, and availability of physicians. This overall burden must lead the health system in Morocco to consider this serious health problem and to try to establish a general approach to deal with it, using different ways of communication like the internet [33]; the TV and the programs of teaching health maintenance, the school programs for children; the sun protection guidelines and the SC screening programs not only for dermatologists, but for all the health care professionals.

This study is not without limitations, especially concerning our choice of participants; all the sections of the population were represented in the study sample, but the percentage of these sections was not equal. Although participants were chosen randomly and we tried to have a representative sample of all categories of the population, 78.3% of our participants were young (between 18 and 45 years old) and having an academic degree in 51% of cases.

Conclusion

Due to the lack of knowledge or the underestimation of SCs in our population, as we proved it in our study, efforts are needed to promote SC's surveillance and screening in Morocco, in addition to the establishment of effective campaigns of SC sensitization.

Abbreviations

BCC: Basal cell carcinoma; EL: Educational level; NMSC: Non-melanoma skin cancers; SC: Skin cancer; SCC: Squamous cell carcinoma; SEL: Socio economic level

Acknowledgements

We are indebted to all patients who participated in this study and gave their consent. We thank all volunteer investigators and the medical staff of the department of Dermatology and clinical epidemiology for their enormous help. Special thanks to the psychiatrist « Dr.M Jaafari » for his help in the questionnaire elaboration.

Funding

The authors declare that they have no fundings.

Authors' contributions

Conception and design: KA, AM. Acquisition, analysis and interpretation of data: KA, BH, GS. Drafting the article: KA; BH. Revising it critically for important intellectual content: KA, ES, MFZ. All authors read and approved the final manuscript.

Competing interests

The authors declare that they have no competing interests.

Author details

[1]Department of dermatology, University Hospital Hassan II, 202 Hay Mohamadi, Fez, Morocco. [2]Department of clinical epidemiology and scientific research, University Hospital Hassan II, Fez, Morocco.

References

1. Cakir BO, Adamson P, Cingi C. Epidemiology and Economic Burden of Nonmelanoma Skin Cancer. Facial Plastic Clinics of North America. 2012; 20(4):419–22.
2. Benchikhi H, Naciri-Bennani B, Tarwate M, Hali F, Khadir K, Zouhair K, et al. Évolution de la répartition des cancers cutanés vus dans le service de dermatologie de Casablanca entre les périodes 1971–1991 et 1992–2011. Ann Dermatol Vénéréol. 2012;139(12):838–9.
3. Lakjiri S, Inani K, Gallouj S, Meziane M, Mikou W, Mernissi FZ. Les mélanomes : expérience de CHU Hassan II, Fès. Ann Dermatol Vénéréol. 2013; 140(Supplement 1):S106.
4. Roebuck H, Moran K, MacDonald DA. PhD, Shumer S, McCune R L. Assessing skin cancer prevention and detection educational needs : an andragogical approach. J Nurs Pract. 2015;11(4):409–16.
5. Kyle J, Hammitt J, Lim H, et al. Economic evaluation of the U.S. Environmental Protection Agency's SunWise program: sun protection education for young children. Am Acad Pediatr. 2008;121:1074–84.
6. de Boz J, Fernández-Morano T, Padilla-Espana L, Aguilar-Bernier M, Rivas-Ruiz F, de Troya-Martín M. Skin Cancer Prevention and DetectionCampaignat Golf Courses on Spain's Costa del Sol. Actas Dermosifiliogr. 2015;106:51–60.
7. Housman TM, Feldman SR, Williford PM, Feischer AB, Goldman ND, Acostamiedo JM, et al. Skin cancer is among the most costly of all cancers to treat for the Medicare population. J Am Acad Dermatol. 2003;48:425–9.
8. Housman TM, Feldman SR, Williford PM, Feischer AB, Goldman ND, Acostamiedo JM, et al. Skin cancer is among the most costly of all cancers to treat for the Medicare population. J Am AcadDermatol. 2003;48:425–9.8-Montague M, Borland R, Sinclair C. Slip! Slop! Slap! andSunsmart, 1980–2000: Skin Cancer Control and 20 Years of Population-Based Campaigning. Health Educ Behav. 2001;28:290–305.
9. Aceituno-Madera P, Buendía-Eisman A, Arias-Santiago S, Serrano-Ortega S. Evolución de la incidencia del cáncer de piel en el periodo 1978–2002. Actas Dermosifiliogr. 2010;101:39–46.
10. Van der Leest RJ, de Vries E, Bulliard JL, Paoli J, Peris K, Stratigos AJ, et al. The Euromelanoma skin cancer prevention campaign in Europe: Characteristics and results of2009 and 2010. J Eur Acad Dermatol Venereol. 2011;25:1455–65.
11. Geller AC, Greinert R, Sinclair C, Weinstock MA, Aitken J, Boniol M, et al. A nationwide population-based skin cancer screening in Germany: Proceedings of the first meeting of the International Task Force on Skin Cancer Screening and Prevention (September 24 and 25, 2009). Cancer Epidemiol. 2010;34:355–8.
12. Mc Carthy WH. The Australian experience in sun protection and screening for melanoma. J Surg Oncol. 2004;86:236–45.
13. Anton WR, Janda M, Baade PD, Anderson P. Primary prevention of skin cancer: A review of sun protection in Australia and internationally. Health Promot Int. 2004;19:369–78.

14. Diepgen TL, Mahler V. The epidemiology of skin cancer. Br J Dermatol. 2002;146(Suppl61):1–6.

15. Gandhi SA, Kampp J. Skin Cancer Epidemiology, Detection, and Management. Med Clin North Am. 2015;99(6):1323–35.

16. Bickers DR, Lim HW, Margolis D, et al. The burden of skin diseases: 2004 a jointproject of the American Academy of Dermatology Association and the Society forInvestigative Dermatology. J Am Acad Dermatol. 2006;55(3):490–500.

17. Alberg AJ, Herbst RM, Genkinger JM, Duszynski KR. Knowledge,attitudes, and behaviors towards skin cancer Maryland youths. J Adolesc Health. 2002; 31(4):372–7.

18. Kaminska-Winciorek G, Wydmanski J, Gajda M, Tukiendorf A. Melanoma awareness and prevalence of dermoscopic examination among internet users: a cross-sectional survey. Postepy Dermatol Alergol. 2016;33(6):421–8.

19. Korta DZ, Saggar V, Wu TP, Sanchez M. Racial differences in skin cancer awareness and surveillance practices at a public hospital dermatology clinic. JAAD. 2014;70(2):312–7.

20. Gordon R. Skin cancer: an overview of epidemiology and risk factors. Semin Oncol Nurs. 2013;29(3):160–9.

21. Harth Y, Schemer A, Friedman-Birnbaum R. Awarness to photodamage versus the actual use of sun protection methods by young adults. J Eur Acad Dermatol Venereol. 1995;4(3):260–6.

22. Cooley JH, Quale LM. Skin cancer preventive behavior and sun protection recommendations. Semin Oncol Nurs. 2013;29(3):223–6.

23. Agbai ON, Buster K, Sanchez M, et al. Skin cancer and photoprotection in people of color: a review and recommendations for physicians and the public. JAAD. 2014;70(4):748–62.

24. Miller KA, Huh J, Unger JB, Richardson JL, Allen MW, Peng DH, Cockburn MG. Patterns of sun protective behaviors among Hispanic children ina skin cancer prevention intrvention. Prev Med. 2015;81:303–8.

25. Natalie Schuz, MichaelEid. Sun Exposure and Skin Cancer Prevention. International Encyclopedia of the Social & Behavioral Sciences, 2nd edition, Volume 23: 696–700.

26. E Senel, I Süslü.Knowledge, attitudes, and behaviors regarding sun protection, effects of the sun, and skin cancer among Turkish high school students and teachers. Dermatol Sin. 2015;33(4):187–90.

27. SunWise. The U.S. EPA's SunWise program: a roadmap. 2014. http://www2.epa. gov/sunwise/us-epas-sunwise-program-roadmap/. Accessed 16 May 2014.

28. McGuire S, Secrest A, Andrulonis R, Ferris L. Surveillance of patients for early detection of melanoma: patterns in dermatologist vs. patient discovery. Arch Dermatol. 2011;258(6):673–8.

29. Siegel V. Exploring the role of the nurse in skin cancer prevention. Dermatol Nurs. 2010;4(12):18–22.

30. Coups EJ, Stapleton JL, Hudson SV, Medina-Forrester A, Rosenberg SA, Gordon M, Natale-Pereira A, Goydos JS. Skin cancer surveillance behaviors among US Hispanic adults. JAAD. 2013;68(4):576–84.

31. Emmons KM, Geller AC, Puleo E, Savadatti SS, Hu SW, Gorham S, Werchniak AE. Dana-Farber skin cancer screening Group. Skin cancer education and early detection at the beach: a randomized trial of dermatologist examination and biometric feedback. JAAD. 2011;64(2):282–9.

32. Christos PJ, Oliveria SA, Masse LC, McCormick LK, Halpern AC. Skin cancer prevention and detection by nurses: attitudes, perceptions, and barriers. J Cancer Educ. 2004;19(1):50–7.

33. Heckman C, Darlow S, Munshi T, Caruso C, Ritterband L, Raivitch S, Fleisher L, Manne S. Development of an Internet Intervention to Address Behaviors Associated with Skin Cancer Risk among Young Adults. Internet Interv. 2015; 2(3):340–50.

Magnitude and associated factors of Atopic dermatitis among children in Ayder referral hospital, Mekelle, Ethiopia

Abraham Getachew Kelbore[1]*, Workalemahu Alemu[2], Ashenafi Shumye[3] and Sefonias Getachew[4]

Abstract

Background: Atopic Dermatitis (AD) is now a day's increasing in prevalence globally. A Prevalence of 5–25 % have been reported in different country. Even if its prevalence is known in most countries especially in developing countries there is scarcity with regard to prevalence and associated risk factors of AD among children in Ethiopia settings. The aim of this study was to determine the magnitude and associated factors of atopic dermatitis among children in Ayder referral hospital, Mekelle, Ethiopia.

Methods: A facility-based cross-sectional study design was conducted among 477 children aged from 3 months to 14 years in Ayder referral hospital from July to September, 2014. A systematic random sampling technique was used to identify study subjects. Descriptive analysis was done to characterize the study population. Bivariate and multivariate logistic regression was used to identify factors associated with AD. The OR with 95 % CI was used to show the strength of the association and a P value < 0.05 was used to declare the cut of point in determining the level of significance.

Results: Among the total respondents, 237 (50.4 %) were males and 233 (49.6 %) were females. The magnitude of the atopic dermatitis was found to be 9.6 % (95 % CI: 7.2, 12.5). In multivariate logistic regression model, those who had maternal asthma (AOR: 11.5, 95 % CI:3.3–40.5), maternal hay fever history (AOR: 23.5, 95 % CI: 4.6–118.9) and atopic dermatitis history (AOR: 6.0, 95 % CI:1.0–35.6), Paternal asthma (AOR: 14.4, 95 % CI:4.0–51.7), Paternal hay fever history (AOR: 13.8, 95 % CI: 2.4–78.9) and personal asthma (AOR: 10.5, 95 % CI:1.3–85.6), and hay fever history (AOR: 12.9, 95 % CI:2.7–63.4), age at 3 months to 1 year (OR: 6.8, 95 % CI: 1.1–46.0) and weaning at 4 to 6 months age (AOR: 3.9, 95 % CI:1.2–13.3) were a significant predictors of atopic dermatitis.

Conclusion: In this study the magnitude of atopic dermatitis was high in relation to other studies conducted so far in the country. Maternal, paternal, personal asthma, hay fever histories, maternal atopic dermatitis history, age of child and age of weaning were independent predicators of atopic dermatitis. Hence, the finding alert a needs of strengthening the national skin diseases prevention and control services in particular in skin care of children related to atopic dermatitis and others. In avoiding early initiation of supplementary feeding specially with personal and families with atopic problem needs further attention of prevention activities.

Keyword: Atopic dermatitis, Cross sectional study, Magnitude, Institutional based study

* Correspondence: kelbore2005@gmail.com
[1]Mekelle University, Tropical Dermatology, Mekelle, North Ethiopia
Full list of author information is available at the end of the article

Background

Atopic dermatitis (AD) is a chronic non-contagious disease that affects the skin. It is characterized primarily by intense itching and the development of papules, scaly lesions, fissures, and crusting [1]. This is one of the most common allergic diseases and manifests as a chronic recurrent dermatitis with itching.

The etiology of AD is multifactorial. Researchers suspect that AD might be caused by environmental factors acting in people who are genetically predisposed to the disease. Heredity is an important biological risk factor in the development of immune sensitization and allergy [2]. Recent data have suggested that loss-of-function genetic variants in the filaggrin gene are associated with AD. Filaggrin plays a role in maintaining the epidermal skin barrier function, whereby it helps to retain moisture in the skin and limits penetration by allergens. These functions can be impaired in filaggrin loss-of-function mutations, this resulting in dry, scaly skin, which increases risk of allergic sensitization and disease [3, 4].

Early life event factors also play a role in the clinical manifestation of AD in children. These may therefore contribute to the increased permeability to foreign proteins in early life and can explain the enhanced antigen uptake in quantities sufficient to influence the immune system this relative intestinal permeability may render the neonate susceptible to pathogen invasion and allergen sensitization [5, 6].

Additionally gastric acid production and enzyme secretion are reduced during the first 4 weeks of life. It is accompanied by immature or disordered intestinal peristaltic activity. The gut-associated lymphoid tissues are incompletely developed at birth. Absorption of large molecules from the gastro intestinal tract (GIT) may lead to immune system dysfunction and, as a result, to the development of AD [5, 7].

The diagnosis of AD is made clinically because there is no laboratory marker or definitive test that can be used to diagnose the condition. Diagnostic criteria for AD were originally developed in an attempt to standardize the type of patient enrolled in research studies. In 1994 a UK Working Party published a minimum list of criteria for AD, which were derived from the Hanifin and Rajka criteria [7, 8].

Studies on the natural history of AD document up to 60 % spontaneous clearing by puberty [9, 10]. AD may recur in adults and the risk is associated with a family history, early onset, severity and persistence of childhood AD and the presence of mucosal atopy.

AD affects up to 20 % of children and 3–5 % of adults in the Western world [11]. The prevalence of AD appear to have risen substantially in many countries in recent decades, a phenomenon that has been attributed variously to changes in lifestyle, nutrition, and other environmental factors. According to the results from a cross-sectional questionnaire survey conducted on random samples of schoolchildren aged 6 to 7 years and 13 to 14 years from centers in 56 countries throughout the world, the prevalence of AD for children aged 6 to 7 years ranged between 2 % (Iran) and 16 % (Japan, Sweden) and for those aged 13 to 14 years ranged between 1 % (Albania) and 17 % (Nigeria). Higher prevalence of AD symptoms was reported in Australia and Northern Europe, and lower prevalence was reported in Eastern and Central Europe and Asia [12].

In Ethiopia in 2005 the prevalence of AD among children age between 1 to 5 years is 4.4 %, which is identified from a cross sectional survey conducted at rural Jimma south west of a country [13].

AD causes various physical problems due to frequent skin damage and itchy sensation, which decrease quality of life. In younger patients, the disease can be sufficiently serious as to disrupt friendships, learning performance, and family relationships, thus negatively influence the overall quality of life in addition to the physical problems. AD has increased in prevalence in many countries in recent decades, but the risk factors for AD in developing countries are unknown [14, 15].

Besides avoiding irritants and moisturizing the skin with emollients, local anti-inflammatory treatment with topical corticosteroids is the mainstay treatment for infants with AD. Parents often fear the side effects and this may lead to non-compliance [16].

The prognosis is reasonable with a recovery rate of 40 % at age two and 65 % in adolescence. AD can be the starting point of the 'allergic march', the natural progression of allergic disorders such as asthma and allergic rhinitis. Children with AD have a chance of approximately 40 % to develop asthma [17].

Breastfeeding (BF) and the developing of AD is controversial issue, Human colostrum contains large quantities of secretory IgA (sIgA). Secretory IgA neutralizes infectious agents while at the same time limiting the damaging effects of tissue inflammation that can occur with other antibody types also that can prevent allergen absorption by limiting contact between ingested antigen and the intestinal mucosal membrane [18]. But different studies reports do not support protective effect of BF [19].

Identifying risk factors related to AD is very crucial to prevent the occurrence, recurrence and complications of the diseases among children with strengthening the National Health Service programs on prevention and control of skin diseases. Several risk factors have been identified in the associated with AD among children, of which the three most important are– family history of atopic diseases, early initiation of food, early exposure to antibiotics [1, 2]. In a case of AD various potential socio demographic, environmental, early life event and personal associated risk factors were also investigated in different countries in the world. However, a virtual consensus among AD researchers regarding the fact that family history of atopic diseases, socioeconomic status of family, early use of antibiotics, early exposure to solid foods is a risk factor for AD among children, age, sex, duration of exclusive breast feeding(EBF), have no clear association with AD [2, 13, 14].

Now a day's the prevalence of AD is increasing in worldwide especially in developing countries of urban area. However, the prevalence and risk factors association with development of AD among children poorly known specifically in Ethiopia [20]. But to the best of our knowledge no study has been done on the magnitude and associated factors of AD among children in Ayder referral hospital, Mekelle in Tigray region. And this study was the first to identify the magnitude and factors associated with AD among children age between 3 months and 14 years who visit dermatology and pediatrics outpatient unit.

Methods
Study area and period
This study was conducted in dermatology and Pediatric Outpatient department units of Ayder referral hospital at Mekelle, Ethiopia. Mekelle is the capital city of the Tigray national regional state which is located at 783 km distance north of Addis Ababa. The town had six hospitals (3 private and 3 public), one referral hospital, five health centers, two private higher dermatologic clinics and thirteen higher clinics [21].

Ayder referral and teaching hospital is one of the hospitals which are serving at the Tigray regional state at the north part of Ethiopia since 2007. Presently, the hospital provides various clinical and referral services including dermatological services ranging from primary to specialized care and serves patients referred from different health facilities in Tigray and neighboring regions. It has 500 health professionals working in the hospital with a total of 480 beds for inpatient services [22].

The study was conducted in Ayder referral and teaching hospital from July to September, 2014.

Study design, study population and sampling
A facility based cross sectional study design was used and children whose age range from 3 months to 14 years who visited the dermatology and pediatrics OPD during the study period were involved.

The sample size was determined by using single population proportion formula with confidence interval 95 % and 3 % margin of error by taking the prevalence rate of AD among children 11.5 % from a study conducted in Mobile Dermatology clinic in Ankober, central Ethiopia [23] and taking the non-respondent rate of 10 % the final sample size becomes 477.

Sampling procedure
Systematic sampling technique was used to identify the study subjects. In average a minimum of 40 children visit on Monday, Tuesday and Thursday at the Dermatology and Pediatric OPDs of the hospital for treatment seek. On Wednesday and Friday up to 20–25 children visits are expected in the OPDs. In total 165 patients seek the treatment per week (within 5 working days). In this study we included every 2nd child patient coming to the OPDs according to their visit.

Data collection and quality control
A structure interview questioner was used in the local language once translated from the English version. Additional data was reviewed from clinical examination card of the child patients. The interview was conducted among the mothers or care givers of the children during both OPD visits.

Five trained master of tropical dermatology students were involved in the data collection process and three of them involved as interviewer and the rest two involved in clinical examination and supervision process. The interview was collected using a structured questioner based on the given guide line. The interviewer approached the patient's mother in a polite and respected manner and kept the confidentiality of patient data.

The socio demographic factors, environmental factors, early life event factors, personal disease associated factors were assessed and skin physical examination was done according to American Academy of dermatology modified paediatrics diagnostic criteria of AD among children. A Pre-test was carried out before actual data collection and some modifications were taken according to the findings. Data completeness and consistency was checked during the collection time and during data entry and cleaning process by doing simple frequency. Ethical clearance was obtained from the Ethical review committee of the College of health science of Mekelle University. Accordingly, permission letter were secured from medical director at Ayder referral hospital. Child Patient identification variables were not used in the study. The studies not inflict harm on or expose children to unnecessary risk as a result of examining of children and interviewing their mothers. Informed consent was obtained verbally from mothers or care givers of children during the interview. When interview and physical examination completed those children who have the problem were linked to the facility for the treatment.

Data analysis
A descriptive analysis using Proportion and frequency, mean, standard deviation, were used. Bivariate logistic regression was applied to see the association between each independent variable with dependent variable and multiple

logistic regression model was used to identify independent predictors. Variable found to be significant at *P value <0.05* in the bivariate analysis were entered to multiple logistic regression. We used the enter approach in for inclusion into the multivariate model while the Hosmer-Lemeshow statistic was used for model diagnostics. Statistical significance was declared at *P value < 0.05* and the entered and analysis of the data was performed using SPSS version 20 statistical software package.

Operational definitions used in the study

Atopic dermatitis: patient must have Essential futures with or without important and associated features list according to American Academy of dermatology modified pediatrics AD diagnostic criteria [24].

    Essential features; are Pruritus and Eczematous changes which must present and, are sufficient for diagnosis: Typical and age-specific patterns and Chronic or relapsing course.

    Important features: Early age at onset, personal or family atopic history, IgE sensitivity and dryness of skin.

    Associated features: Keratosis pilaris/Ichthyosis/Palmar hyper linearity, atypical vascular responses, Perifollicular accentuation/Lichenification/Prurigo Ocular/periorbital changes and Perioral/periauricular lesions.

Result

Socio-demographic characteristics

In this study a total of 477 children patients, who were enrolled based on the inclusion criteria, are studied. Only 7 children patient's parents refused to participate, that makes the response rate 98.5 %. Of these participants, 237 (50.4 %) were males and 233 (49.6 %) females, and 341 (72.6 %) were from the urban and 129 (27.4 %) from rural area. The overall mean and standard deviation of age for study participants were 6.63 and (±3.983).

    About 133 (28.7 %) fathers of the children attended tertiary school and 111 (23.9 %) of them attended Primary school. whereas, 141 (30.1 %) mothers of the children attend Primary school and 124 (26.4 %) were illiterate. Most of children fathers were 148 (32.0 %) civil servant by occupation. Near to two third 291 (62.2 %) of the children mothers were house wife and 81 (17.3 %) of them were civil servant.

    One hundred ninety five (41.5 %) of the family earn a monthly income of less than or equal to 1000 birr and the rest 133 (28.3 %) lie between 1001 and 2000 birr (Table 1).

Environmental factors

Near to one third of the respondents 169 (36 %) described that the surrounding environment in their living home was open spaces or field and 155 (33 %) mentioned as garden. Among the respondents, 195 (41.5 %) of them had less than or equal to four family sizes and 275 (58.5 %) of them had greater than four. Interview on the number of

Table 1 Socio-demographic Characteristics of children in Ayder referral hospital, Mekelle, Ethiopia, 2014

Variable	Category	Frequency	Percent
Sex of child	Male	237	50.4
	Female	233	49.6
Age in category	0.25–1 year	44	9.4
	1⁺–5 years	168	34.5
	5⁺–10 years	162	35.7
	10⁺–14 years	96	20.4
Residence	Urban	341	72.6
	Rural	129	27.4
Father educational status	Illiterate	50	10.8
	Read & write	55	11.9
	Primary school	115	24.8
	High school	111	23.9
	Tertiary school completed	133	28.7
Mother educational status	Illiterate	124	26.4
	Read & write	28	6.0
	Primary school	141	30.1
	High school	93	19.8
	Tertiary school completed	83	17.7
Occupation of Father	Farmer	107	23.2
	Merchant	111	24.0
	Civil servant	148	32.0
	Other	88	20.8
Mother occupation	Civil servant	81	17.3
	Housewife	291	62.2
	Merchant	62	13.2
	Other	34	7.3
Monthly family income	<1000	195	41.5
	1001–2000	133	28.3
	2001–3000	65	13.8
	≥3001	77	16.4

child siblings shows that 200 (42.6 %) of the respondents had one or no sibling, 222 (47.2 %) had two to three siblings and rest had four or more siblings. Pipe water is the main (84 %) source of drinking water among the respondents of the study. A total of 144 (30.6 %) of the respondents uses insecticide at their home and 56 (11.9 %) of the respondents had exposure to second hand smoking in their living home (Table 2).

Early life event factors among children

All of the children had history of breast feeding. Almost near to half 224 (47.7 %) of the children were breast feed for 12 months and above. Three hundred ten (66 %) children have started additional food after age of 6 months and 117 (24.9 %) started at 4 to 6 months age. Animal milk 246 (53.2 %), and packed food and other 160 (34.6 %) were the type of food children exposed before the age of 6 months (Table 3).

Characteristics of personal and family disease factors

History of asthma is interviewed among the family members and 36 (7.7 %) mothers of the child, 33 (7.0 %) fathers of the child, 11 (2.3 %) siblings and 12 (2.6 %) children themselves had asthma. Among the respondents

Table 2 The characteristics of home environmental factors among children in Ayder referral hospital, Mekelle, Ethiopia, 2014

Variable	Category	Frequency	Percent
Home surrounding description	Open spaces or fields nearby	169	36.0
	Many parks or gardens	76	16.2
	Few parks or gardens	155	33.0
	No parks or gardens	70	14.9
People living in the house	<4	195	41.5
	>4	275	58.5
Number of siblings	0–1	200	42.6
	2–3	222	47.2
	4 or more	48	10.2
House type	Single and detached	390	83
	Apartment	80	17
Roof of house	Corrugated	437	93
	Thatched	33	7
Floor of house	Mud	211	44.9
	Cement	259	55.1
Is their carpeted room/s	Yes	144	30.6
	No	326	69.4
Source of water	Pipe	399	84.9
	Well	50	10.6
	River	11	2.3
	Spring	10	2.1
Wood as fuel for cooking	Never	43	9.1
	Some times	133	28.3
	Every day	294	62.6
Electricity fuel for cooking	Never	245	52.1
	Some times	137	29.1
	Every day	88	18.7
Kerosene fuel for cooking	Never	396	84.3
	Some times	57	12.1
	Every day	17	3.6
Animals living in the house	Yes	301	64.0
	No	169	36.0
Pets contact at 1 year of age	Yes	245	53.6
	No	212	46.4
Pets contact after 1 year	Yes	173	38.0
	No	282	62.0
Indoor smoking Exposure	Yes	56	11.9
	No	414	88.1
Use of insecticide	Yes	144	30.6
	No	326	69.4

Table 3 The characteristics of early life event factors among children in Ayder referral hospital Mekelle, Ethiopia, 2014

Variable	Category	Frequency	Percent
Duration of breast feeding	<4 months	16	3.4
	4–6 months	93	19.6
	7–12 months	125	26.6
	≥12 months	224	47.7
	Do not remember	12	2.6
Exclusive breast feeding duration	<6 months	80	17.3
	≥6 months	370	80.3
	Do not remember	11	2.4
Age first started weaning	<4 months	20	4.3
	4–6 months	117	24.9
	≥6 months	310	66.0
	Never	12	2.6
	Do not remember	11	2.3
Type of food 1st initiated	Animal milk	246	53.2
	Packed food	160	34.6
	Other	56	12.1
Vaccination status for any	Yes	455	96.8
	No	15	3.2
DPT Vaccination	Yes	455	96.8
	No	15	3.2
Polio Vaccination	Yes	455	96.8
	No	15	3.2
Child Antibiotic use	Yes	257	54.7
	No	213	45.3
Fruit intake	Never	71	15.1
	Once per week	293	62.3
	More than once per week	106	22.6
Vegetable intake	Never	61	13
	Once per week	247	52.5
	More than once per week	162	34.5

of AD were detected among mothers with house wife status, civil servant, and merchant by occupation. And most of the 19 (4 %) AD diagnosed cases among children were the family monthly income is greater than or equal to 3001birr (~150$). On this study as the age of children increases AD diagnosis were decreased (Fig. 1).

Distribution of AD among children with home environment and early event factors

AD was diagnosed among children whose home surrounding were 20 (4.3 %) open fields followed by few parks and gardens 17 (3.6 %). Children from family size less than four were more diagnosed for AD than those who have greater or equal to four family size. And on segment of children who have one or no siblings 22 (4.7 %) were more diagnosed for AD with followed by two to three siblings 19 (4 %) and above four siblings 4 (0.9 %) (Fig. 2).

Distribution of AD among children with personal and family disease related characters

Children who have AD had maternal history of atopic diseases had asthma, hay fever and dermatitis 37.78, 20

52 (11.1 %) of the children had family history of atopy (Table 4).

Magnitude and distribution of AD with socio demographic characteristics

Out of 470 children, 45 of them were diagnosed with AD according to Atopic dermatitis diagnostic (AAD) criteria with a magnitude of 9.6 % (95 % CI: 7.2, 12.5). Among these, 25 (5.3 %) of them were male and the rest 20 (4.3 %) were females. AD was higher among Urban children residence 36 (7.7 %) than rural 9 (1.9 %) children. Among this 20 (4.3 %), 15 (3.2 %), 5 (1.1 %) cases

Table 4 Personal and family disease related factors with AD diagnosed according to AAD diagnostic criteria, Mekelle, Ethiopia, 2014

Variable	Category	Frequency	Percent (%)
Family history of atopy	Yes	52	11.1
	No	418	88.9
Child mother ever had	Asthma	36	7.7
	Hay fever	12	2.6
	Atopic dermatitis	9	1.9
	None	413	87.9
Child father ever had	Asthma	33	7.0
	Hay fever	17	3.6
	Atopic dermatitis	4	.9
	None	416	88.5
Child siblings ever had	Asthma	11	2.3
	Hay fever	17	3.6
	Atopic dermatitis	6	1.3
	None	436	92.8
Child had ever had	Asthma	12	2.6
	Hay fever	18	3.8
	None	440	93.6

and 11.1 % respectively. The paternal history of atopic diseases shows that asthma (33 %), hay fever (17.78 %), and dermatitis (6 %). Among Children's who had AD 5 (11.1 %) of them have Personal history of asthma and 6 (13.3 %) had hay fever history. Among AD children 80% of them had family atopy history (Fig. 3).

Factors associated with atopic dermatitis among children

Comparison of variables that were statistically significant with AD according to AAD diagnostic criteria for AD on crude analysis were adjusted using enter method multivariate logistic analysis model (Table 5). The variables that showed significant association in binary logistic regression model were age, mother education level, father occupation, family monthly income, indoor smoking exposure, use of insecticide at home, exclusive breast feeding, age of weaning, mother atopic diseases, father atopic diseases, siblings atopic diseases status, and personal atopic history.

According to the multiple logistic regression, the odds of AD were 6.9 times higher among children whose age is 3 months to 1 year old than those with age 10–14 years old. (AOR: 6.9, 95 % CI: 1.0–46.1).

The odds of AD were also higher among children those who had history of mother history asthma, allergic rhinitis or hay fever and atopic dermatitis than those children who had no mother history asthma, allergic rhinitis or hay fever and atopic dermatitis. (AOR: 11.5, 95 % CI: 3.3–40.508), (AOR: 23.5, 95 % CI: 4.6, 118.9) and (AOR: 6, 95 % CI: 1.0–35.6) respectively.

The odds of AD were 14 times higher among children those who had history of paternal asthma (AOR: 13.9, 95 % CI: 2.4–79.0). AD was significantly associated with paternal history of Allergic rhinitis or hay fever (AOR: 14.4, 95 % CI: 4.0–51.7).

Personal history of asthma (AOR: 10.5, 95 % CI: 1.3–85.5), allergic rhinitis or hay fever (AOR: 13.0, 95 % CI: 2.7–63.4), weaning (4–6 month) (AOR: 4.0, 95 % CI: 1.2–13.3) were the variables significantly associated with AD among the children.

Discussion

Atopic dermatitis is one of the most inflammatory skin disease observed among children now a day with increasing prevalence in the world 5–20 % [25]. However, studies on the prevalence and associated risk factor of AD among children are scarce in our country except a few studies conducted. Determining country specific magnitude and Identifying factors related to AD is crucial to halt the occurrence, recurrence and complication of AD by strengthening the national skin diseases prevention and control program. In case of AD among children, various prevalence, demographic, environmental and family and personal diseases factors have been investigated in different countries in the world so far; however, the magnitude and risk factors identified vary based on the (place) countries of studies conducted.

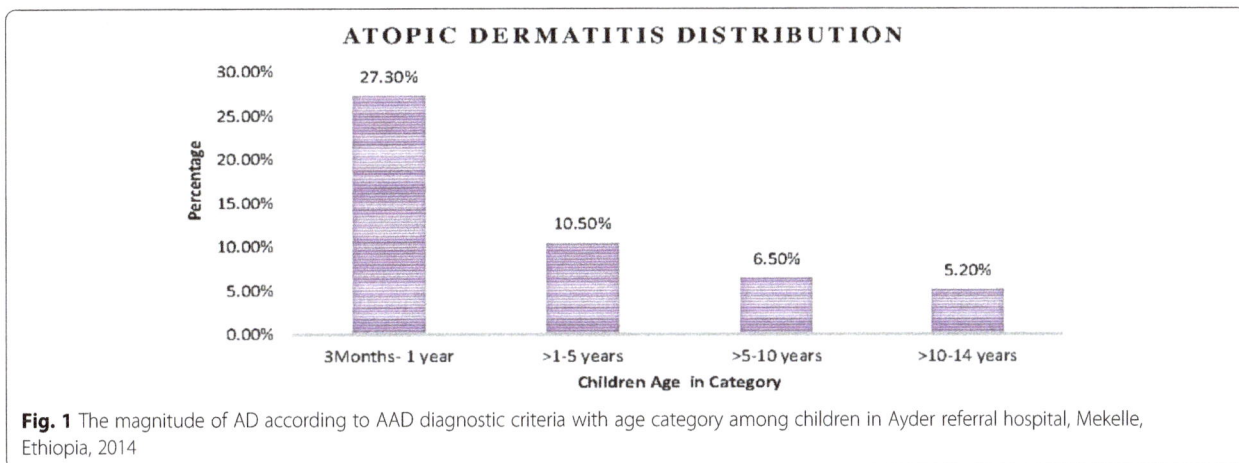

Fig. 1 The magnitude of AD according to AAD diagnostic criteria with age category among children in Ayder referral hospital, Mekelle, Ethiopia, 2014

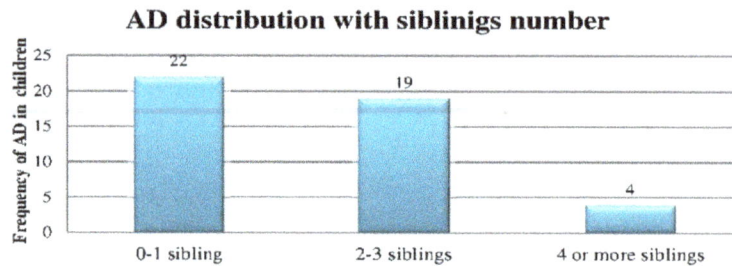

Fig. 2 Distribution of AD with number of siblings among children in Ayder referral hospital, Mekelle, Ethiopia, 2014

This study identified a magnitude of 9.6 % AD based on the AAD diagnostic criteria. The finding is slightly higher than studies conducted in the country at Ankober mobile clinic which was 4.67 % [23], and at Jimma 4.4 % [13]. However, it is less compared to studies from America 11 % [26], Argentina 41.1 % [27] and Japan 18.6 % [28] but still higher from the Tunisian study of 0.65 % [29]. The difference in the proportion of AD reported among the studies might be due to the geographical difference, use of different diagnostic criteria for diagnosis and the age group considered, study season and period. The possible reason for the higher magnitude compared to studies conducted in Ethiopia could be due to the study setting since the study is done at Ayder hospital which is the only referral hospital providing dermatologic services to patients at Mekelle town in the north part of Ethiopia.

The study identified higher chance of AD among children who had maternal history of asthma, hay fever and atopic dermatitis compared to those children who had no maternal history of asthma, hay fever and atopic dermatitis.

A children who had paternal history of asthma and hay fever was more likely exposed to AD compared to those children who had no paternal history of asthma and hay fever. Personal histories of asthma and hay fever or allergic rhinitis were also the most predicting risk factor for AD.

Maternal, Paternal and personal atopic diseases history is the significantly associated factor with AD in this study and it is consistent with studies done in New Zealand [2], Taiwan [30], Iran [31, 32], Yerevan [33], and South Africa

Cape Town [34]. However, it is inconsistent with studies done at rural part of Ethiopia in Jimma area and study from Tunisia [13, 21] which showed no significant association. This difference might be due to methodological differences between the studies, such as different in study design, control of confounding effect and might have information bias which introduced during data collection.

This study was consistent with what has been identified about familial association of AD with atopic family or siblings. So AD is strongly associated with family atopic history factors as documented previously [2].

In children's age 3 months to 1 year old the odds of AD were almost 7 times higher among children than whose age was 10–14 years old children and it is similar with study done in Korea [35] infants aged up to 1 year 26.5 % were diagnosed with AD. The study revealed that the rate of diagnosis dramatically reduced with increasing age: 11.6, 9.2, and 4.6 % in those aged 3, 5, and 10 years, respectively.

The reduction of AD while age increase after the first year may be the magnitude of AD is greatly affected by changes in the environment in which the overall physical immaturity is expected to be an important factor to influence. Speculated that, immaturity of skin barrier function, mucosal immunity, systemic immunity and digestive enzymes are considered to be factors that influence the development of AD symptoms in infancy [4, 5].

According to this study the odds of AD were about four times higher among children who had early weaning at age 4 to 6 months when compared to those children who had weaning after six months. This is in agreement with study conducted in Sweden [36], Yerevan [33], and Iran [31] and systemic review in European countries [34] which showed a significant association to AD. However, it is in contrary to the findings from Tunisia [29] and Ethiopia at Jimma [13].

This difference can be justified with the use of different age classification across the studies, the study setting and the sample size considered and operationalization of certain variables used in study. The association between early weaning and AD can be explained by the Permeability of foreign proteins of GIT barrier increased

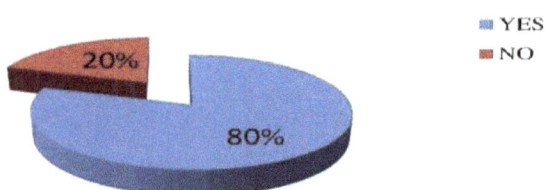

Fig. 3 Family history of atopy distribution with AD among children in Ayder referral hospital, Mekelle, Ethiopia, 2014

Table 5 Factors associated with atopic dermatitis among children in Ayder referral hospital, Mekelle, Ethiopia, 2014

Variable	Atopic dermatitis		COR (95 % CI)	AOR (95 % CI)
	Yes	No		
Age in category				
0.25–1 year	12	32	6.825(2.231–20.883)	**6.886 (1.028–46.097)****
1–5 years	17	145	2.134(0.761–5.983)	1.810(0.403–8.123)
5–10 years	11	168	1.275(0.429–3.786)	0.619(0.132–2.917)
10–14 years	5	91	1	1
Mother educational level				
Illiterate	4	46	1	1
Read & write	2	53	1.286(0.252–6.548)	0.165(0.013–2.134)
Primary school	8	107	0.743(0.243–2.273)	0.813(0.168–3.945)
High school	7	104	1.791(0.641–5.000)	2.165(0.397–11.819)
Tertiary school completed	24	109	5.661(2.81–14.052)	2.421(0.363–16.134)
Occupation of Father				
Farmer	6	101	1	1
Merchant	5	106	1.259(0.373–4.256)	1.090 (0.137–8.697)
Civil servant	26	122	0.279(0.11–0.704)	0.866(0.110–6.835)
Other	8	88	0.653(0.218–1.956)	0.841(0.137–5.166)
Monthly family income				
≤ 1000	14	181	1	1
1001–2000	6	127	0.611(0.229–1.632)	0.531(0.093–3.039)
2001–3000	6	59	1.315(0.483–3.576)	0.828(0.145–4.722)
≥ 3001	19	58	4.235(1.999–8.975)	1.799(0.313–10.343)
Indoor smoking Exposure				
Yes	11	45	1	1
No	34	379	0.367(0.174–0.774)	0.845(0.208–3.432)
Use of insecticide				
Yes	27	117	1	1
No	18	308	0.253(0.134–0.477)	0.631(0.210–1.898)
Exclusive breast feed				
< 6 months	13	67	2.199(1.090 4.435)	1.453(0.380 5.558)
> 6 months	30	340	1	1
Age first started weaning				
< 4 months	1	19	0.806(0.102–6.348)	0.571(0.034–9.715)
4–6 months	22	95	3.547(1.840–6.835)	**3.965(1.184–13.283)****
> 6 months	19	291	1	1
Child mother ever had				
Asthma	12	24	8.104(3.619–18.15)	**11.466(3.246–40.508)****
Hay fever	5	7	11.577(3.420–39.192)	**23.492(4.642–118.88)****
Atopic dermatitis	4	5	12.967(3.269–51.433)	**5.988(1.007–35.602)****
None	24	389	1	1
Child father ever had				
Asthma	16	17	17.703(7.863–39.859)	**13.879(2.439–78.990)****
Hay fever	6	11	10.260(3.459–30.432)	**14.432(4.028–51.705)****
Atopic dermatitis	2	2	18.81(2.524–140.172)	5.653(0.794–40.230)
None	21	395	1	1

Table 5 Factors associated with atopic dermatitis among children in Ayder referral hospital, Mekelle, Ethiopia, 2014 *(Continued)*

Child siblings ever had				
Asthma	2	9	2.327(0.48511.164)	7.154 (0.515–99.432)
Hay fever	2	15	1.396(0.308–6.337)	0.685 (0.037–12.566)
Atopic dermatitis	3	3	10.474(2.043–53.700)	2.600(0.223–30.315)
None	38	398	1	1
Child ever had				
Asthma	5	7	8.529(2.570–28.313)	**10.495 (1.287–85.552)****
Hay fever	6	12	5.971(2.109–16.902)	**12.962 (2.650–63.401)****
None	34	406	1	**1**

NB. ** *P* < 0.05 (significant association)

during early life period due to the immaturity of digestive system and may render the neonate susceptible to allergen invasion and sensitization [5, 6].

This study found no effect of several risk factors that have long been linked to AD, including sex, residence, education status and occupation of parents, family monthly income, home surrounding, family size, number of siblings, type of house, presence of carpeted rooms at home, source of water, types of fuel used for cooking at home, use of insecticides at home, exposure to indoor smoking, living animals at home, pets contact at 1 year of age and after 1 year, breast-feeding duration, exclusive breast-feeding, vaccination status, antibiotic use, siblings atopic diseases history. However, in other studies variables such as; residence in urban area [37], parent's education and occupational status, family monthly income, family size, number of siblings [38, 39], breast feeding duration, exclusive breast feeding [28, 33, 36], use of insecticides, exposure to indoor smoking [40] and siblings atopic history [31, 41] were significantly associated with AD among children.

Thus, as it has been explained above, this study is not resistance to some of the differences observed in the empirical literatures related to factors associated with AD. Within the context of this study, some of the results go against some studies and conform to others. Surprisingly, we found some of the variables which had been significant factors of AD in other studies, not statistically significant factors of AD in Ayder referral hospital Mekelle. Nonetheless, based on the availability of resources, the author believes that, the study can be further developed in order to determine magnitude and associated factors of AD at the national level.

Conclusion

The study found substantially high magnitude of Atopic dermatitis compared to other studies done in the country so far.

Factors such as age of a child, maternal history of asthma, allergic rhinitis/hay fever, Atopic dermatitis, paternal history of asthma and hay fever, personal asthma and hay fever history, Children who started weaning at age of 4 to 6 months were independent predictors of AD among children.

– Hence, these needs great attention through strengthening institutional as well as house hold interventions, targeted towards awareness, prevention and treatment of AD through national skin diseases prevention and control services. Training of health professional particularly health extension workers helps to create awareness about the disease among the communities. Provision of health education to parents coming to the outpatient visit time specifically for those children who have family history of atopic disease is very recommendable. The facility and community based health education still have to address education on care of skin of children and on avoiding early initiation of supplementary feeding to a child and further research work can be recommended to see clear picture at regional or national level.

Competing interests
The authors declare that they have no competing interests.

Authors' contributions
AG: Initiated the research, wrote the research proposal, conducted the research, did data entry and analysis and wrote the manuscript. MD: Involved in the write up of the proposal, write up of the manuscript. AS: Involved in the write up of the proposal, write up of the manuscript. SG: Involved in the write up of the proposal, data analysis and write up of the manuscript. All authors read and approved the final manuscript.

Authors' information
1. Abraham Getachew Kelbore: BSc, MSc. Tropical Dermatology
2. Workalemahu Alemu Belachew MD, Dermatovenereologist, assistant Prof, at college of health science Mekelle University, Mekelle
3. Ashenafi Shumye: BSc, MPH Public Health Department, College of Health Sciences, Mekelle University, Mekelle, Ethiopia
4. Sefonias Getachew Kelbore: BSc, MPH (Epidemiology) school of Public Health, College of Health Sciences, Addis Ababa University, Addis Ababa, Ethiopia

Acknowledgement
We are thankful to all respondents of children parents and care givers for their willing to participate in the study as it is through their cooperation that we have been able to write this report.
We are also grateful for the heads of two units' institutions for allowing us to collect data.
We also would like to thank to Mekelle University for the financial support and technical assistance and approving this study. Our appreciation also extends to study participants and Tropical dermatology students who participated in examining children and data collection, for diligent efforts and hospitality.

Funding
The research was funded through Mekelle university post graduate school, Ethiopia.

Author details
[1]Mekelle University, Tropical Dermatology, Mekelle, North Ethiopia.
[2]Dermatovenereology Department, Mekelle University, Mekelle, North Ethiopia. [3]Public Health Department, Mekelle University, Mekelle, North Ethiopia. [4]Addis Ababa University, School of Public Health, Addis Ababa, Ethiopia.

References
1. Donal Y, Lawerence F, Boguniewic Z. Atopic dermatitis. In: Wolff K, Wella A, Katz S, et al., editors. Fitzpatrick's dermatology in general medicine. New York: McGraw-Hill; 2008. p. 146–50.
2. Friedmann P, Ardern M, Cox N, et al. Atopic dermatitis. In: Burns T, Breathnack S, editors. Rook's text book of dermatology. UK: Black publishing ltd; 2010. p. 1037–46.
3. Van den Oord RA, Sheikh A. Filaggrin gene defects and risk of developing allergic sensitisation and allergic disorders: systematic review and meta-analysis. BMJ. 2009;339:24–33.
4. Palmer CN, Irvine AD, Terron-Kwiatkowski A, et al. Common loss-of-function variants of the epidermal barrier protein filaggrin are a major predisposing factor for atopic dermatitis. Nat Genet. 2006;38(4):441–6.
5. Rautan S, Walker A. Immunophyisiology and nutrition of the gut. In: Duggan C. et al. (ed). Nutrition in pediatrics. Canada: BC Decker; 2008. p. 252–6.
6. Böttcher MF, Jenmalm MC. Breastfeeding and the development of atopic disease during childhood. Clin Exp Allergy. 2002;32:159–61.
7. Williams HC, Burney PG, Hay RJ, et al. The U.K. Working Party's Diagnostic Criteria for Atopic Dermatitis. I. Derivation of a minimum set of discriminators for atopic dermatitis. Br J Dermatol. 1994;131(3):383–96.
8. Hanifin JM, Rajka G. Diagnostic features of atopic dermatitis. Acta Dermato-Venereologica. 1980;(Suppl 92):44–7.
9. Williams HC. Atopic dermatitis. N Engl J Med. 2005;352:2314–24.
10. National Institute for Health and Clinical Excellence. Atopic dermatitis in children. Management of atopic dermatitis in children from birth up to the age of 12 years. NICE clinical guideline 57. London: NICE; 2007.
11. Asher MI, Montefort S, Bjorksten B, et al. Worldwide time trends in the prevalence of symptoms of asthma, allergic rhinoconjunctivitis, and eczema in childhood: ISAAC Phases One and Three repeat multicountry cross-sectional surveys. Lancet. 2006;368:733–43.
12. The International Study of Asthma and Allergies in Childhood (ISAAC) Steering Committee. Worldwide variation in prevalence of symptoms of asthma, allergic rhinoconjunctivitis, and atopic eczema: ISAAC. Lancet. 1998;351:1225–32.
13. Haileamlak A, Dagoye D, Williams H, et al. Early life risk factors for atopic Dermatitis in Ethiopian children. J Allergic Clin Immunol. 2005;115:370–6.
14. Diepgen T. Is the prevalence of atopic dermatitis increasing? In: Williams HC, editor. Atopic dermatitis. Cambridge: Cambridge University Press; 2000. p. 96–112.
15. Park CK, Park CW, Lee CH. Quality of life and the family impact of atopic dermatitis in children. Korean J Dermatol. 2007;45:429–38.
16. Charman CR, Morris AD, Williams HC. Topical corticosteroid phobia in patients with atopic eczema. Br J Dermatol. 2000;142(5):931–6.
17. Gustafsson D, Sjoberg O, Foucard T. Development of allergies and asthma in infants and young childrenwith atopic dermatitis–a prospective follow-up to 7 years of age. Allergy. 2000;55(3):240–5.
18. Jackson KM, Nazar AM. Breastfeeding, the Immune Response, and Long-term Health. J Am Osteopath Assoc. 2006;106:203–7.
19. Ludvigsson JF, Mostrom M, Ludvigsson J, et al. Exclusive breast feeding and risk of atopic dermatitis in infants. Pediatr Allergy Immunol. 2005;16:201–8.
20. Dagoye D, Bekele Z, Woldemichael K, Nida H, Yimam M, Venn AJ, et al. Domestic risk factors for wheeze in urban and rural Ethiopianchildren. Q J Med. 2004;97:1–11.
21. Central Statistical Agency [Ethiopia], ICF International. Ethiopia Demographic and Health Survey 2011. Addis Ababa, Ethiopia, Calverton, Maryland, USA: Central statistical agency and ICF International; 2012.
22. Tigray Regional State. Bureau of Plan and Finance Five Years (2010/11–2014/15) Growth & Transformation Plan, Mekelle, E.C; 2003
23. Nigusse S, Beraldo M, Shibeshi D, et al. A Mobile Community Dermatologic Clinic in Ankober Woreda, Central Ethiopia. Comm Dermatol J. 2013;8:1–12.
24. Simpson EL, Hanifin JM. Atopic dermatitis. Med Clin North Am. 2006;90(1):149–67.
25. ISAAC, 1998. International Study of Asthma and Allergies in Childhood (ISAAC), Phase Three Manual. Available at: http://isaac.auckland.ac.nz/Phasethr/Phs3Frame.html. Accessed on 20 May 2014.
26. Shaw TE, Currie GP, Koudelka CW, Simpson EL. Eczema prevalence in the United States: data from the 2003 National Survey of Children's Health. J Invest Dermatol. 2011;131:67.
27. New-Dei-Cas I, Dei-Cas P, Acuña K. Atopic dermatitis and risk factors in poor children from Great Buenos Aires, Argentina. Clin Exp Dermatol. 2009;34(3):299–303.
28. Miyake Y, Tanaka K, Sasaki S, et al. Breastfeeding and atopic eczema in Japanese infants: The Osaka Maternal and Child Health Study. Pediatr Allergy Immunol. 2009;20:234–41.
29. Amouri M, Masmoudi A, Borgi N, et al. Atopic dermatitis in Tunisian school children. Pan Afr Med J. 2011;9:34.
30. Wang IJ, Guo YL, Hwang KC, Hsieh WS, Chuang YL, Lin SJ, et al. Genetic and environmental predictors for pediatric atopic dermatitis. Acta Pediatric Taiwan. 2006;47(5):238–42.
31. Farajzadeh S, Shahesmaeili A, Bagargan N, et al. Relationship between duration of breastfeeding and development of atopic dermatitis. J Pakisan Association Dermatologists. 2011;21:80–6.
32. Yang YM, Tsai CL, Lu CY. Exclusive breastfeeding and incident atopic dermatitis in childhood: a systematic review and meta-analysis of prospective cohort studies. Br J Dermatol. 2009;161(2):373–83.
33. Sahakyan A. Risk Factors Associated with the Development of Atopic Dermatitis among Children in Yerevan:A case- control study college of health science, Yerevan, 2003.
34. Obihara CC, Marals BJ, Gie RP, et al. The Association of Prolonged Breastfeeding and Allergic Disease in Poor Urban. Children Eur Respir J. 2005;25:970–7.
35. Lee S, Kim J, Han Y. Atopic dermatitis organizer guild line for children. Asia Pack Allergy. 2011;1:53–63.
36. Kull I, Maria B, Wahlgren C, et al. Breast-feeding reduces the risk for childhood eczema. J Allergy Clin Immunol. 2005;116:657–61.
37. Schram ME, Tedja Am Spijker R, et al. Is there a rural/urban gradient in the prevalence of dermatitis? A systematic review. Br J Dermatol. 2010;162:964–73.
38. Flohr C, Pascoe D, Williams HC. Atopic dermatitis and the "hygiene hypothesis": too clean to be true? Br J Dermatol. 2005;152:202–16.
39. Shams K, Grindlay DJC, Williams HC. What"s new in atopic dermatitis? An analysis of systematic reviews published in 2009–2010. Clin Exp Dermatol. 2011;36:573–8.
40. Obeng BB, Hartgers F, Boakye D, Yazdanbakhsh M. Out of Africa: what can be learned from the studies of allergic disorders in Africa and Africans? Curr Opinion Allergy Clin Immunol. 2008;8:391–7.
41. Purvis DJ, Thompson JMD, Clark PM, et al. Risk Factors for Atopic Dermatitis in New Zealand Children at 3.5 Years of Age. Br J Dermatol. 2005;152:742–9.

Expert Consensus on The Management of Dermatophytosis in India (ECTODERM India)

Murlidhar Rajagopalan[1,12]* , Arun Inamadar[2], Asit Mittal[3], Autar K. Miskeen[4], C. R. Srinivas[5], Kabir Sardana[6], Kiran Godse[7], Krina Patel[8], Madhu Rengasamy[9], Shivaprakash Rudramurthy[10] and Sunil Dogra[11]

Abstract

Background: Dermatophytosis management has become an important public health issue, with a large void in research in the area of disease pathophysiology and management. Current treatment recommendations appear to lose their relevance in the current clinical scenario. The objective of the current consensus was to provide an experience-driven approach regarding the diagnosis and management of tinea corporis, cruris and pedis.

Methods: Eleven experts in the field of clinical dermatology and mycology participated in the modified Delphi process consisting of two workshops and five rounds of questionnaires, elaborating definitions, diagnosis and management. Panel members were asked to mark "agree" or "disagree" beside each statement, and provide comments. More than 75% of concordance in response was set to reach the consensus.

Result: KOH mount microscopy was recommended as a point of care testing. Fungal culture was recommended in chronic, recurrent, relapse, recalcitrant and multisite tinea cases. Topical monotherapy was recommended for naïve tinea cruris and corporis (localised) cases, while a combination of systemic and topical antifungals was recommended for naïve and recalcitrant tinea pedis, extensive lesions of corporis and recalcitrant cases of cruris and corporis. Because of the anti-inflammatory, antibacterial and broad spectrum activity, topical azoles should be preferred. Terbinafine and itraconazole should be the preferred systemic drugs. Minimum duration of treatment should be 2–4 weeks in naïve cases and > 4 weeks in recalcitrant cases. Topical corticosteroid use in the clinical practice of tinea management was strongly discouraged.

Conclusion: This consensus guideline will help to standardise care, provide guidance on the management, and assist in clinical decision-making for healthcare professionals.

Keywords: Dermatophytosis, Consensus, Tinea, Delphi, naïve, Recalcitrant, Combination therapy

Background

Superficial fungal infections are caused by dermatophytes, non-dermatophytic moulds and commensal yeasts [1]. Dermatophytes, the most common causative agents, are assuming high significance in developing countries like India [1].These organisms metabolise keratin and cause a range of pathologic clinical presentations, including tinea pedis, tinea corporis, tinea cruris, etc. [2] Although usually painless and superficial, these fungi can behave in an invasive manner, causing deeper and disseminated infection and should not be neglected

[3]. The lesions may become widespread and may have significant negative social, psychological, and occupational health effects, and can compromise the quality of life significantly [4].

Currently, dermatologists across India are inundated with cases of dermatophytosis presenting with unusual large lesions, ring within ring lesions, multiple site lesions (tinea cruris et corporis), and corticosteroid modified lesions, making diagnosis a difficult bet [5]. This changed face of dermatophytosis has created a real panic among dermatologists. In addition, chronicity of the disease has plagued the patients unlike any other dermatological condition in the country [5]. The recent prevalence of dermatophytosis in India ranges from 36.6–78.4% [6] (Table 1).

* Correspondence: docmurli@gmail.com
[1]Department of Dermatology, Apollo Hospital, Chennai, India
[12]Department of Dermatology, Apollo Hospital, Greams Road No: 21, Greams Lane, Off Greams Road, Chennai, India
Full list of author information is available at the end of the article

Table 1 Epidemiology of dermatophytosis in India

Author (Year)	Area	Sample size	Clinical subtype	Predominant dermatophyte isolate	M:F	Common age group affected
Bhatia et al (2014) [55]	North India	202	Tinea corporis (39.1%)	*T.mentagyrophyte* (63.5%) *T. rubrum* (31%)	5.7:1	21–50 years
Kucheria et al (2015) [56]	North India	100	Tinea corporis (31%)	*T. rubrum* (46.4%) *T. mentagyrophyte* (30.35%)	1.3:1	21–30 years
Naglot et al (2015) [6]	North-east India	632	Tinea corporis (34.82%)	*T. rubrum* (50.15%) *T. mentagyrophyte* (30.35%)	4.4:1	21–40 years
Putta et al (2016) [57]	West India	80	Tinea corporis (41.25%)	*T.mentagyrophyte* (37.74%) *T. tonsurans* (28.3%)	1.5:1	21–40 years
Ramaraj et al (2016) [58]	South India	210	Tinea corporis (63.27%)	*T. rubrum* (48.95%) *T.mentagyrophyte* (44.75%)	4:3	21–40 years
Gupta et al (2014) [1]	Central India	100	Tinea unguium (52.0%)	*T. rubrum* (41%)	3.7:1	> 60 years

The isolation of the dermatophyte species shows minor geographic variations, as evident in studies conducted in different parts of India (Table 1).

Despite the increasing prevalence of cutaneous dermatophytosis across the world, and especially in the tropics, research in this area has often been neglected; hence it continues to be prevalent worldwide, and poses a therapeutic challenge to practitioners [2]. The American Academy of Dermatology guidelines on the management of tinea cruris and corporis were published two decades ago, while the recent guidelines by the British Association of Dermatology focused only on tinea capitis and onychomycosis [7–9]. Also, the treatment recommendations in the standard textbooks of dermatology appear to have lost their relevance in the current clinical scenario [10]. Thus, the management of dermatophytosis in India is in need of an evidence-based, experience-driven, practical approach from the experts in the field [10, 11]. It was therefore decided to set up an Indian Expert Forum Consensus Group with the objective of laying down recommendations for the diagnosis and management of dermatophytosis in India.

Issues

The current face of dermatophytosis in India has possibly been an outcome of a complex and intrigued interplay between host, fungus, drug and environment, contributed by multiple factors, including more humid and warmer climate, the absurd use of topical corticosteroid-based combinations, the increased use of broad spectrum antibiotics, the increasing burden of immune-compromised population, the widespread use of antifungals in the agricultural industry, and the questionable role of antifungal drug resistance [10–12].

It is important to recognise that, in India, registries of all diseases, including fungal diseases are not maintained. It is difficult to predict the climatic, geographical or therapeutic changes in the incidence and prevalence of the fungal infection. Much of what is discussed is assumption, which is why creating a consensus is difficult. The theoretical aspects of pharmacokinetics need not match the clinical response to the drug in different individuals. This factor can be decided only with a good registry. These alarming aspects regarding dermatophytosis and their impact on the quality of life, warrant timely address.

Scope and objectives

Dermatophytosis management has become an important public health issue with a large void in research in the area of disease pathophysiology and management [2]. The existing evidence is primarily based on observational cohort studies rather than randomised controlled trials (RCT). Properly designed RCTs will be required to address these need gaps [10, 11]. There are published guidelines on tinea capitis and unguium [8, 9]. However, these are not applicable for the treatment of other dermatophytosis, like tinea corporis, cruris and pedis, in the current scenario in India.

The scope of this consensus is to bridge this gap and provide an experience-driven approach regarding the diagnosis and treatment for dermatophytosis, including tinea corporis, tinea cruris and tinea pedis.

The consensus was planned around three clinical domains: definitions, laboratory diagnosis and treatment. To our knowledge, this is the first expert consensus developed by the Delphi method for the diagnosis and management of dermatophytosis in India.

This consensus statement was developed using a modified Delphi method - a rigorous process that minimises bias and facilitates a consensual position [13].

Methods

An invitation to participate in the survey was sent by mail in April 2017, to 14 experts working in the field of clinical dermatology and mycology, selected by lead expert Dr. Murlidhar Rajagopalan, according to their clinical experience, their interest in the field as reflected by their international publications, and further, on their experience in generating guidelines.

Eleven experts (listed in the appendix) including eight dermatologists, and three mycologists finally participated in five rounds of a web-based modified Delphi Method from April to September 2017, to develop both a consensual statement on the management of dermatophytosis in the current alarming situation of increased incidence, as well as the prevalence of dermatophytosis in India (Fig. 1).

The literature on dermatophytosis was first reviewed using key-words like "tinea infection", "superficial fungal infections" etc. to retrieve relevant articles on epidemiology, pathophysiology, and management for exploration in the modified Delphi. All experts answered each round (five rounds, 10 questions each) by e-mail. Questions for the rounds were first tested for feasibility and clarity by four non-participants, prior to diffusion to the expert panel (EP). Each Delphi round was delivered by e-mail. E-mail reminders were sent until all members of the EP answered each round of questions. The process was supervised by a lead expert.

The results were analysed after each round, and summary reports describing aggregated group responses were sent to participants in order to allow them to review their answers to the next-round questionnaire. Questions exhibiting a low rate of similar response, after two rounds, were removed to address another field of interest.

The first set of questionnaire was designed to reach a consensus on the definitions for the terminologies including dermatophytosis, chronic dermatophytosis, recurrent dermatophytosis, relapse, trichophytonrubrum syndrome, recalcitrant, and body surface area (BSA). The next two sets of questionnaires were based on a laboratory diagnosis exploring the potential role of KOH mount, fungal culture, dermoscopy and molecular techniques to know their implication in the disease management. The fourth and fifth set of questionnaires were based on understanding the current practice in the management of varied tinea presentations. The participants were also asked to justify their choices.

More than 75% of concordance in response was necessary to reach consensus. Experts arrived at this relatively low figure for consensus based on Delphi after testing the initial questionnaires with very high variability in response. This required restructuring of the questions and redefining what is concordance for the purpose of this survey. However, in the final round of voting when the entire process was reviewed and votometers were used to record opinions on well-defined problems, a concordance of more than 85% was reached in 90% of the responses. Finally, the experts were asked to revise the ranking with written comments on the questions which did not reach the 75% consensus.

Results

The expert panel first achieved consensus on the definitions for the terminologies, as listed in Table 2, during the first Delphi round.

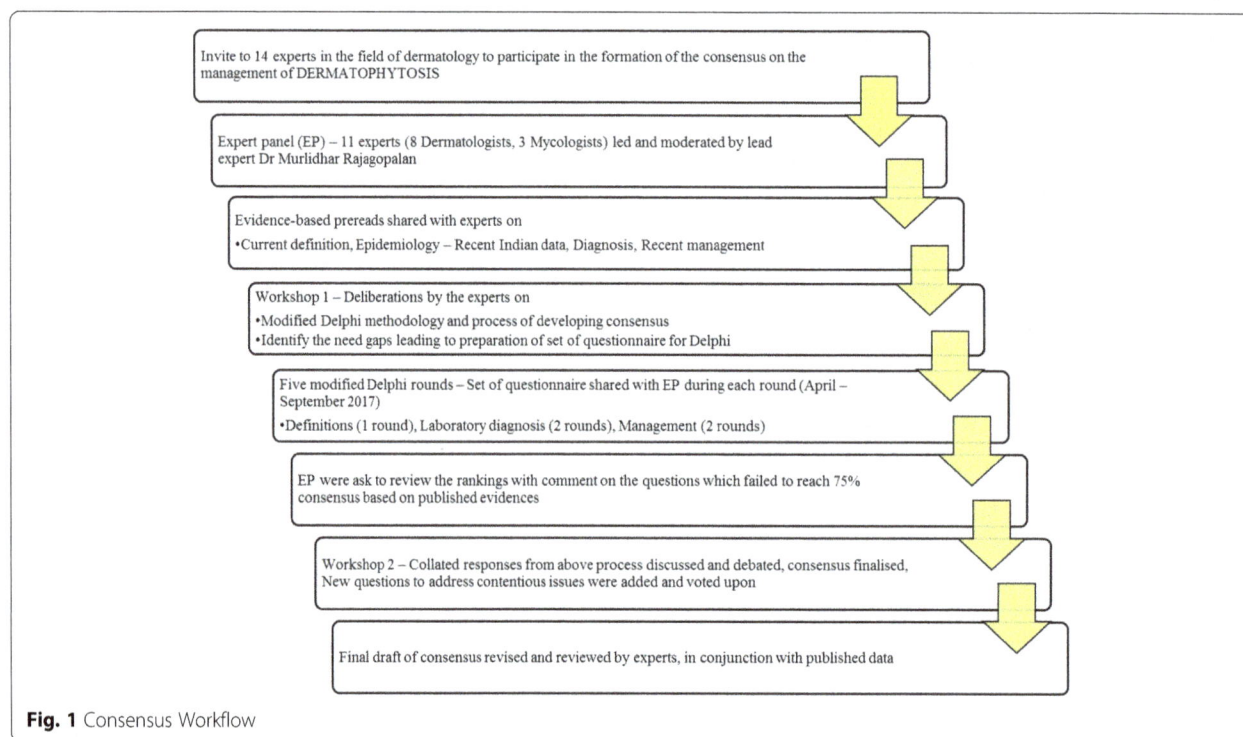

Fig. 1 Consensus Workflow

Table 2 Definitions

Term	Definition
Dermatophytosis	Dermatophytosis (ringworm or tinea) is an infection of the skin or skin derivatives, caused by fungi known as dermatophytes leading to erythema, small papules, plaques, vesicles, fissures, and scaling having ring-like morphology. Dermatophytes are filamentous fungi prone to invade and multiply in keratinised tissue, i.e. skin, hair and nails.
Naïve infection	A given subject is not previously exposed to a particular infection of a given disease or treatment for that disease.
Chronic Dermatophytosis	Dermatophytosis is considered to be chronic when the patients who have suffered from the disease for more than 6 months to 1 year, with or without recurrence, in spite of being adequately treated.
Recurrent Dermatophytosis	Dermatophytosis is considered to be recurrent when there is re-occurrence of the disease (lesions) within few weeks (< 6 weeks) after completion of the treatment.
Relapse	Relapse denotes the occurrence of dermatophytosis (lesions), after a longer period of infection-free interval (6–8 weeks) in a patient who has been cured clinically.
Trichophyton Rubrum Syndrome	Trichophyton Rubrum Syndrome is defined as, (A) Skin lesions at the following four sites: (1) Feet, often involving soles; (2) Hands, often involving palms; (3) Nails; and (4) At least one lesion in another location other than (1) (2) or (3), except for the groin. (B) Positive microscopic analyses of potassium hydroxide preparations of skin scrapings, in all four locations. (C) Identification of *Trichophyton rubrum* by cell culture at three of the four locations at least. For diagnosis of TRS, the criteria (A) and (B) and (C) have to be fulfilled.
BSA	The area of outstretched palm from the wrist to the tip of the fingers can be considered roughly 1% of the body surface area. Less than 3% can be counted mild, 3–10% as moderate, and more than 10% as severe, in terms of the extent of involvement.

For practical purposes, experts suggested the use of the following terminologies:

Recalcitrant tinea infection: This is a generic term that may refer to relapse, recurrence, re-infection, persistence of infection, and chronic infection.

BSA as a clinical assessment tool for dermatophytosis can be a novel concept in defining the severity of the lesions, as shared by all EP members. The application of BSA as a tool in clinical practice will require a further backup through well-designed RCTs.

Questionnaires for Delphi rounds 2 and 3 were based on laboratory diagnoses, which were shared through email to all EP members, post the response to Round 1.

For optimising the laboratory results, the quantity and quality of the material for examination are critical, as agreed by all EP members. Eighty percent of the members agreed for the collection of specimen from the edge of the lesion, as viable hyphae are seen more near the edge of lesion. Scalpel blades and blunt dermal curretes should be used to collect the sample, and it should be transported in dry black strong paper, to avoid the bacterial contamination.

The point of care test recommended by the panel for confirming the diagnosis of dermatophytosis was 10% KOH mount of skin scraping. Further, the EP panel commented on observing the KOH mount, 15–30 min after preparation, to improvise the sensitivity. The adequacy of the sample, and the appropriateness of the collecting tool and expertise will decide the sensitivity and specificity of the diagnosis.

Even though the fungal culture is gold standard in the diagnosis of dermatophytosis, experts were against its routine use in clinical practice to confirm the diagnosis. But fungal culture should be considered in recalcitrant and multisite tinea (tinea cruris et corporis) cases.

EP members identified dermoscopy as an adjunctive tool for the management of dermatophytosis, highlighting the involvement of vellus hair on dermoscopy examination, as an indicator for systemic therapy.

MALDI-TOF (matrix-assisted laser desorption ionisation-time of flight) mass spectrometry (MS was perceived as a promising experimental technique, and not as a practical tool in the real world by all the experts. A prerequisite of culture is mandatory while considering MALDI-TOF, as it cannot be performed on direct clinical samples. Diagnostic tools for tinea unguium and tinea capitis were out of the scope of this discussion.

Questionnaires for Delphi rounds 4 and 5 were based on the management of dermatophytosis, which were shared through email to all EP members, post the response to Round 3.

Experts highlighted the importance of factors, including the site of the infection, the skin area involved (dry/sebum rich), previous antifungal exposure, and the age of the patients while choosing antifungal therapy.

Interdigital is the most common presentation of tinea pedis. The reservoir effect of tinea pedis and its role in the infections of other anatomical sites were emphasised by the members. Bacterial coinfection is commonly associated with tinea pedis, and occasionally found in cases of tinea cruris and corporis. A majority of the experts recommended the use of combination (topical and systemic) antifungal therapy, as empiric treatment in the management of naïve and recalcitrant cases of tinea pedis. Experts favoured the use of topical azoles in tinea pedis management as many non-dermatophyte species cause tinea pedis. However, they believed that the choice of the topical antifungal is also influenced by the clinical subtype of the disease, e.g. ciclopiroxolamine in the management of recalcitrant tinea pedis. In case of systemic antifungal agents, experts favoured terbinafine (250 mg once daily) in naïve cases of tinea pedis whereas itraconazole (200 mg - 400 mg/day, in divided dose) was preferred in recalcitrant and severe cases. The minimum duration of the treatment should be 2–4 weeks in naïve tinea pedis and more than 4 weeks in recalcitrant cases.

The majority of the experts recommended the use of topical therapy in the management of naïve cases of tinea cruris and corporis (localised lesion) while combination therapy is recommended in recalcitrant tinea cruris. However, the choice of topical antifungal agents varied according to the region and personal experience of the individuals. Experts also commented on the fact that in case of naïve tinea corporis with extensive skin involvement or lesions with papules, combination therapy should be favoured. Experts recommended that topical azoles should be the empiric agent of choice in the management of naïve and recalcitrant cases, while no consensus was formed for systemic antifungal agent of choice. In case of systemic antifungal agents, experts preferred either terbinafine (250 mg once daily) or itraconazole (100 mg – 200 mg/day) in naïve cases whereas itraconazole (200 mg - 400 mg/day) was preferred in recalcitrant cases. The minimum duration of the treatment should be 2–4 weeks in naïve tinea cruris and more than 4 weeks in recalcitrant cases.

In case of tinea incognito, where corticosteroids had been used, experts recommended abrupt stoppage of corticosteroids except in settings of steroids induced rosacea, where it is withdrawn in few days. The panel recommended Itraconazole 100 mg–200 mg, twice daily, for the treatment of tinea incognito. The duration of the therapy should be 4–6 weeks or more, in tinea incognito.

Experts recommended that the treatment should be continued for 2 weeks, post clinical cure for topical agents, whereas systemic therapy should be continued in recalcitrant cases only.

Looking at the current explosion of dermatophytosis in India, experts unanimously rejected the role of topical corticosteroid in the management of dermatophytosis.

Doubling of the dose in case of systemic antifungal agents is not required in case of naïve tinea cases, while in the case of recalcitrant tinea infections, doubling the dose is strongly favoured for terbinafine (500 mg/day), while a consensus could not be reached for doubling the dose of itraconazole.

Though there are multiple agents used as supplemental treatment for tinea infections, the role of 6% salicylic acid, antihistamines and moisturisers was agreed upon by the experts. However, these agents are not recommended in all cases. Bacterial super infections need to be treated with appropriate antibacterial agents.

Baseline liver function tests (LFTs) and periodic monitoring are required before starting the systemic antifungal therapy in recalcitrant cases, and in the elderly, especially with prolonged use of itraconazole, while it is not mandatory in naïve cases.

In the paediatric age group, there was no specific recommendation for topical antifungal agents, but fluconazole and terbinafine were preferred as the systemic choice of agents. In the case of pregnant females, topical agents should be preferred, while systemic therapy should be avoided, as far as possible.

Discussion

As discussed earlier, the standard recommendations from current guidelines are no longer relevant in the current Indian context [10]. Hence it was agreed mutually between the experts of clinical dermatology and mycology to develop the experience-based consensus statement.

There are no standard definitions for the various terminologies like relapse, recurrence, persistence and chronic infections, which add to the confusion in the management of dermatophytosis in real world settings. Through Delphi process, experts could arrive at workable explanations of various terminologies for better understanding the clinical profile of dermatophytosis (Table 2).

Laboratory diagnosis

The evolving clinical presentation poses difficulty of clinical differentiation of dermatophytosis from other non-mycotic dermatitis. This often necessitates a laboratory diagnosis to initiate appropriate treatment [14, 15]. As shown in the results, the quality and quantity of the clinical sample are imperative for isolation of dermatophytes as reappraised by Pihet et al. in a recent review [15]. For better yield of results, the edge of the lesion is the most prolific site for skin scrapings [15, 16]. This is in accordance with the current Delphi results. Various instruments were suggested in literature for collecting skin scrapings like scalpel blades, dermal blunt curretes or edge of slide [15–17]. However, based on the Delphi results, experts did not favour any specific instrument for sample collection.

The point of care test for the rapid detection of dermatophytosis is microscopic examination of 10% KOH mount of skin scrapings, as agreed upon by the experts.

The importance of KOH as a simple, rapid, inexpensive and efficient screening technique was highlighted previously by Kurade et al., Pihet et al., McKay et al. [15–17] Hence it is advisable to perform a microscopic examination of 10% KOH mount of skin scrapings in every case, for a better treatment outcome.

Fungal culture provides the definitive identification of fungal species, but its routine application is deferred as it often lacks the sensitivity, prolonged turnaround time (TAT) and paucity of availability [15, 18]. The experts were of the same opinion. However, they recommended the use of culture in special situations, including recalcitrant and multisite tinea (tinea cruris et corporis) cases.

Therapeutic implication of the involvement of vellus hair was recognised by Gomez – Moyano et al. in their large series on tinea of vellus hair [19]. The expert panel also recognised the importance of the identification of vellus hair involvement by dermoscopy and the role in management, as reflected in the consensus shown in the results.

L'Ollivier C et al. recently highlighted the role of the MALDI-TOF MS procedure as a first-line, accurate, economical and faster identification technique for clinical dermatophyte species in routine laboratory [20]. The expert mycologist felt that the routine use of MALDI-TOF MS may not always help in the management as culture is a prerequisite and is available only at a few tertiary level centres across India.

The therapeutic implication of knowing dermatophyte antifungal sensitivity was well recognised by the experts. The current recommendations by "Clinical & Laboratory Standards Institute (CLSI)" lack the consistent correlation between in vitro antifungal sensitivity data and clinical outcome, with lack of MIC breakpoints to categorise the isolate as susceptible, intermediate, or resistant to a particular antifungal agent [21]. Hence, the routine use of antifungal sensitivity is not feasible in real world settings [21].

The clinical appearance of lesions with a history of prior treatment, along with the knowledge of pharmacological properties of antifungal agents will help guide the choice of therapy [22]. Further to this, experts have identified the skin area involved (dry/sebum-rich) and the age of the patients, as additional factors influencing the choice of treatment. An ideal topical treatment should have a high cure rate, low relapse rate, and short duration of action, and should cause minimal adverse effects. In addition, it is important to find a treatment regimen that is satisfactory to the person with the condition, to ensure compliance.

Tinea pedis
Tinea pedis usually begins from interdigital spaces with patterns like hyperkeratotic dry, scaly, macerated, oozing and erosive lesions [23]. Clinical pattern of tinea pedis is not pathogen specific since many non-dermatophyte species are recognised as etiological agents of tinea pedis [23]. Topical therapy is the mainstay treatment option in patients with tinea pedis [2, 24–26]. The necessity to treat tinea pedis topically arises from the fact that interdigital maceration, fissures and desquamation of the stratum corneum may serve as portals of entry for secondary bacterial infections and also as a reservoir for dermatophytosis of other sites as agreed upon by the experts [27, 28]. In macerated, erosive interdigital tinea pedis, often complicated by secondary bacterial infection, antimycotic solutions, gels, or sprays are preferable. By contrast, a cream or ointment is preferable for the treatment of dry and scaly hyperkeratotic tinea pedis [29]. Agents with broad-spectrum antimycotic activity covering dermatophytes, yeasts and molds need to be used in tinea pedis as suggested by the experts [30]. In addition to their antimycotic effects, imidazole also exhibits good antimicrobial effects against Gram-positive bacteria and favoured as the choice of agent by the experts [29, 30]. Other topical agents which are useful in tinea pedis are allylamines, ciclopiroxolamine, amorolfine, etc.

As per Cochrane review systemic therapy is usually used for chronic or failure of topical therapy in tinea pedis [31]. Systemic therapy is also preferable in severe disease forms, such as moccasin and hyperkeratotic tinea pedis [29]. The current therapeutic regimen includes terbinafine 250 mg daily for 2 weeks, or itraconazole 200 mg daily, for 4 weeks [2, 29, 30]. Looking at the current scenario, experts favoured the role of combination therapy in all patients with tinea pedis. However, there are no comparative studies available on the combination of systemic and topical therapy versus monotherapy [2]. Experts commented that while using combination therapy, drugs from different classes should be preferred for wider coverage and to prevent emergence of resistance. In naïve cases, terbinafine 250 mg/day should be preferred while in recalcitrant cases or severe disease forms, itraconazole 200 mg – 400 mg/day in divided dose is the drug of choice. According to experts, the minimum duration of therapy in naïve tinea pedis should be 2–4 weeks, while in case of recalcitrant cases it should be 4 weeks.

Tinea cruris and corporis
As the dermatophytes causing tinea cruris and corporis infection are limited to the superficial keratinised tissue, topical treatments are the most appropriate to use in patients with naïve tinea cruris and corporis, provided the infection is not widespread [32, 33]. Experts were of the same opinion, and recommended the use of topical antifungal agents in naïve cases. The superiority of one

class of topical antifungal over another has not been well established in clinical trials [34]. However, looking at the current scenario, experts favoured the use of topical azoles over allylamines in virtue of antibacterial, anti-inflammatory and broad spectrum antimycotic properties [33]. Topical antifungal treatments are normally well-tolerated and tend not to cause adverse effects.

Extensive superficial lesions or lesions with papules and pustules require oral therapy [2, 35–37]. As discussed earlier, experts favoured the use of combination therapy in such patients and patients with recalcitrant infection. According to experts, terbinafine (250 mg once daily) and itraconazole (100 mg – 200 mg/day) are equally effective in treating naïve cases. In case of recalcitrant cases, experts recommended the use of itraconazole (200 mg – 400 mg/day, in divided dose) along with appropriate topical therapy. According to experts, the minimum duration of therapy in naïve cases should be 2–4 weeks, while in recalcitrant cases, it should be 4 weeks.

Tinea cruris, in most cases, results from autoinoculation in patients with pre-existing tinea pedis [23]. Concomitant tinea pedis, if present, should be treated to reduce risk for recurrence [38]. Other interventions that may be helpful include daily use of desiccant powders in the inguinal area and avoidance of tight-fitting clothing and non-cotton underwear [10, 39]. The role of examining and treating close contacts, and avoidance of body contact sports, were also emphasised as an important input to be counselled when treating a patient with tinea infections.

Tinea incognito

Tinea incognito is a mycotic infection of the skin that has been modified by improper use of steroids and topical immunomodulators such as calcineurin inhibitors in a way that renders it no longer diagnostic [40, 41]. As some high-potency topical steroids are easily accessible as over-the-counter (OTC) products and non-dermatologists can also prescribe topical steroids freely without any fungal examination, the incidence of this form of tinea seems to be gradually increasing [41]. A classic feature is that the inflammatory lesion and the formation of scales may be suppressed, but symptoms relapse when application of the steroid creams is stopped. Alternatively, the lesions may present as marked purulent folliculitis and a diffuse inflammatory response [40–42]. Experts believe that in tinea incognito, oral antifungal therapy is essential and topical corticosteroids should be stopped abruptly. Itraconazole 200 mg – 400 mg daily, for 4–6 weeks or longer, should be the drug of choice as per experts.

Role of topical corticosteroids

A global expert panel meeting on the topical treatment of superficial dermatophytoses, by reviewing numerous meta-analyses, arrived at the conclusion that corticosteroid-based combination therapy has an important role in inflammatory dermatophytosis [43]. Though the experts recognised that corticosteroids may have some role in inflammatory dermatophytosis, looking at the current scenario they vetoed the use of topical corticosteroids in any type of dermatophytosis in India. The experts felt that this would give impetus to prescription of steroids in infective dermatoses, a problem which is already plaguing the country.

Practice recommendations

As per the recommendation in the American Academy of family physicians (AAFP), topical antifungals should be continued for at least 1 week post clinical resolution [22]. However, experts recommended that topical antifungal agents should be continued for 2 weeks post clinical cure, which is in accordance with the recent review on the current scenario of dermatophytosis in India [44]. The continuation of systemic therapy for 2 weeks after clinical resolution in recalcitrant cases, is also recognised by the experts. Since some systemic antifungal drugs can cause hepatotoxicity, it is advisable to do baseline LFTs to rule out impaired liver function and periodic follow-up, if the treatment duration exceeds 4 weeks.

Systemic antifungals in current context

With the current situation of dermatophytosis in India, a radical change in prescription practices has been observed. A majority of dermatologists in India are using a combination of oral antifungals, higher doses of antifungals [30, 45], a longer duration of treatment, and other therapies not even approved for dermatophytosis, for the management of recalcitrant cases, and these tend to benefit the individual patients more [10, 11, 30]. Experts are of same opinion and further recognised the role of a higher dose of terbinafine, however deserted the use of high dose itraconazole due to its non-linear pharmacokinetics.

Experts felt the need to use other systemic antifungals like Griseofulvin (250 mg – 500 mg twice daily) and fluconazole (150 mg–300 mg/week) in patients with whom treatment with terbinafine or itraconazole had failed. However, the delayed clinical response time, a requiring longer duration of the therapy, should be considered before starting the therapy [46].

Adjuvant therapy

Dermatophytoses are usually associated with several-fold increase in epidermal cell proliferation, leading to epidermal thickening with hyperkeratosis and scaling of the skin [47]. As scales impede the absorption of topical antifungal drugs, the sole use of topical antifungal agents may be ineffective, especially in recalcitrant cases [48]. Keratolytics, by their dual effect, can help in increasing levels of topical antifungals, and removing the stratum corneum where fungi lie [30, 38]. Experts recognised these pathological features and recommended the use of topical salicylic acid 3–6%, as it causes softening of the horny layer and the shedding of scales, but it is not to be used in intertriginous areas or the face.

In dermatophytosis, there is significant increase in transepidermal water loss and specific ultrastructural changes, such as disturbed formation of extracellular lipid bilayers leading to disturbed skin barrier function [47]. This may lead to chronicity of the disease. Considering these facts, experts suggested the use of moisturisers as adjuvant therapy in the management of dermatophytosis. Pruritus being the common symptom of dermatophytosis, experts justified the use of antihistamines, as an adjuvant therapy in acute cases.

Elderly patients
In elderly patients, the treatment should be individualised. The patient's need, site and extent of involvement, the presence of comorbidities and the possibility of drug interactions should be considered before starting the treatment [39, 49]. A healthy elderly patient can be treated as per recommendations applied to a young adult. Topical therapy should be favoured in elderly patients; systemic therapy is required only in cases of the failure of topical therapy, extensive lesions and recalcitrant cases. Since systemic triazole drugs (itraconazole, fluconazole) are capable of multiple drug interactions, oral terbinafine should be preferred [39, 49].

Paediatric age group
Dermatophytosis is relatively less common in the paediatric age group. In one Indian study, only 3.1% prevalence of dermatophytosis has been reported [50]. However, in recent years, an exponential increase in dermatophytosis in the paediatric age group has been noted [39]. Experts favoured the use of topical agents in this age group, owing to rapid turnover of skin, which may contribute to a relatively better clinical response to topical therapy alone. Systemic therapy is advised only in extensive lesions or recalcitrant cases. Experts recommended use of fluconazole and terbinafine in paediatric age group. While fluconazole can be used during infancy, terbinafine is recommended only after 2 years of age.

Pregnant females
Topical antifungals are minimally or not absorbed systemically, and therefore can be prescribed at any stage of pregnancy [39, 51–53]. Regarding systemic therapy, terbinafine is pregnancy category B, however, data on its use in pregnancy is not present; also, whether terbinafine crosses the placental barrier is unknown [39, 50]. Other systemic antifungals should be avoided during pregnancy. Though clinical studies with itraconazole have not detected any increased risk during pregnancy, considering the risk conveyed by the azole family in humans, the drug should still be avoided during pregnancy [51]. Effective contraception for 2 months, after taking oral itraconazole before conception, is suggested [54]. The experts discussing the consensus agreed with these recommendations without change.

General measures
Stress on the importance of regularity of medication and adherence to the advice of the physician. Avoid use of tight clothing. Sharing of bed linen, towels and clothes should be avoided. Undergarments, socks, and caps should be regularly washed and dried in the sun and ironed. Patients should be assessed for associated conditions like excessive sweating or obesity which may lead to recurrence. Hence in such patients, frequent change of clothing, use of absorbent powders and deodorants (decrease perspiration), and weight loss should be encouraged.

In case of tinea pedis, medicated powders can be used prophylactically. Use of occlusive footwear and use of slippers in public washrooms should be avoided. Foul smelling and macerated lesions point towards secondary bacterial infection, and should be treated appropriately, using either systemic or topical antibacterial agent.

Entire management pearls are summarised in Table 3.

Conclusions
Although our work has been an attempt to bridge the gaps between the existing recommendations against the current problem in the field of dermatophytosis, in future, the maintenance of registry, the measurement of herd immunity, measuring skin levels of drug and correlation with blood levels, and response to therapy using different dose schedules with special reference to special situations like recalcitrant, relapse, immunocompromised states or patients with comorbidities will be useful for improving therapeutic outcomes.

Priorities for future research to improve the outcome of dermatophytosis management:

- Improved diagnostic tests, with high accuracy, rapid turnaround time, and prognostic value like BSA that can guide antifungal therapy in real time.
- Direct detection of species causing infection and antifungal resistance from clinical specimen.
- Better risk prediction models, including genetic risk factors to target surveillance and prophylaxis.
- Mechanisms to ensure the attainment of maximal antifungal effect as quickly as possible (e.g. combination therapy, therapeutic drug monitoring).

Table 3 Dermatophytosis (Tinea Corporis, Cruris and Pedis) management pearls in Indian settings

Diagnosis

1. Microscopic examination of 10% KOH mount should be the point of care testing for dermatophytosis.
   a) Skin scrapings should be collected from the edge of the lesions.
   b) Transportation should be in dry black strong paper.
2. Sensitivity and specificity of diagnosis depend on
   a) Adequacy of the sample
   b) Appropriateness of the sample collection
   c) Personnel expertise
3. Fungal culture should be reserved in
   a) Recalcitrant and multisite tinea cases.
4. Dermoscopy examination helps to delineate vellus hair involvement
   a) Vellus hair involvement requires systemic therapy.

Management

1. The choice of the antifungal depends on
   a) Pharmacological properties
   b) History of prior exposure to antifungals
   c) The site and extent of the lesion
   d) Skin area involved (dry/sebum rich), and the age of patient
2. Naive and recalcitrant tinea pedis cases to be treated empirically with a combination of topical and systemic antifungals.
3. Naïve tinea cruris and corporis (localised lesion) cases to be treated empirically with topical antifungals alone. For extensive lesions and recalcitrant cases, a combination of topical and systemic antifungals should be used.
4. Topical azoles should be the drug of choice, since they exert anti-inflammatory, antibacterial and broad spectrum antimycotic activity.
5. Preferred systemic agents for naïve tinea cases are terbinafine 250 mg daily or itraconazole 100 mg–200 mg daily, and in recalcitrant cases, itraconazole 200 mg–400 mg daily. A higher dose of systemic antifungals can be considered in certain cases including deep inflammatory, multisite lesions, non-responders, T. rubrum syndrome.
6. The minimum duration of treatment should be 2–4 weeks in naïve cases and > 4 weeks in recalcitrant cases.
7. Systemic therapy should be considered in villous hair involvement.
8. Abrupt withdrawal of corticosteroids should be practised in tinea incognito, with Itraconazole, 200 mg – 400 mg daily, for a minimum duration of 4–6 weeks or more.
9. Topical corticosteroid use in clinical practice of tinea management is strongly discouraged.
10. Adjuvant therapies like antihistamines, salicylic acid and moisturisers play important role in the management.
11. Baseline LFTs and periodic monitoring to be considered during systemic therapy and the elderly.
12. Empiric therapy of choice in paediatric age group is topical antifungals alone. Systemic agents like fluconazole and terbinafine to be reserved for extensive lesions and recalcitrant cases.
13. In the elderly, and patients with comorbid conditions, the treatment should be individualised.
14. In pregnancy, topical antifungals are the agents of choice in any trimester.

Management of Trichophyton Rubrum Syndrome

1. Identify predisposing host environmental factors
2. Establish the diagnosis:
   a) Clinically (Involvement of two or more noncontagious sites, hands, feet, nails, absence of deeper lesions)
   b) Investigation: KOH positivity from all sites, culture positive from at least one site
3. Check for factors such as concomitant HIV infection, use of immunosuppressive etc.
   Their presence may suggest other diagnosis.
4. Antifungals are to be used for a longer period, and can go up to 3 months. Sometimes

Table 3 Dermatophytosis (Tinea Corporis, Cruris and Pedis) management pearls in Indian settings *(Continued)*

They may have to be combined with other antifungals. Some options are:
   a. Itraconazole 200 mg/ day, for 4–6 weeks. Therapy may be extended till complete clinical resolution.
   b. Combination of Itraconazole 200 mg/day and Terbinafine 250 mg/day for 4–6 weeks or extended periods.
   c. Itraconazole 200 mg twice a day × 7 days/month, for 3–5 months, depending on the clinical response.
   d. Topical Luliconazole/Sertaconazole once/twice a day, for 6 weeks or Topical Terbinafine/Amorolfine, twice daily, for extended periods.
5. Taking care of fomites/household contacts.
6. Fungal Culture and antifungal susceptibility tests, if facility is available.
7. If nails are involved, onychomycosis should be suspected and treated accordingly.
8. Assuring patient compliance for the need of continuous therapy till complete clearance of infection from all sites, use of a topical drug in a proper manner and quantity, etc.

- Novel immunomodulatory treatments to maximise antifungal effect and minimise immune-mediated damage.
- Collaborative national and international programmes for dermatophytosis management.

Acknowledgements
We acknowledge our sincere gratitude to the team of the medical services department of Glenmark Pharmaceuticals Limited for help in data collation, analysis and preparation of the manuscript of this expert consensus.

Funding
This consensus was carried out with the grant from Glenmark Pharmaceuticals Limited, as an unrestricted educational grant.

Disclaimer
Adherence to these guidelines will not ensure successful treatment in every situation. Further, these guidelines should not be deemed inclusive of all proper methods of care or exclusive of other methods of care reasonably directed to obtaining the same results. The ultimate judgment regarding the propriety of any specific procedure must be made by the physician in light of all the circumstances presented by the individual patient.

Authors' contributions
MR designed the methodology for the consensus. Evidence based pre-reads were presented by SD, SR and MR to all panellists. SR, MR and AKM. contributed in the development of questionnaire for lab diagnosis while CRS, AI, AM, KG, KS and KP helped in development of questionnaires based on management of dermatophytosis. All panellists actively participated and involved in the synthesis of the consensus and in drafting, reviewing and editing the manuscript. All authors read and approved the final version of the manuscript.

Competing interests

The authors declare that they have no competing interests. The design or procedure of the consensus and the content of the paper are in no way influenced by the grant provider.

Author details

[1]Department of Dermatology, Apollo Hospital, Chennai, India. [2]Department of Dermatology, SBMP Medical College, BLDE Deemed University, Bijapur, India. [3]Department of Dermatology, R.N.T. Medical College and Hospital, Udaipur, India. [4]Dr Miskeen's Central Clinical Microbiology Lab, Thane, India. [5]Department of Dermatology, PSG Hospitals, Peelamedu, Coimbatore, India. [6]Department of Dermatology, Venereology and Leprosy Dr. Ram Manohar Lohia Hospital and Post Graduate Institute of Medical Education and Research, New Delhi, India. [7]Department of Dermatology, Padmashree Dr D Y Patil University, Navi Mumbai, India. [8]Department Of Dermatology, GMERS Medical College & Hospital, Sola, Ahmedabad, India. [9]Department of Dermatology (Mycology), Madras Medical College, Chennai, India. [10]Mycology Division, Department of Medical Microbiology, Postgraduate Institute of Medical Education & Research (PGIMER), Chandigarh, India. [11]Department of Dermatology, Postgraduate Institute of Medical Education & Research (PGIMER), Chandigarh, India. [12]Department of Dermatology, Apollo Hospital, Greams Road No: 21, Greams Lane, Off Greams Road, Chennai, India.

References

1. Gupta CM, Tripathi K, Tiwari S, Rathore Y, Nema S, Dhanvijay AG. Current trends of Clinico mycological profile of Dermatophytosis in Central India. IOSR-JDMS. 2014;13(10):23–6.

2. Sahoo AK, Mahajan R. Management of tinea corporis, tinea cruris, and tinea pedis: a comprehensive review. Indian Dermatol Online J. 2016;7(2):77–86.

3. Bristow IR, Spruce MC. Fungal foot infection, cellulitis and diabetes: a review. Diabet Med. 2009;26(5):548–51.

4. Jerajani H, Janaki C, Kumar S, Phiske M. Comparative assessment of the efficacy and safety of Sertaconazole (2%) cream versus terbinafine cream (1%) versus Luliconazole (1%) cream in patients with Dermatophytoses: a pilot study. Indian J Dermatol. 2013;58(1):34–8.

5. Dogra S, Narang T. Emerging atypical and unusual presentations of dermatophytosis in India. Clin Dermatol Rev. 2017;1:12–8.

6. Naglot A, Shrimali DD, Nath BK, Gogoi HK, Veer V, et al. Recent trends of Dermatophytosis in Northeast India (Assam) and interpretation with published studies. Int J CurrMicrobiol App Sci. 2015;4(11):111–20.

7. Drake LA, Dinehart SM, Farmer ER, Goltz RW, Graham GF, Hardinsky MK, et al. Guidelines of care for superficial mycotic infections of the skin: tinea corporis, tinea cruris, tinea faciei, tinea manuum, and tinea pedis. Guidelines/Outcomes Committee American Academy of Dermatology. J Am Acad Dermatol. 1996;34(2 Pt 1):282–6.

8. Ameen M, Lear JT, Madan V, MohdMustapa MF, Richardson M. British Association of Dermatologists' guidelines for the management of onychomycosis 2014. Br J Dermatol. 2014;171(5):937–58.

9. Fuller LC, Barton RC, MohdMustapa MF, Proudfoot LE, Punjabi SP, Higgins EM. British Association of Dermatologists' guidelines for the management of tinea capitis 2014. Br J Dermatol. 2014;171(3):454–63.

10. Verma S, Madhu R. The great Indian epidemic of superficial dermatophytosis: an appraisal. Indian J Dermatol. 2017;62(3):227–36.

11. Dogra S, Uprety S. The menace of chronic and recurrent dermatophytosis in India: is the problem deeper than we perceive? Indian Dermatol Online J. 2016;7(2):73–6.

12. Zhan P, Liu W. The changing face of Dermatophytic infections worldwide. Mycopathologia. 2017;182(1–2):77–86.

13. Mitchell RB, Hussey HM, Setzen G, Jacobs IN, Nussenbaum B, Dawson C, et al. Clinical consensus statement: tracheostomy care. Otolaryngol Head Neck Surg. 2013;148(1):6–20.

14. Hainer BL. Dermatophyte infections. Am Fam Physician. 2003;67(1):101–8.

15. Pihet M, Le Govic Y. Reappraisal of conventional diagnosis of dermatophytes. Mycopathologia. 2017;182(1–2):169–80.

16. Kurade SM, Amladi SA, Miskeen AK. Skin scraping and a potassium hydroxide mount. Indian J Dermatol VenereolLeprol. 2006;72(3):238–41.

17. McKay M. Office techniques for dermatologic diagnosis. In: Walker HK, Hall WD, Hurst JW, editors. Clinical methods, the history, physical, and laboratory examinations. Boston: Butterworths; 1990. p. 540–3.

18. Feuilhade de Chauvin M. New diagnostic techniques. J Eur Acad Dermatol Venereol. 2005;19(s1):20–4.

19. Gómez-Moyano E, Crespo-Erchiga V. Tinea of vellus hair: an indication for systemic antifungal therapy. Br J Dermatol. 2010;163(3):603–6.

20. L'Ollivier C, Cassagne C, Normand AC, Bouchara JP, Contet-Audonneau N, Hendrickx M, et al. A MALDI-TOF MS procedure for clinical dermatophyte species identification in the routine laboratory. Med Mycol. 2013;51(7):713–20.

21. Yadav A, Urhekar AD, Mane V, Danu MS, Goel N, Ajit KG. Optimization and isolation of dermatophytes from clinical samples and in vitro antifungal susceptibility testing by disc diffusion method. Res Rev. 2013;2(3):19–34.

22. Weinstein A, Berman B. Topical treatment of common superficial tinea infections. Am Fam Physician. 2002;65(10):2095–102.

23. Nenoff P, Krüger C, Schaller J, Ginter-Hanselmayer G, Schulte-Beerbühl R, Tietz HJ. Mycology - an update part 2: dermatomycoses: clinical picture and diagnostics. J Dtsch Dermatol Ges. 2014;12(9):749–77.

24. Crawford F, Hollis S. Topical treatments for fungal infections of the skin and nails of the foot. Cochrane Database Syst Rev. 2007;3:CD001434.

25. Durdu M, Ilkit M, Tamadon Y, Tolooe A, Rafati H, Seyedmousavi S. Topical and systemic antifungals in dermatology practice. Expert Rev Clin Pharmacol. 2017;10(2):225–37.

26. Moriarty B, Hay R, Morris Jones R. The diagnosis and management of tinea. BMJ. 2012;345:e4380.

27. MargaridoLda C. Oral treatments for fungal infections of the skin of the foot. Sao Paulo Med J. 2014;132(2):127.

28. Müller DP, Hoffmann R, Welzel J. Microorganisms of the toe web and their importance for erysipelas of the leg. J Dtsch Dermatol Ges. 2014;12(8):691–5.

29. Nenoff P, Krüger C, Paasch U, Ginter-Hanselmayer G. Mycology - an update part 3: dermatomycoses: topical and systemic therapy. J Dtsch Dermatol Ges. 2015;13(5):387–410.

30. Sardana K, Mahajan K, Mrig PA. Fungal Infections: Diagnosis and treatment. First edition, CBS Publishers and Distributors; 2017. p 266–317.

31. Bell-Syer SE, Khan SM, Torgerson DJ. Oral treatments for fungal infections of the skin of the foot. Cochrane Database Syst Rev. 2012;10:CD003584.

32. El-Gohary M, van Zuuren EJ, Fedorowicz Z, Burgess H, Doney L, Stuart B et al. Topical antifungal treatments for tinea cruris and tinea corporis. Cochrane Database Syst Rev 2014;(8):CD009992. http://cochranelibrary-wiley.com/doi/10.1002/14651858.CD009992/full.

33. Van Zuuren EJ, Fedorowicz Z, El-Gohary M. Evidence-based topical treatments for tinea cruris and tinea corporis: a summary of a Cochrane systematic review. Br J Dermatol. 2015;172(3):616–41.

34. Rotta I, Ziegelmann PK, Otuki MF, Riveros BS, Bernardo NL, Correr CJ. Efficacy of topical antifungals in the treatment of dermatophytosis: a mixed treatment comparison meta-analysis involving 14 treatments. JAMA Dermatol. 2013;149:341–9.

35. Lesher JL Jr. Oral therapy of common superficial fungal infections of the skin. J Am Acad Dermatol. 1999;40(6 Pt 2):S31–4.

36. Bourlond A, Lachapelle JM, Aussems J, Boyden B, Campaert H, Conincx S, Decroix J, Geeraerts C, Ghekiere L, Porters J, Speelman G, Tennstedt D, Kint T, Vandaele R, Haute V, Lint L, Willocx D. Double-blind comparison of Itraconazole with Griseofulvin in the treatment of tinea Corporis and tinea Cruris. Int J Dermatol. 1989;28(6):410–2.

37. Cole GW, Stricklin G. A comparison of a new oral antifungal, terbinafine, with griseofulvin as therapy for tinea corporis. Arch Dermatol. 1989;125:1537–9.

38. Goldstein AO, Goldstein BG. Dermatophyte (Tinea) Infections. Post TW, ed. UpToDate. Waltham: UpToDate Inc. http://www.uptodate.com/contents/dermatophyte-tinea-infections?source=search_result&selectedTitle=1%7E150. Assessed 10 Oct 2017.

39. Kaul S, Yadav S, Dogra S. Treatment of dermatophytosis in elderly, children, and pregnant women. Indian Dermatol Online J. 2017;8:310–8.

40. Solomon BA, Glass AT, Rabbin PE. Tinea incognito and "over-the-counter" potent topical steroids. Cutis. 1996;58:295–6.

41. Dutta B, Rasul ES, Boro B. Clinico-epidemiological study of tinea incognito with microbiological correlation. Indian J Dermatol Venereol Leprol. 2017;83:326–31.

42. Jacobs JA, Kolbach DN, Vermeulen AH, Smeets MH, Neuman HA. Tinea incognito due to Trichophyton rubrum after local steroid therapy. Clin Infect Dis. 2001;33:142-4.

43. Schaller M. Dermatomycoses and inflammation: the adaptive balance between growth, damage, and survival. J Mycol Med. 2015;25:e44–58.

44. Verma S, Madhu R. The great Indian epidemic of superficial dermatophytosis: an appraisal. Indian J Dermatol. 2017;62:227–36.

45. Babu PR, Pravin AJ, Deshmukh G, Dhoot D, Samant A, Kotak B. Efficacy and safety of terbinafine 500 mg once daily in patients with dermatophytosis. Indian J Dermatol. 2017;62:395–9.

46. Rengasamy M, Chellam J, Ganapati S. Systemic therapy of dermatophytosis: practical and systematic approach. Clin Dermatol Rev. 2017;1:S19–23.

47. Jensen JM, Pfeiffer S, Akaki T, Schröder JM, Kleine M, Neumann C, Proksch E, Brasch J. Barrier function, epidermal differentiation, and human beta-defensin 2 expression in tinea corporis. J Invest Dermatol. 2007;127(7):1720–7.

48. Shi TW, Zhang JA, Tang YB, Yu HX, Li ZG, Yu JB. A randomized controlled trial of combination treatment with ketoconazole 2% cream and adapalene 0.1% gel in pityriasisversicolor. J Dermatolog Treat. 2015;26(2):143–6.

49. Baran R, Hay RJ, Garduno JI. Review of antifungal therapy, part II: treatment rationale, including specific patient populations. J Dermatolog Treat. 2008; 19(3):168–75.

50. Maulingkar SV, Pinto MJ, Rodrigues S. A clinico-mycological study of dermatophytoses in Goa, India. Mycopathologia. 2014;178:297–301.

51. Pilmis B, Jullien V, Sobel J, Lecuit M, Lortholary O, Charlier C. Antifungal drugs during pregnancy: an updated review. J Antimicrob Chemother. 2015; 70:14–22.

52. Murase JE, Heller MM, Butler DC. Safety of dermatologic medications in pregnancy and lactation. Part I Pregnancy J Am Acad Dermatol. 2014;70: 401–15.

53. Patel VM, Schwartz RA, Lambert WC. Topical antiviral and antifungal medications in pregnancy: a review of safety profiles. J Eur Acad Dermatol Venereol. 2017;31(9):1440–6.

54. Narang T, Mahajan R, Dogra S. Dermatophytosis: fighting the challenge: conference proceedings and learning points. September 2-3, 2017, PGIMER, Chandigarh, India. Indian Dermatol Online J. 2017;8:527–33.

55. Bhatia VK, Sharma PC. Epidemiological studies on Dermatophytosis in human patients in Himachal Pradesh, India. Springer Plus. 2014;3:134.

56. Kucheria M, Gupta SK, Chhina DK, Gupta V, Hans D, Singh K. Clinico-mycological profile of Dermatophytic infections at a tertiary care hospital in North India. Int J Com Health and Med Res. 2016;2(2):17–22.

57. Putta SD, Kulkarni VA, Bhadade AA, Kulkarni VN, Walawalkar AS. Prevalence of dermatophytosis and its spectrum in a tertiary care hospital, Kolhapur. Indian J Basic Appl Med Res. 2016;5(3):595–600.

58. Ramaraj V, Vijayaraman RS, Rangarajan S, Kindo AJ. Incidence and prevalence of dermatophytosis in and around Chennai, Tamilnadu, India. Int J Res Med Sci. 2016;4:695–700.

Treatment of plaque psoriasis with an ointment formulation of the Janus kinase inhibitor, tofacitinib: a Phase 2b randomized clinical trial

Kim A. Papp[1], Robert Bissonnette[2], Melinda Gooderham[3], Steven R. Feldman[4], Lars Iversen[5], Jennifer Soung[6], Zoe Draelos[7], Carla Mamolo[8], Vivek Purohit[8], Cunshan Wang[8] and William C. Ports[8*]

Abstract

Background: Most psoriasis patients have mild to moderate disease, commonly treated topically. Current topical agents have limited efficacy and undesirable side effects associated with long-term use. Tofacitinib is a small molecule Janus kinase inhibitor investigated for the topical treatment of psoriasis.

Methods: This was a 12-week, randomized, double-blind, parallel-group, vehicle-controlled Phase 2b study of tofacitinib ointment (2 % and 1 %) applied once (QD) or twice (BID) daily in adults with mild to moderate plaque psoriasis. Primary endpoint: proportion of patients with Calculated Physician's Global Assessment (PGA-C) clear or almost clear and ≥2 grade improvement from baseline at Weeks 8 and 12. Secondary endpoints: proportion of patients with PGA-C clear or almost clear; proportion achieving Psoriasis Area and Severity Index 75 (PASI75) response; percent change from baseline in PASI and body surface area; change from baseline in Itch Severity Item (ISI). Adverse events (AEs) were monitored and clinical laboratory parameters measured.

Results: Overall, 435 patients were randomized and 430 patients received treatment. The proportion of patients with PGA-C clear or almost clear and ≥2 grade improvement from baseline at Week 8 was 18.6 % for 2 % tofacitinib QD (80 % confidence interval [CI] for difference from vehicle: 3.8, 18.2 %) and 22.5 % for 2 % tofacitinib BID (80 % CI: 3.1, 18.5 %); this was significantly higher vs vehicle for both dosage regimens. No significant difference vs vehicle was seen at Week 12. Significantly more patients achieved PGA-C clear or almost clear with 2 % tofacitinib QD and BID and 1 % tofacitinib QD (not BID) at Week 8, and with 2 % tofacitinib BID at Week 12. Pruritus was significantly reduced vs vehicle with 2 % and 1 % tofacitinib BID (starting Day 2), and 2 % tofacitinib QD (starting Day 3). Overall, 44.2 % of patients experienced AEs, 8.1 % experienced application site AEs, and 2.3 % experienced serious AEs. The highest incidence of AEs (including application site AEs) was in the vehicle QD group.

Conclusions: In adults with mild to moderate plaque psoriasis, 2 % tofacitinib ointment QD and BID showed greater efficacy than vehicle at Week 8, but not Week 12, with an acceptable safety and local tolerability profile.

Keywords: Psoriasis, Topical, Tofacitinib, CP-690,550, Physician's Global Assessment, Psoriasis Area and Severity Index, PASI, Dermatology Life Quality Index, Pruritus, Itch

* Correspondence: william.c.ports@pfizer.com
[8]Pfizer Worldwide Biopharmaceuticals, Global Innovative Pharma Business, Groton, CT, USA
Full list of author information is available at the end of the article

Background

The World Health Organization has described psoriasis as a 'chronic, non-communicable, painful, disfiguring and disabling disease for which there is no cure' [1]. The majority of people with plaque psoriasis (75–90 %) are considered to have relatively limited mild to moderate disease [2, 3]. Many treatments are available for mild to moderate psoriasis, including topical treatment with corticosteroids, often in combination with vitamin D analogues [4–6]. The use of mid to high potency corticosteroids can be limited by local and systemic adverse effects, particularly on the face and intertriginous areas [5, 7, 8]. Irritation or burning can also occur with vitamin D analogues [9–11]. Topical therapy is also used in combination with phototherapy or systemic therapy in patients with moderate to severe psoriasis [12].

A substantial proportion of patients with psoriasis are dissatisfied with their current treatment [13]. The limited efficacy of non-steroidal topical monotherapy or low potency corticosteroids and the safety issues associated with long-term use of mid to high potency topical corticosteroids suggest an unmet need exists for additional topical therapeutic options.

Tofacitinib (CP-690,550) is a small molecule Janus kinase (JAK) inhibitor; inhibition of JAK1 and JAK3 by tofacitinib blocks signaling of multiple cytokines implicated in immune response and inflammation. The oral formulation of tofacitinib is effective in patients with moderate to severe plaque psoriasis [14–16]. An ointment formulation of tofacitinib investigated for the topical treatment of psoriasis in a Phase 2a study showed the ointment (2 % twice daily [BID]) was effective with acceptable tolerability for mild to moderate psoriasis [17].

The primary objective of this Phase 2b study was to further characterize the efficacy and safety of tofacitinib ointment (2 % and 1 %) applied once daily (QD) or BID over 12 weeks in adult patients with mild or moderate chronic plaque psoriasis, compared with the corresponding vehicle.

Methods

Study design and treatment

This randomized, double-blind, parallel-group, vehicle-controlled study (NCT01831466), conducted at 52 centers in the United States, Canada, Denmark, and Poland, was initiated in May 2013 and completed in September 2014. Patients were randomized 1:1:1 to receive 1 % (10 mg/g) tofacitinib ointment, 2 % (20 mg/g) tofacitinib ointment or corresponding vehicle. Randomization was stratified by baseline severity of psoriasis as defined by the Calculated Physician's Global Assessment (PGA-C). Investigators, study staff and sponsor remained blinded to treatment and randomization information until after the conclusion of the study. Investigator sites were assigned to either QD or BID regimen, but not both; neither investigators nor patients were blinded to regimen.

Tofacitinib ointment was provided in 60 g tubes at a strength of 2 % (maximum feasible concentration) and 1 %; the matching vehicle contained the same inactive ingredients as tofacitinib ointment. Treatments were administered topically at a target application coverage of 3 mg/cm^2 to a treatment area corresponding to 2 to 20 % of the patient's body surface area (BSA). Patients were instructed to treat all treatment-eligible psoriatic areas identified at baseline for 12 weeks, regardless of clearing or improvement in psoriasis. On study visit days, showering or bathing, but not moisturizing, was permitted prior to attending, and study drug was applied in the clinic after study assessments were completed. After the final study treatment, the treatment areas were left untreated during the 4-week follow-up period.

Use of shampoo containing tar, salicylic acid or low or least potent corticosteroid products (eg hydrocortisone and hydrocortisone acetate ≤1 %) was permitted on hair-bearing scalp only throughout the study. The proprietary ointment formulation contained standard excipients for a topical formulation.

Patients

Key inclusion criteria

Subjects were aged ≥18 years with chronic plaque psoriasis for ≥6 months, were required to have a PGA-C score of mild (2) or moderate (3), and have plaque psoriasis covering 2–20 % of their BSA on the trunk and/or limbs, with ≥1 % BSA involvement on the trunk and/or limbs (excluding palms, soles, elbows, knees and below the knees).

Key exclusion criteria

Exclusion criteria included non-plaque forms of psoriasis; drug-induced psoriasis; evidence of skin conditions that would interfere with the evaluation of psoriasis; history of infection requiring hospitalization or treatment with oral or topical antimicrobial therapy within 2 weeks prior to baseline; hepatitis B/C or HIV infection; history of lymphoproliferative disorder or malignancy, except adequately treated or excised basal/squamous cell carcinoma, or cervical carcinoma in situ; evidence of tuberculosis infection; treatment with ustekinumab within the previous 4 months or other biologic agents (excluding etanercept) within the previous 2 months; phototherapy or treatment with etanercept or conventional systemic treatments that could affect psoriasis, such as oral or injectable corticosteroids, retinoids, methotrexate, and cyclosporine, within 4 weeks prior to the first study dose.

Topical treatments that could affect psoriasis (eg corticosteroids, tars, keratolytics, anthralin, vitamin D analogues, and retinoids) were discontinued for ≥2 weeks prior to the first study dose.

Assessments

Clinical signs of plaque psoriasis (erythema, induration and scaling) were scored separately according to a 5-point severity scale: clear (0), almost clear (1), mild (2), moderate (3), and severe (4). These PGA subscores were then summed, averaged, and rounded to the nearest whole number to determine the PGA-C score and category [18]. Evaluation of the PGA-C excluded the scalp (even if the hairless scalp was being treated with study drug), palms, soles, and nails.

The primary endpoint was the proportion of subjects achieving a PGA-C response of clear (0) or almost clear (1) with ≥2 grade improvement from baseline at Week 8 and Week 12, independently. Secondary endpoints included Week 8 and Week 12 assessments of the proportion of patients achieving a PGA-C response of clear (0) or almost clear (1); the proportion of patients achieving a ≥75 % improvement from baseline in Psoriasis Area and Severity Index (PASI75); the percent change from baseline in PASI; and the percent change from baseline in affected BSA.

Evaluation of patient-reported outcomes included change from baseline in itch severity and in the Dermatology Life Quality Index (DLQI). The severity of itch was assessed via the Itch Severity Item (ISI), a single item instrument in which the patient records itching over the previous 24 h on a numerical rating scale of 0 (no itching) to 10 (worst possible itching) [19]. ISI was recorded in the clinic during Visit 1 (baseline/Day 1) and at Visits 3–7 (Weeks 2, 4, 8, 12, and 16), as well as once per day between Visit 1 and the day before Visit 3 by the patient in a diary prior to application of study treatment. Patients in the BID treatment group recorded the ISI before applying either the morning or evening treatment, but at the same time throughout this period.

Safety endpoints included the incidence of treatment-emergent adverse events (AEs), serious AEs (SAEs), and application site AEs, plus the proportion of patients who discontinued due to application site AEs. Physical examination, monitoring of vital signs, and clinical laboratory assessments (including hematology, fasting serum chemistry, fasting lipid panels, and urinalysis) were performed.

Pharmacokinetic (PK) endpoints included tofacitinib PK concentrations for pre-dose and post-dose samples. Pre-dose blood samples were collected at baseline and at Weeks 2, 4, 8, and 12 (0 h). At selected sites, three PK samples were also collected at Week 4 post-dose between 30 min and 1 h, between 2 and 3 h, and between 4 and 10 h.

Statistical analysis

This was an estimation study. A sample size of 70 subjects per treatment group was selected, such that the 80 % confidence interval (CI) width of the difference between tofacitinib and vehicle was approximately 19 %, assuming a 21 % vehicle response and a 36 % response in tofacitinib. Additionally, this sample size would yield approximately 76 % power to establish the superiority of each strength and regimen of tofacitinib to its respective vehicle for the primary endpoint at the 0.10 (one-sided) significance level. No adjustment for multiple comparisons was made.

Patients with mild or moderate psoriasis at baseline (as defined by PGA-C) who were randomized and received at least one dose of study medication (tofacitinib or vehicle) were included in the analyses. Data at Week 8 and Week 12 were evaluated separately.

For the primary endpoint, standard error (SE) and two-sided 80 % CI were calculated using the normal approximation to the binomial proportions. A stratified analysis was conducted by summarizing the difference in proportions adjusted for the baseline PGA-C disease severity using the Cochran-Mantel-Haenszel approach [20, 21]. Patients with missing values were considered non-responders.

PASI75 and PGA-C response of clear or almost clear were analyzed using a marginal logistic regression model fit by pseudo-likelihood (generalized linear mixed model for repeated measures). Response proportions were estimated from the model and odds ratios for treatment contrasts along with 80 % CI were determined. Continuous variables (eg percent change from baseline in PASI and BSA, and change from baseline in ISI) were analyzed using a linear mixed model for repeated measures. Least squares mean (LSM), difference in LSM, SE, and two-sided 80 % CI were calculated. All analyses used observed data without imputation. Separate models were fit for the QD and BID data.

For comparisons in response proportions between the active treatment and corresponding vehicle, statistical significance was declared if the lower limit of the two-sided 80 % CI for the response difference was >0 for the primary efficacy endpoint, and if the lower limit of the two-sided 80 % CI for the odds ratio was >1 for the secondary PGA-C and PASI75 endpoints. For comparisons in LSMs between active treatment and corresponding vehicle, statistical significance was declared if the upper limit of the two-sided 80 % CI was <0 for percent change from baseline in PASI and BSA and change from baseline in ISI. No adjustment for multiple comparisons was made.

All statistical analyses were performed using SAS Software [22].

Results

Patients

Overall, 435 patients were randomized (Fig. 1). In the QD treatment groups, 218 patients received either 2 % tofacitinib, 1 % tofacitinib, or vehicle ($n = 70, 74, 74$, respectively). In the BID treatment groups, 212 patients received either 2 % tofacitinib, 1 % tofacitinib, or vehicle ($n = 71, 70, 71$, respectively). Baseline demographics were generally similar across the treatment groups, with the exception of geographical distribution between the dosing regimens (Table 1).

Efficacy

Only those treatment groups and time points that were statistically significant are described within the text.

Primary endpoints

At Week 8 only, significantly more patients receiving 2 % tofacitinib QD and 2 % tofacitinib BID achieved a PGA-C response of clear or almost clear and ≥2 grade improvement from baseline compared with the corresponding vehicle. Response rate was 18.6 % and 8.1 % for 2 % tofacitinib QD and vehicle QD, respectively, and 22.5 % and 11.3 % for 2 % tofacitinib BID and vehicle BID, respectively. The difference (80 % CI) between response to active treatment and vehicle was 10.8 % (3.1, 18.5) and 11.0 % (3.8, 18.2) for 2 % tofacitinib BID and QD administration, respectively (Fig. 2a–b). At Week 12, no statistically significant differences versus vehicle were seen for 2 % or 1 % tofacitinib by either dosing regimen (Fig. 2a–b).

Secondary endpoints

The proportion of patients achieving a PGA-C response of clear or almost clear was significantly greater for the 2 % tofacitinib QD (35.9 %), 2 % tofacitinib BID (41.8 %) and 1 % tofacitinib QD (23.4 %) treatment groups compared with vehicle (QD 13.8 %, BID 25.2 %) at Week 8, and for the 2 % tofacitinib BID (39.7 %) treatment group compared with vehicle (27.3 %) at Week 12 (Table 2).

At Week 8 and Week 12, significantly more patients receiving 2 % tofacitinib QD (17.9 % and 23.0 %, respectively) achieved a PASI75 response vs vehicle (8.3 % and 8.8 %, respectively) (Table 2). The percent change from baseline in PASI was also significantly greater for the 2 % tofacitinib QD treatment group compared with vehicle at Week 8 and Week 12 (Table 2); the differences (80 % CI) vs corresponding vehicle were –9.2 % (–17.1, –1.4) and –12.3 % (–21.8, –2.8) at Weeks 8 and 12, respectively. The percent change from baseline in BSA was also significantly greater for the 2 % tofacitinib QD treatment group compared with vehicle at Week 12 (Table 2); the difference (80 % CI) vs corresponding vehicle was –20.0 % (–31.4, –8.7).

Patient-reported outcomes

2 % and 1 % tofacitinib BID significantly reduced pruritus compared with vehicle BID as early as Day 2 (the day following the initial dose); these improvements were sustained through Day 14 (Fig. 3a). Numerically greater improvements in ISI were also seen in the 2 % and 1 % tofacitinib QD treatment groups compared with vehicle QD; these improvements were statistically significant for 2 % tofacitinib QD on Days 3–14 (Fig. 3b). Significant improvements in pruritus were maintained for 2 % BID, 1 % BID, and 2 % QD from Week 2 through Week 12 (except Week 8 and 12 for 2 % QD).

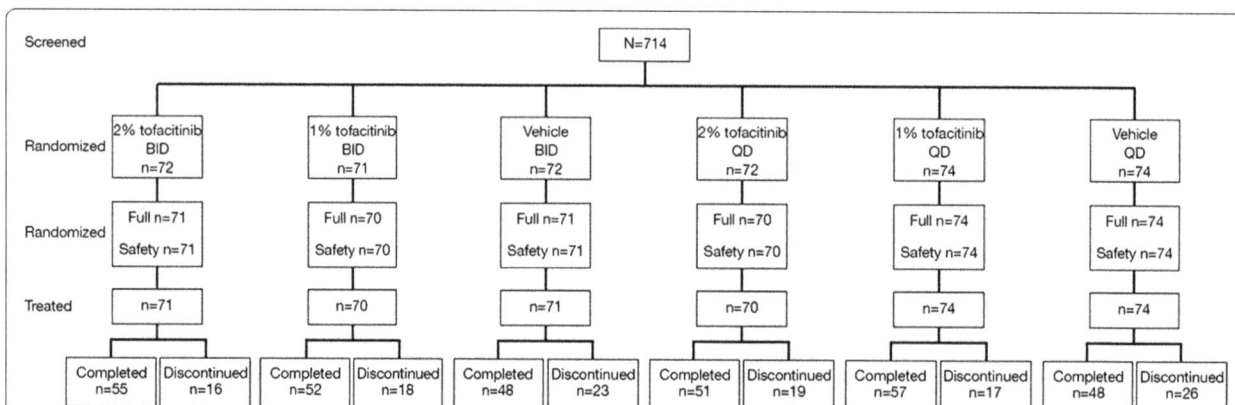

Fig. 1 Patient disposition. Note that the 714 subjects includes subjects with mild, moderate, and severe psoriasis; subjects randomized are those that met the mild to moderate psoriasis eligibility criteria. Following database release, it was discovered that five subjects were randomized, but did not have any record of study drug dosing and were assessed in the clinical database as non-treated subjects; as a consequence, these subjects were excluded from all analyses. *BID* twice daily, *QD* once daily

Table 1 Baseline patient demographics and disease characteristics

	2 % tofacitinib BID N = 71	1 % tofacitinib BID N = 70	Vehicle BID N = 71	2 % tofacitinib QD N = 70	1 % tofacitinib QD N = 74	Vehicle QD N = 74
Age (years)						
Mean (SD)	47.6 (15.6)	50.4 (14.5)	48.8 (15.0)	50.7 (13.2)	47.8 (14.0)	48.9 (13.9)
Range	18.0–74.0	18.0–77.0	21.0–84.0	21.0–77.0	20.0–85.0	20.0–74.0
Male (%)	60.6	67.1	57.7	52.9	67.6	56.8
BMI (kg/m^2)						
Mean (SD)	31.8 (7.9)	29.6 (5.6)	30.2 (8.3)	28.9 (7.8)	31.0 (7.2)	31.1 (6.5)
Range	17.2–58.4	19.2–51.4	17.0–79.8	16.4–68.6	17.6–50.4	20.6–47.4
Race (%)						
White	93.0	85.7	94.4	90.0	91.9	97.3
Black	1.4	4.3	1.4	1.4	2.7	2.7
Asian	4.2	7.1	2.8	5.7	2.7	0.0
Other	1.4	2.9	1.4	2.9	2.7	0.0
Geographical region (%)						
Canada	15.5	30.0	26.8	27.1	23.0	33.8
Denmark	1.4	1.4	0.0	1.4	1.4	1.4
Poland	14.1	12.9	15.5	32.9	39.2	28.4
United States	69.0	55.7	57.7	38.6	36.5	36.5
PGA-C (%)						
Mild	28.2	30.0	29.6	32.9	27.0	27.0
Moderate	71.8	70.0	70.4	67.1	73.0	73.0
PASI score						
Mean (SD)	9.5 (5.1)	8.5 (3.3)	8.5 (3.6)	9.9 (4.1)	10.1 (4.4)	9.6 (3.8)
Range	2.4–29.0	3.0–18.0	2.4–18.0	2.0–19.8	2.8–19.8	3.2–17.1
BSA (%)						
Mean (SD)	7.6 (4.6)	6.4 (3.8)	6.5 (4.1)	7.8 (4.3)	8.4 (4.9)	8.0 (4.5)
Range	2.0–19.0	1.5–17.0	2.0–20.0	2.0–19.0	2.4–20.0	2.0–19.0
ISI score[a]						
Mean (SD)	5.8 (2.6)	5.3 (2.4)	5.4 (2.6)	6.0 (2.7)	5.7 (2.9)	5.4 (3.0)
Range	0.0–10.0	1.0–10.0	0.0–10.0	0.0–10.0	0.0–10.0	0.0–10.0
DLQI						
Mean (SD)	10.6 (5.9)	8.6 (5.5)	9.3 (6.0)	12.2 (7.4)	10.9 (7.0)	10.2 (6.5)
Range	0.0–25.0	1.0–25.0	1.0–24.0	1.0–29.0	1.0–29.0	0.0–26.0

[a]Two patients were missing baseline ISI scores (1 in 2 % tofacitinib QD; 1 in 1 % tofacitinib BID)

BID twice daily, *BMI* body mass index, *BSA* body surface area, *DLQI* Dermatology Life Quality Index, *ISI* Itch Severity Item, *PASI* Psoriasis Area and Severity Index, *PGA-C* Calculated Physician's Global Assessment, *QD* once daily, *SD* standard deviation

At Week 8, 2 % tofacitinib BID and QD significantly improved DLQI more than their respective vehicles (Additional file 1: Figure S1). At Week 12, 2 % tofacitinib QD and 1 % tofacitinib QD significantly improved DLQI more than the vehicle (Additional file 1: Figure S1).

Safety
All adverse events
Overall, 44.2 % of patients experienced treatment-emergent AEs, most of which were mild or moderate in severity (Table 3). The highest incidence of treatment-emergent AEs was in the vehicle QD group, with 54.1 % of patients in this group reporting one or more treatment-emergent AE. The most frequently reported AEs by Medical Dictionary for Regulatory Activities (MedDRA; version 17.1) preferred term were nasopharyngitis (6.7 %), upper respiratory tract infection (4.9 %), and psoriasis (4.9 %).

A total of 11 SAEs were experienced by 10 (2.3 %) patients. No SAEs were reported in the 2 % tofacitinib

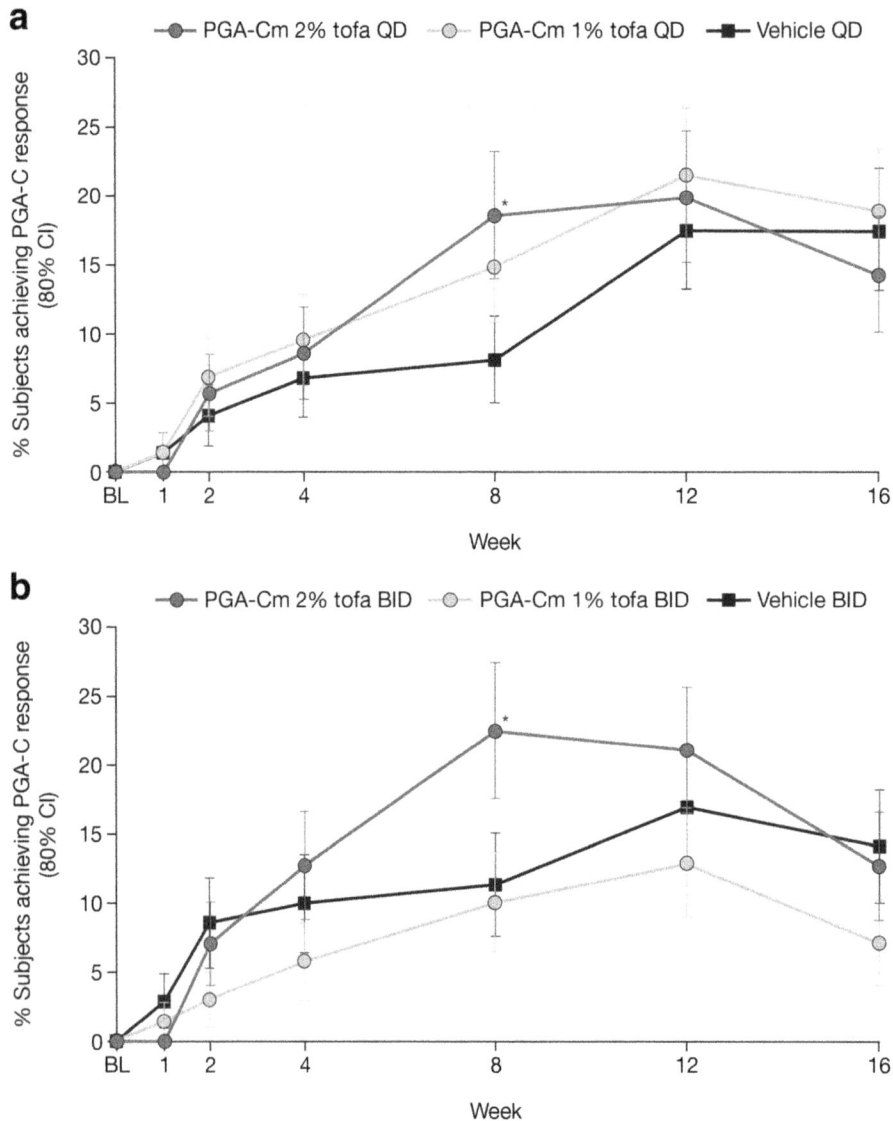

Fig. 2 PGA-C response of clear (0)/almost clear (1) and ≥2 grade improvement at Week 16. *Lower limit 80 % CI of difference tofacitinib versus vehicle >0. Proportion (SE) of patients achieving a PGA-C response of clear (0) or almost clear (1) and ≥2 grade improvement from baseline through to Week 16 for patients applying 2 % tofacitinib, 1 % tofacitinib, or vehicle, once daily (**a**) or twice daily (**b**). Patients who were discontinued or with missing values were considered non-responders. *BID* twice daily, *BL* baseline, *CI* confidence interval, *PGA-C* Calculated Physician's Global Assessment, *PGA-Cm* Calculated Physician's Global Assessment of patients with mild to moderate plaque psoriasis at baseline, *QD* once daily, *SE* standard error, *tofa* tofacitinib

QD or BID treatment groups; SAEs were reported in five patients in the 1 % tofacitinib BID group, in two patients in each of the 1 % tofacitinib QD and vehicle BID groups, and in one patient in the vehicle QD group (Additional file 1: Table S1). No SAEs were assessed by the investigator as treatment-related, with the exception of one SAE of psoriatic arthropathy in the vehicle BID treatment group.

Overall, 21 (4.9 %) patients discontinued from the study due to AEs, most commonly psoriasis, which was reported by six (1.4 %) patients. Seven patients discontinued due to AEs in the vehicle QD group, six with 2 % tofacitinib QD,

four with vehicle BID, three with 1 % tofacitinib QD, and one with 1 % tofacitinib BID (patient was discontinued from the study due to a fatal myocardial infarction as described below).

One death (due to myocardial infarction) occurred in a 53-year-old white male receiving 1 % tofacitinib BID. His final application of tofacitinib ointment was on Study Day 74 and he died on Study Day 86. Relevant medical history included prior myocardial infarction and stent placement, dyslipidemia, hypertension, and 18-year history of tobacco use. The event was considered unrelated to study treatment by the investigator.

Table 2 Secondary efficacy endpoints

Endpoint	Week	2 % tofacitinib BID	1 % tofacitinib BID	Vehicle BID	2 % tofacitinib QD	1 % tofacitinib QD	Vehicle QD
PGA-C, clear (0) or almost clear (1) Responders, % (n/N) Odds ratios (80 % CI)	8	41.8 (26/61) 2.13[b] (1.29, 3.54)	20.9 (14/64) 0.79 (0.45, 1.36)	25.2 (16/55)	35.9 (23/60) 3.52[b] (1.97, 6.28)	23.4 (16/67) 1.92[b] (1.06, 3.48)	13.8 (9/58)
	12	39.7 (24/58) 1.75[b] (1.06, 2.90)	28.4 (18/57) 1.06 (0.62, 1.78)	27.3 (17/55)	36.1 (19/53) 1.36 (0.81, 2.28)	32.9 (22/62) 1.18 (0.71, 1.97)	29.3 (17/52)
PASI75 Responders, % (n/N) Odds ratios (80 % CI)	8	15.2 (10/61) 2.06 (0.96, 4.45)	9.1 (6/64) 1.15 (0.50, 2.66)	8.0 (5/55)	17.9 (11/60) 2.40[b] (1.14, 5.05)	7.2 (5/67) 0.85 (0.36, 2.01)	8.3 (5/58)
	12	20.3 (12/58) 1.42 (0.76, 2.64)	14.4 (9/57) 0.94 (0.48, 1.83)	15.2 (9/55)	23.0 (11/53) 3.11[b] (1.47, 6.55)	12.1 (8/62) 1.44 (0.65, 3.19)	8.8 (5/52)
PASI, % change from baseline LSM, % (N) Difference[a] (80 % CI)	8	−31.8 (61) −8.3 (−17.3, 0.6)	−26.7 (64) −3.2 (−12.1, 5.7)	−23.5 (55)	−28.3 (60) −9.2[b] (−17.1, −1.4)	−25.5 (67) −6.4 (−14.1, 1.3)	−19.1 (58)
	12	−33.9 (58) −6.5 (−17.1, 4.1)	−32.6 (57) −5.2 (−15.7, 5.3)	−27.4 (55)	−33.4 (53) −12.3[b] (−21.8, −2.8)	−27.0 (62) −5.9 (−15.2, 3.3)	−21.1 (52)
BSA, % change from baseline LSM, % (N) Difference[a] (80 % CI)	8	−22.1 (61) −4.2 (−13.1, 4.7)	−20.9 (64) −3.0 (−11.8, 5.8)	−17.9 (55)	−12.5 (60) −8.0 (−16.7, 0.7)	−10.1 (67) −5.7 (−14.2, 2.8)	−4.5 (58)
	12	−31.2 (58) −4.5 (−13.8, 4.9)	−26.0 (57) 0.8 (−8.5, 10.0)	−26.7 (55)	−22.8 (53) −20.0[b] (−31.4, −8.7)	−12.3 (62) −9.5 (−20.6, 1.6)	−2.8 (52)

[a]Difference active – vehicle; [b]meets specification for statistical significance

PASI excluded the scalp, palms, and soles from the assessment/scoring, even if these areas were being treated with study drug. BSA excluded the head, neck, palms, and soles, even if these areas were being treated with study drug

PGA-C and PASI75 responses were analyzed using a Generalized Mixed Model for Repeated Measures without imputation for missing values; percent changes from baseline in PASI and BSA were analyzed using a Mixed Model for Repeated Measures without imputation for missing values; QD and BID data were analyzed separately

BID twice daily, BSA body surface area, CI confidence interval, LSM least squares mean, PASI Psoriasis Area and Severity Index, PGA-C Calculated Physician's Global Assessment, QD once daily

Application site adverse events

Application site AEs were reported in 35 of the 190 (18.4 %) patients who experienced treatment-emergent AEs (8.1 % of total study population); no application site AEs were serious (Table 3). The highest incidence was in the vehicle QD group (Table 3). The most frequently reported application site AEs by MedDRA preferred term were psoriasis (reported by 18 [4.2 %] patients), pruritus (9 [2.1 %]), and application site pain (3 [0.7 %]).

A total of 12 (2.8 %) patients discontinued the study due to application site AEs; seven were from the vehicle QD group, three from the 2 % tofacitinib QD group, and one from each of the vehicle BID and 1 % tofacitinib QD groups. The most common application site AE leading to discontinuation was psoriasis, which was reported by six (1.4 %) patients.

Laboratory assessments

Thirteen patients met the criteria for laboratory safety monitoring (Table 4); no patients met the laboratory monitoring criteria for discontinuation.

Pharmacokinetics

Tofacitinib concentrations were above the lower limit of quantification of 0.01 ng/mL in most plasma samples, with the largest percentage of samples in the concentration range of 0.1 to <1.0 ng/mL (Additional file 1: Table S2). There was a general trend toward higher concentrations with higher dose strength (2 % vs 1 %) but no clear

difference between the dosing regimens (BID vs QD). Across tofacitinib treatment groups, 83.3 %–97.4 % of plasma tofacitinib concentrations were <1.0 ng/mL. The maximum observed plasma concentration of 9.7 ng/mL occurred at Week 12 in the 2 % tofacitinib QD group. Based on the post-dose PK obtained in a limited number of patients, the PK had a flat profile with limited fluctuation in concentrations between doses, as would be expected after topical application. Total exposure based on area under the plasma concentration time profile from time zero to the time tau (AUC_{tau}) in patients with post-dose PK was higher with the higher dose strength, while the relationship between exposure and dose regimen was not clear (Additional file 1: Table S3).

Discussion

Partial inhibition of JAK signaling by tofacitinib results in a multi-tiered intervention in the cycle of psoriasis pathogenesis, with direct impact on dysregulated keratinocytes, reduction in inflammatory infiltrate and, ultimately, normalization of the interleukin (IL)-23/Th17 axis [23]. Oral tofacitinib is effective in patients with moderate to severe plaque psoriasis [14–16], and evidence of efficacy has been seen in the patient with mild to moderate plaque psoriasis with a 2 % topical formulation of tofacitinib applied BID [17].

The current study assessed the efficacy and safety of two dose strengths (2 % and 1 %) of tofacitinib ointment applied either QD or BID in adult patients with mild to moderate plaque psoriasis. Greater efficacy response was

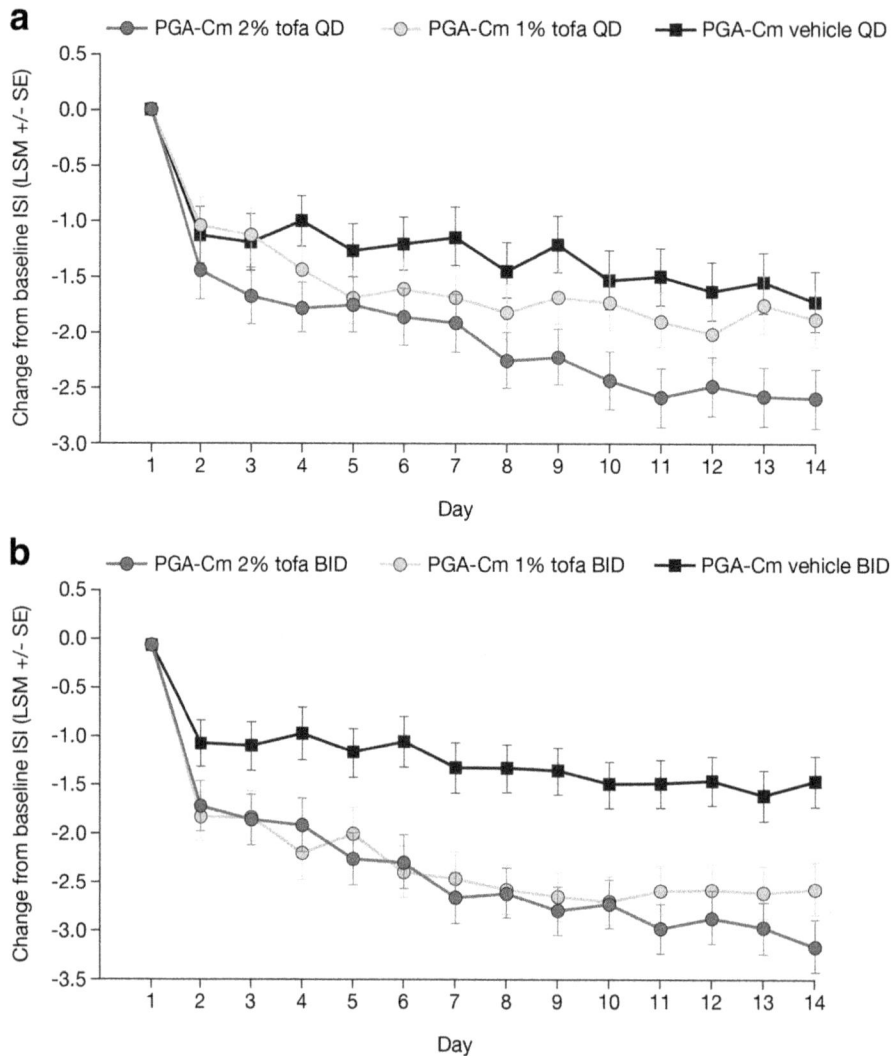

Fig. 3 Change from baseline in Itch Severity Item score through Week 2. Least squares mean (SE) change from baseline in Itch Severity Item score through Week 2 for patients applying 2 % tofacitinib, 1 % tofacitinib, or vehicle, once daily (**a**) or twice daily (**b**). Changes from baseline in ISI were analyzed using a Mixed Model for Repeated Measures without imputation for missing values; QD and BID data were analyzed separately. *BID* twice daily, *ISI* Itch Severity Item, *LSM* least squares mean, *PGA-Cm* Calculated Physician's Global Assessment of patients with mild to moderate plaque psoriasis at baseline, *QD* once daily, *SE* standard error, *tofa* tofacitinib

Table 3 Summary of adverse events, patients discontinued due to adverse events and deaths

	2 % tofacitinib BID	1 % tofacitinib BID	Vehicle BID	2 % tofacitinib QD	1 % tofacitinib QD	Vehicle QD
	N = 71	N = 70	N = 71	N = 70	N = 74	N = 74
Number of AEs	47	51	54	66	65	62
Patients with treatment-emergent AEs, n (%)	30 (42.3)	30 (42.9)	28 (39.4)	34 (48.6)	28 (37.8)	40 (54.1)
Patients with application site AEs, n (%)	4 (5.6)	0 (0.0)	4 (5.6)	8 (11.4)	7 (9.5)	12 (16.2)
Patients with SAEs, n (%)	0 (0.0)	5 (7.1)	2 (2.8)	0 (0.0)	2 (2.7)	1 (1.4)
Patients discontinued due to AEs, n (%)	0 (0.0)	1 (1.4)[a]	4 (5.6)	6 (8.6)	3 (4.1)	7 (9.5)
Deaths, n (%)	0 (0.0)	1 (1.4)[a]	0 (0.0)	0 (0.0)	0 (0.0)	0 (0.0)

[a]Patient had an AE of myocardial infarction and subsequently died; the patient is counted as a discontinuation due to AE and as a death
Categories of adverse events experienced include treatment-emergent, application site and serious adverse events
AE adverse event, *BID* twice daily, *QD* once daily, *SAE* serious adverse event

Table 4 Patients with laboratory values meeting pre-specified protocol criteria* for safety monitoring

Criterion, % (n/N)	2 % tofacitinib BID	1 % tofacitinib BID	Vehicle BID	2 % tofacitinib QD	1 % tofacitinib QD	Vehicle QD
Any criterion	2.9 (2/70)	2.9 (2/70)	1.4 (1/69)	5.8 (4/69)	4.1 (3/73)	1.4 (1/73)
Hemoglobin[a]	1.5 (1/68)	0.0 (0/70)	0.0 (0/69)	0.0 (0/67)	4.1 (3/73)	1.4 (1/72)
Neutrophil count[b]	0.0 (0/68)	0.0 (0/69)	0.0 (0/69)	1.5 (1/67)	0.0 (0/73)	0.0 (0/72)
Lymphocyte count[c]	0.0 (0/68)	0.0 (0/70)	0.0 (0/69)	0.0 (0/67)	0.0 (0/73)	0.0 (0/71)
Platelet count[d]	0.0 (0/68)	0.0 (0/69)	0.0 (0/69)	0.0 (0/67)	0.0 (0/73)	0.0 (0/72)
Serum creatinine[e]	1.4 (1/69)	0.0 (0/70)	0.0 (0/69)	1.5 (1/67)	0.0 (0/73)	0.0 (0/72)
AST/ALT[f]	0.0 (0/69)	2.9 (2/70)	1.4 (1/69)	1.5 (1/67)	0.0 (0/73)	0.0 (0/72)
CPK[g]	0.0 (0/69)	0.0 (0/70)	1.4 (1/69)	3.0 (2/67)	0.0 (0/73)	0.0 (0/72)

*[a]Any hemoglobin value >2 g/dL (>20 g/L) below baseline; [b]Absolute neutrophil count $<1.2 \times 10^9$/L (<1200/mm^3); [c]Absolute lymphocyte count $<0.5 \times 10^9$/L (<500 lymphocytes/mm^3); [d]Platelet count $<100 \times 10^9$/L (<100,000/mm^3); [e]Serum creatinine increase >50 % over the average of screening and baseline values OR absolute increase in serum creatinine >0.5 mg/dL (>44.2 μmol/L) over the average of screening and baseline values; [f]Any AST and/or ALT elevation ≥3 times the ULN, regardless of the total bilirubin; [g]Any CPK >5xULN

ALT alanine aminotransferase, *AST* aspartate aminotransferase, *BID* twice daily, *CPK* creatine phosphokinase, *QD* once daily, *ULN* upper limit of normal

generally observed with 2 % tofacitinib than 1 % tofacitinib, and overall no clear distinction in efficacy was seen between BID and QD dosing.

Greater efficacy of tofacitinib compared with vehicle was seen for more primary and secondary efficacy endpoints at Week 8 than Week 12. While it appeared that the PGA-C response of clear or almost clear and ≥2 grade improvement from baseline plateaued after Week 8, the vehicle treatment group PGA-C responses continued to improve after Week 8, thereby decreasing the difference between tofacitinib and vehicle at Week 12. Explanation for the increase in vehicle responses between Week 8 and Week 12 was not evident after thorough review of the study data for potential contributing factors, although it is possible this could be related to the small sample size of the study.

Patients were required to achieve a ≥2 grade improvement from baseline in PGA-C in addition to having a PGA-C score of clear or almost clear to be considered a responder for the primary efficacy endpoint. This is a much more challenging threshold than the achievement of a PGA-C score of clear or almost clear alone, when a patient need only change from mild (2) to almost clear (1) to be considered a responder. This more stringent criterion is used, as a change from the low end of the mild range to the high end of the almost clear range may not represent a clinically meaningful change.

The clinical significance of objective changes in disease severity were confirmed by the improvement in patient-reported measures. Improvements in health-related quality of life, as indicated by DLQI, reflected the changes seen in PGA-C and PASI. Greater improvements in pruritus were seen compared with vehicle in both tofacitinib BID dosing groups from Day 2 of dosing and for 2 % tofacitinib QD from Day 3. The improvements in pruritus from baseline were likely clinically meaningful (defined as a LSM decrease from baseline in

ISI of 2 points based on analyses conducted with oral tofacitinib therapy for psoriasis) [19] and were seen with 1 % tofacitinib BID from Day 4 through Day 14, with 2 % tofacitinib BID from Day 5 through Day 14, and with 2 % tofacitinib QD from Day 8 through Day 14 (Fig. 3a).

Previous studies have shown oral tofacitinib improved patient-reported pruritus in moderate to severe psoriasis [19, 24, 25]. This is a direct effect, independent from improvements in clinician-reported signs of psoriasis severity [24], with a statistically significant improvement occurring as early as the second day of dosing [26]. Topical tofacitinib also improves pruritus in patients with atopic dermatitis [27].

A very rapid reduction in ISI was seen on initiation of treatment, with a significant reduction in pruritus with both 2 % and 1 % tofacitinib BID compared with vehicle BID as early as the day following the initial dose. Although pruritus is a common feature of psoriasis, the underlying pathogenesis is not understood. Impaired innervation and neuropeptide imbalance in psoriatic skin may be involved; other potential mechanisms include increased expression of IL-2, the opioid system, prostanoids, IL-31, serotonin, proteases and/or vascular abnormalities [28, 29]. Tofacitinib inhibition of JAK may suppress pruritus by blocking signaling via IL-31 [30, 31] and reducing expression of IL-2 [32]. As neuropeptides have a role in the pathogenesis of both psoriasis and pruritus, increased expression of substance P receptor, high-affinity nerve growth factor receptor or calcitonin gene-related peptide receptor may be involved [29].

Overall, topically administered tofacitinib had an acceptable safety profile, with no clinically meaningful differences in the incidence of AEs or SAEs between tofacitinib and vehicle treatment groups. The incidence of AEs coding to the MedDRA Infections and Infestations system organ class was higher in patients receiving vehicle than patients receiving tofacitinib. None of the side effects associated with topical application of potent corticosteroids were observed.

The range of observed plasma concentrations of tofacitinib from the PK analysis showed significant overlap between the dose strengths and regimens. Both AUC_{tau} and maximum observed plasma concentration were higher in patients with QD administration than with BID administration, which was not expected. In addition to dose strength and regimen, PK exposure is likely related to the treatment BSA and/or ointment application rate and this may be contributing to the lack of clear differentiation between the regimens.

In Phase 3 studies of oral tofacitinib in patients with moderate to severe psoriasis, serious infections and herpes zoster infections were associated with tofacitinib treatment [14, 15]. Based on an exposure-response analysis of oral tofacitinib psoriasis data, an average tofacitinib exposure of 12.4 ng/mL was not associated with increased incidence rates of serious infections and herpes zoster infections when compared to patients treated with placebo (unpublished observations). In the current study, more than 83 % of tofacitinib levels measured in plasma from patients in all active treatment groups were <1.0 ng/mL, which represents a >12-fold margin to the exposure levels for oral tofacitinib with no increased incidence rates for serious and herpes zoster infections relative to placebo observed in the oral tofacitinib Phase 3 psoriasis program.

Study limitations

To form the basis for further clinical development, this Phase 2b estimation study used the 2-sided 80 % confidence interval as the pre-specified confidence level per study protocol, whereas in a Phase 3 trial the more rigorous 95 % confidence interval or 0.05 significance level would be used. The stringent eligibility criteria of a Phase 2b clinical study generally exclude some patients who may have been considered for topical treatment outside of the clinical trial environment. The numbers of patients included in the study (~70 per treatment group) is a relatively small sample size. Caution is therefore needed in extrapolating findings to real-world clinical practice. No active comparator to tofacitinib was included so efficacy was not assessed relative to another agent with a known therapeutic effect in psoriasis. No formal statistical comparison was made between QD and BID application, as study sites were assigned to either QD or BID regimens, not both. As such, the dosing regimens essentially represent two separate sub-studies.

Conclusions

This small Phase 2b study demonstrated that topical treatment with the JAK inhibitor tofacitinib in an ointment formulation provided improvement in the clinical signs of psoriasis for patients with mild to moderate chronic plaque psoriasis. Based on the prespecified primary efficacy endpoint, which assesses clinical signs, tofacitinib as a 2 % ointment formulation applied either QD or BID showed significantly greater efficacy compared with vehicle at Week 8, but not at Week 12, and not as a 1 % ointment formulation. Acceptable safety and local tolerability profiles for both QD and BID dosing regimens were observed during 12 weeks of treatment.

Abbreviations

AE: Adverse event; ALT: Alanine aminotransferase; AST: Aspartate aminotransferase; AUC_{tau}: Area under the plasma concentration time profile from time zero to the time tau; BID: Twice daily; BMI: Body mass index; BSA: Body surface area; CI: Confidence interval; CPK: Creatine phosphokinase; DLQI: Dermatology Life Quality Index; IL: Interleukin; ISI: Itch Severity Item; JAK: Janus kinase; LSM: Least squares mean; MedDRA: Medical Dictionary for Regulatory Activities; PASI: Psoriasis Area and Severity Index; PASI75: Psoriasis Area and Severity Index 75; PGA-C: Calculated Physician's Global Assessment; PGA-Cm: Calculated Physician's Global Assessment of patients with mild to moderate plaque psoriasis at baseline; PK: Pharmacokinetic; QD: Once daily; SAE: Serious adverse event; SD: Standard deviation; SE: Standard error; ULN: Upper limit of normal

Acknowledgments

The authors would like to thank the investigators and staff who managed this clinical study, the patients who participated in the study, and Shahbaz Khan, MD, who provided clinical support.
This study was sponsored by Pfizer Inc. Medical writing and editorial support under the direction of the authors was provided by Carole Evans of Complete Medical Communications and funded by Pfizer Inc.

Funding

This study was sponsored by Pfizer Inc. Study design, data collection, analysis and interpretation of results were funded by Pfizer Inc. Pfizer employees participated in study design, data analysis and interpretation.

Authors' contributions

KP, RB, MG, SRF, LI, JS and ZD were all investigators on the study. All authors were involved in data interpretation; and manuscript drafting, reviewing and development. All authors read and approved the final manuscript.

Competing interests

KA Papp has been a consultant for AbbVie, Amgen, Anacor, Active Biotech, Allergan, Astellas, AstraZeneca, Basilea, Bayer, Baxter, Biogen-Idec, Boehringer Ingelheim, Celgene, Dermira, Eli Lilly, Forward Pharma, Galderma, Genentech, GSK, Incyte, Janssen, Kyowa Hakko Kirin, Kythera, Leo Pharma Inc., MedImmune, Merck (MSD), Merck-Serono, Novartis, Pfizer Inc, Regeneron, Rigel, Roche, Takeda, UCB, Valeant, and Xenon; a speaker for AbbVie, Amgen, Allergan, Astellas, AstraZeneca, Basilea, Bayer, Baxter, Biogen-Idec, Boehringer

Ingelheim, Celgene, Dermira, Eli Lilly, Galderma, Genentech, Janssen, Leo Pharma Inc., MedImmune, Merck (MSD), Merck-Serono, Novartis, Pfizer Inc, Regeneron, UCB, and Valeant; and an investigator for AbbVie, Amgen, Anacor, Active Biotech, Allergan, Astellas, AstraZeneca, Basilea, Bayer, Baxter, Biogen-Idec, Boehringer Ingelheim, Celgene, Dermira, Eli Lilly, Forward Pharma, Galderma, Genentech, GSK, Incyte, Janssen, Kyowa Hakko Kirin, Kythera, Leo Pharma Inc., MedImmune, Merck (MSD), Merck-Serono, Novartis, Pfizer Inc, Regeneron, Rigel, Roche, Takeda, UCB, and Valeant.

R Bissonnette has participated in advisory boards for AbbVie, Amgen, Janssen, and Merck. He has received consulting support and/or speaking support from AbbVie, Amgen, Celgene, Eli Lilly and Company, Galderma, Incyte, Janssen, Leo Pharma, Merck, and Novartis. He is an investigator for and his institution receives grant support from AbbVie, Amgen, Eli Lilly, GSK-Stiefel, Merck, Novartis, Pfizer Inc, Kineta, Incyte, Janssen, and Leo Pharma.

M Gooderham has received research, speaking and/or consulting support from a variety of companies including AbbVie, Amgen, Boehringer Ingelheim, Celgene, Galderma, Janssen, Kyowa Hakko Kirin, Leo Pharma Inc., Lilly, MedImmune, Merck, Novartis, Pfizer Inc, Regeneron, and Roche.

SR Feldman has received research, speaking and/or consulting support from a variety of companies including Galderma, GSK/Stiefel, Leo Pharma, Baxter, Boehringer Ingelheim, Mylan, Celgene, Pfizer Inc, Valeant, AbbVie, Cosmederm, Anacor, Astellas, Janssen, Lilly, Merck, Merz, Novartis, Qurient, National Biological Corporation, Caremark, Advance Medical, Suncare Research, Informa, UpToDate and National Psoriasis Foundation. He is founder and majority owner of www.DrScore.com, and founder and part-owner of Causa Research, a company dedicated to enhancing patients' adherence to treatment. He has participated in advisory boards for AbbVie, Boehringer Ingelheim, Merck Novartis, and Pfizer Inc; has served as a consultant for AbbVie, Amgen, Celgene, Galderma Laboratories, Lilly, Mylan, Novartis, and Pfizer Inc, and is a member of speakers' bureaus for Celgene, Galderma, and Janssen.

L Iversen has served as a consultant and/or paid speaker for and/or participated in clinical trials sponsored by companies that manufacture drugs used for the treatment of psoriasis, including AbbVie, Almirall, Amgen, Celgene, Centocor, Eli Lilly, Janssen-Cilag, Leo Pharma, Merck (MSD), Novartis, and Pfizer Inc.

J Soung has received research, speaking and/or consulting support from a variety of companies including Janssen, Eli Lilly, Amgen, AbbVie, Merz, Pfizer Inc, Galderma, Valeant, National Psoriasis Foundation, Cassiopea, Celgene, Actavis, Actelion, and GSK.

Z Draelos received a financial grant from Pfizer Inc as an investigator to conduct the research described in this paper.

C Mamolo, V Purohit, C Wang, and W Ports are employees and shareholders of Pfizer Inc.

Author details
[1]K Papp Clinical Research and Probity Medical Research Inc, Waterloo, ON, Canada. [2]Innovaderm Research, Montreal, QC, Canada. [3]SKiN Centre for Dermatology and Probity Medical Research Inc, Peterborough, and Queens University, Kingston, ON, Canada. [4]Wake Forest Baptist Health, Winston-Salem, NC, USA. [5]Aarhus University Hospital, Aarhus, Denmark. [6]Southern California Dermatology, Santa Ana, CA, USA. [7]Dermatology Consulting Services, High Point, NC, USA. [8]Pfizer Worldwide Biopharmaceuticals, Global Innovative Pharma Business, Groton, CT, USA.

References
1. World Health Assembly 67. Psoriasis 2014. http://apps.who.int/gb/ebwha/pdf_files/WHA67/A67_R9-en.pdf. Accessed 27 Jan 2016.
2. Stern RS, Nijsten T, Feldman SR, Margolis DJ, Rolstad T. Psoriasis is common, carries a substantial burden even when not extensive, and is associated with widespread treatment dissatisfaction. J Investig Dermatol Symp Proc. 2004;9:136–9.
3. Yeung H, Takeshita J, Mehta NN, Kimmel SE, Ogdie A, Margolis DJ, et al. Psoriasis severity and the prevalence of major medical comorbidity: a population-based study. JAMA Dermatol. 2013;149:1173–9.
4. van de Kerkhof PC, Reich K, Kavanaugh A, Bachelez H, Barker J, Girolomoni G, et al. Physician perspectives in the management of psoriasis and psoriatic arthritis: results from the population-based multinational assessment of psoriasis and psoriatic arthritis survey. J Eur Acad Dermatol Venereol. 2015;29:2002–10.
5. Menter A, Korman NJ, Elmets CA, Feldman SR, Gelfand JM, Gordon KB, et al. Guidelines of care for the management of psoriasis and psoriatic arthritis. Section 3. Guidelines of care for the management and treatment of psoriasis with topical therapies. J Am Acad Dermatol. 2009;60:643–59.
6. Papp K, Gulliver W, Lynde C, Poulin Y, Ashkenas J. Canadian guidelines for the management of plaque psoriasis: overview. J Cutan Med Surg. 2011;15:210–9.
7. National Clinical Guideline Centre (UK). Psoriasis: Assessment and Management of Psoriasis. London: Royal College of Physicians (UK); 2012 Oct. National Institute for Health and Clinical Excellence: Guidance. 2012. https://www.nice.org.uk/guidance/cg153. Accessed 27 Jan 2016.
8. van de Kerkhof PC, Kragballe K, Segaert S, Lebwohl M. Factors impacting the combination of topical corticosteroid therapies for psoriasis: perspectives from the international psoriasis council. J Eur Acad Dermatol Venereol. 2011;25:1130–9.
9. Brodell RT, Bruce S, Hudson CP, Weiss JS, Colon LE, Johnson LA, et al. A multi-center, open-label study to evaluate the safety and efficacy of a sequential treatment regimen of clobetasol propionate 0.05% spray followed by Calcitriol 3 mg/g ointment in the management of plaque psoriasis. J Drugs Dermatol. 2011;10:158–64.
10. Barnes L, Altmeyer P, Forstrom L, Stenstrom MH. Long-term treatment of psoriasis with calcipotriol scalp solution and cream. Eur J Dermatol. 2000;10:199–204.
11. Mason AR, Mason J, Cork M, Dooley G, Edwards G. Topical treatments for chronic plaque psoriasis. Cochrane Database Syst Rev. 2009:CD005028.
12. Menter A, Korman NJ, Elmets CA, Feldman SR, Gelfand JM, Gordon KB, et al. Guidelines of care for the management of psoriasis and psoriatic arthritis: section 6. Guidelines of care for the treatment of psoriasis and psoriatic arthritis: case-based presentations and evidence-based conclusions. J Am Acad Dermatol. 2011;65:137–74.
13. Armstrong AW, Robertson AD, Wu J, Schupp C, Lebwohl MG. Undertreatment, treatment trends, and treatment dissatisfaction among patients with psoriasis and psoriatic arthritis in the United States: findings from the national psoriasis foundation surveys, 2003–2011. JAMA Dermatol. 2013;149:1180–5.
14. Papp KA, Menter MA, Abe M, Elewski B, Feldman SR, Gottlieb AB, et al. Tofacitinib, an oral Janus kinase inhibitor, for the treatment of chronic plaque psoriasis: results from two, randomised, placebo-controlled, Phase 3 trials. Br J Dermatol. 2015;173:949–61.
15. Bissonnette R, Iversen L, Sofen H, Griffiths CEM, Foley P, Romiti R, et al. Tofacitinib withdrawal and retreatment in moderate-to-severe chronic plaque psoriasis: a randomized controlled trial. Br J Dermatol. 2015;172:1395–406.
16. Bachelez H, van de Kerkhof PCM, Strohal R, Kubanov A, Valenzuela F, Lee JH, et al. Tofacitinib versus etanercept or placebo in moderate-to-severe chronic plaque psoriasis: a phase 3 randomised non-inferiority trial. Lancet. 2015;386:552–61.
17. Ports WC, Khan S, Lan S, Lamba M, Bolduc C, Bissonnette R, et al. A randomized phase 2a efficacy and safety trial of the topical Janus kinase inhibitor tofacitinib in the treatment of chronic plaque psoriasis. Br J Dermatol. 2013;169:137–45.
18. Cappelleri JC, Bushmakin AG, Harness J, Mamolo C. Psychometric validation of the physician global assessment scale for assessing severity of psoriasis disease activity. Qual Life Res. 2013;22:2489–99.
19. Mamolo CM, Bushmakin AG, Capelleri JC. Application of the Itch Severity Score in patients with moderate-to-severe plaque psoriasis: clinically important difference and responder analyses. J Dermatolog Treat. 2015;26:121–3.
20. Cochran WG. Some methods of strengthening the common $X2$ tests. Biometrics. 1954;10:417–51.
21. Mantel N, Haenszel W. Statistical aspects of the analysis of data from retrospective studies of disease. J Natl Cancer Inst. 1959;22:719–48.
22. SAS Institute Inc. SAS/STAT® 9.3 User's Guide. Cary, North Carolina: SAS Institute Inc; 2011.
23. Krueger J, Clark JD, Suárez-Fariñas M, Fuentes-Duculan J, Cueto I, Wang CQ, Tan H, Wolk R, Rottinghaus ST, Whitley MZ, Valdez H, von Schack D, O'Neil SP, Reddy PS, Tatulych S, for the A3921147 Study Investigators. Tofacitinib attenuates pathologic immune pathways in psoriasis: a randomized Phase 2 study. J Allergy Clin Immunol. 2016;137:1079-90.
24. Bushmakin AG, Mamolo C, Cappelleri JC, Stewart M. The relationship between pruritus and the clinical signs of psoriasis in patients receiving tofacitinib. J Dermatolog Treat. 2015;26:19–22.

25. Luger T, Cappelleri J, Bushmakin A, Mallbris L, Mamolo C. Clinically meaningful improvement in pruritus with tofacitinib: results from a phase 3 program [abstract]. In: The 23rd World Congress of Dermatology Abstracts and Proceedings Vancouver. 2015. http://derm2015.org/program/abstract-volume/. Accessed 27 Jan 2016.

26. Mamolo C, Harness J, Tan H, Menter A. Tofacitinib (CP-690,550), an oral Janus kinase inhibitor, improves patient-reported outcomes in a phase 2b, randomized, double-blind, placebo-controlled study in patients with moderate-to-severe psoriasis. J Eur Acad Dermatol Venereol. 2014;28:192–203.

27. Bissonnette R, Papp KA, Poulin Y, Gooderham M, Raman M, Mallbris L, Wang C, Purohit Y, Mamolo C, Papacharalambous J, Ports WC. Topical tofacitinib for atopic dermatitis: A Phase 2a randomised trial. Br J Dermatol. 2016. Epub ahead of print.

28. Chang SE, Han SS, Jung HJ, Choi JH. Neuropeptides and their receptors in psoriatic skin in relation to pruritus. Br J Dermatol. 2007;156:1272–7.

29. Reich A, Szepietowski JC. Mediators of pruritus in psoriasis. Mediators Inflamm. 2007;2007:64727.

30. Cornelissen C, Luscher-Firzlaff J, Baron JM, Luscher B. Signaling by IL-31 and functional consequences. Eur J Cell Biol. 2012;91:552–66.

31. Sonkoly E, Muller A, Lauerma AI, et al. IL-31: a new link between T cells and pruritus in atopic skin inflammation. J Allergy Clin Immunol. 2006;117:411–7.

32. Flanagan ME, Blumenkopf TA, Brissette WH, Brown MF, Casavant JM, Shang-Poa S, et al. Discovery of CP-690,550: a potent and selective Janus Kinase (JAK) inhibitor for the treatment of autoimmune diseases and organ transplant rejection. J Med Chem. 2010;53:8468–84.

Persistence rates and medical costs of biological therapies for psoriasis treatment in Japan: a real-world data study using a claims database

Rosarin Sruamsiri[1,2], Kosuke Iwasaki[3], Wentao Tang[3] and Jörg Mahlich[4,5*] [iD]

Abstract

Background: Biological therapies (BTs) including infliximab (IFX), adalimumab (ADL), secukinumab (SCK) and ustekinumab (UST) are approved in Japan for the treatment of psoriasis. Although the persistence rates and medical costs of BTs treatment have been investigated in multiple foreign studies in recent years, few such studies have been conducted in Japan and the differences between patients who adhered to treatment and those who did not have not been reported. This study is aimed at investigating the persistence rates and medical costs of BTs in the treatment of psoriasis in Japan, using the real-world data from a large-scale claims database.

Methods: Claims data from the JMDC database (August 2009 to December 2016) were used for this analysis. Patient data were extracted using the ICD10 code for psoriasis and claims records of BT injections. Twelve-month and 24-month persistence rates of BTs were estimated by Kaplan-Meier methodology, and 12-month-medical costs before and after BT initiation were compared between persistent and non-persistent patient groups at 12 months.

Results: A total of 205 psoriasis patients treated with BTs (BT-naïve patients: 177) were identified. The 12-month/24-month persistence rates for ADL, IFX, SCK, and UST in BT-naïve patients were 46.8% ± 16.6%/46.8 ± 16.6%, 53.0% ± 14.9%/41.0% ± 15.5%, 55.4%/55.4% (95% CI not available) and 79.4% ± 9.9%/71.9% ± 12.2%, respectively. Statistically significant differences in persistence were found among different BT treatments, and UST was found to have the highest persistence rate. The total medical costs during the 12 months after BT initiation in BT-naïve patients were (in 1000 Japanese Yen): 2218 for ADL, 3409 for IFX, 465 for SCK, 2824 for UST (average: 2828). Compared with the 12-month persistent patient group, the total medical costs in the persistent group was higher (Δ:+ 118), but for some medications such as IFX or UST cost increases were lower for persistent patients.

Conclusions: UST was found to have the highest persistence rate among all BTs for psoriasis treatment in Japan. The 12-month medical costs after BT initiation in the persistent patient group may not have increased as much as in the non-persistent patient group for some medications.

Keywords: Psoriasis, Biological therapy, Persistence, Medical costs, Real-world data, Claims database

* Correspondence: mahlich@dice.hhu.de; joerg.mahlich@gmail.com
[4]Health Economics and Outcomes Research, Janssen-Cilag GmbH, Johnson & Johnson Platz 1, Neuss 41470, Germany
[5]Düsseldorf Institute for Competition Economics (DICE), University of Düsseldorf, Düsseldorf, Germany
Full list of author information is available at the end of the article

Background

Psoriasis is a chronic autoimmune disease characterized by inflammatory plaques of the skin and known to have a significantly negative impact on patients' quality of life (QoL) [1, 2]. The estimated prevalence of psoriasis in Japan has been reported in previous studies to be 0.34%–0.44% in 2010–2012, and this is expected to increase annually [3, 4].

Biological therapies (BTs) using monoclonal antibodies have been developed to treat psoriasis and to relieve psoriatic symptoms while improving patients' QoL. In Japan, four BTs are for treating psoriasis: infliximab (IFX) and adalimumab (ADL) were approved in 2010, ustekinumab (UST) was approved in 2011, and secukinumab (SCK) was approved in 2014.

Despite the documented benefits of BTs in the treatment of psoriasis, persistence to BT (i.e., the duration of time from initiation to discontinuation of therapy) may vary considerably depending on country, patient characteristics and specific drug used for treatment. The medical costs of BT psoriasis treatment in a hospital setting also need to be investigated.

Multiple previous studies analyzing the persistence rate of BTs in psoriasis patients have been conducted in the European Union (EU) [5–9] and the United States (US) [10–13], indicating the related high level of interest and activity. These studies used patient registries, claims databases, or hospital-based patient cohorts. Overall, the EU studies reported higher 12-month persistence rates for BTs (53%–90%) than US studies (25%–66.7%), suggesting a certain level of outcome heterogeneity among different countries.

Consequently, results from studies in other countries may not reflect the experience in Japan. Few previous studies have been conducted to investigate the use of BT in psoriasis in Japan. Umezawa (2013) [14] analyzed the persistence to ADL, IFX, and UST, using a patient cohort from Jikei University School of Medicine. However, it is not clear to what degree the results are representative of the general population of psoriasis patients across Japan.

Therefore, this study is aimed at investigating the BT psoriasis treatment persistence rates as well as comparing medical costs between patients who were persistent with BT treatment and those who did not, based on data from a large-scale, real-world (RW) claims database in Japan.

Methods

Data source

We utilized the JMDC (Japan Medical Data Center Co., Ltd.) database which contains claims and annual examination data of employees and their dependents from the employees' insurance program in Japan [15]. This database includes approximately 2.7 million members and represents approximately 2.1% of the total Japanese population. The JMDC database has been used to investigate a wide range of conditions in Japan such as schizophrenia, rheumatoid arthritis, or cardiovascular disease [16–18].

The time span of our analysis was August 2009 to December 2016. As patient data were anonymized by the database provider, no informed consent was necessary.

Study population and study design

For the analysis of persistence rates, the study population was identified based on the International Classification of Diseases, 10th revision (ICD-10) [19] and claims records of BT injections. Patients who had both a diagnosis of psoriasis as ICD 10: L40 at any time and claims records that documented the receipt of a BT via injection at any location (i.e. at a clinic or as self-injection at home) were selected for analysis. Patients with a diagnosis of rheumatoid arthritis, inflammatory bowel disease, ankylosing spondylitis, and juvenile arthritis were excluded. ICD-10 codes for these diseases are listed in Appendix A (see Additional file 1).

Among the patients selected for analysis, BT-naïve patients were further identified as those who had no record of BT prescription within one year before the BT index date in the database. BT-naïve patients were used for primary analysis of persistence rates, while the total patient group, including both BT-naïve and BT-experienced patients, was also used for secondary analysis.

For the analysis of medical costs, the index date was defined as the first claim for a BT. Among patients selected for the analysis of persistence rates, only those who had at least 24 months of follow-up data (12 months both pre- and post-BT initiation) in the database were eligible for a calculation and comparison of medical costs pre- and post- BT initiation.

Similar to the analysis for persistence rates, the BT-naïve patient group was used for primary analysis of medical costs while the total patient group, including both BT-naïve and BT-experienced patients, was also used for secondary analysis.

Outcomes

Primary outcome of this study was the persistence rate for BT over time. We used the Kaplan-Meier method to estimate the 12-month and 24-month persistence rates for ADL, IFX, SCK, and UST treatment in the BT-naïve group and the total patient group. The persistence period was defined as the time from treatment initiation (index date) until discontinuation of the index BTs (Fig. 1a).

Patients were categorized as discontinuing the index BT based on whichever of the following occurred first: (1) a period of 90 consecutive days without the index BT (non-BT refill period) for ADL, IFX, SCK, or 150 days

a Measurement of non-BT refill period

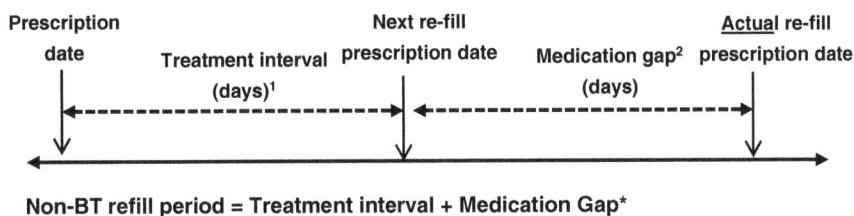

Prescription date ... Treatment interval (days)[1] ... Next re-fill prescription date ... Medication gap[2] (days) ... Actual re-fill prescription date

Non-BT refill period = Treatment interval + Medication Gap*

[1]The treatment interval of individual prescription was defined as 30 days for ADL, IFX, SCK, and 90 days for UST. It was based on the approved dosage and regimen of each BT, which was shown in Appendix A.

[2]Medication Gap: 60 days for ADL, IFX, SCK, and UST.

b Measurement of medical costs

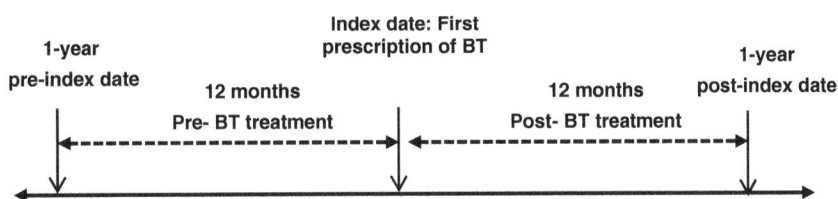

1-year pre-index date ... 12 months Pre- BT treatment ... Index date: First prescription of BT ... 12 months Post- BT treatment ... 1-year post-index date

Fig. 1 Measurement of non-BT refill period and medical costs. Legends: **a** Measurement of non-BT refill period. [1]The treatment interval per individual prescription was defined as 30 days for ADL, IFX, SCK, and 90 days for UST. It was based on the approved dosage and treatment regimen for each BT, which is shown in Appendix A. [2]Medication Gap: 60 days for ADL, IFX, SCK, and UST. **b** Measurement of medical costs

for UST was found; or (2) the patient switched from the index BT to other treatment(s) during follow-up. This definition of persistence was consistent with the one employed in other studies with BTs for psoriasis treatment using claims data [10, 12].

The non-BT refill period was defined as the sum of the treatment interval and medication gap. The treatment interval was defined as 30 days for ADL, IFX, SCK, and 90 days for UST, based on the approved dosage and regimen of each BT (see Appendix B, Additional file 1). A medication gap of 60 days was used for all BTs.

In addition, for patients who have a 12 month-follow-up period both pre- and post- BT initiation, the persistence rates (number of persistent patients during 12 months after BT initiation/number of total patients) were calculated. The definition of the non-BT refill period was the same as the one used for the Kaplan-Meier analysis. The medication gap used in the base case was 60 days, but was varied in the sensitivity analyses. The gap definitions used in the base case and sensitivity analysis are presented in Appendix C (see Additional file 1).

Only patients who had at least 12-months of follow-up data pre- and post- BT initiation were selected for the analysis of medical costs. Medical costs were determined and compared for the 12 months before the index date (first initiation of BTs) and the 12 months after the index date in the BT-naïve/total patient group (Fig. 1 b).

These patients were split into two more groups. Patients who continued BT for a 12-month period were allocated to the persistence group, while others were allocated to the non-persistence group. The differences in medical costs between these two groups were also analyzed.

The analysis of medical costs included the following items: outpatient medical costs, inpatient medical costs, costs of drugs other than BTs, and overall costs. Costs of BTs were included in outpatient medical costs or inpatient medical costs. All costs were calculated based on Japanese Yen (JPY).

Statistical analysis

Descriptive statistics were used to analyze the characteristics of patients receiving BTs, along with the medical costs they caused pre- and post- BT initiation.

Kaplan-Meier curves were plotted to show the persistence to different BTs. The log-rank and Wilcoxon rank sum tests were used to assess the differences in persistence rates for different BTs in the whole group and BT-naïve patient groups. A *p* value of ≤0.05 was considered statistically significant. The analysis was undertaken using SAS software (ver. 9.4; SAS Institute Inc. Cary, NC, USA).

Results

Study population

The patient flow diagram for the analysis is shown in Fig. 2. 28,006 patients with a diagnosis of psoriasis were identified from 250,189 claims with ICD-10: L40. A total of 3093 patients who used BTs were identified from 57,111 claims of BT injections. Overall, 381 patients who used BTs and had a diagnosis of psoriasis were extracted. A total of 208 patients who had received a diagnosis of rheumatoid arthritis, inflammatory bowel disease, ankylosing spondylitis, or juvenile arthritis were excluded. In the end, 173 patients were selected for the analysis.

Table 1 shows the patient characteristics of each treatment group in total and stratified by BT-naïve/experienced status. Patients who had received more than one BT in the past were counted in each separate BT group. By counting each patient separately for each BT received, a total of 205 patients were identified for analysis, and patients in each BT group were not mutually exclusive. Among them, 177 patients were BT-naïve, while the other 28 patients were BT-experienced. The mean age of the total, BT-naïve, and BT-experienced patient group was 47.1 years, 47.3 years, and 46.2 years, respectively. The percentage of female patients in the total, BT-naïve, and BT-experienced group was 18.1%, 19.8%, and 7.1%, respectively.

In Table 1, the respective numbers of total, BT-naïve and BT-experienced patients for each of the specific treatment groups are reported as well and were as follows: 42, 37, and 5 in the ADL group; 52, 48, and 4 in the IFX group; 21, 13, and 8 in the SCK group; and 90, 79, and 11 in the UST group. Among the 205 patients who received BTs, 77 patients provided 12-month data both pre- and post- BT initiation; 42 of 77 patients

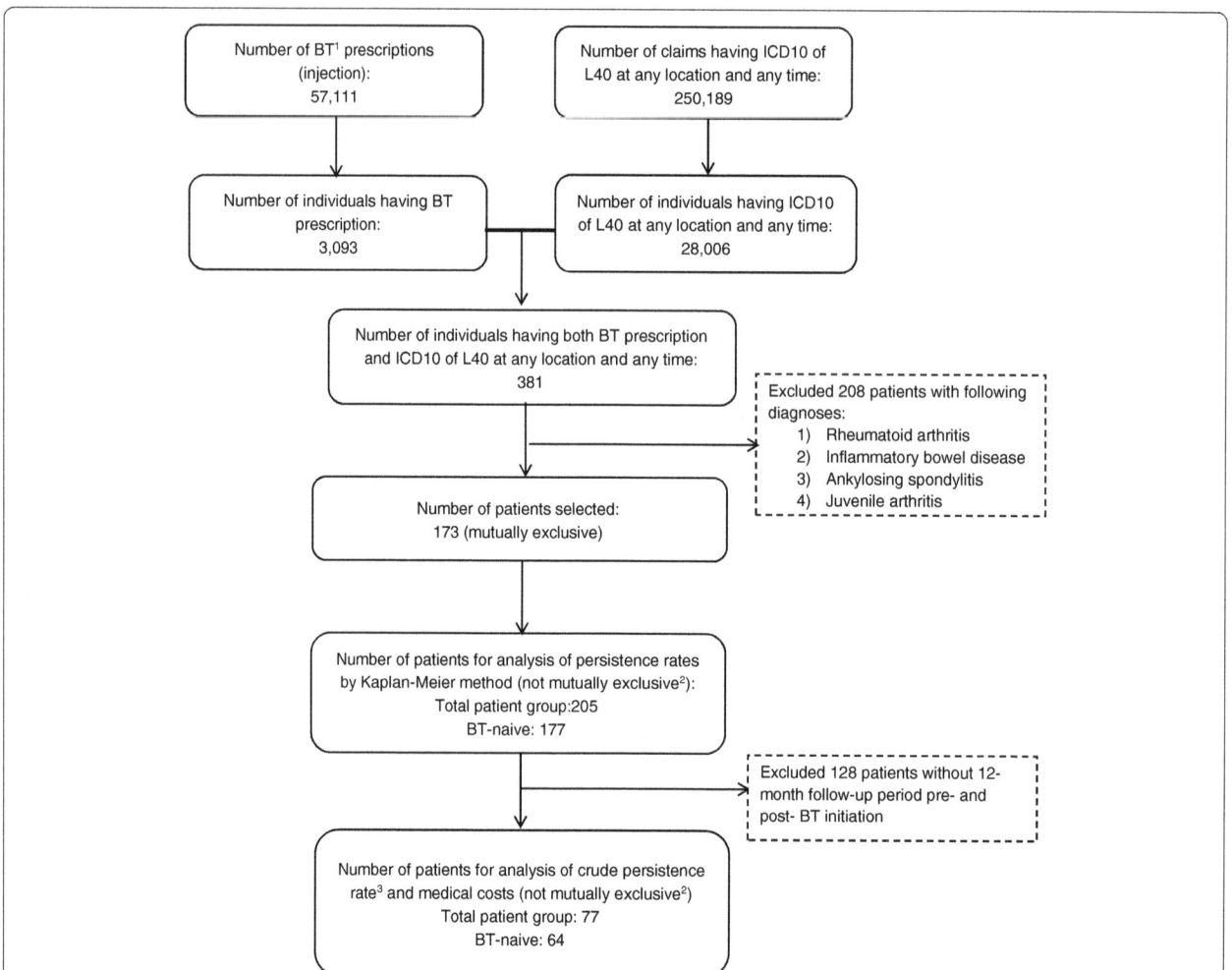

Fig. 2 Cascade figure of patient flow. Legends: [1]BT: biological therapies; [2]for the purpose of analysis, multiple cycles of any BT treatment administered to one patient were counted as different patients. [3]number of persistent patients during 12-month after BT initiation/number of total patients

Table 1 Demographics of total patient population

	Total					BT-naïve					BT-experienced				
	ADL	IFX	SCK	UST	Sub total	ADL	IFX	SCK	UST	Sub total	ADL	IFX	SCK	UST	Sub total
Number of patients	42	52	21	90	205	37	48	13	79	177	5	4	8	11	28
Average Age	50.0	46.2	45.4	46.8	47.1	50.9	46.0	46.2	46.5	47.3	43.4	47.5	44.3	48.4	46.2
% Female	7.1%	21.2%	33.3%	17.8%	18.1%	8.1%	20.8%	46.2%	20.3%	19.8%	0.0%	25.0%	12.5%	0.0%	7.1%

ADL Adalimumab, *IFX* Infliximab, *SCK* Secukinumab, *UST* Ustekinumab

continued the BT they initiated for 12 months, while the other 35 patients discontinued within 12 months of starting treatment.

Table 2 shows the prevalence of comorbidities in the overall group of 205 patients. Hyperlipidemia and hypertension were the most common co-morbidities.

Persistence rates

Figure 3 presents the Kaplan Meier curves, using a non-BT refill period of 90 days for ADL, IFX and SCK, and 150 days for UST, for both the BT-naïve patient group and the total patient group.

The 12/24-month persistence rates for each BT are shown in Table 3.

In the total patient group, the 12-month persistence rates (±95% CI) for ADL, IFX, SCK, and UST were 45.9% ± 15.5%, 53.1% ± 14.7%, 74.2% (95% CI for SCK not available) and 79.8% ± 9.1%, respectively. The 24-month persistence rates were 45.9% ± 15.5% (ADL), 41.1% ± 15.4% (IFX), 74.2% (95% CI for SCK not available), and 73.4% ± 10.9% (UST). Statistically significant differences were found in the persistence rates among different BTs, either by log-rank test or Wilcoxon test (both $p < 0.001$). UST was found to have a significantly higher persistence rate in the pairwise comparisons with ADL and IFX (all p values ≤0.001 in either the log-rank test or Wilcoxon test), while no statistically significant difference was found between UST and SCK (log-rank test $p = 0.254$; Wilcoxon test $p = 0.163$). The proportions of patients who maintained persistent during the 12-month period after initiating BT - as relative to the total number

of patients calculated in the base case and sensitivity analyses - are shown in Appendix D (see Additional file 1).

For BT-naïve patients, the 12-month persistence rates ±95% confidence intervals (CI) for ADL, IFX, SCK, and UST were 46.8 ± 16.6, 53.0 ± 14.9%, 55.4% (95% CI for SCK not available), and 79.4% ± 9.9%, respectively. The 24-month persistence rates were 46.8% ± 16.6% (ADL), 41.0% ± 15.5% (IFX), 55.4% (95% CI for SCK not available), and 71.9% ± 12.2% (UST). Statistically significant differences were found in the persistence rates among different BTs, either by the log-rank test or Wilcoxon test (both $p < 0.001$). UST was found to have a significantly higher persistence rate not only in the pairwise comparisons with ADL and IFX (all p values ≤0.001 in either log-rank test or Wilcoxon test), but also in the pairwise comparisons with SCK (log-rank test $p = 0.006$, Wilcoxon test $p = 0.004$).

Medical costs

Overall, 77 patients (BT-naïve patients: 64) providing data for the 12-month periods pre- and post-BT initiation were analyzed for medical costs. Table 4 outlines the medical costs pre- and post-BT treatment initiation in BT-naïve patients and the total patient group (all cost data presented in 1000 JPY units). Costs included inpatient medical costs, outpatient medical cost, costs of drugs other than BTs, and total costs. As only two patients with a secukinumab treatment fulfilled the inclusion criteria for cost analysis, we will not report the cost assessment for this treatment. Among all patients, 12-month total costs before biologic treatment initiation

Table 2 Comorbidity characteristics of total patient population

	ADL	IFX	SCK	UST	Total
Number of patients	42 (100%)	52 (100%)	21 (100%)	90 (100%)	205 (100%)
Obesity	0 (0%)	0 (0%)	0 (0%)	1 (1.1%)	1 (0.5%)
Diabetes without complication/comorbidity	2 (4.8%)	4 (7.7%)	0 (0%)	6 (6.7%)	12 (5.9%)
Diabetes with complication/comorbidity	0 (0%)	2 (3.8%)	1 (4.8%)	4 (4.4%)	7 (3.4%)
Hypertension	6 (14.3%)	11 (21.2%)	4 (19.0%)	28 (31.1%)	49 (23.9%)
Hyperlipidemia	8 (19.0%)	13 (25.0%)	5 (23.8%)	20 (22.2%)	46 (22.4%)
Subsequent/old myocardial infarction	0(0%)	1 (1.9%)	0(0%)	1 (1.1%)	2 (1.0%)
Heart failure	2 (4.8%)	4 (7.7%)	0 (0%)	8 (8.9%)	14 (6.8%)

ADL Adalimumab, *IFX* Infliximab, *SCK* Secukinumab, *UST* Ustekinumab, *DLMOL* Disorders of lipoprotein metabolism and other lipidemias

a BT-naïve patient group (177 patients)

b Total patient group (205 patients)

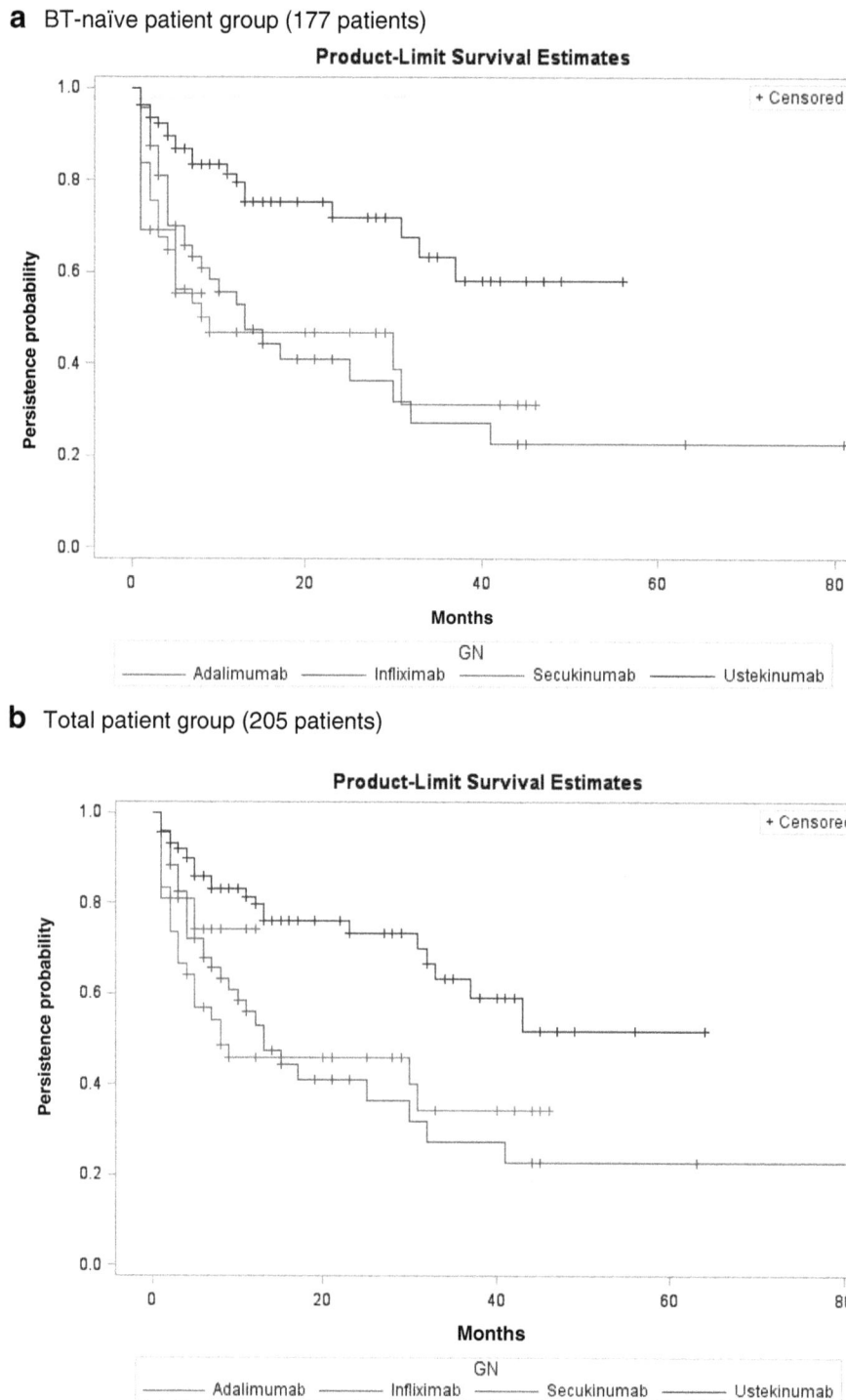

Fig. 3 Kaplan-Meier Curves of BT persistence in the BT-naïve and the total patient groupLegends: **a** BT-naïve patient group (number: 177 patients). **b** Total patient group (number: 205 patients).

was ¥886,000 per patient. First year cost increase after initiation of biologic treatment was ¥1,907,000.

Among the 64 BT-naïve patients, total medical cost per patient during the 12 months after BT initiation averaged 2828,000 JPY. Compared to the 12 months before

BT initiation, the increase in medical costs was 2,187,000 JPY. Among the 64 BT-naïve patients, 33 patients (33/64, 51.6%) who continued BT treatment over 12 months constituted the persistent group, while the remaining 31 patients (31/64, 48.4%) who discontinued

Table 3 12/24-month persistence rates and 95% confidence intervals (CI) for BTs psoriasis therapy

	Total				BT-naïve			
	ADL	IFX	SCK	UST	ADL	IFX	SCK	UST
Number of patients	42	52	21	90	37	48	13	79
12-month persistence rate ± 95% CI	45.9% ± 15.5%	53.1% ± 14.7%	74.2% (95% CI not available)	79.8% ± 9.1%	46.8% ± 16.6%	53.0% ± 14.9%	55.4% (95% CI not available)	79.4% ± 9.9%
24-month persistence rate ± 95% CI	45.9 ± 15.5%	41.1% ± 15.4%	74.2% (95% CI not available)	73.4% ± 10.9%	46.8 ± 16.6%	41.0% ± 15.5%	55.4% (95% CI not available)	71.9 ± 12.2%
p-value of log-rank test (versus UST)	< 0.001	< 0.001	0.254	–	< 0.001	< 0.001	0.006	–
p-value of wilcoxon test (versus UST)	< 0.001	0.001	0.163	–	< 0.001	0.001	0.004	–

ADL Adalimumab, *IFX* Infliximab, *SCK* Secukinumab, *UST* Ustekinumab. 95% CI of SCK was not available because of too small number of patients

formed the non-persistent group. Tables 5 and 6 show the medical costs in the persistent and the non-persistent group.

In the persistent group, the total medical costs during the 12 months after BT initiation averaged at 2,897,000 JPY. Compared with the 12 months before BT initiation the medical cost increase was 2,244,000 JPY on average. In the non-persistent group, total medical costs during the 12 months after BT initiation were 2,755,000 JPY on average. Compared with 12 months before BT initiation the increase in medical costs was 2,126,000 JPY.

The results of the medical cost comparison between the persistent and non-persistent groups are shown in Table 7. Only among patients receiving ADL the 12-month cost increase after BT initiation was smaller in the non-persistent than in the persistent group (Δ:-812). This difference was mainly due to the outpatient medical cost differences including drug costs for BTs (Δ:-1514). At the same time, costs of drugs other than BTs also showed differences (Δ: + 498). Among

patients receiving IFX or UST the 12-month medical cost increase after BT initiation was larger in the non-persistent group than in the persistent group (Δ: + 362 for IFX, + 43 for UST). Similar results comparing the persistent and non-persistent groups were also found by the analysis of the total group of 77 patients. Compared with the persistent group, the 12-month medical costs after BT initiation in the non-persistent group decreased most for patients who received ADL (Δ:-599). Among patients receiving UST, a slight decrease was observed (Δ:-164). Among patients receiving IFX, 12-month medical costs after BT initiation increased for the non-persistent group (Δ: + 101).

Discussion
Persistence rates
Our analysis using RWD from Japan (both in the BT-naïve patient group and the total patient group) found the BT persistence rates among psoriasis patients to be higher than those reported in the US studies [10–

Table 4 Characteristics and medical costs of patients with 12 month-follow-up period pre- and post-BT initiation

		Total				BT-naïve			
		ADL	IFX	UST	Sub total	ADL	IFX	UST	Subtotal
Number of patients		18	20	37	77	14	19	30	64
Average Age		47.7	46.5	46.2	46.8	49.6	47.3	46.3	47.5
%Female		11.1%	20.0%	16.2%	15.6%	14.3%	21.1%	20.0%	18.8%
Cost (pre)		¥760	¥950	¥900	¥886	¥365	¥916	¥603	¥641
In 1000 JPY unit	IP	¥18	¥343	¥254	¥235	¥0	¥361	¥162	¥188
	OP	¥513	¥301	¥425	¥405	¥133	¥261	¥216	¥210
	RX	¥229	¥306	¥221	¥246	¥232	¥294	¥225	¥244
Cost increase		¥1538	¥2429	¥1865	¥1907	¥1853	¥2494	¥2221	¥2187
In 1000 JPY unit	IP	¥95	¥601	- ¥37	¥156	¥146	¥633	¥21	¥228
	OP	¥1077	¥1958	¥2011	¥1754	¥1379	¥1974	¥2296	¥1965
	RX	¥366	- ¥130	- ¥109	- ¥2	¥328	- ¥113	- ¥96	- ¥5

ADL Adalimumab, *IFX* Infliximab, *UST* Ustekinumab, pre:12 months pre-initiation, cost increase: increase from pre to post 12 months post-initiation, *JPY* Japanese Yen, *IP* inpatient medical costs, *OP* outpatient medical cost, *RX* costs of drugs other than BTs

Table 5 Characteristics and medical costs of patients in the persistent group

		Total				BT-naïve			
		ADL	IFX	UST	Sub total	ADL	IFX	UST	Sub total
Number of patients		6	6	29	42	4	6	23	33
Average Age		50.8	44.7	45.0	46.0	54.0	44.7	44.8	45.9
%Female		16.7%	16.7%	17.2%	16.7%	25.0%	16.7%	21.7%	21.2%
Cost (pre)		¥1092	¥1062	¥925	¥988	¥360	¥1062	¥597	¥653
In 1000 JPY unit	IP	¥55	¥603	¥315	¥340	¥0	¥603	¥201	¥250
	OP	¥876	¥398	¥418	¥473	¥263	¥398	¥211	¥251
	RX	¥161	¥61	¥192	¥175	¥97	¥61	¥186	¥152
Cost increase		¥1606	¥2246	¥1875	¥1883	¥2433	¥2246	¥2211	¥2244
In 1000 JPY unit	IP	- ¥55	- ¥174	- ¥147	- ¥140	¥0	- ¥174	- ¥98	- ¥100
	OP	¥1365	¥2446	¥2114	¥2054	¥2461	¥2446	¥2380	¥2402
	RX	¥295	- ¥26	- ¥91	- ¥30	- ¥27	- ¥26	- ¥71	- ¥57

ADL Adalimumab, *IFX* Infliximab, *UST* Ustekinumab, pre:12 months pre-initiation, cost increase: increase from pre to post 12 months post-initiation, *JPY* Japanese Yen, *IP* inpatient medical costs, *OP* outpatient medical cost, *RX* costs of drugs other than BTs

12] but lower than the persistence rates reported in the EU studies [5–9, 20]. Regarding UST, the 12-month persistence rates reported in the two US studies by Chastek (2016) [10] and Gu (2016) [11] were 43.3 and 25%, respectively. These rates were obviously lower than those reported in the EU studies (78.6–90%) and the rates as per our analysis (79.4). The main reason for such differences may be that Chastek (2016) and Gu (2016) defined a non-BT refill period of 45 days, which was shorter than the non-BT refill periods used in the EU studies and our study. The defined length of the non-BT refill period was 90 days or 180 days in the EU studies, while it was 150 days for UST, and 90 days for the other BTs in our study. As UST's approved label defines a longer interval between injections than the labels of other BTs, using a shorter non-BT refill period is considered to have a greater impact on UST's persistence rate. Using different non-BT refill periods for different BTs as per each drug's approved label, which were factored into our analysis of Japanese RWD data, is considered more appropriate for analyzing the persistence rate. This was also suggested in another US study by Doshi (2016) [12], which defined non-BT refill period as the sum of treatment interval as per regimen and a medication gap of 90 days for all BTs. The 12-month persistence rate for UST used by Doshi (2016) increased conspicuously to 65% compared with Chastek (2016) and Gu (2016). However, even the UST adherence rate reported by

Table 6 Characteristics and medical costs of patients in the non-persistent group

		Total				BT-naïve			
		ADL	IFX	UST	Sub total	ADL	IFX	UST	Subtotal
Number of patients		12	14	8	35	10	13	7	31
Average Age		46.1	47.3	50.5	47.8	47.9	48.5	51.1	49.1
%Female		8.3%	21.4%	12.5%	14.3%	10.0%	23.1%	14.3%	16.1%
Cost (pre)		¥595	¥902	¥808	¥762	¥367	¥848	¥621	¥629
In 1000 JPY unit	IP	¥0	¥231	¥32	¥108	¥0	¥249	¥36	¥122
	OP	¥332	¥259	¥448	¥324	¥81	¥198	¥232	¥166
	RX	¥263	¥412	¥328	¥330	¥286	¥401	¥353	¥341
Cost increase		¥1504	¥2507	¥1828	¥1937	¥1620	¥2608	¥2254	¥2126
In 1000 JPY unit	IP	¥170	¥933	¥362	¥511	¥204	¥1005	¥414	¥577
	OP	¥932	¥1749	¥1638	¥1395	¥946	¥1756	¥2021	¥1499
	RX	¥402	- ¥175	- ¥172	¥31	¥470	- ¥153	- ¥181	¥50

ADL Adalimumab, *IFX* Infliximab, *UST* Ustekinumab, pre:12 months pre-initiation, cost increase: increase from pre to post 12 months post-initiation, *JPY* Japanese Yen, *IP* inpatient medical costs, *OP* outpatient medical cost, *RX* costs of drugs other than BTs

Table 7 Comparison of medical costs of BT-naïve patients between the persistent (P) and non-persistent (NP) group

		ADL			IFX			UST			Total		
		P	NP	Δ	P	NP	Δ	P	NP	Δ	P	NP	Δ
Number of patients		4	10		6	13		23	7		33	31	
Cost (pre)		¥360	¥367	¥7	¥1062	¥848	- ¥214	¥597	¥621	¥24	¥653	¥629	- ¥24
In 1000 JPY unit	IP	¥0	¥0	¥0	¥603	¥249	- ¥354	¥201	¥36	- ¥165	¥250	¥122	- ¥128
	OP	¥263	¥81	- ¥182	¥398	¥198	- ¥200	¥211	¥232	¥21	¥251	¥166	- ¥85
	RX	¥97	¥286	¥189	¥61	¥401	¥340	¥186	¥353	¥167	¥152	¥341	¥189
Cost (increase)		¥2433	¥1621	- ¥812	¥2246	¥2608	¥362	¥2211	¥2254	¥43	¥2244	¥2126	-¥118
In 1000 JPY unit	IP	¥0	¥204	¥204	-¥174	¥1005	¥1179	-¥98	¥414	¥512	-¥100	¥577	¥677
	OP	¥2460	¥946	- ¥1514	¥2446	¥1756	-¥690	¥2380	¥2021	-¥359	¥2402	¥1499	-¥903
	RX	-¥27	¥471	¥498	-¥26	-¥153	-¥127	-¥71	-¥180	-¥109	-¥57	¥50	¥107

P persistent, *NP* non-persistent, Δ costs of NP minus costs of P, *ADL* Adalimumab, *IFX* Infliximab, *UST* Ustekinumab, pre:12 months pre-initiation, increase: increase from pre to post 12 months post-initiation, *JPY* Japanese Yen, *IP* inpatient medical costs, *OP* outpatient medical cost, *RX* costs of drugs other than BTs

Doshi (2016) was still lower by comparison than the one reported in the EU studies and our study. This difference may be a result of the older patient group (mean age: 60.7 years) analyzed by Doshi (2016), compared with the EU studies and our study (mean age: approximately 50 years and younger). Other possible reasons such as differences in the health insurance systems, prescription preferences, and cultural factors were not covered in this study but may need to be discussed in future studies. Regarding ADL and IFX, the 12-month persistence rates demonstrated in our study were closer to the rates reported in the US studies and, by comparison, lower than those reported in the EU studies. Such differences were especially large among patients receiving ADL, so that our study found 12-month persistence rate for ADL of 46.8%, while that in the EU studies ranged from 64.6 to 79.7%. The 12-month persistence rate for IFX in our study was 53.0%, while that in the EU studies ranged from 63.6 to 70.9%. The causes of such differences with ADL and IFX treatment were unclear, as the possible differences between Japan and the EU with respect to treatment outcomes [21], incidence of anti-IFX and anti-ADL antibodies [22, 23], and prescription patterns of ADL and IFX were considerable. Moreover, the Japanese study by Umezawa (2013) reported much higher persistence rates than our study, namely 73.3, 79.7 and 96.7% for IFX, ADL and UST, respectively [14]. This study was a cohort study conducted in one hospital, while our study was based on a RWD database, which was considered as more representative of the patients with psoriasis across Japan, and the persistence rates of our study were closer to the reports from other studies.

Medical costs

Although the psoriasis treatment outcomes were considered to have been improved by the introduction of BTs, the high costs of these drugs remain an important issue

[24]. Several studies have discussed the costs of BTs and found a negative association between the patient motivation to initiate BT and its costs [25]. In general, it was evident that inpatient costs were generally higher after initiation of biologic therapy. Part of this cost increase might be due to hospitalizations for adverse events, e.g. infections, that patients experience when taking the new medication [26].

In our analysis of BT-naïve patients, the increases in the 12-month medical costs after BT initiation compared with those before BT initiation were highest in patients with IFX and lowest in patients with ADL. However, the 12-month medical costs after BT initiation were considered to be influenced by the persistence rates for the different BTs. When comparing the 12-month medical costs after BT initiation in the persistent and non-persistent groups, we found the most conspicuous cost decrease for ADL in the non-persistent group compared with the persistent group, namely from 2793 to 1988 JPY (Δ: -28.8%). Conversely, the costs for UST and IFX increased in the non-persistent group compared with the persistent group (Δ: + 2.4% for UST, + 4.5% for IFX). This finding suggested that the medical costs for patients who discontinued BTs within 12 months may not decrease by much but instead have the potential to increase compared to the costs for patients who were persistent with the BTs. Similar analyses of a period longer than 12 months are expected to be performed in future studies. The costs for drugs other than BTs increased for all non-persistent patients compared with the costs for persistent patients (Δ: + 687 for ADL; + 213 for IFX; and + 58 for UST), suggesting an increase in alternative treatments after patients discontinued BTs. Moreover, some patients were found to discontinue BTs due to the adverse events they experienced during the treatment. The treatment for adverse events may also contribute in part to the increase in drug costs not related to BTs.

This study is not an economic cost effectiveness evaluation of specific treatments, which was performed elsewhere. According to Igarashi et al. (2013), annual costs (2013) for ADL were 23,995 USD in the first and 23,107 USD in the second year. For IFX the costs were 38,860 USD and 32,593 USD, for UST they were 26,660 and 23,087. PASI 75 response rates were 83% for IFX, 74% for UST, and 59% for ADL. In the first year of induction treatment, the lowest cost per responder was for UST, followed by ADL and IFX. In the subsequent year of maintenance treatment, the cost per responder for UST remained the lowest [27].

A more recent study of Imafuku et al. (2018), however, reported annual treatment costs amounting to 15,668 USD for ADL (40 mg), 25,522 USD for IFX, 19,541 USD for UST (45 mg), and 10,423 USD for SEC. Assumed PASI 75 response rates in that study were 64% for IFX, 64% for UST, and 74% for ADL. Costs per responder were therefore lowest for ADL and SCK [28].

Limitations

There are several limitations to this study. First of all, evidence quality generated from the claims data analyses is generally limited due to the limited parameters available in the claims database. In this study, we were unable to filter by disease severity and disease activity of psoriasis at the time of BT initiation. Secondly, it was difficult to determine the treatment outcomes from claims data. We were unable to determine the reasons for discontinuation of treatment, which could have included adverse events, lack of efficacy, or even clinical remission. However, compared with the persistent group, no conspicuous decrease in the total medical costs, or increase in the costs of drugs other than BTs in the non-persistent group, were observed, suggesting that a clinical remission may not have been the main reason for the discontinuation of BTs within 12 months. Thirdly, the generalizability of these findings should be approached with caution. As our data were generated from the JMDC database, we cannot rule out the existence of bias towards younger patients. The results may, therefore, not be very representative of the patients with psoriasis aged older than 65 years of age in Japan.

Also, due to our study's relatively small sample size, we were not able to test determinants of treatment discontinuation. Data from a large UK registry-reported multivariate analysis showed that being female, an active smoker, and – surprisingly – a higher baseline dermatology life quality index were predictors of discontinuation [29]. For second-line biologic therapy it was shown that being female, having multiple comorbidities and a high Psoriasis Area and Severity Index when switching to second-line biologic therapy were general predictors for discontinuation [30]. Finally, we need to acknowledge

the differences in baseline covariates across different BTs, in particular with respect to gender. The variation of female patients across different biologic agents might be related to different perceptions of evidence availability in female psoriasis patients who are pregnant or lactating [31]. As women tend to discontinue their treatment more often than men, this is a potential source of a bias.

Conclusions

Our analysis using claims data of psoriasis patients in Japan revealed an adherence rate for UST that is closer to the results found by the EU studies and higher than the results found by the US studies. On the other hand, the adherence rates for ADL and IFX were found to be closer to the results obtained in the US studies and lower than the results in the EU studies.

Like most other studies have revealed our study also found UST to have the highest adherence rate among all BTs for psoriasis treatment, in both the BT-naïve patient group or the total patient group. The 12-month medical costs after BT initiation for adherent patients may not have increased as much as in the non-adherent patient group. Factors associated with a longer BT adherence period, which may lead to a better clinical outcome and possible cost-savings for patients are expected to be explored in future studies.

Abbreviations

ADL: Adalimumab; BTs: Biological therapies; CI: Confidence interval; EU: European Union; ICD: International Classification of Diseases; IFX: Infliximab; JMDC: Japan Medical Data Center Co., Ltd.; JPY: Japanese Yen; QoL: Quality of life; RWD: Real-world data; SCK: Secukinumab; US: United States; UST: Ustekinumab

Funding

Data were acquired by Janssen Pharmaceutical KK. The funding body provided support in the form of salaries for authors [JM, RS], but did not have any additional role in the study design, data collection and analysis, decision to publish, or preparation of the manuscript.

Authors' contributions

RS, KI, and JM designed the study. WT conducted the analysis. WT, KI, and JM drafted the manuscript. All authors revised the manuscript for intellectual content, read and approved the final manuscript.

Ethics approval and consent to participate

This was a retrospective study carried out using claims data from the commercial JMDC database; the authors were not involved in the collection of these data and data were anonymized before addition to the research database. Retrieval of the data from this database occurred in an unlinked fashion. As the data had been anonymized, the Ethical Guidelines for

Epidemiological Research (Ministry of Education, Culture, Sports, Science and Technology, and Ministry of Health, Labor and Welfare of Japan), which require ethics approval and informed consent, are not applicable to this study. Based on the Ethical Guidelines on Biomedical Research Involving Human Subjects (Ministry of Education, Culture, Sports, Science and Technology, and Ministry of Health, Labor and Welfare of Japan), pharmacoepidemiological studies conducted on medical databases qualify as research carried out on pre-existing material and information that do not require any interventions or interactions with patients. For such studies, including this study, obtaining written informed consent from patients is not mandatory. The authors had permission from JMDC to access the database.

Competing interests

JM, and RS were affiliated with Janssen Pharmaceutical KK at the time the study was conducted, a company that develops and markets drugs for the treatment of psoriasis. KI and WT received honoraria from Janssen KK.

Author details

[1]Health Economics, Janssen Pharmaceutical KK, 5-2, Nishi-kanda 3-chome Chiyoda-ku, Tokyo 101-0065, Japan. [2]Center of Pharmaceutical Outcomes Research, Naresuan University, Phitsanulok, Thailand. [3]Milliman, Tokyo, Japan. [4]Health Economics and Outcomes Research, Janssen-Cilag GmbH, Johnson & Johnson Platz 1, Neuss 41470, Germany. [5]Düsseldorf Institute for Competition Economics (DICE), University of Düsseldorf, Düsseldorf, Germany.

References

1. Bhosle MJ, Kulkarni A, Feldman SR, Balkrishnan R. Quality of life in patients with psoriasis. Health Qual Life Outcomes. 2006;4:35.

2. Darjani A, Heidarzadeh A, Golchai J, et al. Quality of life in psoriatic patients: a study using the short Form-36. Int J Prev Med. 2014;5(9):1146–52.

3. Kubota K, Kamijima Y, Sato T, et al. Epidemiology of psoriasis and palmoplantar pustulosis: a nationwide study using the Japanese national claims database. BMJ Open. 2015;5:e006450.

4. Terui T. Nakagawa H, et al.a survey of the status of psoriasis conducted using information obtained from health insurance claims provided by health insurance societies. J Clin Ther Med (Rinsyo-iyakku). 2014;30(3):279–85. (in Japanese)

5. Zweegers J, van den Reek JM, et al. Body mass index predicts discontinuation due to ineffectiveness and female sex predicts discontinuation due to side-effects in patients with psoriasis treated with adalimumab, etanercept or ustekinumab in daily practice. A prospective, comparative, long-term drug-survival study from the BioCAPTURE registry. Br J Dermatol. 2016;175(2):340–7.

6. Arnold T, Schaarschmidt ML, et al. Drug survival rates and reasons for drug discontinuation in psoriasis. J Dtsch Dermatol Ges. 2016;14(11):1089–99.

7. Dávila-Seijo P, Dauden E, et al. Survival of classic and biological systemic drugs in psoriasis: results of the BIOBADADERM registry and critical analysis. J Eur Acad Dermatol Venereol. 2016;(30):1942–50.

8. Iskandar IYK, Ashcroft DM, et al. Patterns of biologic therapy use in the management of psoriasis: cohort study from the British Association of Dermatologists biologic interventions register (BADBIR). Br J Dermatol. 2017; 176(5):1297–307.

9. Pogácsás L, Borsi A, et al. Long-term drug survival and predictor analysis. J Dermatol. 2017;28(7):635–41.

10. Chastek B, White J, et al. A retrospective cohort study comparing utilization. Adv Ther. 2016;33(4):626–42.

11. Gu T, Shah,N, et al. Comparing biologic cost per treated patient across indications. Drugs - Real World Outcomes 2016.3:369–381.

12. Doshi JA, Takeshita J, et al. Biologic therapy adherence, discontinuation, switching, and restarting among patients with psoriasis in the US Medicare population. J Am Acad Dermatol. 2016;74(6):1057–65.

13. Menter A, Papp KA, et al. Drug survival of biologic therapy in a large, disease-based registry of patients with psoriasis: results from the psoriasis longitudinal assessment and registry (PSOLAR). J Eur Acad Dermatol Venereol. 2016;30(7):1148–58.

14. Umezawa Y, Nobeyama Y, et al. Drug survival rates in patients with psoriasis after treatment. J Dermatol. 2013;40:1008–13.

15. Japan Medical Data Center. [Online]. Available from: https://www.jmdc.co.jp/en/.

16. Kuwabara H, Saito Y, Mahlich J. Adherence and re-hospitalizations in patients with schizophrenia: evidence from Japanese claims data. Neuropsychiatr Dis Treat. 2015;11:935–40.

17. Guelfucci F, Kaneko Y, Mahlich J, Sruamsiri R. Cost of depression in Japanese patients with rheumatoid arthritis: evidence from administrative data. Rheumatology and Therapy. 2018;5(1):171–83.

18. Davis K, Meyers J, Zhao Z, McCollam P, Murakami M. High-risk atherosclerotic cardiovascular disease in a real-world employed Japanese population: prevalence, cardiovascular event rates, and costs. Atheroscler Thromb. 2015;22(12):1287–304.

19. International Classification of Diseases (Japanese version). [Online]. Available from: http://www.dis.h.u-tokyo.ac.jp/byomei/icd10/.

20. Egeberg A, Ottosen M, Gniadecki R, Broesby-Olsen S, Dam T, Bryld L, Rasmussen M, Skov L. Safety, efficacy and drug survival of biologics and biosimilars for moderate-to-severe plaque psoriasis. Br J Dermatol. 2018; 178(2):509–19.

21. Di Lernia V, Ricci C, et al. Clinical predictors of non-response to any tumor necrosis factor (TNF) blockers: a retrospective study. J Dermatolog Treat. 2014;25(1):73–4.

22. Matsumoto Y, Maeda T, Tsuboi R, Okubo Y. Anti-adalimumab and anti-infliximab antibodies developed in psoriasis vulgaris patients reduced the efficacy of biologics: report of two cases. J Dermatol. 2013;40:389–92.

23. Hsu L, Snodgrass BT, et al. Antidrug antibodies in psoriasis: a systematic review. Br J Dermatol. 2014;170(2):261–73.

24. Fujita Y. The latest treatment for psoriasis-focused on biological therapies. Home Health Care for the People with Intractable Diseases (Nanbyo to Zaitaku Kea). 2015;21(3):29–33. (in Japanese)

25. Umezawa Y, Mabuchi T, et al. A study of questionnaire regarding biological treatment in patients with psoriasis. Hifuka no Rinsyo 2008.50(3):339–344 (in Japanese).

26. Yiu Z, Exton L, Jabbar-Lopez Z, et al. Risk of serious infections in patients with psoriasis on biologic therapies: a systematic review and meta-analysis. J Invest Dermatol. 2016;136(8):1584–91.

27. Igarashi A, Kuwabara H, Fahrbach K, Schenkel B. Cost-efficacy comparison of biological therapies for patients with moderate to severe psoriasis in Japan. J Dermatolog Treat. 2013;24(5):351–5.

28. Imafuku S, Nakano A, Dakeshita H, Li J, Betts KA, Guerin A. Number needed to treat and costs per responder among biologic treatments for moderate-to-severe plaque psoriasis in Japan. J Dermatolog Treat. 2018;29(1):24–31.

29. Warren R, Smith C, Yiu Z, Ashcroft D, Barker J, Burden A, Lunt M, McElhone K, Ormerod A, Owen C, Reynolds N, Griffiths C. Differential drug survival of biologic therapies for the treatment of psoriasis: a prospective observational cohort study from the British Association of Dermatologists biologic interventions register (BADBIR). J Invest Dermatol. 2015;135(11):2632–40.

30. Iskandar I, Warren R, Lunt M, Mason K, Evans I, McElhone K, Smith CH, Reynolds N, Ashcroft D, Griffiths C. Differential drug survival of second-line biologic therapies in patients with psoriasis: observational cohort study from the British Association of Dermatologists biologic interventions register (BADBIR). J Invest Dermatol. 2018;138:775e784.

31. Porter ML, Lockwood SJ, Kimball AB. Update on biologic safety for patients with psoriasis during pregnancy. Int J Women's Dermatol. 2017;3(1):21–5.

A multicenter, randomized, open-label pilot trial assessing the efficacy and safety of etanercept 50 mg twice weekly followed by etanercept 25 mg twice weekly, the combination of etanercept 25 mg twice weekly and acitretin, and acitretin alone in patients with moderate to severe psoriasis

Joo-Heung Lee[1*], Jai-Il Youn[2], Tae-Yoon Kim[3], Jee-Ho Choi[4], Chul-Jong Park[3], Yong-Beom Choe[5], Hae-Jun Song[6], Nack-In Kim[7], Kwang-Joong Kim[8], Jeung-Hoon Lee[9] and Hyun-Jeong Yoo[10]

Abstract

Background: Etanercept, a soluble tumor necrosis factor receptor, and acitretin have been shown to be effective in treating psoriasis. Acitretin is widely used in Korea. However, the combination of etanercept plus acitretin has not been evaluated among Korean patients with psoriasis. The objective of this study was to investigate the efficacy and safety of combination therapy with etanercept and acitretin in patients with moderate to severe plaque psoriasis.

Methods: Sixty patients with psoriasis were randomized to receive etanercept 50 mg twice weekly (BIW) for 12 weeks followed by etanercept 25 mg BIW for 12 weeks (ETN-ETN); etanercept 25 mg BIW plus acitretin 10 mg twice daily (BID) for 24 weeks (ETN-ACT); or acitretin 10 mg BID for 24 weeks (ACT). The primary efficacy measurement was the proportion of patients achieving 75 % improvement in Psoriasis Area and Severity Index (PASI 75) at week 24. Secondary end points included 50 % improvement in PASI (PASI 50) at week 24 and clear/almost-clear by Physician Global Assessment (PGA) at each visit through week 24.

Results: The proportions of patients achieving PASI 75, PASI 50, and PGA clear/almost-clear at week 24 in the ETN-ETN (52.4, 71.4, and 52.4 %, respectively) and ETN-ACT groups (57.9, 84.2, and 52.6 %, respectively) were higher than in the ACT group (22.2, 44.4, and 16.7 %, respectively). The incidence of adverse events was similar across all arms. This was an open-label study with a small number of patients.

Conclusion: In Korean patients with moderate to severe plaque psoriasis, etanercept alone or in combination with acitretin was more effective than acitretin. All treatments were well tolerated throughout the study.

Keywords: Psoriasis, Etanercept, Acitretin, Combination therapy, Efficacy, Safety, Korean patients

* Correspondence: joosoo@skku.edu
[1]Department of Dermatology, Samsung Medical Center, Sungkyunkwan University School of Medicine, 50 Irwon-dong, Gangnam-gu, Seoul, Korea
Full list of author information is available at the end of the article

Background

Psoriasis is a chronic autoimmune condition that affects 1 to 3 % of the general population worldwide [1–3]. Psoriasis has been associated with an increased risk for arthritis [4, 5], diabetes [4, 6, 7], cardiovascular disease [4, 8], depression [4, 9], and poor quality of life (QoL) [4, 10]. Although there is as yet no cure [1–3], there are several effective treatments available to manage the disease [11–16].

In clinical trials, etanercept, a tumor necrosis factor-alpha (TNFα) inhibitor, has been shown to be effective in managing psoriasis including improvements in Psoriasis Area Severity Index (PASI) scores [17–19], Physician's Global Assessment (PGA) [18, 19], and QoL [19, 20]. Acitretin, a systemic retinoid, is also effective for the management of psoriasis [21]. Acitretin is frequently used in combination with other agents (e.g., phototherapy and vitamin D), since acitretin monotherapy is often only moderately effective [21–24]. Since acitretin is not an immunosuppressive agent, combination treatment with etanercept may have a synergistic effect with a low risk of toxicity [21, 24]. This has been demonstrated in a pilot study in which the combination of acitretin and low-dose etanercept was as effective as high-dose etanercept, and both were significantly more effective than acitretin alone [25]. The purpose of the current study was to evaluate combination therapy of etanercept plus acitretin among Korean patients with psoriasis.

Methods

Patients

This study was reviewed and approved by local Institutional Review Boards (Appendix) and was conducted in compliance with the ethical principles originating in or derived from the Declaration of Helsinki and in compliance with Good Clinical Practice Guidelines. All patients provided signed informed consent.

Patients were eligible for study enrolment if they were at least 18 years of age and had active, clinically stable moderate to severe plaque psoriasis involving ≥10 % body surface area (BSA) or PASI ≥10. Exclusion criteria included evidence of skin conditions (e.g., eczema) other than psoriasis that would interfere with evaluations of the effect of study medication on psoriasis; any rheumatologic disease; prior exposure to biologic therapies, including etanercept, within 24 weeks of baseline visit; previous history of phototherapy or any systemic or topical therapy, including acitretin, for psoriasis within the previous 28 days before baseline visit; uncontrolled hypertension or diabetes mellitus; any severe hematologic, cardiovascular, renal, hepatic, or pulmonary disorders; known contraindication or hypersensitivity to etanercept or acitretin or their excipients; women who were pregnant, expecting to become pregnant, or breast-feeding

during the study period; patients with any clinically relevant concurrent medical conditions such as active or chronic infections, including human immunodeficiency virus, hepatitis B virus and hepatitis C virus infections, and active or recent (within 2 years) tuberculosis; history of cancer (or carcinoma in situ) other than resected cutaneous basal cell or squamous cell carcinoma within the past 5 years before the screening visit; or patients who had received any investigational drug within 3 months of screening visit.

Study design

In this multicenter, randomized, open-label trial, patients were randomly assigned to one of three treatment groups: (a) etanercept 50 mg twice weekly (BIW) for 12 weeks followed by etanercept 25 mg BIW for a further 12 weeks (ETN–ETN); (b) etanercept 25 mg BIW and acitretin 10 mg twice daily (BID) for 24 weeks (ETN-ACT); (c) acitretin 10 mg BID for 24 weeks (ACT; Fig. 1). This study was conducted in compliance with the ethical principles of the Declaration of Helsinki and the International Conference on Harmonization Good Clinical Practice Guidelines and registered on ClinicalTrials.gov, identifier NCT00936065.

The primary endpoint was proportion of patients achieving ≥75 % improvement from baseline in PASI score (PASI 75) at week 24. Secondary endpoints included the proportion of patients achieving either PASI 75 or PASI 50 (≥50 % improvement from baseline) at each visit through week 24, PGA status of "clear/almost-clear", and change in percent of BSA involvement from baseline over time.

Statistical analysis

The sample size was calculated assuming 20 patients per group with a response rate of 35–65 % which would yield a confidence interval below ± 21.9 %. Further assuming the response rate difference for primary efficacy endpoints is 20 % (i.e., 40 vs. 60 %), the 95 % confidence interval would be approximately ± 30 %.

Statistical analysis was performed using SAS software, version 9.13. Efficacy evaluation was performed on the modified intent-to-treat (mITT) and per protocol (PP) population sets. The mITT population included all randomly assigned patients who received at least one dose of test medication and had both baseline and on-therapy PASI evaluations. The PP population included those members of the mITT population who had no major protocol violations that could potentially alter the interpretation of the efficacy analysis.

For the outcomes at each visit, the proportions of responders and the 95 % confidence interval (CI) were determined and the differences between treatment groups were assessed using Fisher exact test or Chi-square test with multiple comparisons, if necessary. Kaplan-Meier

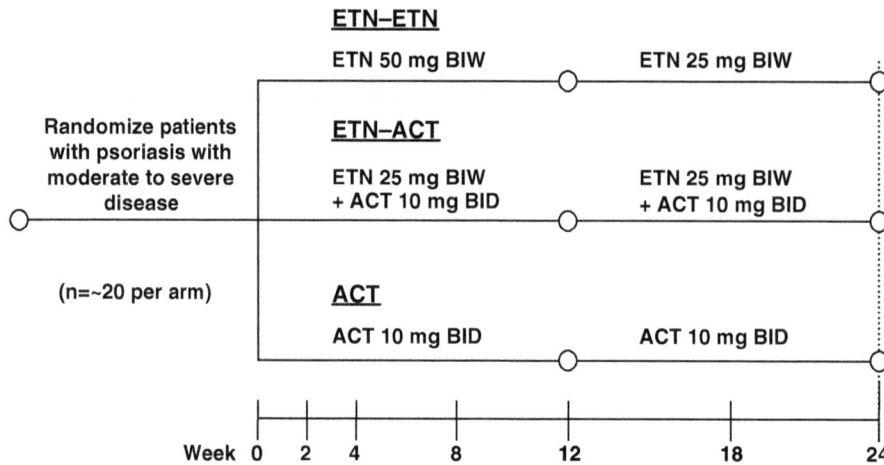

Fig. 1 Study design. *ACT*, acitretin; *BID*, twice daily; *BIW*, twice weekly; *ETN*, etanercept

estimations for time to first occurrence of each event were determined and the log-rank test was used for statistical testing. For these analyses, no imputation was applied and the patients who did not experience the event were censored at the time of last observation.

Basic descriptive statistics are presented for other measures and the statistical significance of the change from baseline within the treatment groups was assessed using the paired t-test or the Wilcoxon signed-rank test. Differences in change from baseline between the treatment groups were assessed using one-way analysis of variance (ANOVA) or the Kruskal-Wallis test.

Results

All results of this study have been posted on Clinical-Trials.gov, NCT00936065.

Patients

Of the 60 patients enrolled in this study and randomized to the three treatment arms, 45 completed the study (Fig. 2). One patient withdrew from the study after randomization but before receiving any study medication. Reasons for study discontinuation included patient request ($n = 6$), protocol violation ($n = 4$), unsatisfactory response ($n = 2$), adverse event (AE; $n = 2$), and lost to follow-up ($n = 1$). The baseline demographics were similar across all treatment arms (Table 1).

Efficacy

The proportion of patients achieving PASI 75 by week 24 in the ETN–ETN and the ETN-ACT groups was numerically more than twice that observed for the ACT group

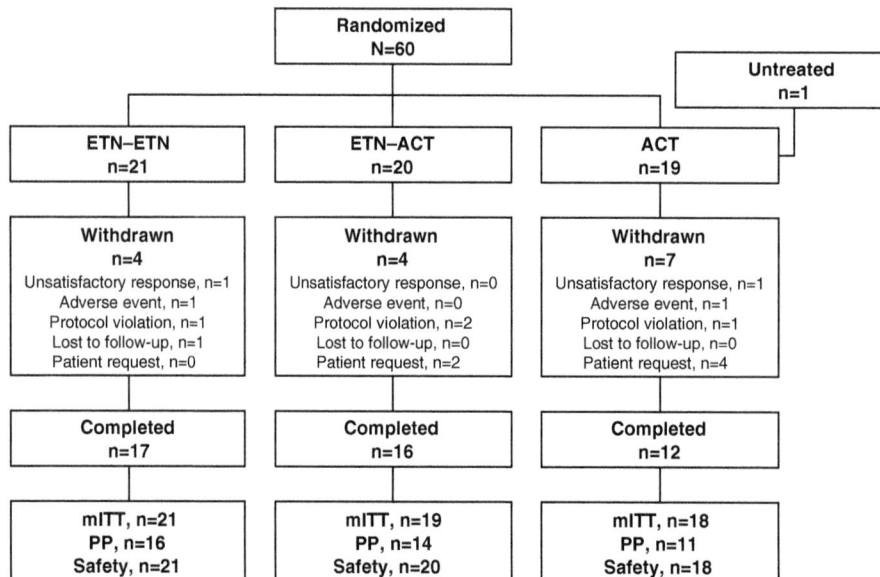

Fig. 2 Patient disposition. *ACT*, acitretin; *ETN*, etanercept; *mITT*, modified intent-to-treat population; *PP*, per-protocol population

Table 1 Baseline demographics for the mITT population

Characteristic	ETN 50 mg–ETN 25 mg (n = 21)	ETN 25 mg–ACT 10 mg (n = 19)	ACT 10 mg (n = 18)	Total (N = 58)
Mean age, y (SD)	38.6 (9.5)	35.5 (8.8)	42.4 (12.0)	38.8 (10.3)
Mean height, cm (SD)	169.5 (9.3)	171.7 (5.5)	170.9 (6.8)	170.6 (7.4)
Mean weight, kg (SD)	74.1 (16.0)	74.0 (11.6)	74.2 (9.8)	74.1 (12.7)
Gender, n (%)				
Male	16 (76.2 %)	17 (89.5 %)	15 (83.3 %)	48 (82.8 %)
Cigarette status, n (%)				
Prior cigarette usage	5 (23.8 %)	5 (26.3 %)	3 (16.7 %)	13 (22.4 %)
Current cigarette usage	10 (47.6 %)	11 (57.9 %)	10 (55.6 %)	31 (53.5 %)
No	6 (28.6 %)	3 (15.8 %)	5 (27.8 %)	14 (24.1 %)
Alcohol status, n (%)				
Ex-drinker	2 (9.5 %)	2 (10.5 %)	2 (11.1 %)	6 (10.3 %)
Current-drinker	13 (61.9 %)	13 (68.4 %)	11 (61.1 %)	37 (63.8 %)
No	6 (28.6 %)	4 (21.1 %)	5 (27.8 %)	15 (25.9 %)
Prior therapies for psoriasis, n (%)				
Methotrexate	2 (9.5 %)	1 (5.3 %)	0	3 (5.2 %)
Cyclosporine	2 (9.5 %)	2 (10.5 %)	1 (5.6 %)	5 (8.6 %)
PUVA	0	3 (15.8 %)	0	3 (5.2 %)
Other[a]	12 (57.1 %)	12 (63.2 %)	10 (55.6 %)	34 (58.6 %)

Abbreviations: *ACT* acitretin, *CS* clinically significant, *ETN* etanercept, *mITT* modified intent-to-treat population, *NCS* not clinically significant, *PUVA* psoralen plus ultraviolet A radiation therapy, *SD* standard deviation
[a]Includes systemic antimycobacterials, medication for treating alimentary tract and metabolism conditions, cardiovascular drugs, respiratory drugs, dermatologicals, and systemic hormonal preparations

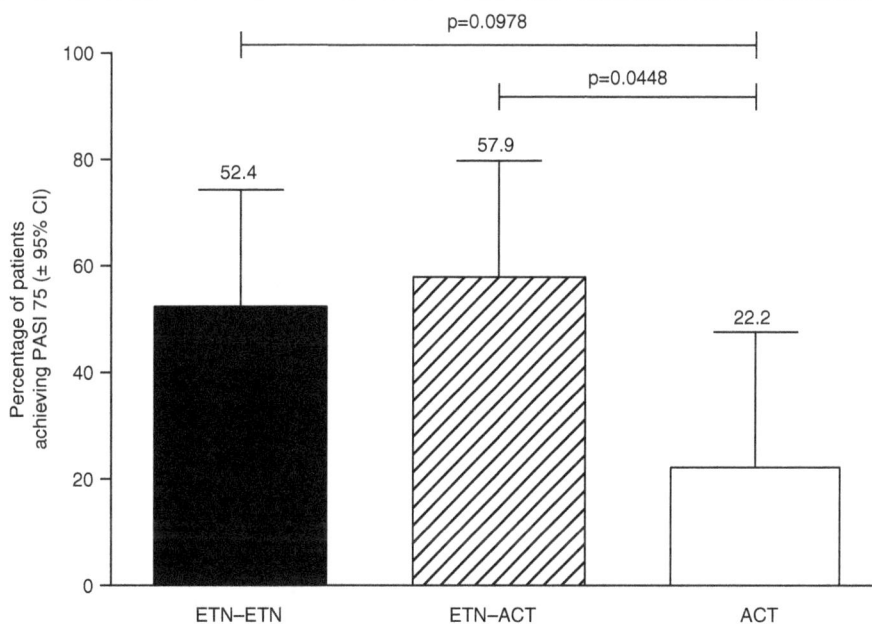

Fig. 3 Proportion of patients achieving PASI 75 at week 24. *ACT*, acitretin; *ETN*, etanercept; *PASI*, Psoriasis Area Severity Index

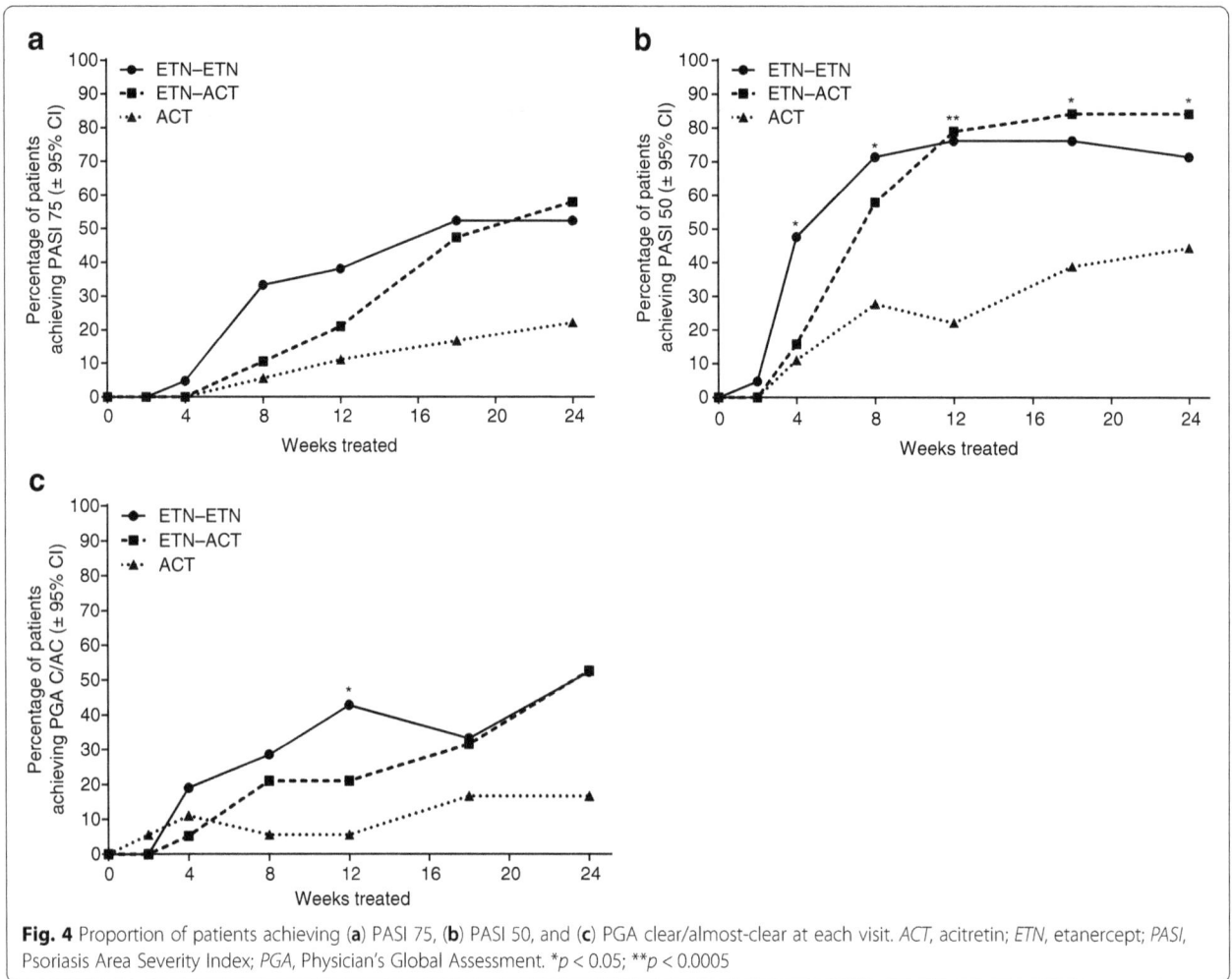

Fig. 4 Proportion of patients achieving (a) PASI 75, (b) PASI 50, and (c) PGA clear/almost-clear at each visit. *ACT*, acitretin; *ETN*, etanercept; *PASI*, Psoriasis Area Severity Index; *PGA*, Physician's Global Assessment. *$p < 0.05$; **$p < 0.0005$

(Fig. 3); however, only the pairwise comparison between the ETN-ACT and ACT groups showed statistical significance ($p = 0.0448$).

The proportion of patients achieving PASI 75 increased at each visit for all treatment arms (Fig. 4a). Of the three treatment arms, patients in the ETN–ETN group demonstrated the greatest PASI 75 response during the first 18 weeks, after which their response was comparable to that observed for the ETN-ACT group. The PASI 75 responses demonstrated by both of these groups was numerically greater than double that observed for the ACT group. However, statistically significant treatment difference was not shown at any time point.

The proportion of patients achieving PASI 50 increased for all treatment arms (Fig. 4b). The change from baseline was statistically significant for all treatment arms. A greater proportion of patients in the ETN–ETN and ETN-ACT treatment arms achieved PASI 50 at all visits than did patients in the ACT arm.

The proportion of patients achieving PGA clear/almost-clear increased for all treatment arms (Fig. 4c). Patients in

the ETN–ETN treatment arm demonstrated the greatest improvements up to week 12, after which improvements were similar to those of patients in the ETN-ACT treatment arm. The proportion of patients achieving PGA clear/almost-clear in the ETN–ETN and ETN-ACT arms was more than triple that for the ACT arm.

The median time to achieve PASI 75 for patients in the ETN–ETN arm was 126 days compared with 146 days for patients in the ETN-ACT arm (Table 2). The median time to achieve PASI 50 was the same for patients in the ETN–ETN and the ETN-ACT arms (56 days) and much shorter than for patients in the ACT arm (126 days). The difference was statistically significant among the three treatment arms (PASI 75: $p = 0.0448$ and PASI 50: $p = 0.0033$). Additionally, the median time to achieve PGA clear/almost-clear was comparable between the ETN–ETN and ETN-ACT treatment arms (167 and 165 days, respectively). The median time to achieve PASI 75 and PGA clear/almost-clear could not be determined for patients in the ACT arm.

Table 2 Median time to response

Response	Median time to response, days (95 % CI)			p value
	ETN 50 mg–ETN 25 mg (n = 21)	ETN 25 mg–ACT 10 mg (n = 19)	ACT 10 mg (n = 18)	
PASI 75	126 (56, 146)	146 (124, NA)	NA (127, NA)	0.0448
PASI 50	56 (28, 56)	56 (54, 84)	126 (56, NA)	0.0033
PGA clear/almost-clear	167 (55, 172)	165 (59, NA)	NA (87, NA)	0.3536

Abbreviations: *ACT* acitretin, *CI* confidence interval, *ETN* etanercept, *NA* not available, *PASI* Psoriasis Area Severity Index, *PGA* Physician's Global Assessment

After 24 weeks of treatment, mean reduction in percent BSA involvement from baseline was greatest in the ETN–ETN treatment arm (–17.5 %) compared with the ETN-ACT treatment arm (–16.9 %) and the ACT treatment arm (–10.3 %) at all visits (Fig. 5). The treatment difference was statistically significant at weeks 4, 8, 12, and 18, whereas the biggest reduction from baseline was at week 24 in all three treatment groups.

Safety

Safety was evaluated on all patients who received at least one dose of study medication. Across the three treatment arms, 38 (64.4 %) patients reported 85 AEs, and 27 (45.8 %) patients reported 46 treatment-related AEs during the study. The overall incidence of AEs was similar in the three treatment arms (Table 3). The most common AEs reported across any treatment arm (Table 4) were pruritus (n = 6, 10.2 %), alopecia (n = 5, 8.5 %), and dry lips (n = 5, 8.5 %). One patient in the ACT arm reported a serious AE (severe back pain), which was determined by the investigator not to be related to the study treatment. No life-threatening treatment-emergent AEs occurred during the study nor were there any changes in laboratory tests, vital signs, or physical observations that were considered clinically important (Table 3).

Discussion

Psoriasis is a chronic autoimmune disease and is often associated with joint inflammation in psoriatic arthritis, a comorbidity that affects between 10 and 30 % of all people with psoriasis [2, 3, 26]. Severe cases of psoriasis have been shown to affect health-related QoL to an extent similar to the effects of other chronic diseases such as depression, hypertension, congestive heart failure, or type 2 diabetes [27].

In multiple trials, etanercept has been shown to be effective in improving the disease severity of psoriasis and patient QoL [17–20]. However, treatment with high doses of etanercept can be expensive [28]. In this context, even though acitretin monotherapy is often only moderately effective [21–24], acitretin is widely used to treat psoriasis and is considered a standard of care in Korea. Furthermore, acitretin has been reported to have malignancy chemoprevention characteristics [21, 29]. Since acitretin is not an immunosuppressive agent and may act synergistically with biologic agents (e.g., etanercept), with a low risk

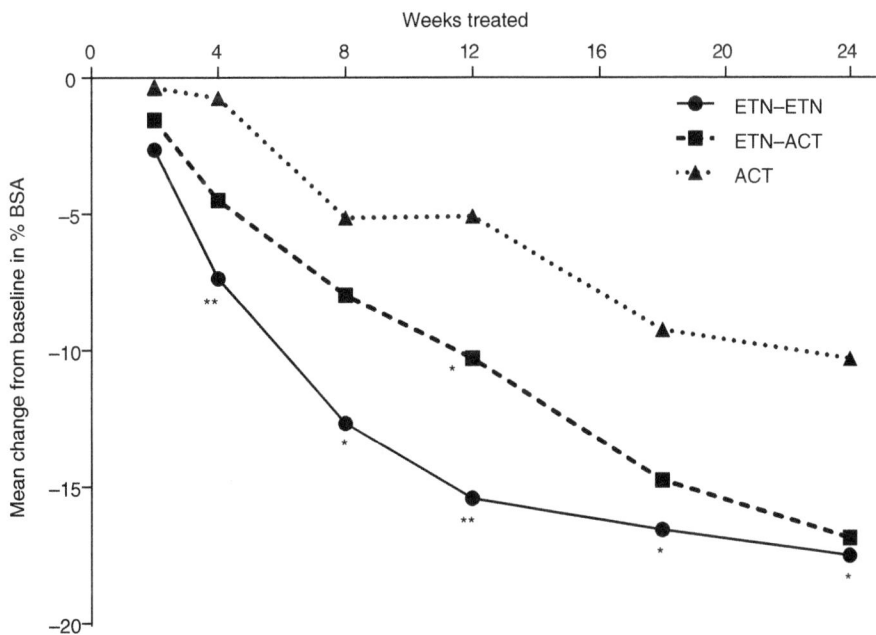

Fig. 5 Change from baseline in percent BSA involvement of psoriasis at each visit. *ANCOVA*, analysis of covariance; *ACT*, acitretin; *BSA*, body surface area; *ETN*, etanercept. *p < 0.05; **p < 0.005 (treatment difference tested by ANCOVA)

Table 3 Summary of treatment-emergent adverse events

	All Causality TEAEs				Treatment-Related AE			
	ETN–ETN (n = 21)	ETN–ACT (n = 20)	ACT (n = 18)	Total (N = 59)	ETN–ETN (n = 21)	ETN–ACT (n = 20)	ACT (n = 18)	Total (N = 59)
Patients with TEAEs, n (%)	14 (66.7 %)	14 (70.0 %)	10 (55.6 %)	38 (64.4 %)	9 (42.9 %)	10 (50.0 %)	8 (44.4 %)	27 (45.8 %)
Total number of TEAEs	22	38	25	85	11	22	13	46
Patients with SAEs, n (%)	0 (0.0 %)	0 (0.0 %)	1 (5.6 %)	1 (1.7 %)	0 (0.0 %)	0 (0.0 %)	0 (0.0 %)	0 (0.0 %)
Total number of SAEs	0	0	1	1	0	0	0	0
Permanent discontinuation due to AE, n (%)	1 (4.8 %)	0	1 (5.6 %)	2 (3.4 %)	–	–	–	–

Abbreviations: ACT acitretin, *AE* adverse event, *ETN* etanercept, *SAE* serious adverse event, *TEAE* treatment-emergent adverse event

of toxicity, a combination of etanercept and acitretin could be a viable treatment option for patients with psoriasis while keeping treatment affordable and potentially having additional beneficial effects. The results of a pilot study [25], a case series [30], and a posthoc review of clinical treatment practice [24] have suggested that the combination of etanercept and acitretin is effective and safe for the treatment of psoriasis. However, the efficacy and safety of this combination to treat Korean patients with psoriasis have not been determined until now.

The data presented here demonstrate that the combination of etanercept 25 mg BIW + acitretin 10 mg BID appears to be as effective for the treatment of psoriasis in Korean patients as etanercept 50 mg BIW for 12 weeks followed by etanercept 25 mg BIW.

Table 4 Incidence of TEAEs in ≥10 % of patients in any treatment arm

System organ class	ETN 50 mg– ETN 25 mg (n = 21)	ETN 25 mg– ACT 10 mg (n = 20)	ACT 10 mg (n = 18)	Total (N = 59)
Skin and subcutaneous tissue disorders				
Pruritus	3 (14.3 %)	2 (10.0 %)	1 (5.6 %)	6 (10.2 %)
Alopecia	–	4 (20.0 %)	1 (5.6 %)	5 (8.5 %)
Skin exfoliation	–	2 (10.0 %)	1 (5.6 %)	3 (5.1 %)
Gastrointestinal disorders				
Dry lip	–	3 (15.0 %)	2 (11.1 %)	5 (8.5 %)
Cheilitis	–	2 (10.0 %)	2 (11.1 %)	4 (6.8 %)
Chapped lips	–	1 (5.0 %)	2 (11.1 %)	3 (5.1 %)
Investigations				
Alanine aminotransferase increased	1 (4.8 %)	2 (10.0 %)	–	3 (5.1 %)
Blood bilirubin increased	–	2 (10.0 %)	–	2 (3.4 %)
Musculoskeletal and connective tissue disorders				
Myalgia	–	–	2 (11.1 %)	2 (3.4 %)
Vascular disorders				
Hypertension	–	2 (10.0 %)	–	2 (3.4 %)

Abbreviations: ACT acitretin, *ETN* etanercept, *TEAE* treatment-emergent adverse event

Furthermore, based on the numerical proportion of patients achieving efficacy endpoints (i.e., PASI 75, PASI 50, PGA clear/almost-clear, and reduction in disease-related BSA), and time to achieve these efficacy endpoints (i.e., time to achieve PASI 75, PASI 50, and PGA clear/almost-clear), both of these treatments appear to be more effective than acitretin 10 mg BID alone. In particular, the PASI 75 response rate at week 24 for the combined treatment arm (57.9 %) and the etanercept 50 mg–etanercept 25 mg arm (52.4 %) was numerically more than twice the rate of the acitretin 10 mg arm (22.2 %), although the differences were not statistically significant. However, unadjusted pairwise comparison showed a significant difference between the combined treatment group and acitretin 10 mg group ($p = 0.0448$). Furthermore, the proportion of patients achieving PGA clear/almost-clear in the ETN–ETN and ETN-ACT arms was more than triple that for the ACT arm. It is possible that due to the small number of patients, statistical significance was not achieved between the ETN–ETN and ETN-ACT arms and the ACT arm. Our results are consistent with an earlier Italian, randomized, controlled, pilot trial that showed PASI 75 response at week 24 was achieved by 45 % of the patients in the etanercept 25 mg BIW group, 44 % of the patients treated with etanercept 25 mg + acitretin, and 30 % of the patients in the acitretin 0.4 mg-kg^{-1} daily group. However, etanercept 25 mg BIW is not commonly effective in treating plaque psoriasis. Consequently, in our study, we treated patients at a higher initial dose of etanercept (50 mg BIW) and adjusted the dose downward to 25 mg BIW as the patients improved – a treatment regimen that we believe better reflects the real-world conditions.

These data demonstrate that the combination of etanercept with acitretin is just as effective as etanercept alone at week 24. However, patients treated with etanercept alone achieved the efficacy outcome endpoints faster than did patients receiving the combination. Treatment with etanercept alone may be preferred by patients wanting a more rapid resolution of their disease whereas treatment with the combination of these two drugs may be preferable for others without sacrificing efficacy or safety. The treating physician will need to consider these options in consultation with the patient to determine the optimum treatment regimen.

All treatments appeared to be safe and well tolerated by the patients. The incidence and severity of AEs appeared to be similar across all treatment arms. No life-threatening AEs were reported and no patient-reported SAEs that were related to study treatment. For patients with skin diseases, these results are important in terms of satisfaction with treatment and improvement of signs and symptoms of the disease, and could potentially affect their QoL.

Conclusions

In this study, the treatment of psoriasis with the combination therapy of etanercept and acitretin substantially reduced the severity of disease in Korean patients over a period of 24 weeks. These results suggest that etanercept could be added to acitretin to treat Korean patients with psoriasis, especially when the disease is resistant or responding inadequately to topical treatment or phototherapy. Combination therapy of etanercept and acitretin, and etanercept alone, are both effective and well tolerated; however, the choice of treatment may depend on finding a balance between the costs of the treatment versus the rapidity with which patients desire to experience the benefits of the treatment.

Appendix

Site ID	Institution	PI	IRB No.
1002	Hallym University Medical Center	Kwang-Joong Kim	2010-S003
1003	The Catholic University of Korea Seoul St. Mary's Hospital	Tae-Yoon Kim	KC09MSMV0185
1004	Samsung Medical Center	Joo-Heung Lee	2009-08-101
1005	Asian Medical Center	JeeHo Choi	2009-0645
1006	Bucheon St. Mary's Hospital	ChulJong Park	HC09BSMV0091
1007	Konkuk University Hospital	YongBeom Choe	KUH1120010
1008	Korea University Medical Center, Guro Hospital	HaeJun Song	GR09163-001
1009	Kyung Hee University Medical Center	NackIn Kim	KMC IRB 0922-05
1010	Seoul National University Hospital	Jai-Il Yoon	H-0911-041-301
1011	Chungnam National University Hospital	JeungHoon Lee	0912-128

Abbreviations

ACT, acitretin; AE, adverse event; ANCOVA, analysis of covariance; ANOVA, analysis of variance; BID, twice daily; BIW, twice weekly; BSA, body surface area; CI, confidence interval; ETN, etanercept; mITT, modified intent-to-treat population; NA, not available; PASI, Psoriasis Area and Severity Index; PGA, Physician's Global Assessment; PP, per-protocol population; PUVA, psoralen plus ultraviolet A radiation therapy; QoL, quality of life; SAE, serious adverse event; SD, standard deviation; TEAE, treatment-emergent adverse event; TNFα, tumor necrosis factor alpha

Acknowledgements

Medical writing support was provided by Mukund Nori, PhD, MBA, CMPP, of Engage Scientific Solutions and was funded by Pfizer.

Funding

This study was funded by Pfizer Pharmaceuticals Korea Limited; etanercept is a product of Pfizer.

Authors' contributions

All authors participated in study design, data collection, data interpretation, development, review, and final approval of the manuscript.

Competing interests

Hyun-Jeong Yoo is an employee of Pfizer Pharmaceuticals Korea Limited; etanercept is a product of Pfizer. All other authors report no competing interests.

Author details

[1]Department of Dermatology, Samsung Medical Center, Sungkyunkwan University School of Medicine, 50 Irwon-dong, Gangnam-gu, Seoul, Korea. [2]Department of Dermatology, National Medical Center, Seoul, Korea. [3]Department of Dermatology, College of Medicine, The Catholic University of Korea, Seoul, Korea. [4]Department of Dermatology, Asian Medical Center, University of Ulsan College of Medicine, Seoul, Korea. [5]Department of Dermatology, Konkuk University School of Medicine, Seoul, Korea. [6]Department of Dermatology, College of Medicine, Korea University, Seoul, Korea. [7]Department of Dermatology, College of Medicine, Kyung Hee University, Seoul, Korea. [8]Department of Dermatology, Hallym University Sacred Heart Hospital, Seoul, Korea. [9]Department of Dermatology, School of Medicine, Chungnam National University, Daejeon, Korea. [10]Pfizer Pharmaceuticals Korea Limited, Seoul, Korea.

References

1. Parisi R, Symmons DPM, Griffiths CEM, Ashcroft DM. Global Epidemiology of Psoriasis: A Systematic Review of Incidence and Prevalence. J Invest Dermatol. 2013;133(2):377–85.
2. Science of Psoriasis: Statistics [https://www.psoriasis.org/sites/default/files/psoriasis_fact_sheet.pdf].
3. Facts about psoriasis [http://www.worldpsoriasisday.com/web/page.aspx?refid=130].
4. Griffiths CE, Barker JN. Pathogenesis and clinical features of psoriasis. Lancet. 2007;370(9583):263–71.
5. Ibrahim G, Waxman R, Helliwell PS. The prevalence of psoriatic arthritis in people with psoriasis. Arthritis Rheum. 2009;61(10):1373–8.

6. Qureshi AA, Choi HK, Setty AR, Curhan GC. Psoriasis and the risk of diabetes and hypertension: a prospective study of US female nurses. Arch Dermatol. 2009;145(4):379–82.

7. Wolf N, Quaranta M, Prescott NJ, Allen M, Smith R, Burden AD, Worthington J, Griffiths CE, Mathew CG, Barker JN, et al. Psoriasis is associated with pleiotropic susceptibility loci identified in type II diabetes and Crohn disease. J Med Genet. 2008;45(2):114–6.

8. Ahlehoff O. Psoriasis and Cardiovascular Disease: epidemiological studies. Dan Med Bull. 2011;58(11):B4347.

9. Kurd SK, Troxel AB, Crits-Christoph P, Gelfand JM. The risk of depression, anxiety, and suicidality in patients with psoriasis: a population-based cohort study. Arch Dermatol. 2010;146(8):891–5.

10. Dubertret L, Mrowietz U, Ranki A, van de Kerkhof PC, Chimenti S, Lotti T, Schäfer G. European patient perspectives on the impact of psoriasis: the EUROPSO patient membership survey. Br J Dermatol. 2006;155(4):729–36.

11. Menter A, Gottlieb A, Feldman SR, Van Voorhees AS, Leonardi CL, Gordon KB, Lebwohl M, Koo JY, Elmets CA, Korman NJ, et al. Guidelines of care for the management of psoriasis and psoriatic arthritis: Section 1. Overview of psoriasis and guidelines of care for the treatment of psoriasis with biologics. J Am Acad Dermatol. 2008;58(5):826–50.

12. Gottlieb A, Korman NJ, Gordon KB, Feldman SR, Lebwohl M, Koo JY, Van Voorhees AS, Elmets CA, Leonardi CL, Beutner KR, et al. Guidelines of care for the management of psoriasis and psoriatic arthritis: Section 2. Psoriatic arthritis: overview and guidelines of care for treatment with an emphasis on the biologics. J Am Acad Dermatol. 2008;58(5):851–64.

13. Menter A, Korman NJ, Elmets CA, Feldman SR, Gelfand JM, Gordon KB, Gottlieb A, Koo JY, Lebwohl M, Lim HW, et al. Guidelines of care for the management of psoriasis and psoriatic arthritis. Section 3. Guidelines of care for the management and treatment of psoriasis with topical therapies. J Am Acad Dermatol. 2009;60(4):643–59.

14. Menter A, Korman NJ, Elmets CA, Feldman SR, Gelfand JM, Gordon KB, Gottlieb AB, Koo JY, Lebwohl M, Lim HW, et al. Guidelines of care for the management of psoriasis and psoriatic arthritis: section 4. Guidelines of care for the management and treatment of psoriasis with traditional systemic agents. J Am Acad Dermatol. 2009;61(3):451–85.

15. Menter A, Korman NJ, Elmets CA, Feldman SR, Gelfand JM, Gordon KB, Gottlieb A, Koo JY, Lebwohl M, Lim HW, et al. Guidelines of care for the management of psoriasis and psoriatic arthritis: Section 5. Guidelines of care for the treatment of psoriasis with phototherapy and photochemotherapy. J Am Acad Dermatol. 2010;62(1):114–35.

16. Menter A, Korman NJ, Elmets CA, Feldman SR, Gelfand JM, Gordon KB, Gottlieb A, Koo JY, Lebwohl M, Leonardi CL, et al. Guidelines of care for the management of psoriasis and psoriatic arthritis: section 6. Guidelines of care for the treatment of psoriasis and psoriatic arthritis: case-based presentations and evidence-based conclusions. J Am Acad Dermatol. 2011; 65(1):137–74.

17. Papp KA, Tyring S, Lahfa M, Prinz J, Griffiths CE, Nakanishi AM, Zitnik R, van de Kerkhof PC, Melvin L. A global phase III randomized controlled trial of etanercept in psoriasis: safety, efficacy, and effect of dose reduction. Br J Dermatol. 2005;152(6):1304–12.

18. van de Kerkhof PC, Segaert S, Lahfa M, Luger TA, Karolyi Z, Kaszuba A, Leigheb G, Camacho FM, Forsea D, Zang C, et al. Once weekly administration of etanercept 50 mg is efficacious and well tolerated in patients with moderate-to-severe plaque psoriasis: a randomized controlled trial with open-label extension. Br J Dermatol. 2008;159(5):1177–85.

19. Strohal R, Puig L, Chouela E, Tsai TF, Melin J, Freundlich B, Molta CT, Fuiman J, Pedersen R, Robertson D. The efficacy and safety of etanercept when used with as-needed adjunctive topical therapy in a randomised, double-blind study in subjects with moderate-to-severe psoriasis (the PRISTINE trial). J Dermatolog Treat. 2013;24(3):169–78.

20. Thaci D, Galimberti R, Amaya-Guerra M, Rosenbach T, Robertson D, Pedersen R, Yang S, Kuligowski M, Boggs R. Improvement in aspects of sleep with etanercept and optional adjunctive topical therapy in patients with moderate-to-severe psoriasis: results from the PRISTINE trial. J Eur Acad Dermatol Venereol. 2013;28(7):900–6.

21. Dunn LK, Gaar LR, Yentzer BA, O'Neill JL, Feldman SR. Acitretin in dermatology: a review. J Drugs Dermatol. 2011;10(7):772–82.

22. Claes C, Kulp W, Greiner W, von der Schulenburg JM, Werfel T. Therapy of moderate and severe psoriasis. GMS Health Technol Assess. 2006;2:Doc07.

23. Monfrecola G, Baldo A. Retinoids and phototherapy for psoriasis. J Rheumatol Suppl. 2009;83:71–2.

24. Smith EC, Riddle C, Menter MA, Lebwohl M. Combining systemic retinoids with biologic agents for moderate to severe psoriasis. Int J Dermatol. 2008; 47(5):514–8.

25. Gisondi P, Del Giglio M, Cotena C, Girolomoni G. Combining etanercept and acitretin in the therapy of chronic plaque psoriasis: a 24-week, randomized, controlled, investigator-blinded pilot trial. Br J Dermatol. 2008;158(6):1345–9.

26. Committee for Medicinal Products for Human Use (CHMP). Guideline on clinical investigation of medicinal products indicated for the treatment of psoriasis. London: European Medicines Agency; 2004.

27. Sampogna F, Chren MM, Melchi CF, Pasquini P, Tabolli S, Abeni D. Age, gender, quality of life and psychological distress in patients hospitalized with psoriasis. Br J Dermatol. 2006;154(2):325–31.

28. D'Souza LS, Payette MJ. Estimated cost efficacy of systemic treatments that are approved by the US Food and Drug Administration for the treatment of moderate to severe psoriasis. J Am Acad Dermatol. 2015;72(4):589–98.

29. Bettoli V, Zauli S, Virgili A. Retinoids in the chemoprevention of non-melanoma skin cancers: why, when and how. J Dermatolog Treat. 2013; 24(3):235–7.

30. Conley J, Nanton J, Dhawan S, Pearce DJ, Feldman SR. Novel combination regimens: biologics and acitretin for the treatment of psoriasis– a case series. J Dermatolog Treat. 2006;17(2):86–9.

Features of human scabies in resource-limited settings: the Cameroon case

Emmanuel Armand Kouotou[1,2,3], Jobert Richie N Nansseu[4,5*], Isidore Sieleunou[6], Defo Defo[2,7], Anne-Cécile Zoung-Kanyi Bissek[2,3] and Elie Claude Ndjitoyap Ndam[2,3]

Abstract

Background: The persistent high prevalence of human scabies, especially in low- and middle-income countries prompted us to research the sociodemographic profile of patients suffering from it, and its spreading factors in Cameroon, a resource-poor setting.

Methods: We conducted a cross-sectional survey from October 2011 to September 2012 in three hospitals located in Yaoundé, Cameroon, and enrolled patients diagnosed with human scabies during dermatologists' consultations who volunteered to take part in the study.

Results: We included 255 patients of whom 158 (62 %) were male. Age ranged from 0 to 80 years old with a median of 18 (Inter quartile range: 3–29) years. One to eight persons of our patients' entourage exhibited pruritus (mean = 2.1 ± 1.8). The number of persons per bed/room varied from 1 to 5 (mean = 2.1 ± 0.8). The first dermatologist's consultation occurred 4 to 720 days after the onset of symptoms (mean = 77.1 ± 63.7). The post-scabies pruritus (10.2 % of cases) was unrelated to the complications observed before correct treatment (all p values > 0.05), mainly impetiginization (7.1 %) and eczematization (5.9 %).

Conclusion: Human scabies remains preponderant in our milieu. Populations should be educated on preventive measures in order to avoid this disease, and clinicians' knowledges must be strengthened for its proper diagnosis and management.

Keywords: Human scabies, Contagiousness, Post-scabies pruritus, Cameroon

Background

Human scabies, an ectoparasitosis transmitted to humans through direct or indirect skin contact, is caused by *Sarcoptes scabiei hominis*, a mite infecting only human beings [1]. This skin infection has been described to occur as cyclic epidemics [2]. It has also been shown to be associated with poverty, overpopulation, poor personal hygiene, and war-centric pandemics [1–3]. In fact, the disease is particularly rampant in overcrowded places without adequate sanitation such as school milieu, nursing homes and prisons [2, 4]. The diagnosis of scabies is based on identification of the mite using dermoscopy and/or skin scrapings/microscopy. But in resource-constrained areas where

these technologies may scarcely be available, the diagnosis of scabies will be essentially based on anamnesis and clinical findings, hence the need for an experienced clinician who will make the right diagnosis [3, 4]. The management of this pathology integrates treatment of the patient as well as that of his entourage, along with disinfection of clothes and bedding [4].

Evidence from the literature shows that the prevalence of scabies in African countries is persistently high, being as such noticeable among individuals, and in some specific groups and collectivities [3–6]. As a matter of fact, nearly 300 million cases of this skin infection are reported in the world annually [7]. As such, scabies is one of the pathologies mostly encountered in developing and resource-limited countries [8, 9].

Paradoxically, there is dearth of research targeting the features of human scabies in resource-poor countries. The present study was thus undertaken, the purpose of which

---

* Correspondence: jobertrichie_nansseu@yahoo.fr
[4]Sickle Cell Disease Unit, Mother and Child Centre, Chantal Biya Foundation, Yaoundé, Cameroon
[5]Department of Public Health, Faculty of Medicine and Biomedical Sciences, University of Yaoundé I, PO Box 1364, Yaoundé, Cameroon
Full list of author information is available at the end of the article

was to draw up the socio-demographic profile of patients infected with scabies, and to determine its related spreading factors in Cameroon, a low-income country.

Methods
Study design and setting
We conducted a cross-sectional survey from October 2011 to September 2012 in 3 hospitals, all of which are located in Yaoundé the political capital of Cameroon, namely: the Yaoundé Central Hospital, the Biyem-Assi District Hospital and the Elig-Essono Medical Centre. Each of these three health facilities are provided with competent and experienced dermatologists who are lecturers in the main Faculty of Medicine of the country.

Study participants and data collection
Participants were patients, irrespective of their age and sex, who came or were brought on out-patient consultations for dermatologic problems. During the survey period, we consecutively included patients who described night-prevailing pruritus and/or any notion of contamination, and whose physical examination, performed by the dermatologist, revealed characteristic lesions of human scabies.

Data collection used a structured questionnaire recording socio-demographic background (age, sex, profession, educational level, underlying conditions), risk or spreading factors (number of persons living in the room or sleeping on the same bed), duration between onset of symptoms and first consultation, and clinical relevant signs and symptoms.

After the diagnosis was made at this initial consultation, patients were placed on specific medication, namely the benzoate of benzyle to be applied on the whole body two times at a 24 h-interval, after a lukewarm bath and on a humid skin. This operation was to be repeated one week later. Patients and their entourage were treated simultaneously. In cases of impetiginization, an antiseptic and a macrolide were prescribed for seven days before the application of the scabicide, and in cases of eczematization, a topic corticoid was to be applied 24 h after the anti-scabious treatment for 4 to 5 days. Additionally, clothes and bedding were decontaminated by washing them with warm water followed by spraying of an anti-scabious containing pyréthrinoïde. No quarantine measures were applied. Patients were subsequently given a weekly appointment to assess evolution of lesions and response to treatment. Unhappily, dermoscopy and/or skin scrapings/microscopy were not available to confirm the presence of mite. Therefore, we were comforted in our diagnosis in case the response to treatment was good with complete regression of lesions. The post-scabies treatment pruritus was considered as persistent after three completed weeks following an adequate anti-scabious treatment.

Statistical methods
Data were coded and entered using Microsoft Excel 2010 from Windows, and were further analyzed with Epi info version 3.5.3 (Centre for Disease Control, Atlanta, USA). Results are presented as mean ± standard deviation (SD) or median (inter-quartile range IQR) for quantitative variables, and as count (frequency) for qualitative ones. The Chi-2 test served for qualitative variable comparisons and the Student t test (or equivalents) for quantitative ones. Odds ratios (OR) with 95 % confidence intervals (CI) were used to investigate the influence of eczematisation and impetiginization on the persistence of pruritus after treatment. A p value < 0.05 determined statistically significant results.

Ethical considerations
Approvals were obtained from administrative authorities of the different study sites, and an ethical clearance was delivered by the ethical board of the Faculty of Medicine and Biomedical Sciences of the University of Yaoundé I, Cameroon. Patients or their guardians were informed of the various aspects of the study, and we anonymously enrolled only those who volunteered to take part in it after they have signed an informed consent form.

Results
Background characteristics
On the whole, we recruited 255 patients diagnosed with scabies, among whom 158 (62 %) were males, hence a sex ratio of 1.63/1. Participants' ages ranged from 0 to 80 years old, with a median of 18 (IQR 3-29). Table 1 displays our participants' age groups, educational level, profession and health underlying conditions. Patients aged 0-5 years old were the most encountered (30.6 %) followed by those aged 25–35 years (23.1 %, see Table 1). Ninety patients (35.3 %) attended the secondary school, and 46 (18 %) went to the university or college. Forty three point one percent of our respondents were students, and 17 (6.7 %) were civil servants. One patient (0.4 %) presenting with scabies (specifically Norwegian scabies) was mentally retarded, and 4 patients (1.6 %) were known HIV positive subjects (see Table 1).

Spreading factors
When analyzing the spreading factors we have searched for (see Table 2), we found no age difference between males and females. Two hundred and forty two subjects (94.9 %) were currently living with their family members, and almost all our participants were suspected to have been contaminated by their close entourage. The number of persons per room or bed varied from 1 to 5 with a mean of 2.1 ± 0.8, and there was no related difference between men and women ($p = 0.51$). Furthermore, the number of persons exhibiting pruritus in the entourage

Table 1 Characteristics of the study population with regard to their age, educational level, profession and underlying condition

		Number	Percentage (%)
Age (years)	<1	30	11.8
	1–5	48	18.8
	6–11	27	10.6
	12–18	25	9.8
	19–24	28	11
	25–35	59	23.1
	36–45	16	6.3
	> 45	22	8.6
Educational level	Never went to school	5	2.0
	Nursery	17	6.7
	Primary	45	17.6
	Secondary	90	35.3
	University/College	46	18.0
	Missing data	52	20.4
Profession	Civil servant	17	6.7
	Driver	6	2.4
	Trader	13	5.1
	Couturier/Hairdresser	11	4.3
	Student	110	43.1
	Teacher	4	1.6
	Manoeuvre	12	4.7
	Housewife	11	4.3
	Other	8	3.1
	Unemployed	11	4.3
	Missing data	52	20.4
Underlying condition	Retarded person		
	Yes	1	0.4
	No	254	99.6
	HIV infection		
	Yes	4	1.6
	No	103	40.3
	Unknown	144	56.5
	Missing data	4	1.6

ranged between 1 and 8 with a mean equal to 2.1 ± 1.8, and was significantly higher among males than females (2.5 ± 2.0 vs 1.9 ± 1.5 respectively, $p = 0.02$; see Table 2). Duration between onset of symptoms and first consultation varied from 4 to 720 days, with a mean of 77.1 ± 63.7. Before this consultation, 195 patients (74.9 %) had already tried a previous treatment without any success (mainly antibiotics, antifungals, antihistaminics or plant-based medicines), this being either prescribed by general practitioners or specialists other than dermatologists, or auto-medications.

Results of physical examination

The main lesions we observed were crusts (82.4 %), papules (69.8 %), and papulo-vesicles (68.6 %; see Table 3). These lesions were predominantly located at interdigital spaces (80 %), under-buttock creases (71.8 %), wrists (70.2 %), and inter-buttock creases (56.5 %; see Table 3). Only one patient (0.4 %) presented with crusted/Norwegian scabies. Two skin related complications were recorded before treatment: impetiginization (7.1 %) and eczematization (5.9 %). Four patients (26.7 %) presenting with eczematization had a history of atopy. After being adequately treated (i.e. anti-scabies + disinfection of clothes and bedding + treatment of the whole entourage) with complete regression of lesions, twenty six (10.2 %) patients presented with persistence of pruritus. While investigating the influence of impetiginization and eczematization on the occurrence of post-scabies pruritus, we found that patients with eczematization before an adequate treatment would have had an odds of 2.1 to develop a post-scabies pruritus than their counterparts, and an odds of 1.1 in case of impetiginization. But these odds are merely descriptive, as they were statistically non-significant ($p = 0.19$ and 0.57 respectively; see Table 4).

Discussion

This hospital-based cross-sectional study among an out-patient population revealed that human scabies may be common in Yaoundé, Cameroon. The number of persons per room/bed as well as the number of persons in the entourage may play a role in the spreading of the disease, though the design of the study precluded us from meticulously investigating such interactions. Further, the dominating lesions were crusts, papules and papulo-vesicles, and

Table 2 Spreading factors compared between males and females

Variable	Sex (mean ± SD)		Total	p
	Female	Male		
Age	2.1 ± 0.7	19.6 ± 18.3	2.1 ± 0.7	0.76
Number of persons per bed/room	2.1 ± 0.7	1.9 ± 0.8	2.1 ± 0.8	0.51
Number of persons with pruritus in the entourage	2.5 ± 2.0	1.9 ± 1.5	2.1 ± 1.8	0.02*
Duration between onset of symptoms and first consultation (days)	79.0 ± 64.9	76.0 ± 63.2	77.1 ± 63.7	0.72

*p value < 0.05

Table 3 Type and location of lesions

	Number (N = 255)	Percentage (%)
Type of lesions		
Vesicles	137	53.7
Papulo-vesicles	175	68.6
Papules	178	69.8
Nodules	65	25.5
Pustules	40	15.7
Crusty lesions	210	82.4
Scabious furrow	55	21.6
Scratch marks	135	52.9
Location of lesions		
Face	25	9.8
Anterior trunk	123	48.2
Posterior trunk	109	42.7
Axilla	136	53.3
Areola	60	25.5
Umbilical	99	38.8
Wrist	179	70.2
Under-buttock creases	183	71.8
Inter-buttock creases	144	56.5
Palms	45	17.6
Interdigital spaces	204	80.0
Glans	118	46.3
Sole	40	15.7
Diffuse	51	20.0

the prevailing sites of lesions were buttocks and wrists. We do suggest therefore that populations, especially those living in resource-limited areas, should be educated on preventive measures such as adopting rigorous personal hygiene, avoiding overcrowding and overpopulation in rooms/houses whenever possible, and promoting or reinforcing hand hygiene. Additionally, there is need to emphasize on scabies training for medical students and introduce regular updates on scabies diagnosis and treatment for health care

Table 4 Factors influencing the persistence of pruritus after treatment

		Persistence of pruritus		OR	95 % CI		p value
		Yes	No				
Eczematization							
	Yes	3	12	2.1	0.7	6.3	0.19
	No	22	210	1	–	–	
Impetinization							
	Yes	2	16	1.1	0.3	4.3	0.57
	No	23	206	1	–	–	

OR Odds ratio, *CI* Confidence interval

workers. Eventually, Governments should work towards poverty reduction to limit overcrowding.

We found a male (62 %) and younger age (median 18 years) predominance, these being consistent with Do Ango-Padonou et al's findings in Benin [10]. More than half of our respondents (59.6 %) had attended the nursery, primary or secondary school, but only 46 (18 %) patients had gone to the university. This finding may be due to the fact that younger children have closer physical contact with more individuals; as such they may be at increased risk of infestation. But further studies are warranted to thoroughly investigate such a concern. On another hand, we recorded 110 students (43.1 %), comparable to the 50.8 % proportion recorded in Bangui and 41.7 % in Dakar [11, 12]. This predominance of students could perhaps be explained by the overcrowding and overpopulation that characterize schools of resource-limited contexts, as there is body of evidence claiming that these are, among others, prevailing risk factors of human scabies [2–4, 6].

Consistent with the literature, results from our study are perhaps suggestive that overcrowding may be a contributive factor leading to the occurrence of scabies [3, 4, 12, 13]. Indeed, we found that 242 (94.9 %) of our patients were currently living with other members of their families, with more than one person sharing the same room/bed, and more than one person exhibiting pruritus in the entourage. It is true however that we must have undertaken a case-control study to underpin such an observation with robust scientific evidence.

We observed a delay of 4 to 720 days from onset of symptoms to the first dermatologist consultation. This may be attributable to the low socio-economic status of our patients as we are in a resource-poor context, and less than 10 % of our participants had a constant salary. Further, shame and/or taboo may delay the consultation, given scabies is perceived to be associated with poor hygiene and sanitation [2–4]. Lastly, non-dermatologist physicians may contribute to this delay if they are not well trained to properly diagnose and manage or refer cases of scabies. Such a long delay we have witnessed from onset of symptoms to diagnosis and adequate treatment is an important contributive factor in the spreading of the disease, the patient remaining contagious during all this period. It may consequently explain the persistently high prevalence of the disease latterly described [6, 13, 14].This constant high prevalence of scabies among resource-limited settings, along with its legendary contagiousness and related complications, makes perhaps this pathology a real public health hazard which may deserve full attention from local health authorities [15].

Evidence from the literature shows that the diagnostic of human scabies may be essentially clinical with a very good sensitivity (96.2 %) and specificity (98.0 %) [15].

The disease may evolve to a chronic stage, this fuelled by a long delay between onset of symptoms and adequate management, presenting thereby with some complications. For instance, we found that 7.1 % and 5.9 % of our patients respectively exhibited impetiginization and eczematization. But Kobangué et al. [11] observed a 2 to 3 times higher prevalence of these complications than ours: 17.2 % and 19.9 % respectively for the former and the latter. Besides, 10.2 % of our respondents exhibited a persistence of pruritus after they have been adequately treated and followed-up. This finding is in line with previous observations and has been attributed to the use of irritating drugs to treat the disease, a very bad observance of the treatment, an acarophobia, or an early and premature re-infestation [16].

While examining the influence of impetiginization and eczematization on the occurrence of post-scabies treatment pruritus, we found that patients with eczematization before any adequate treatment would have been 2.1 times more likely than their counterparts to develop a post-scabies pruritus, and, 1.1 times in case of impetiginization. Regrettably, these findings were not statistically significant ($p = 0.19$ and 0.57 respectively), may be due to the cross-sectional design of the study and the small sample size. Over time, the pruritus, which is sometimes very disabling, alongside the chronic lesions and complications of scabies, may disastrously impact the health condition of patients, dreadfully altering the quality of life of children and adults as well [8, 9].

Unfortunately, the design of this study precluded us from extensively investigating risk factors of scabies in our milieu. In fact, there was no control group (e.g. patients presenting with skin conditions, but without scabies) in order to compare the two groups and sort out some risk factors. Additionally, we are unable to generalize our findings to the entire Cameroonian population as the study was a hospital-based one, restricted in only three hospitals of Yaoundé, and only to dermatologist consultations too. Moreover, the absence of exact and reliable data on the total number of hospital visits or total number of visits due to skin problems hampered an estimation of the caseload of scabies. Another limitation of this study lies in the small sample size which could perhaps explain the absence of associations between variables. Eventually, dermoscopy and/or skin scrapings/microscopy were not available to confirm the presence of mite, and we did not search for proteinuria in patients presenting with impetiginization. Nonetheless, the two dermatologists in charge of the clinical assessment of the disease were very well-trained and experienced clinicians, and the clinical assessment of scabies has been shown with good sensitivity and specificity [16]. Further well-designed studies with large number of patients need to be conducted in order to better assess the burden, risk factors and clinical profile of human scabies in our settings.

Conclusion

To date, human scabies remains a common dermatologic pathology in Yaoundé, Cameroon. There are contributive factors such as an increased number of persons per room/bed or in the close entourage, and a long delay between onset of symptoms and proper diagnosis and management. Populations must be educated and sensitized on its related preventive measures such as adoption of rigorous personal hygiene, avoidance of overcrowding and overpopulation in rooms/houses whenever possible, and promotion or reinforcement of hand hygiene. Additionally, there is need to increase emphasis on scabies training for medical students and introduce regular updates on scabies diagnosis and treatment for health care workers. Eventually, Governments should work towards poverty reduction to limit overcrowding.

Competing interests
The authors declare that they have no competing interests.

Authors' contributions
Study concept and design: EAK, ACZB. Data collection: EAK, DD. Data analysis and interpretation: EAK, IS, JRNN. Drafting: EAK, JRNN. Manuscript critical revision: EAK, ACZB, DD, IS, JRNN, ECNN. All authors read and approved the final manuscript.

Acknowledgments
The authors gratefully acknowledge all the patients who have volunteered to participate in the present study.

Author details
[1]Biyem-Assi District Hospital, Yaoundé, Cameroon. [2]Department of Medicine and Medical Specialties, Faculty of Medicine and Biomedical Sciences, University of Yaoundé I, Yaoundé, Cameroon. [3]Yaoundé General Hospital, Yaoundé, Cameroon. [4]Sickle Cell Disease Unit, Mother and Child Centre, Chantal Biya Foundation, Yaoundé, Cameroon. [5]Department of Public Health, Faculty of Medicine and Biomedical Sciences, University of Yaoundé I, PO Box 1364, Yaoundé, Cameroon. [6]School of Public Health, University of Montréal, Montréal, Canada. [7]Yaoundé Central Hospital, Yaoundé, Cameroon.

References
1. Barete S, Chosidow O, Bécherel P, Caumes E. Ectoparasitoses (poux et gale) et piqûres d'insectes. Encyclopédie Médico-Chirurgicale 8-530-A-10.
2. Revuz J. La gale dans les maisons de retraite. Concours Med. 1994;116:2325–9.
3. Ceulemans B, Tennstedt D, Lachapelle JM. La gale humaine: Réalités d'aujourd'hui. Louvain médical. 2005;124(6):S127–33.
4. Gaspard L, Laffitte E, Michaud M, Eicher N, Lacour O, Toutous-Trellu L. Scabies in 2012. Rev Med Suisse. 2012;8(335):718–22. 724–5.
5. Gallais V, Bourgault-Villada I, Chosidow O. Poux et gale: nouveautés cliniques et thérapeutiques. La Presse médicale (1983) A. 1997;26(35):1682–6.
6. Hegab DS, Kato AM, Kabbash IA, Dabish GM. Scabies among primary schoolchildren in Egypt: sociomedical environmental study in Kafr El-Sheikh administrative area. Clin Cosmet Investig Dermatol. 2015;8:105–11.
7. Hicks MI, Elston DM. Scabies. Dermatol Ther. 2009;22(4):279–92.
8. Hay RJ, Steer AC, Engelman D, Walton S. Scabies in the developing world–its prevalence, complications, and management. Clin Microbiol Infect. 2012;18(4):313–23.
9. Worth C, Heukelbach J, Fengler G, Walter B, Liesenfeld O, Feldmeier H. Impaired quality of life in adults and children with scabies from an impoverished community in Brazil. Int J Dermatol. 2012;51(3):275–82.

10. Do Ango-Padonou F, Adjogan P. Aspects épidémiologiques de la gale humaine en milieu scolaire béninois. Med Afr Noire. 1986;33(12):915–7.

11. Kobangué L, Mballa MD, Abéyé J. Gale sarcoptique: aspects épidémiologiques et cliniques. Ann Dermatol Venereol. 2007;134(S1):98.

12. Niang SO, Kane A, Diallo M, Barry S, Dieng MT, Ly F, et al. Les dermatoses dans les écoles coraniques à Dakar. Ann Dermatol Venereol. 2005;132(HS3):925.

13. Walton SF, Currie BJ. Problems in diagnosing scabies, a global disease in human and animal populations. Clin Microbiol Rev. 2007;20(2):268–79.

14. Bitar D, Thiolet JM, Haeghebaert S, Castor C, Poujol I, Coignard B, et al. La gale en France entre 1999 et 2010: augmentation de l'incidence et implication en santé publique. Ann Dermatol Venereol. 2012;139:428–34.

15. Chosidow O, Sbidian E. La gale: une reconnaissance méritée ! Ann Dermatol Venereol. 2012;139:425–7.

16. Bécherel PA, Barete S, Francès C, Chosidow O. Ectoparasitoses (pédiculoses et gale): stratégie thérapeutique actuelle. Ann Dermatol Venereol. 1999;126:755–61.

Cost and effectiveness of prescribing emollient therapy for atopic eczema in UK primary care in children and adults: a large retrospective analysis of the Clinical Practice Research Datalink

George Moncrieff[1]*, Annie Lied-Lied[2], Gill Nelson[2], Chantal E Holy[3], Rachel Weinstein[4], David Wei[3] and Simon Rowe[5]

Abstract

Background: The Clinical Practice Research Datalink (CPRD) was used to evaluate the overall costs to the National Health Service, including healthcare utilisation, of prescribing emollients in UK primary care for dry skin and atopic eczema (DS&E).

Methods: Primary care patients in the UK were identified using the CPRD and their records were interrogated for the 2 years following first diagnosis of DS&E. Data from patients with ($n = 45,218$) and without emollient prescriptions ($n = 9780$) were evaluated. Multivariate regression models were used to compare healthcare utilisation and cost in the two matched groups (age, sex, diagnosis). Two sub-analyses of the Emollient group were performed between matched groups receiving (1) a colloidal oatmeal emollient (Aveeno-First) versus non-colloidal oatmeal emollients (Aveeno-Never) and (2) Aveeno prescribed first-line (Aveeno-First) versus prescribed Aveeno later (Aveeno-Subsequently). Logistic regression models calculated the odds of prescription with either potent / very potent topical corticosteroids (TCS) or skin-related antimicrobials.

Results: Costs per patient were £125.80 in Emollient ($n = 7846$) versus £128.13 in Non-Emollient ($n = 7846$) matched groups ($p = 0.08$). The Emollient group had fewer visits/patient (2.44 vs. 2.66; $p < 0.0001$) and lower mean per-visit costs (£104.15 vs. £113.25; $p < 0.0001$), compared with the Non-Emollient group. Non-Emollient patients had 18% greater odds of being prescribed TCS and 13% greater odds of being prescribed an antimicrobial than Emollient patients. In the Aveeno-First ($n = 1943$) versus Aveeno-Never ($n = 1943$) sub-analysis, costs per patient were lower in the Aveeno-First compared with the Aveeno-Never groups (£133.46 vs. £141.11; $p = 0.0069$). The Aveeno-Never group had ≥21% greater odds of being prescribed TCS or antimicrobial than the Aveeno-First group. In the Aveeno-First ($n = 1357$) versus Aveeno-Subsequently ($n = 1357$) sub-analysis, total costs were lower in the Aveeno-First group (£140.35 vs. £206.43; $p < 0.001$). Patients in the Aveeno-Subsequently group had 91% greater odds of being prescribed TCS and 75% greater odds of being prescribed an antimicrobial than the Aveeno-First group.

Conclusions: Acknowledging limitations from unknown disease severity in the CRPD, the prescription of emollients to treat DS&E was associated with fewer primary care visits, reduced healthcare utilisation and reduced cost. Prescribing emollients, especially those containing colloidal oatmeal, was associated with fewer TCS and antimicrobial prescriptions.

(Continued on next page)

* Correspondence: georgemoncrieff@hotmail.com
[1]Mayfield Clinic Summertown, Oxford OX2 7DE, UK
Full list of author information is available at the end of the article

(Continued from previous page)

Keywords: Atopic dermatitis, Eczema, Emollient, Healthcare utilisation, Colloidal oatmeal, CPRD, Topical steroid, Antimicrobial

Background

Dry skin and atopic eczema (DS&E), also described as atopic dermatitis (AD), is a common condition characterised by inflammatory flares followed by periods of remission. Prevalence estimates vary across diagnosis codes, age, and country, but in the UK, a range from 6 to 34% seems probable [1, 2].

A 1998 analysis within the UK National Health Service (NHS) estimated the cost of treatment of DS&E to be over £100 million each year [3]. Costs since then are likely to have increased significantly as the number of eczema-related UK general practitioner (GP) visits increased from 3.77 to 4.02 per person per year and the number of eczema-related prescriptions increased 56.6% from 2001 to 2005 [4]. Flares may occur frequently (as often as two or three times per month) and can have a negative effect on quality of life [5]. In one study, individuals with AD on average reported having over nine flares a year, with flares lasting around 2 weeks [6].

Treatment of DS&E typically includes use of emollients, which reduce the number of flares, prolong the interval between flares, and reduce the need for topical corticosteroids (TCS) [7–12]. Emollients were recommended for use as first-line therapy for patients with DS&E by a recent expert consensus group [7].

Evidence also suggests benefits of emollients in avoiding the development of AD. AD is often the first indication of the "atopic march," a progression to other diseases (food allergy, asthma, and allergic rhinitis) that can appear later in life in affected individuals [13]. In a US/UK study in a population of neonates at high risk for developing AD, use of emollients beginning within 3 weeks of birth for 6 months reduced the risk of developing AD by 50% [14], and investigations continue with a large, ongoing clinical trial (Barrier Enhancement for Eczema Prevention [BEEP]) to evaluate the effectiveness of emollient therapy during the first year of life [15]. In a pilot study, use of an emollient for the first 6 months of life was associated with a trend towards reduced AD and food sensitisation at 1 year of age [16]. In Japanese infants at high risk for developing AD, use of emollients from birth to 32 weeks of life reduced the risk of developing AD by 32% [17].

In England, the National Institute for Health and Care Excellence (NICE) provides clinical guidance on the management of atopic eczema and cost-effective treatment options, during and between flares of the condition, in children under 12 years of age. The treatment strategy for atopic eczema is a stepped approach with an emollient prescribed at each step, regardless of the severity of the condition [5]. Although the NICE guidance applies only to children, current advice from the Primary Care Dermatology Society also recommends a similar stepwise approach for the management of atopic eczema in adults [17].

Adding emollients to the treatment of children with DS&E was cost-neutral in prior studies — the added cost of the emollient being offset by a reduction in other treatment costs for DS&E [18–20]. However, despite acceptance by expert clinical groups [21, 22], the value and effectiveness of prescribing some emollients remain to be proven.

In this study, the Clinical Practice Research Datalink (CPRD) database [23] was interrogated to analyse emollient use and healthcare utilisation in patients with DS&E beginning in 2008—a year after publication of NICE guidelines recommending emollient therapy [5, 24]. In addition, our study investigated the use of Aveeno, an emollient that contains active colloidal oatmeal known to be beneficial in the treatment of DS&E [25, 26].

Methods

This was a retrospective group study using data from the CPRD database of anonymised patient medical records. The study protocol (# 16_198R) was approved by the Independent Scientific Advisory Committee (ISAC) for the Medicines & Healthcare Products Regulatory Agency and patient-informed consent was not required for use of this observational dataset. No additional institutional review board approval is required for CPRD studies. The study is registered at http://isrctn.com/ISRCTN91126037.

Group identification

All patients with a DS&E diagnosis code (see Additional file 1: Diagnosis codes) between 2008 and 2012 diagnosed during a regular primary care consultation were identified. The date of the first DS&E diagnosis was referred to as "index" diagnosis.

The group comprised (1) all patients aged 1 year and older at index who had at least 12 months pre- and 2 years post-index complete medical history, and (2) patients less than 1 year of age at index who had complete medical records in the database from birth to at least 2 years post-index. Patients with any diagnosis of DS&E

during the period before index ("washout window") were excluded, thus ensuring as far as possible that all patients had their first diagnosis of DS&E at time of index. The study period started at index and continued for 2 years post-index (Fig. 1).

The period before index was used to analyse presence of comorbidities. Comorbidities analysed during the pre-index period included atopic diseases (asthma, food allergies, and allergic rhinitis) often associated with the "atopic march" [13]. The Charlson Comorbidity Index (CCI), a widely used index originally developed to predict mortality based on the presence of 19 conditions, was also evaluated. The CCI can be used to study burden of disease and is indicative of overall health status [27–29]. All patients with a CCI ≥5 were

excluded from the study as it was determined that their significant comorbidities may act as confounders in the analyses.

During the pre-index and study period, all patients' diagnoses were analysed for coincident skin diseases that could result in significant use of TCS, such as bullous pemphigoid, lupus, lichen planus, and vitiligo (see Additional file 2). Patients with any such diagnosis before or during the study period were excluded from the study, as it might have been difficult to distinguish use of TCS for these conditions versus for DS&E.

From this population, patients with at least two distinct emollient prescriptions within 6 months of index were identified and included in the "Emollient" group. Of the remaining patients, those with at least two

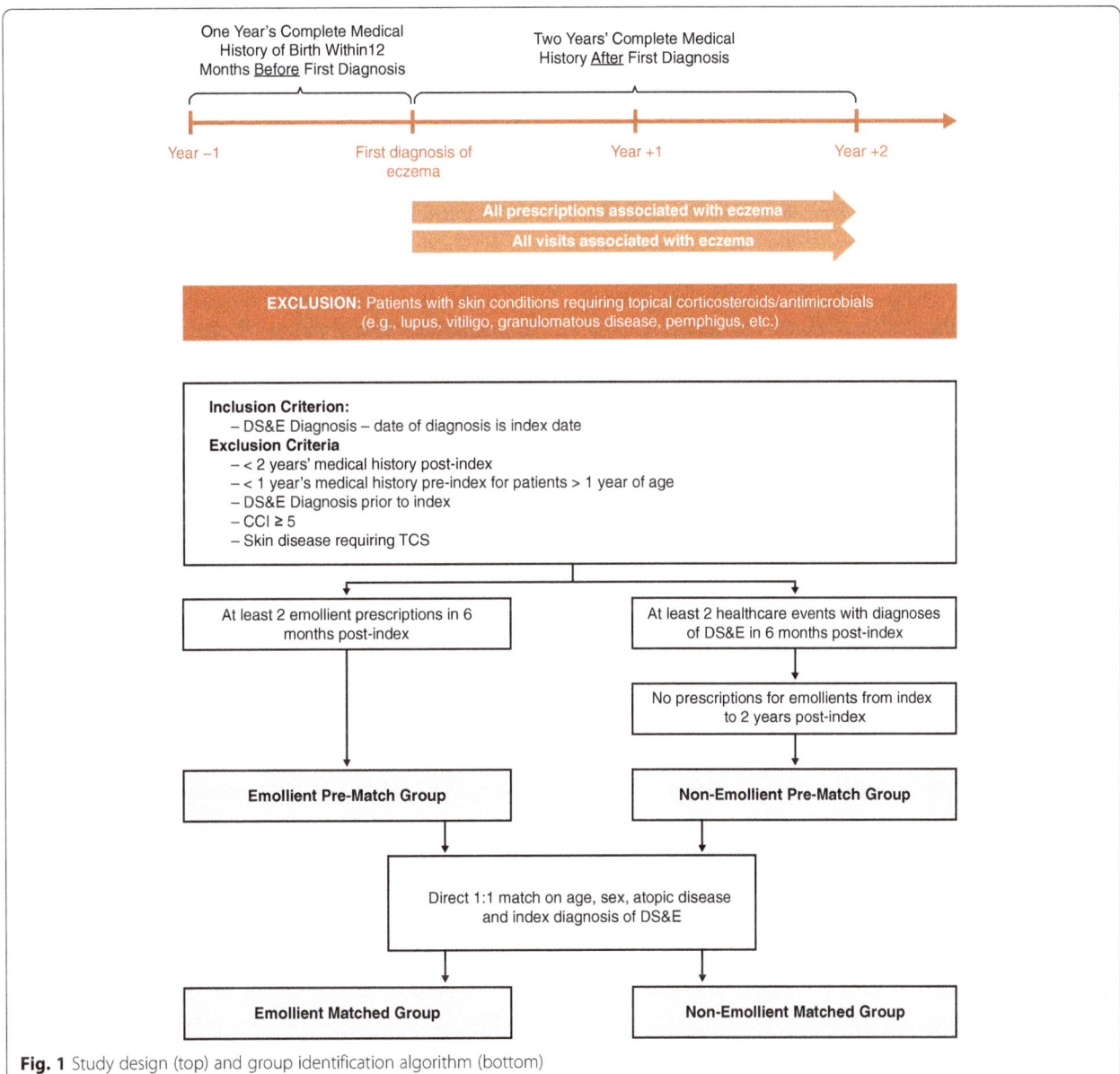

Fig. 1 Study design (top) and group identification algorithm (bottom)

healthcare visits with diagnoses of DS&E within 6 months of index but no emollient prescriptions at any time from index to 2 years post-index were included in the "Non-Emollient" group.

These "Emollient" and "Non-Emollient" groups were further defined as the "Pre-match" groups. Pre-matched groups were then matched using a 1:1 exact matching algorithm based on age, presence of AD (defined as having at least one of the following conditions: food allergy [Y/N], allergic rhinitis [Y/N], asthma [Y/N]), sex, and index diagnosis. The inclusion of index diagnosis in the variables used for matching was particularly important as different index diagnoses may have reflected slightly different disease severities and presentation. Using a direct match with index diagnosis as a variable ensured both investigational and control arms of having similar diagnoses at index. The final cohorts were defined as matched Emollient and matched Non-Emollient groups. A graphical representation of the group identification methodology is shown in Fig. 1.

Outcomes identification

The following outcomes were identified for all patients: (1) Frequency and cost of visits with DS&E diagnoses; (2) total cost of prescriptions provided during visits with DS&E diagnoses, by prescription category, from index to 2 years post-index. The prescription categories were based on version 71 of the British National Formulary chapters and included TCS, antimicrobial-containing prescriptions (topical and oral), emollients, and all other; (3) presence of at least one prescription for potent/very potent TCS provided during visits with DS&E diagnoses; and (4) presence of at least one prescription for an antimicrobial-containing medication during visits with DS&E diagnoses.

Statistical analyses

Descriptive statistics were performed on pre-match and matched groups. Continuous variables were expressed in terms of means, medians, and standard deviations. Proportions of comorbidities in each group were assessed descriptively. Standard t tests were used to assess differences between groups.

To compare healthcare utilisation between the matched groups of Emollient versus Non-Emollient patients, a multivariate regression model (generalised estimating equations [GEE]) was employed, controlling for covariates (age, sex, CCI, and presence of atopic conditions) and adjusting for correlation between clusters, defined in this study as GP practices. GEE models are robust and are designed to cope with outcomes with different distributions, and have the capacity to adjust the correlation within clusters [30].

To estimate the odds of being prescribed either a potent or very potent TCS or an antimicrobial-containing prescription, a logistic regression model was built using all available variables. These odds were calculated for the matched Emollient versus Non-Emollient groups and the c values were captured for each model.

Subgroup analyses

Current guidelines recommend that patients be offered a choice of emollient to choose one agreeable to the individual [5], as emollients that feel agreeable are more likely to be used appropriately and therefore to yield better outcomes. Additional subgroup analyses were performed within the Emollient group and were designed to evaluate whether the prescription of Aveeno-branded products containing colloidal oatmeal, which have been shown previously to be well-liked by patients [31], result in lower healthcare utilisation than other emollients. Two sub-analyses were performed.

1. Aveeno-First versus Aveeno-Never: Patients from the Emollient pre-match group prescribed an Aveeno-branded emollient at time of index were identified and defined as Pre-Match "Aveeno-First." Of the remaining patients, those who were never prescribed an Aveeno-branded emollient at any time during the study period were categorised as Pre-Match "Aveeno-Never." The Aveeno-First and Aveeno-Never pre-match groups were matched using a direct matching algorithm as defined above and compared using the outcomes and statistics as also defined above.

2. Aveeno-First versus Aveeno-Subsequently: Patients who were prescribed an Aveeno-branded product subsequent to another emollient between days 5 and 730 post-index were categorised as pre-match "Aveeno-Subsequently," and included those who may have received Aveeno at a later stage, for example, as a third or fourth choice. The pre-match Aveeno-First and Aveeno-Subsequently groups were matched and outcomes analysed as described above

Cost analysis

Costs of all patient contacts were analysed and "priced" accordingly (e.g., nurse contact had a lower price than GP contact), using costs as outlined in the Personal Social Services Research Unit (PSSRU) Costs of Health and Social Care for 2015 [32]. Prescription costs were estimated using publicly available costs per drug for 2015 [33]. The net ingredient cost (NIC) was obtained for all prescriptions and linked to all prescriptions within CPRD. The total cost for all prescriptions were then calculated by taking the amounts prescribed multiplied by the NIC per quantity. The perspective of this analysis is strictly that of the UK NHS—no other societal or otherwise related costs were included in the total cost of care. All analyses were performed using SAS 9.4 (SAS Institute, Cary, NC).

Results

Emollient versus Non-Emollient

A total of 54,998 patients met the inclusion criteria, with 45,218 patients in the Emollient group and 9780 patients in the Non-Emollient group (Table 1). Percentages of patients with ADs and the age distribution differed significantly between groups. Table 1 shows the 13 most prevalent index diagnoses in each group. The most prevalent diagnosis in both groups was AD/eczema. Many of the differences between the groups most likely represent diseases of children versus adults, with most (55%) of the patients who received emollient prescriptions being < 16 years of age, whereas only 15% of those in the Non-Emollient group were aged < 16 years.

Matching

Direct matching (1:1) to normalise differences between groups in age, presence of atopic disease, sex, and index diagnosis resulted in 7846 patients in both the Non-Emollient and the Emollient matched groups. After matching, differences remained in terms of geographic location and CCI distribution. More patients with CCI = 0 were in the Non-Emollient group versus the Emollient group; however, both groups had the same percentage of females (59.62%), similar age distribution (82.00% ≥19 years of age), the same percentage of patients with AD (allergic rhinitis: 7.18%, asthma: 13.05%, food allergies: 0.25%), and the same index diagnoses. Inter-group differences were within the designed scope of the GEE models.

Healthcare utilisation

Costs to the NHS over the 2-year study period were approximately the same in the Emollient (£125.80) versus Non-Emollient (£128.13) matched groups, with the costs of emollients in the Emollient group offset by lower costs for visits and other prescriptions (Fig. 2). The number of visits was statistically significantly lower in the Emollient (2.44 visits) versus Non-Emollient (2.66 visits) group ($p < 0.0001$), a difference of 9.06% (95% confidence interval [CI]: 7.19–10.97%). The decreased number of primary care visits translated into a significantly decreased overall cost of visits for the Emollient group (£104.15 vs. £113.25 for Non-Emollient, $p < 0.0001$). The difference was estimated at 8.74% (95% CI: 6.96–10.56%). Using the GEE model, total cost of care to the NHS was estimated at £125.98 per patient in the Emollient group versus £127.98 in the Non-Emollient group. The difference suggested a non-statistically significant trend ($p = 0.08$) of 1.58% of increased costs for those in the Non-Emollient group.

Table 1 Study population (before matching)

	Emollient (n = 45,218)	Non-Emollient (n = 9780)
Regional distribution %		
East Midlands	8.91	10.55
London	12.5	8.67
North East	1.75	3.13
North West	11.87	14.66
Northern Ireland	3.7	1.51
Scotland	10.79	9.62
South Central	11.62	13.15
South East Coast	7.95	11.13
South West	7.2	8.26
Wales	12.36	6.56
West Midlands	9.43	10.47
Yorkshire and Humber	1.92	2.27
Age distribution %		
Less than 1 year	13.43	1.17
1 to 5 years	29.24	6.13
6 to 10 years	7.1	3.21
11 to 15 years	5.64	3.64
16 to 18 years	2.87	2.32
19 to 65 years	26.38	63.11
More than 65 years	15.33	20.42
Disease type %		
Atopic dermatitis/eczema	43.62	26.24
Contact dermatitis	2.8	6.95
Dermatitis NOS	6.31	14.39
Dermatitis/dermatoses	1.49	2.84
Eczema NOS	18.36	15.12
Flexural eczema	3.37	1.44
Hand eczema	1.04	1.29
Infantile eczema	13.84	1.55
Infected eczema	2.57	4.54
Itch	2.06	7.46
Pruritus NOS	3.28	9.71
Seborrhoeic dermatitis capitis	0.45	5.62
Skin irritation	0.81	2.85

Note that responses from 1451 subjects for Disease Type were missing and not included in this analysis
NOS, not otherwise specified

Prescribing an emollient was associated with reduced prescriptions of potent or very potent TCS in the matched groups (Fig. 2). The proportion of patients treated with potent/very potent TCS was 42.45% in the Non-Emollient group compared with 37.89% in the Emollient group, and the odds of being prescribed a potent or very potent TCS in the Non-Emollient group

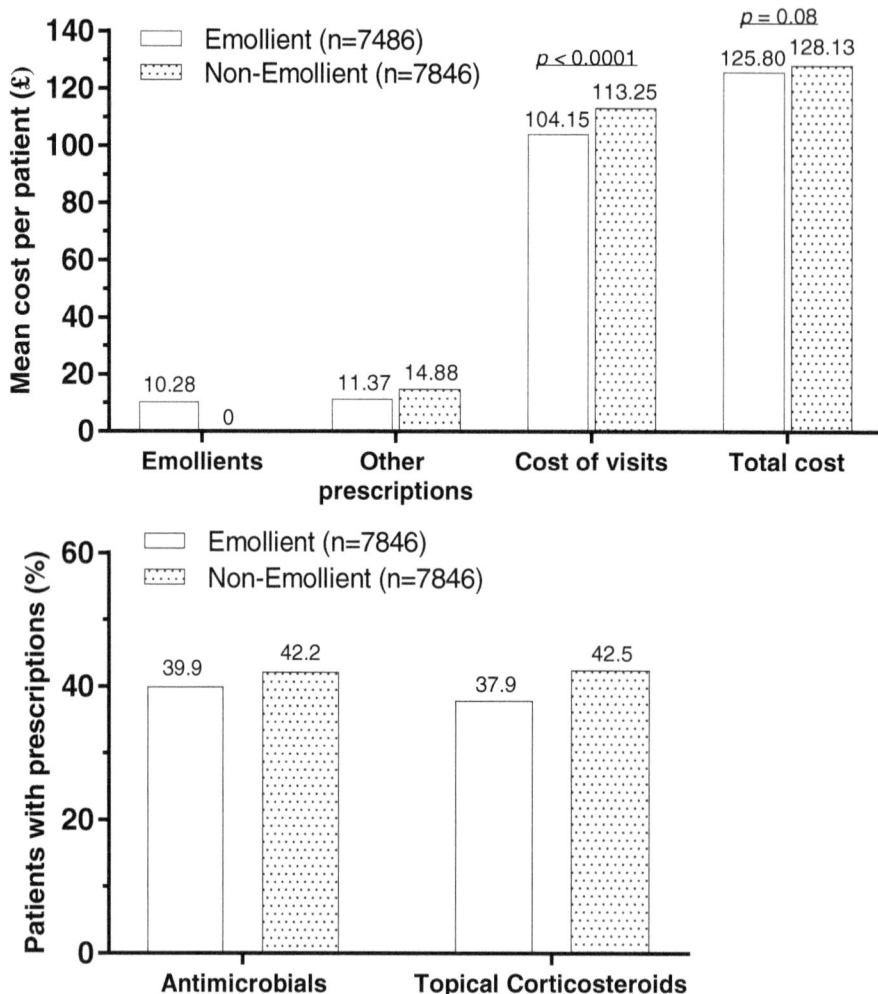

Fig. 2 Costs (top) and medication use (bottom) in matched Emollient versus Non-Emollient groups

was 1.18 (95% CI: 1.10–1.26), indicating an 18% increased odds of treatment compared with the reference Emollient group.

The proportion of patients treated with antimicrobial-containing prescriptions was 42.19% (3310/7846) in the Non-Emollient group compared with 39.96% (3135/7846) in the Emollient group (Fig. 2). The odds of being prescribed an antimicrobial-containing prescription in the Non-Emollient group was 1.13 (95% CI: 1.06–1.21), suggesting a 13% increased odds of treatment versus patients in the reference Emollient group.

Aveeno-First versus Aveeno-Never

Matched groups of 1943 patients each for the Aveeno-First versus Aveeno-Never groups were analysed.

Costs for emollient and/or non-emollient prescriptions did not differ between Aveeno-First and Aveeno-Never

groups (Fig. 3). Additionally, patients in the Aveeno-First group made fewer visits than matched patients in the Aveeno-Never group (2.68 vs. 2.83 visits; $p = 0.0081$), resulting in lower visit costs and statistically significantly lower overall costs ($p = 0.0069$) in the Aveeno-First group.

The percentages of patients treated with potent/very potent TCS were lower in the Aveeno-First (15.64%) versus Aveeno-Never group (18.11%; Fig. 3). The odds ratio of being prescribed a potent or very potent TCS in the Aveeno-Never versus Aveeno-First group was 1.214 (95% CI: 1.007–1.464), suggesting the Aveeno-First group was less likely to receive a prescription for a potent or very potent TCS within 2 years after the diagnosis.

The percentage of patients prescribed skin-condition-related antimicrobial was lower in the Aveeno-First (34.53%) versus Aveeno-Never group (39.42%; Fig. 3). The odds ratio of being prescribed an antimicrobial-containing

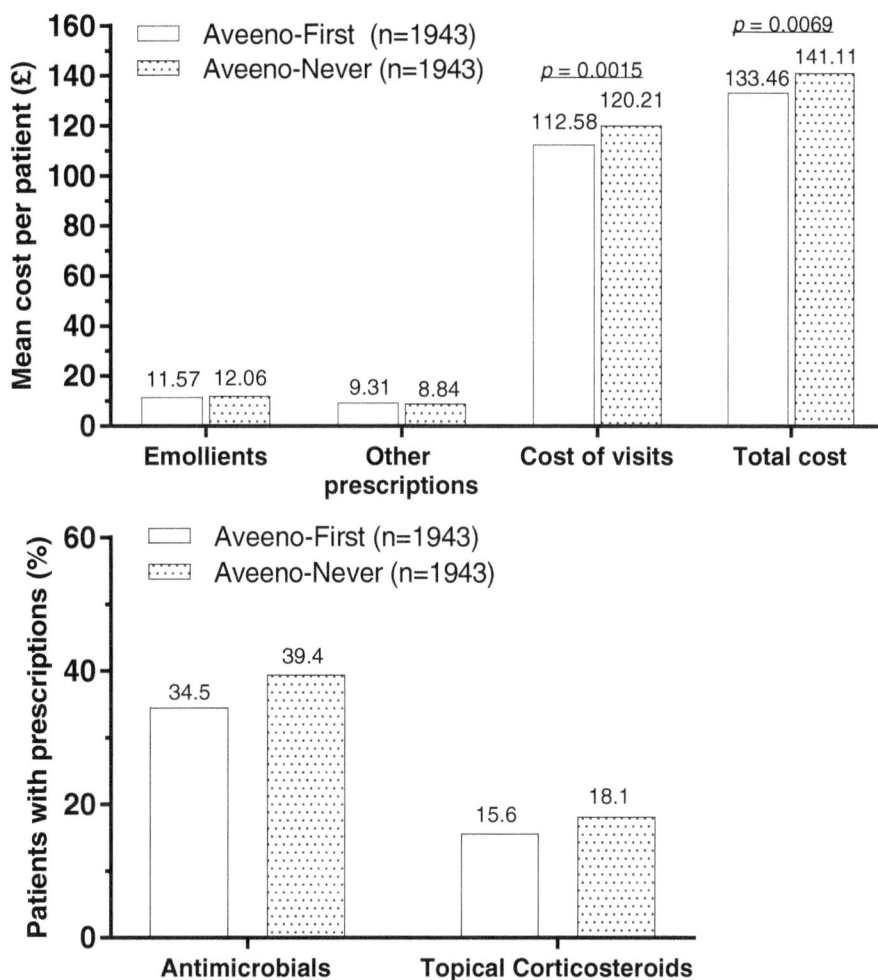

Fig. 3 Cost (top) and medication use (bottom) in matched Aveeno-First versus Aveeno-Never groups

prescription in the Aveeno-Never versus Aveeno-First group was 1.252 (95% CI: 1.090–1.437), suggesting the Aveeno-First group was 25% less likely to receive a prescription for a skin condition-related antimicrobial within 2 years after diagnosis.

Aveeno-First versus Aveeno-Subsequently

The second sub-analysis included 1357 matched patients in each group, namely the Aveeno-First and the Aveeno-Subsequently groups. Delayed prescribing of Aveeno was associated with significantly higher costs for prescriptions and more GP visits within the 2 years following the diagnosis of atopic eczema (2.89 visits for Aveeno-First vs. 4.14 visits for Aveeno-Subsequently, a difference of 43.1%). Prescribing Aveeno as a first-line treatment for DS&E was associated with lower visit costs and lower overall costs than in the Aveeno-Subsequently group within the 2 years following the index diagnosis (Fig. 4).

The percentage of patients prescribed potent or very potent TCS (Fig. 4) was lower in the Aveeno-First group (10.24%) than in the Aveeno-Subsequently group (16.14%), with the odds ratio of being prescribed a potent or very potent TCS in the Aveeno-Subsequently group versus the Aveeno-First group being 1.914 (95% CI: 1.489–2.462). Hence, patients had 91% greater odds of receiving a prescription for a treatment with potent or very potent TCS when not prescribed Aveeno first than when Aveeno was prescribed first.

The percentage of patients treated with skin-condition-related antimicrobials was also lower in the Aveeno-First group (35.96%) than in the Aveeno-Subsequently group (49.08%; Fig. 4). The odds ratio of being prescribed an antimicrobial in the Aveeno-Subsequently group versus the Aveeno-First group was 1.748 (95% CI: 1.495–2.044). Hence, patients who did not receive Aveeno first-line had 75% greater odds of treatment with antimicrobial than when Aveeno was received first-line.

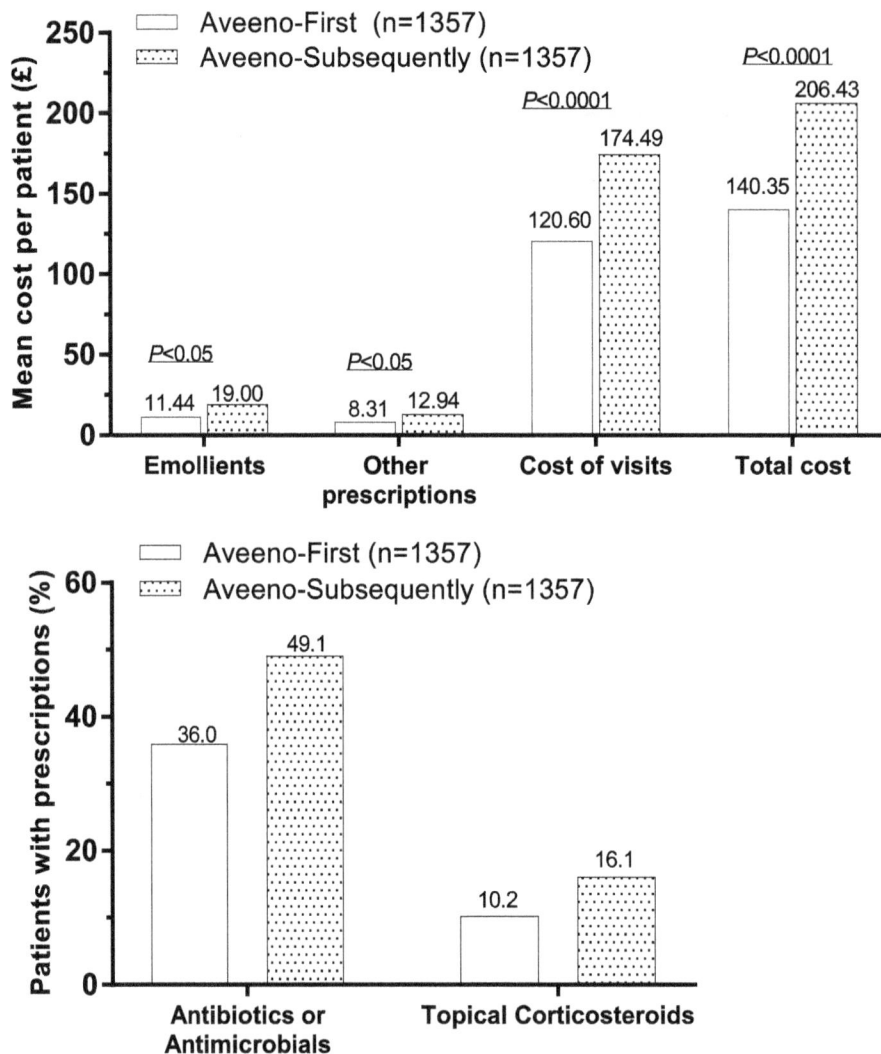

Fig. 4 Cost (top) and medication use (bottom) in matched Aveeno-First versus Aveeno-Subsequently groups

Discussion

This study evaluated the utilisation and costs of primary healthcare resources using data from the CPRD to estimate the value of prescribing emollients for DS&E to patients presenting to their GP in the UK. In examining the component costs of care, including emollients, other medicines prescribed for DS&E, and patient visits, the most important cost driver appeared to be the number and associated cost of patient visits by patients to primary care, with the Emollient and Aveeno-First groups having fewer clinic visits and therefore lower overall costs than the Non-Emollient and Aveeno-Never groups. Reducing repeat visits is particularly relevant to the UK, where the annual GP consultation rate per person increased more than 13% from 2007 to 2014 [34], and has continued to increase to the point that GP practice is in a state of crisis with escalating demand outstripping capacity [35, 36].

Skin disorders, such as eczema, make up a significant portion of the GP's workload in the UK and elsewhere [19, 37], and primary care visits in the UK for skin diseases and eczema have been increasing year on year [4]. A 2014 King's Fund report [38], using data based on a report by Schofield et al. [39], suggested that, with an average of two consultations per episode, the average GP with a patient list size of 1700 would have had 630 consultations for skin conditions per year in 2006 [39]. Reducing patient visits to primary care would not only benefit patients and reduce demand on primary care, but could also help reduce the burden on the entire healthcare service [36, 40].

This study suggests that a policy to prescribe emollients to patients when the diagnosis of DS&E is initially made may save the NHS money, or at least be cost-neutral. Initial analysis identified that more patients with a diagnosis of DS&E received a prescription for an emollient than those who did not (45,218 vs. 9780). The age distribution of Emollient versus Non-Emollient pre-match groups indicated that the Emollient group was substantially younger than the Non-Emollient group. As prescriptions for children under 16 years are dispensed free of charge, they may be more likely to be filled than those incurring a cost to the patient. Hence, non-paediatric patients may be encouraged to purchase an emollient rather than fill a prescription, and thus would incur personal costs to obtain treatment for this condition that would not be recorded in the CPRD. The effect of the patient purchasing an emollient under these conditions would have skewed healthcare system costs away from emollient prescriptions that were reimbursed and reduced the apparent efficacy of treatment and the observed differences seen between Emollient and Non-Emollient groups.

Although emollients are recommended as first-line therapy for DS&E [5, 7, 24], current and future cost pressures on the NHS are likely to put more pressure on primary care providers to avoid issuing prescriptions for emollients [7] or to choose the prescribed emollient primarily on the basis of cost [41]. Furthermore, patients tend to use emollients sub-optimally in insufficient quantity, and too infrequently [7, 9]. Encouraging purchase rather than prescription could exacerbate this tendency and the negative impact on clinical outcomes, potentially increasing health costs for follow-up visits and additional medications in the longer term.

In the Aveeno-First versus Aveeno-Subsequently comparison, visit and prescription costs were significantly greater when the patient did not receive Aveeno as a first-line treatment, suggesting that costs increase when a patient requires repeat healthcare visits to adjust treatment. In DS&E, this study suggests that, rather than reserving Aveeno as a second or third-line therapy, prescribing Aveeno first-line may save NHS primary care costs. In a recent UK study of emollient therapy for eczema in children, four different emollients, including Aveeno, were evaluated [20]. In that study, no significant difference was noted among the costs of the emollients, and similar to the study reported herein, the main cost driver was the cost of a primary care appointment.

This study also indicates a reduction in steroid prescriptions in the Emollient and Aveeno-First groups, and supports previous research suggesting emollient use can reduce the need for a TCS prescription [8–10, 12].

Another important finding was that emollient therapy, and Aveeno in particular, might reduce the need for prescriptions of antimicrobial therapy in eczema. This study appears to be the first report suggesting that emollient therapy can reduce the need for antimicrobial prescriptions, and supports the findings of Francis and co-workers, who reported that oral and topical antibiotics had little or no benefit to reduce eczema severity in children with clinically infected eczema already being treated with emollients and TCS [42, 43]. Reducing antibiotic use will help the GP professional community to contribute to antimicrobial stewardship goals [44, 45], thereby slowing the development of antimicrobial resistance, an area of grave concern [46]. Additional research will be required to confirm these findings.

Limitations

As with all database studies, the findings presented herein assume accurate diagnoses of patients and do not correct for potential errors in coding. Disease types included for initial cohort identification were broad (Table 1); however, the analysis was based on groups matched exactly for index diagnosis. Furthermore, this analysis may be relevant to the UK healthcare system only, as other healthcare systems, such as those in the EU or USA, may not reimburse emollient prescriptions for DS&E and costs will be different in these healthcare systems.

Severity of disease was not available in the CPRD as disease severities are not recorded in the database beyond those captured by normal diagnoses. More severe patients prescribed a TCS may not receive a prescription for an emollient that visit because the prescriber is focussed on using the TCS. Thus, should cases in the Emollient groups (including Aveeno groups) have been less severe, this may have overestimated the effect of the emollient therapy in a group expected to have fewer visits and lower costs. However, we tried to minimise the effect of a severity bias by matching for age and type of disease.

Total costs may have been underestimated because only costs associated with a DS&E diagnosis were considered for this analysis. Personal purchase of emollients by patients was not captured in the CPRD and thus might result in an underestimate of the use of emollients and inaccurate assignment of patients to the Non-Emollient group, which would tend to bias the results towards no effect.

Conversely, prescriptions that were written but not filled cannot be identified and could have resulted in an overestimate of the proportion of emollient users, although some of those with unfilled prescriptions may have selected to purchase an emollient for themselves instead. We tried to reduce the impact of this limitation by requiring two distinct prescriptions for the Emollient group, ensuring that these patients were highly likely to have filled at least one prescription. Each of these scenarios could have influenced the study to reduce the apparent positive impact of prescribing emollients and specifically Aveeno.

Direct matching of groups and age differences between Non-Emollient and Emollient groups may have resulted in groups that do not reflect the overall population of patients with DS&E in the CPRD. In the matched group analysis of the Emollient versus Non-Emollient group, to maximise the size of the Non-Emollient group, the Emollient group had more adults than the overall pre-matched Emollient group. However, in the analyses of Emollient groups, the demographics more closely match those in the overall Emollient population.

Conclusions

In conclusion, this study suggested that prescription of an emollient to treat DS&E may be associated with reduced cost of care, primarily owing to fewer primary care visits and other prescriptions, though disease severity is an unknown and potential confounder in this analysis. Emollient cost was a small fraction of the overall cost of treating eczema in general practice. Furthermore, prescribing emollients was associated with a potential for fewer antibiotic or potent/very potent TCS prescriptions. Timely prescribing of Aveeno to improve the integrity of the skin barrier [47, 48] can result in fewer flares and would probably result in decreased antimicrobial prescribing in UK primary care. Prescribing Aveeno was also associated with overall lower costs compared with prescribing other emollients, and overall costs were lowered most when Aveeno was prescribed first, rather than when prescribed as a second or subsequent choice for patients who may have found other products unsuitable.

Abbreviations

AD: Atopic dermatitis; CCI: Charlson Comorbidity Index; CPRD: Clinical Practice Research Datalink; DS&E: Dry skin and atopic eczema; GEE: Generalised estimating eqs.; GP: General practitioner; ISAC: Independent Scientific Advisory Committee; NHS: National Health Service; NIC: Net ingredient cost; NICE: National Institute for Health and Care Excellence; PSSRU: Personal Social Services Research Unit; TCS: Topical corticosteroids

Acknowledgements

Medical writing and editorial support was provided by Alex Loeb, PhD, CMPP, of Evidence Scientific Solutions, Philadelphia, PA, USA and was funded by Johnson & Johnson Consumer Inc., Skillman, NJ, USA.

Funding

This study was funded by Johnson & Johnson Ltd. (UK).

Authors' contributions

All authors have read and approved the manuscript. GM, SR: Drafting the manuscript and revising it critically for important intellectual content. CH, GN, ALL: Conception and acquisition of data, data analysis, revising manuscript critically for important intellectual content. RW, DW: data analysis, revising manuscript critically for important intellectual content.

Competing interests

CH, GN, ALL, RW, DW are employees of the study sponsor, Johnson & Johnson.
GM and SR have received research funding from Johnson & Johnson.

Author details

[1]Mayfield Clinic Summertown, Oxford OX2 7DE, UK. [2]Johnson & Johnson Ltd (UK), Maidenhead, Berkshire, UK. [3]Johnson & Johnson, Inc, New Brunswick, NJ, USA. [4]Janssen Research and Development, LLC, Titusville, NJ, USA. [5]NHS Wakefield Clinical Commissioning Group, West Yorkshire, UK.

References

1. Odhiambo JA, Williams HC, Clayton TO, Robertson CF, Asher MI. ISAAC phase Three Study Group: global variations in prevalence of eczema symptoms in children from ISAAC Phase Three. J Allergy Clin Immunol. 2009;124(6):1251–8.
2. Abuabara K, Yu AM, Okhovat JP, Allen IE, Langan SM. The prevalence of atopic dermatitis beyond childhood: a systematic review and meta-analysis of longitudinal studies. Allergy. 2017;73(3):696–704.
3. Herd RM, Tidman MJ, Prescott RJ, Hunter JA. The cost of atopic eczema. Br J Dermatol. 1996;135(1):20–3.
4. Simpson CR, Newton J, Hippisley-Cox J, Sheikh A. Trends in the epidemiology and prescribing of medication for eczema in England. J R Soc Med. 2009;102(3):108–17.
5. Atopic eczema in under 12s: diagnosis and management (CG57) [https://www.nice.org.uk/guidance/cg57/resources/atopic-eczema-in-under-12s-diagnosis-and-management-pdf-975512529349].
6. Zuberbier T, Orlow SJ, Paller AS, Taïeb A, Allen R, Hernanz-Hermosa JM, Ocampo-Candiani J, Cox M, Langeraar J, Simon JC. Patient perspectives on the management of atopic dermatitis. J Allergy Clin Immunol. 2006;118(1):226–32.
7. Moncrieff G, Cork M, Lawton S, Kokiet S, Daly C, Clark C. Use of emollients in dry-skin conditions: consensus statement. Clin Exp Dermatol. 2013;38(3):231–8.
8. Msika P, De Belilovsky C, Piccardi N, Chebassier N, Baudouin C, Chadoutaud B. New emollient with topical corticosteroid-sparing effect in treatment of childhood atopic dermatitis: SCORAD and quality of life improvement. Pediatr Dermatol. 2008;25(6):606–12.
9. Cork MJ, Britton J, Butler L, Young S, Murphy R, Keohane SG. Comparison of parent knowledge, therapy utilization and severity of atopic eczema before and after explanation and demonstration of topical therapies by a specialist dermatology nurse. Br J Dermatol. 2003;149(3):582–9.
10. Harcharik S, Emer J. Steroid-sparing properties of emollients in dermatology. Skin Therapy Lett. 2014;19(1):5–10.
11. Johansson SG, Bieber T, Dahl R, Friedmann PS, Lanier BQ, Lockey RF, Motala C, Ortega Martell JA, Platts-Mills TA, Ring J, et al. Revised nomenclature for allergy for global use: report of the Nomenclature Review Committee of the

World Allergy Organization, October 2003. J Allergy Clin Immunol. 2004; 113(5):832–6.

12. van Zuuren EJ, Fedorowicz Z, Christensen R, APM L, BWM A. Emollients and moisturisers for eczema. Cochrane Database Syst Rev. 2017;2. https://doi.org/10.1002/14651858.CD012119.pub2.

13. Bantz SK, Zhu Z, Zheng T. The atopic march: progression from atopic dermatitis to allergic rhinitis and asthma. J Clin Cell Immunol. 2014;5:202.

14. Simpson EL, Chalmers JR, Hanifin JM, Thomas KS, Cork MJ, McLean WH, Brown SJ, Chen Z, Chen Y, Williams HC. Emollient enhancement of the skin barrier from birth offers effective atopic dermatitis prevention. J Allergy Clin Immunol. 2014;134(4):818–23.

15. Chalmers JR, Haines RH, Mitchell EJ, Thomas KS, Brown SJ, Ridd M, Lawton S, Simpson EL, Cork MJ, Sach TH, et al. Effectiveness and cost-effectiveness of daily all-over-body application of emollient during the first year of life for preventing atopic eczema in high-risk children (the BEEP trial): protocol for a randomised controlled trial. Trials. 2017;18(1):343.

16. Lowe AJ, Su JC, Allen KJ, Abramson MJ, Cranswick N, Robertson CF, Forster D, Varigos G, Hamilton S, Kennedy R, et al. A randomized trial of a barrier lipid replacement strategy for the prevention of atopic dermatitis and allergic sensitization: the PEBBLES pilot study. Br J Dermatol. 2018;178(1):e19–21.

17. Horimukai K, Morita K, Narita M, Kondo M, Kitazawa H, Nozaki M, Shigematsu Y, Yoshida K, Niizeki H, Motomura K, et al. Application of moisturizer to neonates prevents development of atopic dermatitis. J Allergy Clin Immunol. 2014;134(4):824–30.

18. Mason JM, Carr J, Buckley C, Hewitt S, Berry P, Taylor J, Cork MJ. Improved emollient use reduces atopic eczema symptoms and is cost neutral in infants: before-and-after evaluation of a multifaceted educational support programme. BMC Dermatol. 2013;13:7.

19. Verboom P, Hakkaart-Van L, Sturkenboom M, De Zeeuw R, Menke H, Rutten F. The cost of atopic dermatitis in the Netherlands: an international comparison. Br J Dermatol. 2002;147(4):716–24.

20. Ridd MJ, Garfield K, Gaunt DM, Hollinghurst S, Redmond NM, Powell K, Wilson V, Guy RH, Ball N, Shaw L, et al. Choice of Moisturiser for Eczema Treatment (COMET): feasibility study of a randomised controlled parallel group trial in children recruited from primary care. BMJ Open. 2016;6(11):e012021.

21. Batchelor JM, Ridd MJ, Clarke T, Ahmed A, Cox M, Crowe S, Howard M, Lawton S, McPhee M, Rani A, et al. The Eczema Priority Setting Partnership: a collaboration between patients, carers, clinicians and researchers to identify and prioritize important research questions for the treatment of eczema. Br J Dermatol. 2013;168(3):577–82.

22. Lindh JD, Bradley M. Clinical effectiveness of moisturizers in atopic dermatitis and related disorders: a systematic review. Am J Clin Dermatol. 2015;16(5):341–59.

23. Herrett E, Gallagher AM, Bhaskaran K, Forbes H, Mathur R, van Staa T, Smeeth L. Data resource profile: clinical Practice Research Datalink (CPRD). Int J Epidemiol. 2015;44(3):827–36.

24. Lewis-Jones S, Mugglestone MA. Guideline Development Group: Management of atopic eczema in children aged up to 12 years: summary of NICE guidance. BMJ. 2007;335(7632):1263–4.

25. Kurtz ES, Wallo W. Colloidal oatmeal: history, chemistry and clinical properties. J Drugs Dermatol. 2007;6(2):167–70.

26. Fowler JF Jr. Colloidal oatmeal formulations and the treatment of atopic dermatitis. J Drugs Dermatol. 2014;13(10):1180–3.

27. Quan H, Li B, Couris CM, Fushimi K, Graham P, Hider P, Januel JM, Sundararajan V. Updating and validating the Charlson comorbidity index and score for risk adjustment in hospital discharge abstracts using data from 6 countries. Am J Epidemiol. 2011;173(6):676–82.

28. Roffman CE, Buchanan J, Allison GT. Charlson Comorbidities Index. J Physiother. 2016;62(3):171.

29. Charlson ME, Pompei P, Ales KL, MacKenzie CR. A new method of classifying prognostic comorbidity in longitudinal studies: development and validation. J Chronic Dis. 1987;40(5):373–83.

30. Hubbard AE, Ahern J, Fleischer NL, Van der Laan M, Lippman SA, Jewell N, Bruckner T, Satariano WA. To GEE or not to GEE: comparing population average and mixed models for estimating the associations between neighborhood risk factors and health. Epidemiology. 2010;21(4):467–74.

31. Dean B, Carmichael A. Emollient packs: providing choice in dermatology. Nurs Pract. 2006;30:52.

32. Curtis L, Burns A: Unit costs of health and social care 2015. University of Kent, Canterbury: Personal Social Services Research Unit (PSSRU); 2015. http://www.pssru.ac.uk/project-pages/unit-costs/2015/. Accessed 21 Sept 2017.

33. Health & Social Care Information Centre. Prescription cost analysis: England 2015. 2016. https://files.digital.nhs.uk/publicationimport/pub20xxx/pub20200/pres-cost-anal-eng-2015-rep.pdf.

34. Hobbs FDR, Bankhead C, Mukhtar T, Stevens S, Perera-Salazar R, Holt T, Salisbury C, National Institute for Health Research School for Primary Care R. Clinical workload in UK primary care: a retrospective analysis of 100 million consultations in England, 2007-14. Lancet. 2016;387(10035):2323–30.

35. International Medical Press. GMC: medical profession at breaking point. 2017. https://www.univadis.co.uk/viewarticle/gmc-medical-profession-at-breaking-point-574740?u=g7Nnk16ewgvMdmxgbnmgSZF1%2BQxifzEMX%2BWttAFi2HUQ0lE2b0tVyTSvUNWAn2cK&utm_source=adhoc%20email&utm_medium=%20weekly%202.5%20specialists&utm_content=1857967&utm_term=. Accessed 15 Jan 2018.

36. General Medical Council: The state of medical education and practice in the UK. In. London, UK. General Medical Council. 2017. https://www.gmc-uk.org/about/what-we-do-and-why/data-and-research/the-state-of-medical-educationand-practice-in-the-uk. Accessed 26 Jan 2018.

37. Kerr OA, Tidman MJ, Walker JJ, Aldridge RD, Benton EC. The profile of dermatological problems in primary care. Clin Exp Dermatol. 2010;35(4):380–3.

38. The King's Fund: How can dermatology services meet current and future patient needs while ensuring that quality of care is not compromised and that access is equitable across the UK? 2014. http://www.bad.org.uk/shared/get-file.ashx?id=2347&itemtype=document. Accessed 27 Sept 2017.

39. Schofield JK, Fleming D, Grindlay D, Williams H. Skin conditions are the commonest new reason people present to general practitioners in England and Wales. Br J Dermatol. 2011;165(5):1044–50.

40. Montgomery HE, Haines A, Marlow N, Pearson G, Mythen MG, Grocott MPW, Swanton C. The future of UK healthcare: problems and potential solutions to a system in crisis. Ann Oncol. 2017;28(8):1751–5.

41. Wiltshire Clinical Commissioning Group: Emollient prescribing guideline for adults in primary care April 2017. 2017. http://www.bcapformulary.nhs.uk/includes/documents/Emollients_Prescribing_Guideline_-April-2017-FINAL.pdf. Accessed 27 Sept 2017.

42. Francis NA, Ridd MJ, Thomas-Jones E, Butler CC, Hood K, Shepherd V, Marwick CA, Huang C, Longo M, Wootton M, et al. Oral and topical antibiotics for clinically infected eczema in children: a pragmatic randomized controlled trial in ambulatory care. Ann Fam Med. 2017;15(2):124–30.

43. Francis NA, Ridd MJ, Thomas-Jones E, Shepherd V, Butler CC, Hood K, Huang C, Addison K, Longo M, Marwick C et al: A randomised placebo-controlled trial of oral and topical antibiotics for children with clinically infected eczema in the community: the ChildRen with Eczema, Antibiotic Management (CREAM) study. Health Technol Assess. 2016;20(19):i-xxiv,1–84.

44. Public Health England, NHS England: Patient safety alert. Stage two: resources. Addressing antimicrobial resistance through implementation of an antimicrobial stewardship programme. 2015. http://www.england.nhs.uk/wpcontent/uploads/2015/08/psa-amr-stewardship-prog.pdf. Accessed 26 Jan 2018.

45. National Institute for Health and Care Excellence (NICE). Antimicrobial stewardship: systems and processes for effective antimicrobial medicine use (NICE guideline). 2015. https://www.nice.org.uk/guidance/ng15/resources/antimicrobial-stewardship-systems-andprocesses-for-effective-antimicrobial-medicine-use-pdf-1837273110469. Accessed June 18, 2018.

46. O'Neill J. Antimicrobial resistance: tackling a crisis for the health and wealth of nations in: Review on Antimicrobial Resistance. Chaired by Jim O'Neill. 2014. https://amrreview.org/sites/default/files/AMR%20Review%20Paper%20-%20Tackling%20a%20crisis%20for%20the%20health%20and%20wealth%20of%20nations_1.pdf. Accessed 15 Jan 2018.

47. Ilnytska O, Kaur S, Chon S, Reynertson KA, Nebus J, Garay M, Mahmood K, Southall MD. Colloidal oatmeal (Avena Sativa) improves skin barrier through multi-therapy activity. J Drugs Dermatol. 2016;15(6):684–90.

48. Lisante TA, Nunez C, Zhang P, Mathes BM. A 1% colloidal oatmeal cream alone is effective in reducing symptoms of mild to moderate atopic dermatitis: results from two clinical studies. J Drugs Dermatol. 2017;16(7):671–6.

Randomized placebo control study of insulin sensitizers (Metformin and Pioglitazone) in psoriasis patients with metabolic syndrome (Topical Treatment Cohort)

Surjit Singh[1*] and Anil Bhansali[2]

Abstract

Background: Increased prevalence of metabolic syndrome (MS) is observed in psoriasis. Metformin has shown improvement in cardiovascular risk factors while pioglitazone demonstrated anti proliferative, anti-inflammatory and anti angiogenic effects. Study objective is to evaluate the efficacy and safety of Insulin sensitizers (metformin and pioglitazone) in psoriasis patients with metabolic syndrome (MS).

Methods: Single centre, parallel group, randomized, study of metformin, pioglitazone and placebo in psoriasis patients with MS.

Results: Statistically significant improvement was observed in Psoriasis Area and Severity Index (PASI), Erythema, Scaling and Induration (ESI) and Physician global assessment (PGA) scores in pioglitazone (p values – PASI = 0.001, ESI = 0.002, PGA = 0.008) and metformin groups (p values – PASI = 0.001, ESI = 0.016, PGA = 0.012) as compared to placebo. There was statistically significant difference in percentage of patients achieving 75 % reduction in PASI and ESI scores in metformin (p value – PASI = 0.001, ESI = 0.001) and pioglitazone groups (p vaue – PASI = 0.001, ESI = 0. 001). Significant improvement was observed in fasting plasma glucose (FPG) and triglycerides levels in metformin and pioglitazone arms. Significant improvement was noted in weight, BMI, waist circumference, FPG, triglycerides and total cholesterol after 12 weeks of treatment with metformin while pioglitazone showed improvement in FPG, triglyceride levels, systolic blood pressure (SBP), diastolic blood pressure (DBP), total cholesterol and LDL cholesterol levels. There was no difference in pattern of adverse drug reaction in three groups.

Conclusion: Insulin sensitizers have shown improvement in the parameters of MS as well as disease severity in psoriasis patients.

Keywords: Psoriasis, Metabolic syndrome, Insulin sensitizers, Metformin, Pioglitazone

Abbreviations: ACE inhibitors, Angiotensin Converting Enzyme Inhibitors; ALT, Alanine Transaminase; AMPK, Adenosine Monophosphate-activated Protein Kinase; ANOVA, Analysis of Variance; AST, Aspartate Transaminase; BMI, Body Mass Index; CVS, Cardiovascular; DBP, Diastolic Blood Pressure; DM, Diabetes Mellitus; ERK1/
(Continued on next page)

* Correspondence: sehmby_ss@yahoo.com; ss.sehmby@gmail.com
[1]Department of Pharmacology, All India Institute of Medical Sciences (AIIMS), Jodhpur 342005, India
Full list of author information is available at the end of the article

(Continued from previous page)
2, Extracellular Signal-related Kinase 1/2; ESI, Erythema, Scaling and Induration; FPG, Fasting Plasma Glucose; HDL, High density lipoprotein; HTN, Hypertension; IL, Interleukin; LDL, Low Density Lipoprotein; LOCF, Last Observation Carry Forward; MS, Metabolic Syndrome; NCEP ATP III, National Cholesterol Education Program's Adult Treatment Panel III; OD, Once Daily; PASI, Psoriasis Area and Severity Index; PFA, Physician Global Assessment; PPAR-γ, Peroxisome Proliferator-activated receptor- γ; SBP, Systolic Blood Pressure; SD, Standard Deviation; TNF-α, Tumor Necrosis Factor- α; TZD, Thiazolidinedione

Background

Psoriasis is a chronic, inflammatory multisystemic disorder with genetic basis affecting 2-3 % of world population and affecting about 0.4 % of Asians [1]. Psoriasis has been found to be associated more commonly with obesity, metabolic syndrome (MS) [1, 2], diabetes mellitus [3] and increased cardiovascular (CVS) mortality and morbidity [4–6]. Metabolic syndrome (MS) is a cluster of risk factors including central obesity, atherogenic dyslipidemia, hypertension and glucose intolerance and is a strong predictor of cardiovascular diseases, diabetes and stroke [7–9]. Many cytokines (e.g. interferon-γ, TNF-α, IL-6, IL-8, IL-12, IL-17, IL-19 and IL-23) involved in the pathogenesis of psoriasis are also known to contribute to the cascade of metabolic syndrome such as hypertension, dyslipidemia and insulin resistance [10]. Prodifferentiating, antiproliferative, anti-inflammatory and antiangiogenic effects of Peroxisome proliferator-activated receptor- γ (PPAR-γ) ligands may potentially have beneficial role in psoriasis [11–13] as exemplified by demonstrated efficacy of Thiazolidinediones (TZDs) in treatment of psoriasis [14–18]. Metformin is an 'insulin sensitiser', lowers glucose levels without increasing insulin secretion. It has shown additional beneficial effects in adults with type 2 diabetes, including weight reduction, decreasing hyperinsulinemia, improving lipid profiles, augmented fibrinolysis and enhanced endothelial function [19–21], that all are usual metabilic abnormalities observed in subjects with MS. Therfore we anticipated that such pharmacological effects observed with metformin might be of use in psoriatic patients with MS. To the best of our knowledge no study till date has evaluated metformin and pioglitazone head to head in patients of psoriasis with MS. Present study was planned as comparative evaluation of safety & efficay of metformin with pioglitazone in placebo controlled setting in patients of psoriasis with MS.

Methods

Clinical trial design

Study was approved by Institute Ethics committee, Post Graduate Institute of Medical Education and Research. This clinical trial was a single centre, parallel group, randomized, open label with blinded endpoint assessment of metformin, pioglitazone and placebo in psoriasis patients with MS satisfying inclusion and exclusion criteria. Our study is a part of larger study in which we evaluated the prevalence of MS in psoriasis. Then psoriasis patients having MS were divided into systemic (moderate to severe psoriasis, randomized into metformin and placebo arms) and topical treatment cohort (mild to moderate psoriasis, randomized into metformin, piolglitazone and placebo arms) and were evaluated for the effect of insulin sensitizers on disease parameters and MS. In this paper, we have discussed the results of topical treatment cohort.

All patients visiting psoriasis clinic at our Institute were screened for MS and other eligibility criteria. Both males and females, > 18 years with plaque psoriasis [mild to moderate disease severity (<10 % of body surface area) [22], on treatment (had taken even a single application of topical therapy in the past) and treatment naïve (no past history of treatment for their disease)] and having MS i.e. the presence of three or more criteria of the modified National Cholesterol Education Program's Adult Treatment Panel III (NCEP ATP III) [23]: waist circumference > 90 cm in men and > 80 cm in women, hypertriglyceridemia ≥ 150 mg/dl, high density lipoprotein (HDL) cholesterol < 40 mg/dl in males and < 50 mg/dl in females, blood pressure ≥ 130/85 mmHg and fasting plasma glucose ≥ 110 mg/dl and willing to provide written informed consent were included in the study. Patients with severe disease, on topical therapy other than coal tar, pregnant or nursing women, significant hepatic impairment (serum bilirubin, AST, ALT and alkaline phosphatase >1.5 times the upper limit of normal), renal insufficiency - serum creatinine ≥1.5 mg/dL (men) or ≥1.4 mg/dL (women) and contraindication to metformin and pioglitazone were excluded from the study.

Clinical examination including psoriasis area and severity index (PASI) [22] scores and erythema, scaling and induration (ESI) scoring [24] was done. Clinical photographs of patients were taken at baseline and post treatment. Baseline investigations were done and eligible patients were randomized in an open label manner to either placebo (empty gelatin capsules), metformin 1000 mg once daily (O.D) or pioglitazone 30 mg O.D groups for a period of 12 weeks, after taking written informed consent. All patients were given standard topical 5 % coal tar ointment in addition to study drugs. The randomization codes were computer generated. Randomization codes were concealed in an opaque envelope. The drug dispensation was done by a person who was not involved with the assessment of the study endpoints. Evaluation for efficacy parameters was done at 0 and 12 weeks. Safety evaluation was also done throughout the study.

Efficacy evaluation

Blinded end points assessment of the efficacy parameters was done at 12 weeks. Psoriasis lesions were evaluated using psoriasis area and severity index (PASI) scores and erythema, scaling and induration (ESI) score [24]. Each component of ESI was graded from 0 to 3; 0 – clear, 1 - mild, 2 - moderate, 3 - severe. The most severe condition was given 9 points whereas absence of disease been given 0 points.

Also all the parameters of MS as defined by modified National Cholesterol Education Program's Adult Treatment Panel III (NCEPIII) criteria [23] were assesed at baseline and 12 weeks. Serum IL-6 and TNF-α levels was done at 0 and 12 weeks in subgroup (10, 7 and 9 patients in placebo, metformin and pioglitazone groups respectively) of patients by Human ELISA kit (RayBiotech, Inc. Georgia. USA).

The primary efficacy end point was mean change in PASI, ESI and PGA scores from baseline after 12 weeks of therapy between three treatment groups given along with standard treatment for psoriasis. The Secondary efficacy end point were number of parameters of MS improved, change in individual parameters of MS, IL -6 and TNF – α from baseline after 12 weeks of treatment with metformin, pioglitazone or placebo. The change in Physician Global Assessment (PGA) from baseline and percentage of patients achieving 75 % reduction in ESI and PGA score in the three treatment groups were other end points.

Sample size calculation

Assuming a standard deviation of 2 in PASI scores, and a difference of 2 in PASI score between drug and placebo arm at 12 weeks to be clinically significant at α = 0.05 and with 80 % power, a sample size of 16 patients per group has been calculated and with a dropout rate of about 20 %, 19 patients will be required to be included in each group.

Statistical analysis

Data was expressed as Mean ± SD (95 % confidence intervals), numbers (percentages) and median (interquartile range). Baseline characteristics between three treatment groups were compared using one way ANOVA for numerical variables and Chi-Square test for categorical variables. Analysis was carried out using intention to treat principle.

Mean changes in PASI, ESI and PGA scores at 12 weeks from baseline between three treatment groups were compared using One way ANOVA followed by post hoc Scheffe. Chi-Square test or Fischer's Exact test was used to compare the categorical variables. Intra group comparison of mean changes in individual parameters of MS and lipid profile was carried out by paired T-test and inter group comparison by One way ANOVA. Difference in changes in serum levels of IL-6 and TNF-α between the groups was done by One way ANOVA.

Results were analyzed as Intention-to-treat analysis with last observation carry forward (LOCF). A two-sided P-value less than 0.05 was considered as statistically significant.

Results

A total of 83 consecutive adult psoriasis patients with MS were screened from June 2010 to April 2011 (Fig. 1). Out of 83 patients, 23 were excluded from the study. 23, 16 and 21 patients were randomized to placebo, pioglitazone and metformin treatment groups respectively. Disposition of patients and reasons for withdrawal were summarized in Fig. 1. Hence, 21 patients in placebo arm, 16 in pioglitazone and 18 patients in metformin arm completed the study. As Intention to treat analysis with last observation carry forward (LOCF) was done, so all the subjects as randomized were included for final analysis.

No significant difference was observed in baseline demographics and MS characteristics among three treatment groups except past history of remission (Table 1).

ESI and PGA scores and parameters of Metabolic Syndrome (MS)

Statistically significant improvement was observed in PASI, ESI and PGA scores in pioglitazone (P values – PASI = 0.001, ESI = 0.002, PGA = 0.008) and metformin groups (P values – PASI = 0.001, ESI = 0.016, PGA = 0.012) as compared to placebo (Fig. 2). There was statistically significant difference in percentage of parameters of MS improved following 12 weeks of treatment in pioglitazone (15 %) and metformin (16.2 %) groups as compared to placebo (3.5 %) (Fig. 3). Statistically significant difference in percentage of patients achieving 75 % reduction in PASI and ESI scores in metformin (p value – PASI = 0.001, ESI = 0.001) and pioglitazone groups (p value – PASI = 0.001, ESI = 0.001) (Fig. 4). Statistically significant improvement is observed in FPG, total cholesterol and triglycerides levels (Table 2) in metformin and pioglitazone arms as compared to placebo. Significant improvement was also observed in percentage of

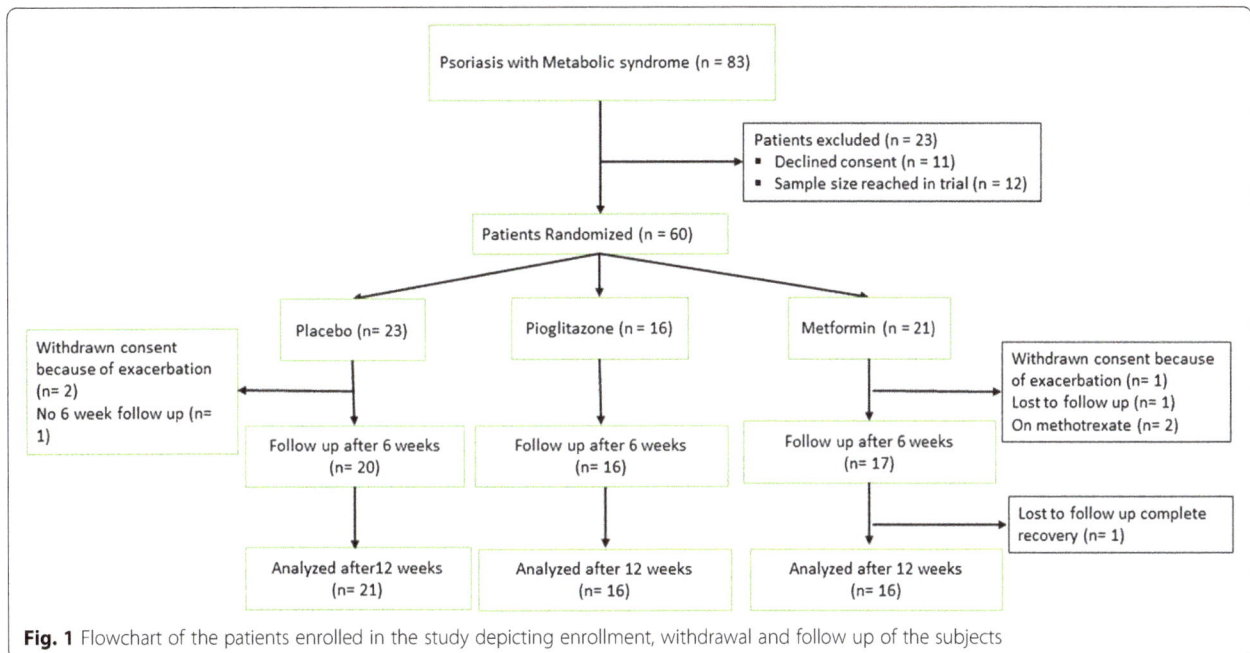

Fig. 1 Flowchart of the patients enrolled in the study depicting enrollment, withdrawal and follow up of the subjects

patients achieving 75 % reduction in PGA scores (Fig. 4) and change in weight and waist circumference in metformin group as compared to placebo (Table 2). Significant improvement was observed in weight, BMI, waist circumference, FPG, triglycerides and total cholesterol after treatment with metformin (Table 2). Similarly improvement was seen in FPG, triglyceride levels, systolic blood pressure (SBP), diastolic blood pressure (DBP), total cholesterol and LDL cholesterol levels after treatment with pioglitazone for 12 weeks (Table 2). No significant change in the IL-6 and TNF-α levels among three groups (Fig. 5).

No significant difference in the mean number of adverse events in three groups except for weight gain between metformin and pioglitazone (Table 3).

Discussion

Baseline characteristics were similar among three treatment groups except for percentage of individuals having remission. The difference observed in baseline characteristic is unlikely to be of clinical significance and could not have accounted for the higher efficacy observed in metformin and pioglitazone groups in comparison to placebo group. All patients were given topical 5 % coal tar treatment. As the compliance achieved is around 90 %, which is ensured by direct questioning and pill count, it is less likely that topical treatment with 5 % coal tar would have resulted in the differences in efficacy among three treatment groups. In our study, metformin and pioglitazone cause significant improvement in PASI, ESI and PGA scores as compared to placebo.

In metformin, pioglitazone and placebo group, 52.4 %, 50 % and 17.4 % of the patients had complete improvement in MS respectively (metformin vs placebo – OR (95 % CI), 5.2 (1.3–20.7), P value = 0.019; pioglitazone vs placebo – (OR (95 % CI) = 4.8 (1.1–20.4), P value = 0.036; metformin vs pioglitazone – (OR (95 % CI) = 0.9 (0.2–3.3), P value = 0.886). Therefore, metformin and pioglitazone beneficial effect on MS parameters might be accounted for the improved efficacy in psoriasis disease itself.

Clinical studies had also demonstrated the proof of efficacy of TZDs in psoriasis. Pioglitazone had demonstrated superior efficacy to placebo group alone as well as in combination therapy with acitretin in psoriasis patients [14, 15]. Two open label studies [16, 17] had demonstrated marked improvement in psoriasis lesions with troglitazone in chronic plaque type psoriasis patients. Robertshaw and Friedman [18] have also demonstrated excellent improvement with pioglitazone in 4 out of 5 patients with chronic plaque type psoriasis in an open label, pilot study.

Study done by Bongartz et al (2005) with pioglitazone 60 mg/day for 12 weeks in psoriatic arthritis patients with tender and swollen joints, demonstrated 60 % of the patients met the psoriatic arthritis response criterion. Mean percentage reduction in PASI was 38 %, along with median tender joint count decreased from 12–4 and median swollen joint count from 5 to 2 (P <0.05 for both) [25]. The observed higher percentage reduction in ESI and PGA scores in our study is thus expected and is a demonstration of pioglitazone efficacy.

Table 1 Baseline characteristics of three treatment groups

Baseline characteristics	Placebo (n = 23)	Metformin (n = 21)	Pioglitazone (n = 16)	p-value
Age (years) Mean (±SD)	46.9 (±10.4)	45.1 (±13.0)	44.0 (±12.9)	0.747
Male/Females, n (%)	14/9 (60.9/39.1)	12/9 (57.1/42.9)	9/7 (56.3/43.7)	0.950
Total duration of disease (years) Mean (±SD)	9.1 (±8.6)	6.0 (±6.9)	6.9 (±11.2)	0.492
Seasonal Exacerbation, n (%)	13 (56.5)	13 (61.9)	6 (37.5)	0.313
Seasonal improvement, n (%)	13 (56.5)	13 (61.9)	5 (31.3)	0.152
Remission, n (%)	21 (91.3)	11 (52.4)	10 (62.5)	0.014
Nail involvement, n (%)	17 (73.9)	13 (61.9)	12 (75.0)	0.602
Joint involvement, n (%)	7 (30.4)	5 (23.8)	4 (25.0)	0.870
DM, n (%)	2 (8.7)	3 (14.3)	3 (18.6)	0.653
HTN, n (%)	11 (47.8)	10 (47.6)	5 (31.3)	0.523
Family H/O Psoriasis, n (%)	4 (17.4)	3 (14.3)	0 (0)	0.225
Alcohol, n (%)	6 (26.1)	8 (38.1)	6 (37.5)	0.643
Smoking, n (%)	3 (13.0)	3 (14.3)	1 (6.3)	0.727
Vegetarian, n (%)	10 (43.8)	11 (52.4)	12 (75.0)	0.144
BMI (kg/m^2), Mean (±SD)	29.5 (±3.7)	27.6 (±3.7)	27.4 (±4.3)	0.151
Waist Circumference (cm), Mean (±SD)	105.3 (±9.1)	99.0 (±9.9)	100.2 (±8.7)	0.70
ESI, Mean (±SD)	5.9 (±1.6)	5.3 (±1.5)	5.4 (±1.3)	0.412
PGA, Mean (±SD)	3.4 (±0.9)	3.1 (±0.8)	3.2 (±0.8)	0.476
FPG (mg/dl), Mean (±SD)	97.6 (±20.8)	101.9 (±35.1)	103.4 (±28.9)	0.797
Total Cholesterol (mg/dl), Mean (±SD)	184.4 (±37.5)	206.9 (±36.2)	207.2 (±42.3)	0.95
Triglycerides (mg/dl), Mean (±SD)	181.8 (±61.3)	194.3 (±63.1)	200.1 (±55.9)	0.623
HDL (mg/dl), Mean (±SD)	45.1 (±13.5)	44.3 (±6.6)	45.0 (±9.7)	0.968
LDL (mg/dl), Mean (±SD)	107.6 (±35.7)	126.1 (±29.1)	123.1 (±42.3)	0.194
SBP (mmHg), Mean (±SD)	130.4 (±11.5)	130.6 (±12.9)	135.6 (±11.5)	0.344
DBP (mmHg), Mean (±SD)	84.7 (±7.9)	85.9 (±7.9)	85.6 (±8.5)	0.875
Calcium channel blockers, n (%)	5 (21.7)	3 (14.3)	3 (18.6)	0.815
Beta blockers, n (%)	2 (8.7)	1 (4.8)	0 (0)	0.471
Angiotensin receptor blockers, n (%)	2 (8.7)	2 (9.5)	0 (0)	0.456
ACE inhibitors, n (%)	1 (4.3)	0 (0)	1 (6.3)	0.543
Diuretics, n (%)	0 (0)	0 (0)	1 (6.3)	0.247
Sulfonylureas, n (%)	2 (8.7)	0 (0)	1 (6.3)	0.403
Anxiolytics, n (%)	1 (4.3)	1 (4.8)	0 (0)	0.684
Lithium, n (%)	1 (4.3)	0 (0)	0 (0)	0.441
Antidepressants, n (%)	1 (4.3)	2 (9.5)	0 (0)	0.413
Insulin, n (%)	0 (0)	1 (4.8)	0 (0)	0.389
Modafinil, n (%)	0 (0)	1 (4.8)	0 (0)	0.389
NSAIDS, n (%)	0 (0)	1 (4.8)	0 (0)	0.389
Ca, Vitamin D, n (%)	0 (0)	1 (4.8)	0 (0)	0.389
Steroids, n (%)	0 (0)	0 (0)	1 (6.3)	0.247
Beta 2 agonists, n (%)	0 (0)	0 (0)	1 (6.3)	0.247

DM diabetes mellitus, *HTN* hypertension, *BMI* body mass index, *ESI* erythema, scaling and Induration, *PFA* physician global assessment, *FPG* fasting plasma glucose, *HDL* high density lipoprotein, *LDL* low density lipoprotein, *SBP* systolic blood pressure, *DBP* diastolic blood pressure, *ACE inhibitors* angiotensin converting enzyme inhibitors
Values are presented as Mean (±SD) or n (%)

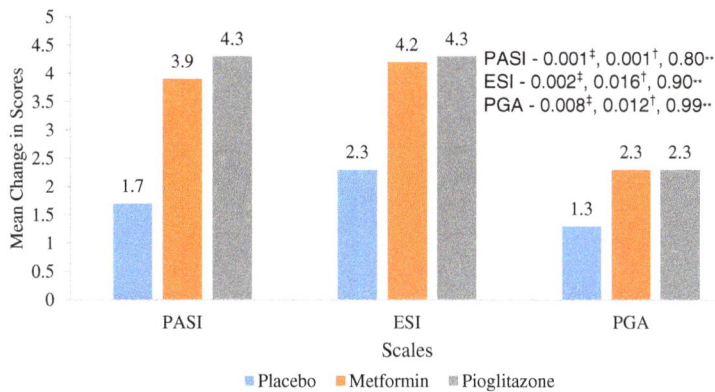

Fig. 2 Mean change in PASI, ESI and PGA scores in three treatment groups from baseline (Intention to treat Analysis). ‖ = Inter-group comparisons for PASI, ESI and PGA scores at 12 weeks as compared to baseline was carried out by One Way ANOVA, post hoc test used Scheffe; † = metformin vs placebo, ‡ = Pioglitazone vs placebo,** = metformin vs pioglitazone. PASI - Psoriasis area and severity index, ESI – Erythema, Scaling and Induration, PGA – Physician Global Assessmenty

To the best of our knowledge, effect of metformin in psoriasis patients with MS as done in our study has not been explored earlier. Our study has demonstrated improved efficacy of metformin in psoriasis disease itself as well as features of MS. A population based case control study Brauchli et al estimated the decreased risk of developing a first-time psoriasis diagnosis with metformin use as compared to matched controls [OR = 0.77 (95 % CI – 0.62–0.96)] [26]. One case of psoriasiform drug eruption associated with metformin usage has been observed, which on dechallenge and rechallenege leads to improvement and reappearance of lesions respectively [27]. In view of the case report, it has to be kept in mind that there can be clinical worsening of psoriasis with the use of metformin for treatment of psoriasis.

The anti-proliferative [16, 28], pro-differentiating [29], anti-inflammatory [11, 12, 30] and anti-angiogenic [31, 32] effects of TZDs seen in other studies may underlie the observed beneficial anti-psoriatic effects of pioglitazone. Metformin act through activation of adenosine monophosphate-activated protein kinase (AMPK) in extracellular signal-related kinase (ERK1/2) signaling pathway leading to cell cycle arrest and therefore inhibition of cell proliferation, hallmark of psoriasis [33]. AMPK activation not only inhibits iNOS, dendritic, T cell and monocyte/macrophage activation but also activates IL-10 and TGF-β, thereby exerting its anti-inflammatory action [34]. The anti-proliferative and anti-inflammatory action of metformin might have resulted in improvement of psoriasis.

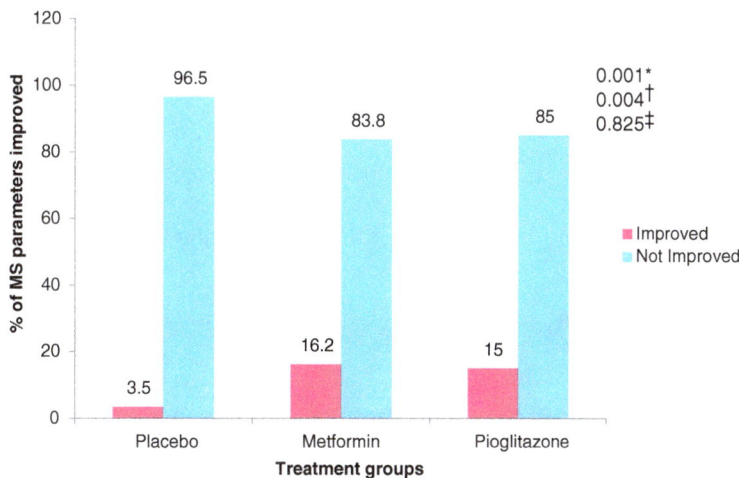

Fig. 3 Percentage of parameters of metabolic syndrome (MS) improved following 12 weeks of treatment in placebo, metformin and pioglitazone groups from baseline (Intention to treat Analysis). Inter-group comparisons for percentage of parameters of metabolic syndrome improved carried out by Chi-square test. * = Placebo vs metformin, † = placebo vs pioglitazone, ‡ = metformin vs pioglitazone; MS = Metabolic syndrome

PASI - 0.001*, 0.528†, 0.001‡
ESI - 0.001*, 0.729†, 0.001‡
PGA - 0.017*, 0.272†, 0.250‡

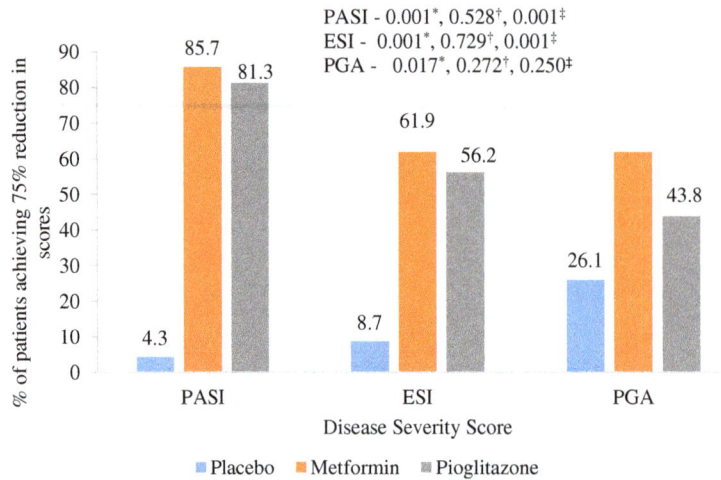

Fig. 4 Percentage of patients achieving 75 % reduction in PASI, ESI and PGA scores in placebo, metformin and pioglitazone groups from baseline (Intention to treat Analysis). Inter-group comparisons for 75 % reduction in PASI, ESI and PGA scores between three treatment groups carried out by Chi-square test. * = placebo vs metformin, † = metformin vs pioglitazone, ‡ = placebo vs pioglitazone. PASI - Psoriasis area and severity index, ESI – Erythema, Scaling and Induration, PGA – Physician Global Assessment

In diabetics, metformin had shown to decrease HbA_{1C}, total and LDL cholesterol, serum triglycerides, fasting insulin levels and improves HDL cholesterol [35–37]. Metformin has shown to improve cardiovascular outcomes by mitigating apoptosis [38]. These results are similar to the results observed in our study. In our study, although an increase in mean weight and BMI was observed with pioglitazone but decrease in mean waist circumference was also observed. Clinical studies had shown despite the weight gain reported in all the studies, which may equal as much as 0.5 kg per month for monotherapy, mean waist to hip ratio remains invariably unchanged. In one study, favorable effect on body fat distribution was demonstrated when patients with type

Table 2 Mean Change in individual parameters of metabolic syndrome after 12 weeks of treatment in three treatment groups from baseline (Intention to treat Analysis)

Treatment	Placebo (n = 23)		Metformin (n = 21)		Pioglitazone (n = 16)		ANOVA with post hoc Tukey's [b]
Parameters	Mean change [Mean ± SD]	p value[a]	Mean change [Mean ± SD]	p value[a]	Mean change [Mean ± SD]	p value[a]	Between groups, df = 2, p value
Weight (kg)	−0.6 ± 3.1	0.338	1.1 ± 1.9	0.016[f]	−0.4 ± 1.7	0.324	0.048[c], 0.970[d], 0.129[e]
BMI (kg/m²)	−0.1 ± 1.4	0.663	0.4 ± 0.7	0.016[f]	−0.2 ± 0.7	0.370	0.186[c], 0.995[d], 0.210[e]
Waist circumference (cm)	−0.9 ± 4.0	0.314	1.9 ± 2.7	0.003[f]	0.9 ± 2.3	0.119	0.013[c], 0.200[d], 0.606[e]
FPG (mg/dl)	2.2 ± 10.0	0.312	15.2 ± 19.2	0.002[f]	20.5 ± 17.4	<0.001[f]	0.021[c], 0.002[d],0.577[e]
Triglycerides (mg/dl)	1.1 ± 43.3	0.903	44.3 ± 45.4	<0.001[f]	53.3 ± 36.9	<0.001[f]	0.004[c], 0.001[d], 0.798[e]
HDL (mg/dl)	−1.7 ± 6.6	0.221	−1.9 ± 4.6	0.060	−1.5 ± 9.6	0.544	0.992[c], 0.994[d], 0.974[e]
SBP (mm Hg)	0.0 ± 8.6	1.000	1.7 ± 6.7	0.257	5.1 ± 6.3	0.005[f]	0.725[c], 0.094[d], 0.354[e]
DBP (mm Hg)	0.3 ± 7.9	0.876	1.7 ± 4.2	0.077	4.1 ± 5.5	0.009[f]	0.546[c], 0.085[d], 0.475[e]
Total Cholesterol (mg/dl)	1.4 ± 29.2	0.816	21.8 ± 25.2	0.001[f]	24.0 ± 29.5	0.005[f]	0.049[c], 0.042[d], 0.970[e]
LDL (mg/dl)	−5.9 ± 28.3	0.324	6.6 ± 20.0	0.146	9.8 ± 11.6	0.004[f]	0.151[c], 0.079[d], 0.898[e]

FPG fasting plasma glucose, *HDL* high density lipoprotein, *SBP* systolic blood pressure, *DBP* diastolic blood pressure, *BMI* body mass index, *LDL* low density lipoprotein
[a] Intra-group comparisons for weight, BMI, individual parameters of lipid profile and metabolic syndrome carried out by Paired *T*-test
[b] Inter-group comparisons for individual parameters carried out by One way ANOVA, post hoc Tukey's test
[c] Metformin vs placebo
[d] pioglitazone vs placebo
[e] metformin vs pioglitazone
[f] statistically significant difference compared to baseline

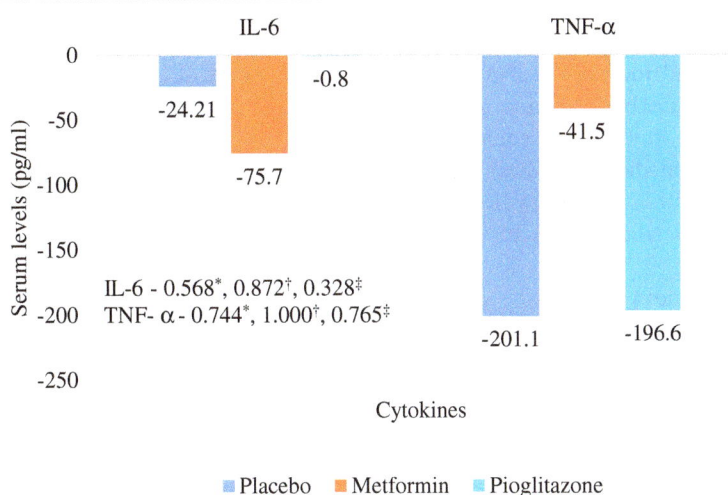

Fig. 5 Mean decrease in levels of IL-6 and TNF-α in three treatment groups from baseline in subgroup of patients (Intention to treat Analysis). Values are expressed as Mean ± SD. Inter-group comparisons for IL-6 and TNF-α carried out by One way ANOVA, *- Metformin vs placebo, †- pioglitazone vs placebo, ‡ - metformin vs pioglitazone, IL-6 – Interleukin-6, TNF-α – Tumor necrosis factor-α

Table 3 Adverse events observed during the study in placebo, metformin and pioglitazone treatment groups in topical treatment arm

Adverse Event	Placebo (N = 23)	Metformin (N = 21)	Pioglitazone (N = 16)	P value (Fischer's Exact test)
Redness	1	1	0	>0.99[a], >0.99[b],>0.99[c]
Pain	1	0	0	>0.99[a], >0.99[b],>0.99[c]
Hyperpigmentation	7	5	4	0.74[a], >0.99[b] > 0.99[c]
Hypopigmentation	0	1	1	0.477[a], 0.41[b] > 0.99[c]
Exacerbation	2	3	0	0.658[a], 0.503[b], 0.243[c]
Hypothyroidism	1	0	0	>0.99[a], >0.99[b]
Edema	0	0	2	0.162[b], 0.180[c]
c/o Weight Gain	0	0	2	0.162[b], 0.180[c]
Anemia	0	0	0	-
Abdominal Pain	0	1	0	0.477[a], >0.99[c]
Headache	0	0	0	-
Gastritis	0	0	0	-
Nausea	0	0	0	-
Vomiting	0	0	0	-
Dizziness	0	0	0	-
Diarrhea	0	1	0	0.477[a], >0.99[c]
Heartburn	0	1	0	0.477[a], >0.99[c]
>3 times SGOT/SGPT	0	0	0	-
Slight increase in SGOT/SGPT	0	0	0	-
Increased TLC	0	0	0	-
Weight gain > 1 kg	8	3	8	0.169[a], 0.509[b], 0.030[c]
Recurrence after 3 months	4	6	5	0.377[a], 0.312[b], 0.860[c]

Inter group comparison between groups was done by Fischer's Exact test; p – value ≤ 0.05 was considered statistically significant
[a] placebo vs metformin
[b] placebo vs pioglitazone
[c] metformin vs pioglitazone

II diabetes were treated with pioglitazone 45 mg/day for 16 weeks [39]. MR imaging revealed that pioglitazone decreased visceral fat area and increased subcutaneous fat mass. With 1H-MR spectroscopy in same group of patients, significant decrease in liver fat content was demonstrated. Thus, thiazolidinedione's (TZDs) have favorable effects on body fat distribution, intra hepatic fat content and adipose tissue metabolism, all resulting in increased insulin sensitivity.

Our study had revealed a mean fall of 20.5 mg/dl in FPG in psoriasis patients with MS with pioglitazone 30 mg/day. PROFIT-J study have shown improvement in glycemic control, DBP and lipid profile [40]. In clinical trials, pioglitazone monotherapy at a dose of 30 mg/day revealed a dose dependent lowering of FPG by 1.0–3.1 mmol/L and HbA$_{1C}$ reductions ranging between 0.3 and 1.08 % from baseline, significant when compared with placebo [41–45]. Pioglitazone increases peripheral insulin sensitivity, enhancing both splanchnic and peripheral glucose uptake, in patients with type II diabetes in randomized, placebo controlled, 12–26 weeks trial [40, 46, 47]. We observed a mean decrease in serum triglycerides, total cholesterol and LDL cholesterol of 53.3, 24 and 9.8 mg/dl respectively, with pioglitazone 30 mg/day. Lipid profiles generally improved in pioglitazone recipients in three placebo controlled 12–26 week trial [41, 42, 48]. Favorable increases in HDL cholesterol were greater in pioglitazone than placebo recipients in three trials [40, 42, 48].

Mean reduction in SBP and DBP of 5.1 and 4.1 mmHg respectively was measured in pioglitazone group in our study, which was significant as compared to baseline. In a review article by Giles et al, the observed magnitude of reduction was 4–5 mmHg in SBP and 2–4 mmHg in DBP, which were sufficient to significantly reduce cardiovascular event rates [49]. The decrease in cardiovascular risk factors namely lipid profile and blood pressure in our study might contribute to the overall decrease in diabetes and cardiovascular mortality in psoriasis patients with MS.

Increased risk of bladder cancer with the long term use of pioglitazone as shown in French cohort study [50], UK nested case control study [51] and interim results of longitudinal study [52]. However, the 10-year final analysis of longitudinal study [52] did not show any statistically significant findings of increased risk of bladder cancer with long term use of pioglitazone [53]. Similarly, no statistically significant association was found in two Taiwanese studies [54, 55]. Infact, TZDs have shown to decrease the risk of breast, brain, colorectal, ear-nose-throat, kidney, liver, lung, lymphatic, prostate, stomach and uterus cancer significantly [56]. FDA although issued a safety warning, has not withdrawn the drug.

There are no significant differences in metformin as compared to pioglitazone with regard to improvement

in psoriasis and MS parameters. But there is significant reduction in weight with the use of metformin and due to controversy of increased risk of bladder cancer associated with pioglitazone; metformin can be preferred over pioglitazone in psoriasis patients with MS.

In subgroup analysis, 10 % of patients in placebo, 14.3 % in metformin and 37.5 % of patients in pioglitazone subgroup had no decline or rather increase in the levels of IL-6 and TNF-α, consistent with the relapse of psoriasis in these patients in next 6 months. Remitting relapsing nature of the disease might be accounted for no significant change in the IL-6 and TNF-α level.

Randomization and placebo control are the strengths of our study. The study also has some limitations. Intermediate dose of pioglitazone (30 mg/day) and metformin (1000 mg/day) was used in the study. Secondly, it was an open label study, although blinded end point assessment was done.

Conclusion
Insulin sensitizers have shown improvement in the parameters of MS as well as psoriasis disease. With further evaluation in clinical studies, Insulin sensitizers can be used for the management of psoriasis patients with MS.

Acknowledgement
Thankful to Dr. Sunil Dogra and Late Dr. Inderjeet Kaur for constant support and excellent academic inputs in the study.

Funding
This study was carried out in Post graduate institute of medical sciences, Chandigarh. This study was part of dissertation for degree of Doctrine of Medicine in Clinical Pharmacology. This study was not supported financially by any pharmaceutical company.

Authors' contribution
SS and AB conceptualize the study design, SS drafted the protocol with the approval of AB. SS collected the data and did statistical analysis. All authors read and approve the final manuscript.

Competing interests
The authors declare that they have no competing interests.

Author details
[1]Department of Pharmacology, All India Institute of Medical Sciences (AIIMS), Jodhpur 342005, India. [2]Department of Endocrinology, Post Graduate Institute of Medical Education and Research (PGIMER), Chandigarh 160012, India.

References

1. Sommer DM, Jenisch S, Suchan M, Christophers E, Weichenthal M. Increased prevalence of the metabolic syndrome in patients with moderate to severe psoriasis. Arch Dermatol Res. 2006;298(7):321–8.
2. Gelfand JM, Yeung H. Metabolic syndrome in patients with psoriatic disease. J Rheumatol Suppl. 2012;89:24–8.
3. Neimann AL, Shin DB, Wang X, Margolis DJ, Troxel AB, Gelfand JM. Prevalence of cardiovascular risk factors in patients with psoriasis. J Am Acad Dermatol. 2006;55(5):829–35.
4. Executive Summary of The Third Report of The National Cholesterol Education Program (NCEP). Expert panel on detection, evaluation, and treatment of high blood cholesterol in adults (Adult Treatment Panel III). JAMA. 2001;285(19):2486–97.
5. Armstrong EJ, Harskamp CT, Armstrong AW. Psoriasis and major adverse cardiovascular events: a systematic review and meta-analysis of observational studies. J Am Heart Assoc. 2013;2(2):e000062.
6. Patel RV, Shelling ML, Prodanovich S, Federman DG, Kirsner RS. Psoriasis and vascular disease-risk factors and outcomes: a systematic review of the literature. J Gen Intern Med. 2011;26(9):1036–49.
7. Wilson PW, D'Agostino RB, Parise H, Sullivan L, Meigs JB. Metabolic syndrome as a precursor of cardiovascular disease and type 2 diabetes mellitus. Circulation. 2005;112(20):3066–72.
8. Eckel RH, Grundy SM, Zimmet PZ. The metabolic syndrome. Lancet. 2005; 365(9468):1415–28.
9. Wannamethee SG, Shaper AG, Lennon L, Morris RW. Metabolic syndrome vs Framingham Risk Score for prediction of coronary heart disease, stroke, and type 2 diabetes mellitus. Arch Intern Med. 2005;165(22):2644–50.
10. Sterry W, Strober BE, Menter A. Obesity in psoriasis: the metabolic, clinical and therapeutic implications. Report of an interdisciplinary conference and review. Br J Dermatol. 2007;157(4):649–55.
11. Ricote M, Li AC, Willson TM, Kelly CJ, Glass CK. The peroxisome proliferator-activated receptor-gamma is a negative regulator of macrophage activation. Nature. 1998;391(6662):79–82.
12. Jiang C, Ting AT, Seed B. PPAR-gamma agonists inhibit production of monocyte inflammatory cytokines. Nature. 1998;391(6662):82–6.
13. Malhotra S, Bansal D, Shafiq N, Pandhi P, Kumar B. Potential therapeutic role of peroxisome proliferator activated receptor-gamma agonists in psoriasis. Expert Opin Pharmacother. 2005;6(9):1455–61.
14. Shafiq N, Malhotra S, Pandhi P, Gupta M, Kumar B, Sandhu K. Pilot trial: Pioglitazone versus placebo in patients with plaque psoriasis (the P6). Int J Dermatol. 2005;44(4):328–33.
15. Mittal R, Malhotra S, Pandhi P, Kaur I, Dogra S. Efficacy and safety of combination Acitretin and Pioglitazone therapy in patients with moderate to severe chronic plaque-type psoriasis: a randomized, double-blind, placebo-controlled clinical trial. Arch Dermatol. 2009; 145(4):387–93.
16. Ellis CN, Varani J, Fisher GJ, Zeigler ME, Pershadsingh HA, Benson SC, et al. Troglitazone improves psoriasis and normalizes models of proliferative skin disease: ligands for peroxisome proliferator-activated receptor-gamma inhibit keratinocyte proliferation. Arch Dermatol. 2000; 136(5):609–16.
17. Pershadsingh HA, Sproul JA, Benjamin E, Finnegan J, Amin NM. Treatment of psoriasis with troglitazone therapy. Arch Dermatol. 1998;134(10):1304–5.
18. Robertshaw H, Friedmann PS. Pioglitazone: a promising therapy for psoriasis. Br J Dermatol. 2005;152(1):189–91.
19. Cohn G, Valdes G, Capuzzi DM. Pathophysiology and treatment of the dyslipidemia of insulin resistance. Curr Cardiol Rep. 2001;3(5):416–23.
20. Mehnert H. Metformin, the rebirth of a biguanide: mechanism of action and place in the prevention and treatment of insulin resistance. Exp Clin Endocrinol Diabetes. 2001;109 Suppl 2:S259–64.
21. Stadtmauer LA, Wong BC, Oehninger S. Should patients with polycystic ovary syndrome be treated with metformin? Benefits of insulin sensitizing drugs in polycystic ovary syndrome–beyond ovulation induction. Hum Reprod. 2002;17(12):3016–26.
22. Van Voorhees AS, Feldman SR, Koo JY, Lebwohl MG, Menter A. The psoriasis and psoriatic arthritis pocket guide: treatment algorithms and management options. National Psoriasis Foundation. Available from: https://www.psoriasis.org/health-care-providers/treating-psoriasis.
23. Misra A, Wasir JS, Pandey RM. An evaluation of candidate definitions of the metabolic syndrome in adult Asian Indians. Diabetes Care. 2005;28(2):398–403.
24. Sharma V, Kaur I, Kumar B. Calcipotriol versus coal tar: a prospective randomized study in stable plaque psoriasis. Int J Dermatol. 2003;42(10):834–8.
25. Bongartz T, Coras B, Vogt T, Scholmerich J, Muller-Ladner U. Treatment of active psoriatic arthritis with the PPARgamma ligand pioglitazone: an open-label pilot study. Rheumatology (Oxford). 2005;44(1):126–9.
26. Brauchli YB, Jick SS, Curtin F, Meier CR. Association between use of thiazolidinediones or other oral antidiabetics and psoriasis: A population based case-control study. J Am Acad Dermatol. 2008;58(3):421–9.
27. Koca R, Altinyazar HC, Yenidunya S, Tekin NS. Psoriasiform drug eruption associated with metformin hydrochloride: a case report. Dermatol Online J. 2003;9(3):11.
28. Demerjian M, Man MQ, Choi EH, Brown BE, Crumrine D, Chang S, et al. Topical treatment with thiazolidinediones, activators of peroxisome proliferator-activated receptor-gamma, normalizes epidermal homeostasis in a murine hyperproliferative disease model. Exp Dermatol. 2006;15(3):154–60.
29. Bhagavathula N, Nerusu KC, Lal A, Ellis CN, Chittiboyina A, Avery MA, et al. Rosiglitazone inhibits proliferation, motility, and matrix metalloproteinase production in keratinocytes. J Invest Dermatol. 2004;122(1):130–9.
30. Buckingham RE. Thiazolidinediones: Pleiotropic drugs with potent anti-inflammatory properties for tissue protection. Hepatol Res. 2005;33(2):167–70.
31. Takagi T, Yamamuro A, Tamita K, Yamabe K, Katayama M, Mizoguchi S, et al. Pioglitazone reduces neointimal tissue proliferation after coronary stent implantation in patients with type 2 diabetes mellitus: an intravascular ultrasound scanning study. Am Heart J. 2003;146(2):E5.
32. Marx N, Wohrle J, Nusser T, Walcher D, Rinker A, Hombach V, et al. Pioglitazone reduces neointima volume after coronary stent implantation: a randomized, placebo-controlled, double-blind trial in nondiabetic patients. Circulation. 2005;112(18):2792–8.
33. Li W, Ma W, Zhong H, Liu W, Sun Q. Metformin inhibits proliferation of human keratinocytes through a mechanism associated with activation of the MAPK signaling pathway. Exp Ther Med. 2014;7(2):389–92.
34. Glossmann H, Reider N. A marriage of two "Methusalem" drugs for the treatment of psoriasis?: Arguments for a pilot trial with metformin as add-on for methotrexate. Dermatoendocrinol. 2013;5(2):252–63.
35. United Kingdom Prospective Diabetes Study (UKPDS). Relative efficacy of randomly allocated diet, sulphonylurea, insulin, or metformin in patients with newly diagnosed non-insulin dependent diabetes followed for three years. BMJ. 1995;310(6972):83–8.
36. UK Prospective Diabetes Study (UKPDS) Group. Effect of intensive blood-glucose control with metformin on complications in overweight patients with type 2 diabetes (UKPDS 34). Lancet. 1998;352(9131) :854–65.
37. Dai X, Wang H, Jing Z, Fu P. The effect of a dual combination of noninsulin antidiabetic drugs on lipids: a systematic review and network meta-analysis. Curr Med Res Opin. 2014;30(9):1777–86.
38. Elmadhun NY, Sabe AA, Lassaletta AD, Chu LM, Sellke FW. Metformin mitigates apoptossis in ischemic myocardium. J Surg Res. 2014;192(1):50–8.
39. Miyazaki Y, Mahankali A, Matsuda M, Mahankali S, Hardies J, Cusi K, et al. Effect of pioglitazone on abdominal fat distribution and insulin sensitivity in type 2 diabetic patients. J Clin Endocrinol Metab. 2002; 87(6):2784–91.
40. Yoshii H, Onuma T, Yamazaki T, Watada H, Matsuhisa M, Matsumoto M, et al. Effects of pioglitazone on macrovascular events in patients with type 2 diabetes mellitus at high risk of stroke: the PROFIT-J study. J Atheroscler Thromb. 2014;21(6):563–73.
41. Aronoff S, Rosenblatt S, Braithwaite S, Egan JW, Mathisen AL, Schneider RL. Pioglitazone hydrochloride monotherapy improves glycemic control in the treatment of patients with type 2 diabetes: a 6-month randomized placebo-controlled dose-response study. The Pioglitazone 001 Study Group. Diabetes Care. 2000;23(11):1605–11.
42. Rosenblatt S, Miskin B, Glazer NB, Prince MJ, Robertson KE. The impact of pioglitazone on glycemic control and atherogenic dyslipidemia in patients with type 2 diabetes mellitus. Coron Artery Dis. 2001;12(5):413–23.
43. Kaneko T, Baba S, Toyota T. Dose finding study of AD-4833 in patients with NIDDM on diet therapy alone: double blind comparative study on four dosages. Jpn J Clin Exp Med. 1997;74:1250–77.
44. Kaneko T, Baba S, Toyota T. Clinical evaluation of an insulin-resistance improving agent, AD-4833, in patients with NIDDM on diet therapy alone: a placebo controlled double blind clinical study. Jpn J Clin Exp Med. 1997;74:1491–514.

45. Chawla S, Kaushik N, Singh NP, Ghosh RK, Saxena A. Effect of addition of either sitagliptin or pioglitazone in patients with uncontrolled type 2 diabetes mellitus on metformin: A randomized controlled trial. J Pharmacol Pharmacother. 2013;4(1):27–32.

46. Kawamori R, Matsuhisa M, Kinoshita J, Mochizuki K, Niwa M, Arisaka T, et al. Pioglitazone enhances splanchnic glucose uptake as well as peripheral glucose uptake in non-insulin-dependent diabetes mellitus. AD-4833 Clamp-OGL Study Group. Diabetes Res Clin Pract. 1998;41(1):35–43.

47. Wallace TM, Levy JC, Matthews DR. An increase in insulin sensitivity and basal beta-cell function in diabetic subjects treated with pioglitazone in a placebo-controlled randomized study. Diabet Med. 2004;21(6):568–76.

48. Herz M, Johns D, Reviriego J, Grossman LD, Godin C, Duran S, et al. A randomized, double-blind, placebo-controlled, clinical trial of the effects of pioglitazone on glycemic control and dyslipidemia in oral antihyperglycemic medication-naive patients with type 2 diabetes mellitus. Clin Ther. 2003;25(4):1074–95.

49. Giles TD, Sander GE. Effects of thiazolidinediones on blood pressure. Curr Hypertens Rep. 2007;9(4):332–7.

50. Neumann A, Weill A, Ricordeau P, Fagot JP, Alla F, Allemand H. Pioglitazone and risk of bladder cancer among diabetic patients in France: a population-based cohort study. Diabetologia. 2012;55(7):1953–1962.doi:10.1007/s00125-012-2538-9.

51. Azoulay L, Yin H, Filion KB, Assayag J, Majdan A, Pollak MN, et al. The use of pioglitazone and the risk of bladder cancer in people with type 2 diabetes: nested case-control study. BMJ. 2012;344:e3645.

52. Lewis JD, Ferrara A, Peng T, Hedderson M, Bilker WB, Quesenberry Jr CP, et al. Risk of bladder cancer among diabetic patients treated with pioglitazone: interim report of a longitudinal cohort study. Diabetes Care. 2011;34(4):916–22.

53. TPC Limited. Takeda Announces Completion of the Post-Marketing Commitment to Submit Data to the FDA, the EMA and the PMDA for Pioglitazone Containing Medicines Including ACTOS. 2014. Available from: https://www.takeda.com/news/2014/20140829_6714.html.

54. Chang CH, Lin JW, Wu LC, Lai MS, Chuang LM, Chan KA. Association of thiazolidinediones with liver cancer and colorectal cancer in type 2 diabetes mellitus. Hepatology. 2012;55(5):1462–72.

55. Tseng CH. Pioglitazone and bladder cancer: a population-based study of Taiwanese. Diabetes Care. 2012;35(2):278–80.

56. Lin HC, Hsu YT, Kachingwe BH, Hsu CY, Uang YS, Wang LH. Dose effect of thiazolidinedione on cancer risk in type 2 diabetes mellitus patients: a six-year population-based cohort study. J Clin Pharm Ther. 2014;39(4):354–60.

Adherence to drug treatments and adjuvant barrier repair therapies are key factors for clinical improvement in mild to moderate acne: the ACTUO observational prospective multicenter cohort trial in 643 patients

Raúl de Lucas[1], Gerardo Moreno-Arias[2], Montserrat Perez-López[3], Ángel Vera-Casaño[4], Sonia Aladren[5], Massimo Milani[5*] and on behalf of ACTUO Investigators study group

Abstract

Background: In acne, several studies report a poor adherence to treatments. We evaluate, in a real-life setting conditions, the impact of compliance to physician's instructions, recommendations and adherence to the treatments on clinical outcome in patients with mild to moderate acne in an observational, non-interventional prospective study carried out in 72 Dermatologic Services in Spain (ACTUO Trial).

Methods: Six-hundred-forty-three subjects were enrolled and 566 patients (88 %) completed the 3 study visits. Study aimed to evaluate the impact of adherence (assessed with ECOB scale) on clinical outcome, as well as how the use of specific adjuvant treatments (facial cleansing, emollient, moisturizing and lenitive specific topical products) influences treatment's adherence and acne severity (0–5 points score). Recommendation of specific adjuvant skin barrier repair products was made in 85.2 %.

Results: Overall, clinical improvement was observed throughout follow-up visits with an increased proportion of patients who reported reductions of ≥50 % on the total number of lesions (2 months: 25.2 %; 3 months: 57.6 %) and reductions of severity scores (2.5, 2.0 and 1.3 at 1, 2 and 3 months after treatment, respectively). Adherence to treatment was associated with a significant reduction on severity grading, a lower number of lesions and a higher proportion of patients with ≥50 % improvement.

Conclusions: Good adherence to medication plus adherence to adjuvants was significantly associated with a higher clinical improvement unlike those that despite adherence with medication had a low adherence to adjuvants. A good adherence to adjuvant treatment was
associated with improved adherence and better treatment outcomes in mild to moderate acne patients.
(ISRCTN Registry: ISRCTN14257026).

Keywords: Acne vulgaris, Emollients, Observational study, Patient adherence, Topical administration

* Correspondence: massimo.milani@isdin.com
[5]Isdin S.A. Medical Department, Provençals 33, Barcelona, Spain
Full list of author information is available at the end of the article

Background

Acne is a common skin chronic disease that very often requires prolonged treatments [1]. With a chronic course [2] and an episodic pattern of presentation [3], Acne vulgaris lesions occur mainly in exposed areas like the face and the presternal region. The effect of the scarring may be notable and the functional, social and emotional impact on the patient's quality of life may be significant [4, 5]. Adherence to doctor prescriptions has a major impact on treatment outcome [6]. Several studies conducted over the past few years suggest that adherence to acne medications is particularly low [3, 7] and has been associated with inadequate response to therapy [8], especially when both topical and systemic treatments are prescribed to the same patient [9]. The treatment plan and the choice of specific active ingredients should take into account not only the individual characteristics of the patient and/or the disease but also their preferences and expectations with treatment as well as questions of convenience [10].The adverse effects of the various therapies available should also be borne in mind in order to increase adherence to the physician's instructions and recommendations, thus promoting what are known as health-related behaviours [7]. Specific systemic and topical acne treatments are very often associated with local side effect such as dry, burning and itching sensations [7] hence poor tolerability further worsens compliance [11].'Based on the evidence and clinical experience obtained with topical treatments and their possible irritant effects [12], adjuvant skin barrier repair therapies such as specific emulsion and detergent products, hydrating and emollients are often prescribed in order to reduce these side effects, all in search of improving adherence to therapeutic strategies [13, 14]. Other factors such as a good and efficient physician-patient relationship are also crucial for improving adherence to therapeutic strategy [15] since this interaction includes specific roles and motivations [16] that might be essential to the healing of many patients, particularly so for patients with chronic disease or disease having a negative impact on quality of life and self-esteem such as acne [17]. Adherence with acne therapies has been evaluated mainly in subjects irrespective to grading severity of the condition (from mild to severe forms) [8, 18] but, so far, few data are available regarding this conduct in patients with mild to moderate forms. We evaluated in a real-life setting condition the impact of adherence to dermatologist instructions and recommendations and adherence to the treatments x(specific anti acne treatments and adjuvant therapies) on the clinical outcome in patients with mild to moderate acne. The participating physicians of the ACTUO trial were practicing experienced Spanish dermatologists working in hospital outpatient dermatology services.

Methods

ACTUO was a multicenter, prospective, observational, epidemiological study of patients with mild to moderate acne treated at 72 dermatology services throughout Spain between October 2011 and November 2012. All study materials were evaluated and approved by a Clinical Research Ethics Committee before the study start. Approval (Ethics Committee of "Centro Medico Teknon" Barcelona Spain) was obtained August 1, 2011.

a) Subjects

A total of 643 subjects with mild to moderate acne, after they provided written informed consent, were enrolled in the study. Eligibility criteria were men and women with mild to moderate acne vulgaris eligible for a specific acne treatment (topical retinoid agents or antiseptics and/or systemic antibiotics) willing to participate in the study. The study was conducted at three visits carried out in a period of three months (V1: baseline, and two follow-up visits: V2 and V3). In all 3 visits, data on acne severity was recorded on the Case Report Form (CRF) by the dermatologist using the global ranking system of the FDA [19] (0: no lesions, 4: severe) and the total number of acne lesions. Acne severity was also evaluated by the patient. In addition, adherence to anti-acne treatments and adjuvant therapies was also assessed trough study.

b) Primary outcome

The main objective of this analysis was to evaluate the impact of adherence to the treatments on the clinical outcome in patients with mild to moderate acne. A secondary outcome was to evaluate the impact of the use of specific adjuvant treatments (facial cleansing products, emollient moisturizing and lenitive specific topical cream products containing mainly rhamnosoft as emollient and antiflammatory agent) on adherence level and entity of the clinical outcome obtained. Acne severity was assessed at each visit with a 5-point score system (from 0 to 4), absolute count of lesions and percentage of patient reaching a ≥50 % reduction in lesion numbers. Adherence to treatment was evaluated at visit 2 and visit 3 by means of validated 4-item questionnaire (ECOB) with a dichotomous classification: good adherence (ECOB score = 4) and poor adherence (ECOB <4). Poor adherence to treatment was defined as a different to expected answer on the ECOB questionnaire. The four questions of ECOB were according to Pawin et al. [20].

The degree of adherence to the adjuvant measures prescribed by the doctor (application of cleansers and moisturizers for facial skin care) was assessed using the data provided by the patients attending all three study visits. It was considered that patients who followed all their doctor's instructions and recommendations in at least three of the four assessments showed compliance with the medical advice. The effects of adherence to adjuvant treatment on the doctor's and patient's final assessments of acne severity was compared in patients "without /practically without lesions" (FDA scores = 0–1) and patients "with lesions" (FDA scores ≥ 2–4). The ACTUO study has evaluated also the impact of acne and acne treatments on quality of life evaluated by means of Cardiff Acne Disability Index [21] (CADI) and Dermatology Life Quality Index (DLQI) [22]. However these data would be presented elsewhere.

c) *Statistical methods*

The FDA ratings made by the physician and patient after three months were grouped into two categories: presence of lesions (FDA ≥2-4), or absence or near absence of lesions (FDA = 0–1). Using the parameters *severity* and *total number of lesions*, improvement was assessed by classifying patients into two groups based on the reduction of acne severity (≥50 % improvement vs. improvement <50 %) and the percentages of reduction of comedones and papules/pustules. Statistical analysis was performed using the statistical software SPSS ver.19. Continuous variables were expressed as mean (SD). Categorical binary variables were expressed as proportions (%). The Mann–Whitney, Wilcoxon and the chi-square tests were used for inference statistical analysis tests. A multivariate logistics regression analysis was performed in order to assess the correlation between improvement of acne severity score, percentage of patients with 50 % or more in acne lesion number reduction, and the following variable: demographic data, adherence to specific treatments and to adjuvant treatments.

Results

Table 1 gives information about patients' characteristics at the time of enrollment. A total of 643 cases were enrolled. A total of 566 patients (88 %) completed the 3-visit study. Data are presented as per protocol analysis. At baseline, adjuvant products were prescribed in 83.8 % of the patients. The application frequency was 1.3/day. Prescription for specific adjuvant products was made for 85.2 % of the patients. Severity of acne assessed by the physician was 2.5 ± 0.6 and mean number of comedones was 18.9 ± 2. Severity acne score was significantly ($p < 0.001$) reduced in comparison with baseline after 1 month (2.0 ± 0.8) and after 3 months (1.3 ± 0.9). At the end of study period patients scoring 0 (complete cure of acne) were 17 %. In general, significant reductions in the severity scores vis-à-vis the baseline visit were observed in both doctor's and patients' assessment (2.1 ± 0.9 at one month and 1.4 ± 0.9 at three months; $p < 0.001$). Figure 1 shows the evolution of acne severity score in the population as a whole.

Percentage of patients showing at least 50 % of lesion reduction was 25.2 % at visit 2 and 57.6 % at visit 3.

According to the ECOB scores, good adherence to treatment was documented in 50.0 % of the patients at visit 2 and in 66.3 % at visit 3. Good adherence to treatment was associated with a significant ($p < 0.05$) acne improvement in comparison with poor adherence group at both control visits. At visit 3 acne severity score was 1.19 ± 0.8 in patients with good adherence to adjuvants vs. 1.4 ± 0.9 in poor adherence group. Good adherence to specific acne treatments (facial cleansers) was documented in 83.6 % at visit 2 and in 89.9 % at visit 3. At the end of study, patients with good adherence to treatment presented a significant improvement of acne both in term of acne severity score (1.2 vs. 1.7; $p = 0.001$) and regarding the proportion of patients whom reduction of lesions was ≥50 % (60.9 % vs. 32.8 %; $p < 0.001$) when compared to those with poor adherence (Fig. 2). In patients for whom the dermatologist had prescribed adjuvant therapies, a good adherence to this treatment was documented in 36.2 %. Adherence to adjuvant treatment improves acne thus it was associated with a significant reduction of score grading severity at visit 3 (1.2 vs. 1.4; $P = 0.002$), with a higher percentage of reduction of average lesions number vs. baseline (50.8 % vs. 43.7 %; $p = 0.015$) and with more patients obtaining a ≥50 % reduction in acne lesions' number (65.9 % vs. 51.5 %; $p = 0.003$) in comparison with the low adherence group (Fig. 2). Adherence to adjuvant treatments was associated with a greater proportion of patients with a complete cure of acne (defined as no or very few acne lesions) at the final visit in comparison with poor-adherers (66.5 % vs. 52.6 %; $p = 0.004$). In particular, good adherence to adjuvant treatments improved the adherence to topical retinoid therapy therefore influencing clinical improvement of acne showing a higher proportion patients with adherence to treatment in adherers to adjuvants when compared to non-adherers (85.5 % vs. 70.7 %; $p < 0.001$). In addition, in patients with a good adherence toadjuvants were significantly more frequently considered with an ≥50 % improvement on clinical outcome in comparison with those that did not adhere to adjuvants (65.9 % vs. 51.5 %; $p = 0.003$).

Multiple logistic regression analysis was performed to identify factors influencing clinical improvement of acne. Adherence to specific treatments, adherence to adjuvant treatments and good adherence to treatment are significantly ($p = 0.001$) correlated with clinical improvement of acne. In accordance with previous studies, sex (women vs. men) and the fact to be accompanied (by parents/tutor or relative) or not at the medical visit are also independent factors affecting improvement clinical outcome of acne. Other analysis allowed observing an association between the patient's assessment of quality of life based on the DLQI scale and the adherence to adjuvant treatment since rates of improvement

Table 1 Sociodemographic data and acne severity at baseline visit

		n	mean (SD)	n (%)
Gender	Male	635	–	240 (37.8 %)
	Female			395 (62.2 %)
Age		617	21.3 (7.2)	
Study level	Primary school	632	–	24 (3.8 %)
	Secondary school			151 (23.9 %)
	Vocational training (school)			51 (8.1 %)
	Pre-university			188 (29.7 %)
	Vocational training (technical college)			30 (4.7 %)
	First cycle university studies			41 (6.5 %)
	Second cycle university studies			146 (23.1 %)
	Others			1 (0.2 %)
Physician's acne evaluation	Without lesions	640	2.47 (0.64)	–
	Practically without lesions			32 (5.0 %)
	Mild			298 (46.6 %)
	Moderate			290 (45.3 %)
	Severe			20 (3.1 %)
Patient's acne evaluation	Without lesions	594	2.10 (0.85)	16 (2.7 %)
	Practically without lesions			126 (21.2 %)
	Mild			245 (41.2 %)
	Moderate			195 (32.8 %)
	Severe			12 (2.0 %)
Lesion location[a]	Facial	637	–	622 (97.6 %)
	Back			212 (33.3 %)
	Shoulders			81 (12.7 %)
	Presternal area			73 (11.5 %)
	Others			2 (0.3 %)
Total number of lesions[a] (Percentages of 568 patients with lesions)	Comedones	546	18.9 (20.4)	532 (93.7 %)
	Papules/pustules	551	11.4 (10.2)	545 (96.0 %)
	Nodules	378	0.9 (1.7)	147 (25.9 %)
Recommendation of specific adjuvant products (facial soaps/cleansers and specific facial care products)	No	640	–	104 (16.3 %)
	Yes			536 (83.8 %)

[a]Non-exclusive categories
N number of patients, SD standard deviation; % = Percentage

on QoL were lower in non-compliers (43 % vs. 56.1 %, $p = 0.007$).

Discussion

Low adherence to treatments is still a relevant problem in the treatment of mild to moderate acne [23]. The definition of strategies to improve adherence with both pharmacological and behavioural treatment remains a major challenge. Suboptimal medication adherence is one of the major reasons for treatment failure in subject with acne vulgaris [24]. Our findings reveal that dermatologists in

Spain frequently prescribe specific adjuvant treatment for acne. They recommend the use of specific products including non-comedogenic soaps and moisturizers in over 80 % of acne patients. The synergy between the effects of drug treatment and adjuvant products can improve comfort during the various stages of treatment and can encourage patients to continue the application of the products. Adherence to adjuvant treatment was associated not only with a 2.4-fold increase in the probability of adherence to pharmacological treatment, but also with a significant reduction in acne severity, in the number of lesions as assessed by both

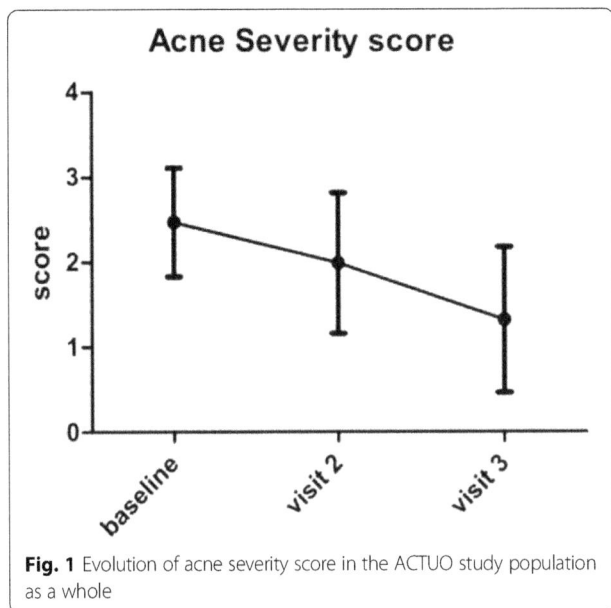

Fig. 1 Evolution of acne severity score in the ACTUO study population as a whole

the treating physician and the patient, and a higher percentage of patients whose severity improved by 50 % or more. In the ACTUO study low adherence to treatment was found in 50 % of the patients (at 1 month) and this result is in line with previous published data. Low adherence to adjuvant treatments was observed in up to 63.8 % of subjects after 3 months. In addition we have to consider that these data derived from a per protocol analysis, not including 12.4 % of patients not attending to control visits which therefore could be considered as"non-complier" by definition. In line with previous experiences [3], we have observed that adherence to pharmacological treatment is a key factor for the improvement of acne both in terms of reduction of severity grading, number of lesions and

percentage of patients obtaining at least a 50 % acne improvement. Good adherence to adjuvant treatments also improves clinical evolution of acne with a greater reduction of severity of grading and number of lesions and with a significant greater percentage of patients obtaining a 50 % or more improvement of acne in comparison with patients with poor adherence to adjuvant treatments. Furthermore, patients with good adherence with drug and those with adherence to adjuvant treatments presented the highest percentage of patients with improvement of acne lesions ≥50 %. In addition, in the present study it was shown that adherence to adjuvant products is the second most important factor (just after adherence to drug treatment) influencing the degree of acne improvement. A good adherence to adjuvant treatment is associated with an improved adherence to acne treatments and with a better treatment outcome in mild to moderate acne patients. Some limitations should be taken in account in evaluating the results of our study. In particular the evaluation of compliance was based on self-reporting questionnaire. This approach however was used in other studies assessing the same outcome and the ECOB questionnaire is considered a validated tool [3, 18]. On the other hand, we believe that the sample size and the study design adopted, quite close to "real life" conditions of acne treatment strategies, could be considered as aspects increasing the external validity and the generalization of the observed results of the ACTUO.

Conclusions

The ACTUO observational study results confirm that adherence to pharmacological treatment and adjuvant therapies are both key factors of acne improvement in terms of reduction of severity, number of lesions and percentage of patients with at least a 50 % acne improvement. In addition,

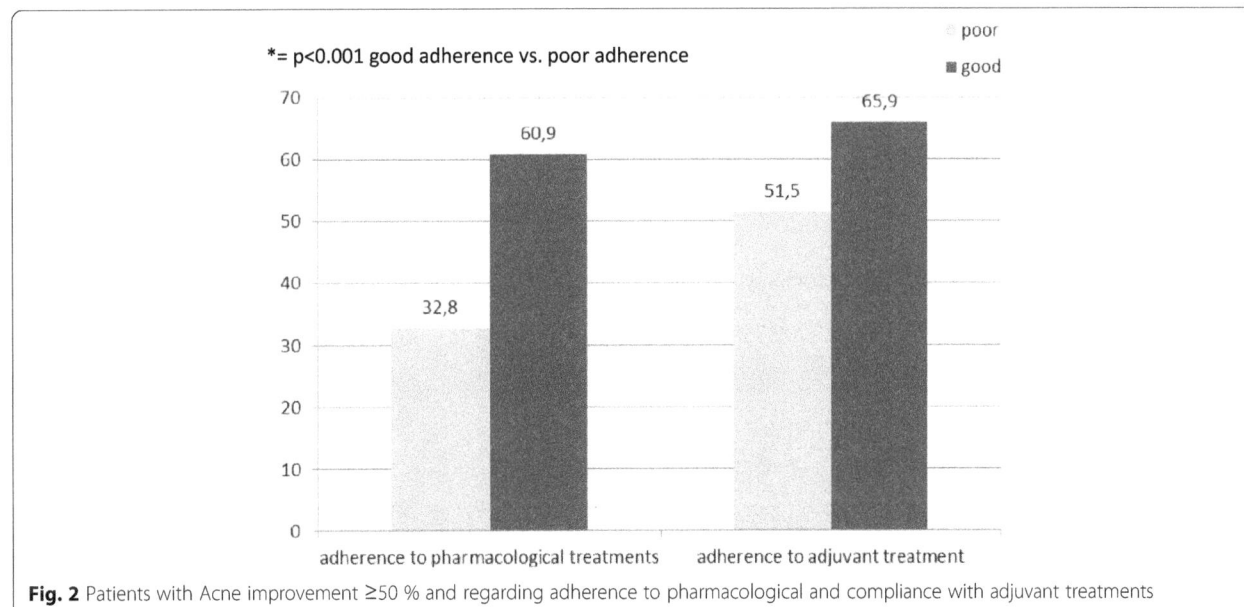

Fig. 2 Patients with Acne improvement ≥50 % and regarding adherence to pharmacological and compliance with adjuvant treatments

adherence to adjuvant treatment with specific cleansers and moisturizers for patients with acne is the second most important factor in achieving symptom improvement, after completion of drug treatment. Good adherence to adjuvant treatment is associated with a 2.2-fold increase in the probability of adherence to topical pharmacological treatment and with significant reductions in the severity and number of acne lesions.

Abbreviations
ECOB: Elaboration de un outil de evaluación de l'observance des traitaments medicamenteux; CRF: Case report form; FDA: Federal Drugs Administration.

Competing interests
Sonia Aladren and Massimo Milani are ISDIN employees. The ACTUO study was supported by an unrestricted grant of ISDIN SA.

Authors' contributions
RDL, GMA, MPL, AVC participated in the study design, coordination and patients enrollment. MM and SA participated in the design of study protocol and data analysis. All authors read and approved the final manuscript.

Acknowledgements
Actuo Study Group Investigators: Abellaneda Fernández, Cristina; Aguayo Leyva, Ingrid Rocío; Alcaraz León, Inmaculada; Alonso García, Ignacio; Arechalde Pérez, Ana; Balbín Carrero, Eva; Ballestero Corominas, Alejandro; Bilbao Badiola, Ibon; Boada García, Aram; Ciudad Blanco, Cristina; De Lucas, Raúl; Del Pozo Hernando, Luis Javier; Del Rio Reyes, Rosa; Eguino Gorrochategui, Patricia; Escalas Taberner, Juan; Espelt Otero, Jorge Luis; Fernández Angel,Isabel; Fernández Casado, Alex; Fernández Torres, Rosa Mª; Gallego Álvarez, Silvia; Galvany Rosell, Loida; Gamo Villegas, Reyes; Ginarte Val, Manuel; Gómez Fernández, Cristina; Gómez Vázquez, Mercedes; Gutiérrez De La Peña, Javier; Hernandez Cano, Natalia; Houmani Houmani, Manmoud; Ibargoyen Esnal, Jesús; Iglesias Sancho, Maribel; Izquierdo Herce, Noelia; Jeremías Torruella, Javier; Latorre Fuentes, José Mª; Llambrich Mañes, Alex; López Ferrer, Ana; Mariscal Polo, Amaia; Márquez Balbas, Gemma; Martin Ezquerra, Gemma; Martin Urda, Maria Teresa; Martinez Escala, Maria Estela; Martinez Fernández, Matilde; Mieras Barceló, Caterina; Molina Ruiz, Ana; Montero Pérez, Iria; Moreno Arias, Gerardo A.; Nadal Llado, Cristina; Naranjo Díaz, Maria José; Nasarre Calvo,Jaume; Navajas Pinedo, Belén; Oleaga Morante, José Manuel; Perelló Llinas, Guillermo; Pérez Losada, Mª Eugenia; Pérez-López, Montserrat; Pérez-Beato De Cos, Mª Paz; Pestoni Porven, Carmela; Poza Magdalena, Olga; Rocamora Duran, Vicenc; Rodriguez Caruncho, Clara; Rodriguez Granados, Mª Teresa; Roe Crespo, Esther; Ruiz Carrascosa, José Carlos; Salgado Boquete, Laura; Sanchez Muros, Virginia; Sanz De Galdeano Palacio,Carmen; Taberner Ferrer, Rosa; Trasobares Marugan, Lidia; Uria García, Mª Carmen Valle Martin, Mª Del Mar; Valle Santana, Pilar; Vázquez García, Juan; Velasco Pastor, Manuel; Vera Casaño, Angel; Vilarrasa Rull, Eva; Waadad Waadad, Tamim.

Author details
[1]Hospital Universitario La Paz, Madrid, Spain. [2]Hospital Quirón Teknon, Barcelona, Spain. [3]Clínica Dermatológica de Moragas, Barcelona, Spain. [4]Hospital Carlos Haya,, Málaga, Spain. [5]Isdin S.A. Medical Department, Provençals 33, Barcelona, Spain.

References
1. Kligman AM. An overview of acne. J Invest Derm. 1974;62:268–87.
2. Bhate K, Williams HC. Epidemiology of acne vulgaris. Br J Dermatol. 2013;168:474–85.
3. Thiboutot D, Gollnick H, Bettoli V, Dréno B, Kang S, Leyden JJ, et al. New insights into the management of acne: an update from the Global Alliance to Improve Outcomes in Acne group. J Am Acad Dermatol. 2009;60:S1–50.
4. Lasek RJ, Chren MM. Acne vulgaris and the quality of life of adult dermatology patients. Arch Dermatol. 1998;134:454–8.
5. Goulden V. Guidelines for the management of acne vulgaris in adolescents. Pediatr Drugs. 2003;5:301–13.
6. Weiden PJ, Rao N. Teaching medication compliance to psychiatric residents: placing an orphan topic into a training curriculum. Acad Psychiatry. 2005;29:203–10.
7. Haider A, Shaw JC. Treatment of acne vulgaris. JAMA. 2004;292:726–35.
8. McDonald HP, Garg AX, Haynes RB. Interventions to enhance patient adherence to medication prescriptions: scientific review. JAMA. 2002;288:2868–79.
9. Dréno B, Layton A, Zouboulis CC, López-Estebaranz JL, Zalewska-Janowska A, Bagatin E, et al. Adult female acne: a new paradigm. J Eur Acad Dermatol Venereol. 2013;27:1063–70.
10. Russell JJ. Topical therapy for acne. Am Fam Physician. 2000;61:357–65.
11. Snyder S. Medical adherence to acne therapy: a systematic review. Am J Clin Dermatol. 2014;15:87.
12. Weiss JS. Current options for the topical treatment of acne vulgaris. Pediatr Dermatol. 1997;14:480–8.
13. Herane MI, Fuenzalida H, Zegpi E, De Pablo C, Espadas MJ, Trullás C, et al. Specific gel-cream as adjuvant to oral insotretinoin improved hydration and prevented TEWL increase – a double blind, randomized, placebo-controlled study. J Cosmet Dermatol. 2009;8:181–5.
14. Del Rosso JQ. Clinical relevance of skin barrier changes associated with the use of oral isotretinoin: the importance of barrier repair therapy in patient management. J Drugs Dermatol. 2013;12:626–31.
15. Renzi C, Picardi A, Abeni D, et al. Association of dissatisfaction with care and psychiatric morbidity with poor treatment compliance. Arch Dermatol. 2002;138:337–42.
16. Tsou AY, Creutzfeldt CJ, Gordon JM. The good doctor: professionalism in the 21st century. Handb Clin Neurol. 2013;118:119–32.
17. Farin E, Gramm L, Schmidt E. Predictors of communication preferences in patients with chronic low back pain. Patient Prefer Adherence. 2013;7:1117–27.
18. Zaghloul SS, Cunliffe WJ, Goodfield MJ. Objective assessment of compliance with treatments in acne. Br J Dermatol. 2005;152:1015–21.
19. US Department of Health and Human Services Food and Drug Administration Center for Drug Evaluation and Research (CDER). Guidance for Industry; AcneVulgaris: Developing Drugs for Treatment. 2005.
20. Pawin H, Beylot C, Chivot M, Faure M, Poli F, Revuz J, et al. Creation of a tool to assess adherence to treatments for acne. Dermatology. 2009;218:26–32.
21. Motley RJ, Finlay AY. Practical use of a disability index in the routine management of acne. Clin Exp Dermatol. 1992;17:1–3.
22. De Tiedra AG, Mercadal J, Badía X, Mascaró JM, Herdman M, Lozano R. Adaptación transcultural al español del cuestionario Dermatology Life Quality Index (DLQI): El índice de calidad de vida en dermatología. Actas Dermatosifilogr. 1998;89:692–700.
23. Jones-Caballero M, Pedrosa E, Peñas PF. Self-reported adherence to treatment and quality of life in mild to moderate acne. Dermatology. 2008;217:309–14.
24. Miyachi Y, Hayashi N, Furukawa F, Akamatsu H, Matsunaga K, Watanabe S, et al. Acne management in Japan: study of patient adherence. Dermatology. 2011;223:174–81.

Variation of mutant allele frequency in *NRAS* Q61 mutated melanomas

Zofia Hélias-Rodzewicz[1,2*], Elisa Funck-Brentano[1,3], Nathalie Terrones[1], Alain Beauchet[4], Ute Zimmermann[1,2], Cristi Marin[1,2], Philippe Saiag[1,3] and Jean-François Emile[1,2*]

Abstract

Background: Somatic mutations of *BRAF* or *NRAS* activating the MAP kinase cell signaling pathway are present in 70% of cutaneous melanomas. The mutant allele frequency of *BRAF* V600E (M%*BRAF*) was recently shown to be highly heterogeneous in melanomas. The present study focuses on the *NRAS* Q61 mutant allele frequency (M%*NRAS*).

Methods: Retrospective quantitative analyze of 104 *NRAS* mutated melanomas was performed using pyrosequencing. Mechanisms of M%*NRAS* imbalance were studied by fluorescence in situ hybridization (FISH) and microsatellite analysis.

Results: M%*NRAS* was increased in 27.9% of cases. FISH revealed that chromosome 1 instability was the predominant mechanism of M%*NRAS* increase, with chromosome 1 polysomy observed in 28.6% of cases and intra-tumor cellular heterogeneity with copy number variations of chromosome 1/*NRAS* in 23.8%. Acquired copy-neutral loss of heterozygosity (LOH) was less frequent (19%). However, most samples with high M%*NRAS* had only one copy of *NRAS* locus surrounding regions suggesting a WT allele loss. Clinical characteristics and survival of patients with either <60% or ≥60% of M%*NRAS* were not different.

Conclusion: As recently shown for M%*BRAF*, M%*NRAS* is highly heterogeneous. The clinical impacts of high M%*NRAS* should be investigated in a larger series of patients.

Keywords: Melanoma, M%*NRAS*, Imbalance, Pyrosequencing, WT allele loss

Background

Cutaneous melanoma is a highly aggressive and treatment-resistant human cancer. The most frequent genetic alterations involve genes of the MAP kinase signaling pathway [1–3]. Activating hot-spot mutations are mainly found in *BRAF* (codon V600) and in *NRAS* (codon Q61, and less frequently in the codons G12 and G13) genes, in 35–50% and 15–25% of cutaneous melanoma, respectively [4, 5]. Among *BRAF* alterations, the *BRAF* V600E mutation in exon 15 is predominant (85%) and due to a substitution of a valine to a glutamic acid (c.1799 T > A, p.V600E) [6, 7]. *BRAF* and *NRAS* mutations are almost always mutually exclusive [8, 9].

Mutant *NRAS* melanomas have been reported to have more aggressive clinical features than other subtypes,

with thicker lesions, elevated mitotic activity, and higher rates of lymph node metastasis [10–12]. Additionally, *NRAS* mutation status was reported as a predictor of poorer outcomes with lower median survival compared to non-*NRAS* mutated melanoma [10, 13].

The discovery of *BRAF* mutations led to the development of targeted treatments [14, 15]. However despite major clinical benefit in melanomas with *BRAF* mutation, secondary resistance occurs in most patients during the first year of treatment. Thus combinations of BRAF and MEK inhibitors have been developed, and were shown to induce longer progression free survivals (PFS) of patients with *BRAF* mutated melanomas [16–18]. By contrast, targeted treatment of patients with *NRAS* mutated melanomas is still a challenge, although an international phase 3 prospective study with the MEK inhibitor binimetinib recently provided promising results [19].

We recently studied the frequency of *BRAF* mutant alleles (M%*BRAF)* and showed that M%*BRAF* is highly

* Correspondence: zofia.helias-ext@aphp.fr; jean-francois.emile@uvsq.fr
[1]Research Unit EA4340 Biomarkers in Cancerology and Hemato Oncology, Versailles SQY University, Paris-Saclay University, 9, Avenue Charles de Gaulle, 92104 Boulogne-Billancourt, France
Full list of author information is available at the end of the article

heterogeneous and frequently increased in *BRAF* mutated melanomas [20]. Interestingly, a recent clinical study showed that the increased *BRAF* V600 mutation level was significantly associated with a better response rate to vemurafenib during the first 10 months of treatment [21]. These observations highlighted the importance of quantitative evaluation of *BRAF* mutation before melanoma treatment.

Although biological and clinical implication of the frequency of mutant alleles of *BRAF* in melanomas are currently under investigation, no data are available concerning the variation of M%*NRAS*. Accordingly, we conducted this study to investigate *NRAS* Q61 mutations and M%*NRAS* in a series of 199 melanomas wild type for *BRAF* V600. The mechanisms of the M%*NRAS* variations were then studied by fluorescence in situ hybridization (FISH) and by amplified fragment length polymorphism (AFLP).

Methods

Patients and samples

Melanoma samples were obtained from the bank of biological resources of Ambroise Paré Hospital in Boulogne-Billancourt. The research was performed in compliance with the ethical principles of the Helsinki Declaration (1964) and with the French ethics laws. Patients were informed and approved the use of their samples for research purpose. Tumor samples collection was declared to the French Ministry of Research (DC 2009–933). Melan-Cohort study was approved by CPP IDF 8 Ethics committee (030209) and registered with https://www.clinicaltrials.gov/ct2/search (NCT00839410). Clinical and survival data were collected from clinical records of the Dermatology Department of Ambroise Paré Hospital.

The frequency of *NRAS* Q61 mutations was evaluated in a consecutive series of melanomas received for diagnosis from March 2013 until May 2015. Additionally, a second series of patients, whose samples were received earlier to March 2013, mutated for *NRAS* were also included for the evaluation of M%*NRAS*. In our previous paper concerning the *BRAF* mutant allele frequency in melanoma [20], we observed a distinct distribution of the percentage of mutated allele according to the percentage of tumor cells. However, the inter-pathologist reproducibility for the evaluation of tumor cell content was substantial for the 80% cut-off (κ = 0.79). Therefore, we excluded samples with less than 80% of melanoma cells from further *NRAS* molecular analysis.

NRAS mutant allele detection and quantification

Before DNA extraction, HES slides were reviewed to confirm the presence of melanoma cells and to select areas with highest density of tumor cells for macrodissection. For microsatellite analysis, DNA from corresponding normal tissue section was extracted. Genomic DNA was extracted from formalin-fixed and paraffin-embedded (FFPE) fragments of melanoma as previously described [22].

Pyrosequencing was performed as already described [23]. Profiles for different *NRAS* mutations were established and confirmed by Sanger sequencing method (Additional file 1: Figure S1). Three different assays for detection of *NRAS* Q61 mutation were designed and primers used for DNA amplification, pyrosequencing, and Sanger method are presented in Table 1. Pyrosequencing Assay 1 allows the quantification of all but one *NRAS* Q61 mutation (c.183A > T p.Q61H) [24]. Pyrosequencing Assay 2 is an edited version of Assay 1, in which the order of injected nucleotides was modified to allow the quantification of all *NRAS* Q61 mutations. Pyrosequencing Assay 3 was developed to rescue some cases with a very bad FFPE DNA quality. For patients with several samples available, the M%*NRAS* used was that obtained from the first metastasis.

Microsatellite analysis

Eight microsatellite markers were selected from the NCBI dbSNP short genetic variations database and analyzed by AFLP. Their positions are showed in Fig. 1, and the primers used in Table 1. No highly heterozygous microsatellite was identified within *NRAS* gene; thus the genetic status of this gene was evaluated on the basis of two microsatellites closed to *NRAS* locus (rs3220698 and rs3220987). PCR reactions were performed with fluorescent-labeled forward primers and the amplified PCR products were analyzed by capillary array electrophoresis on the ABI PRISM 3100 sequencer (Applied Biosystems, Foster City, USA) and GeneScan software (Applied Biosystems). Detection of loss of heterozygosity was performed as detailed in Loss of Heterozygosity Analysis Getting Started Guide. Two independent experiments were performed to confirm LOH results. The probability of one *NRAS* allele loss was evaluated as very high if only one allele was detected in each *NRAS* locus surrounding microsatellites (e.g. Fig. 1, case Y11.136). If only one of *NRAS* surrounding markers presented one microsatellite allele, this probability was evaluated as mean (e.g. Fig. 1, case Y14.711). The analysis was considered as inconclusive if both *NRAS* locus surrounding microsatellites gave non informative results (e.g. Fig. 1, case Y10.1471).

FISH analysis

FISH analysis was performed on tissue microarray (TMA) containing 94 melanomas and on tissue sections from 7 melanoma patients. FISH probe preparation and FISH

Table 1 Primers and pyrosequencing assay information. Primers sequences used for PCR, Sanger sequencing, pyrosequencing and AFLP technique

NRAS Pyrosequencing ASSAY 1	
PCR 124 nt	
Primer F-Biotine	ACACCCCCAGGATTCTTACAGA
Primer R	GCCTGTCCTCATGTATTGGTC
Pyrosequencing primer	CATGGCACTGTACTCTTC
Nucleotide injection order	GTTACGTCAGCTG
NRAS Pyrosequencing ASSAY 2	
PCR 124 nt	
Primer F-Biotine	ACACCCCCAGGATTCTTACAGA
Primer R	GCCTGTCCTCATGTATTGGTC
Pyrosequencing primer	CATGGCACTGTACTCTTC
Nucleotide injection order	GCATACGTCAG
NRAS Pyrosequencing ASSAY 3	
PCR 90 nt	
Primer F-Biotine	ACAAGTGGTTATAGATGGTGA
Primer R	ATGTATTGGTCTCTCATGGCA
Pyrosequencing primer	CATGGCACTGTACTCTTC
Nucleotide injection order	GCATACGTCAGCT
Sanger Sequencing	
Primer F	ACAAGTGGTTATAGATGGTGA
Primer R	ATGTATTGGTCTCTCATGGCA
AFLP primers	
rs3219599 F	TTCAAGGCTGCAGTGAGCTA
rs3219599 R	AGTGGAAGCTAGACACACATTAAGA
s3219653 F	CCAGAGAGACAGAACTGAACAAA
s3219653 R	CAAATTTTGGACCTGCCATG
rs3219587 F	GGGCAAATGGAGGAAAGAGA
rs3219587 R	TAAAAATACCCCCACCCCACT
rs3220698 F	TTAAAAAACGTACTGCCACATTCA
rs3220698 R	GGCAGAAACCAGGAAATGTAGTA
rs3220987 F	GGCTTTTAGCTATGATTTGAGA
rs3220987 R	GACTCAGGAAATAAACAAGGC
rs3220389 F	CGCTGCTCACTCCTCCTCTGA
rs3220389 R	AGTGCTGCTCTCAGTGAACTC
rs3219612 F	AGCACACAATATACTCTCTCAGA
rs3219612 R	ACCTGGGCAAAAGAGTAAGACC
rs3219703 F	AACGAAGGTGTACTGGGACTGGT
rs3219703 R	ACAGGGATGTGAGGGATTTTTTC

technique was performed as already described [20, 25]. All samples were analyzed with RP11-245I3 and RP11-269F19 probes covering *NRAS* and a region of chromosome 1 telomeric to *NRAS* gene (chr1:45.142.760–45.303.288, (2009 GRCh37/hg19)), respectively. Chromosome 1/

NRAS disomie was concluded if two FISH signals for each probe were observed and polysomy if three or more FISH signals were detected in the majority of cell. Chromosome 1/*NRAS* signal ratios 2:1 and 1:2 were described as *NRAS* monosomy and *NRAS* gain, respectively. Innumerable *NRAS* FISH signals were interpreted as amplification. Intra-tumor heterogeneity was defined as a presence of cell populations with different chromosome 1/*NRAS* status; some cells with increase, some with normal and some with loss of *NRAS* allele.

ATGC data analysis

Sequencing data about *NRAS* mutation of 479 cutaneous skin melanomas were extracted from cBioPortal platform as describe by Gao and colleagues [26]. The *NRAS* Q61 mutant allele percentage in 85 melanomas was compared to the data of our series.

Statistical analysis

Overall survival (OS) was defined as the period between the date of the primary melanoma diagnosis to the date of death (all causes) or last follow-up evaluation. Survival was censored at the last follow-up evaluation. Distant metastasis free survival (DMFS) was defined as the period between the date of the primary melanoma diagnosis to the date of onset of stage IV melanoma or death. The date of onset of stage IV melanoma was defined as the date of the clinical examination or imaging procedure that provided an unequivocal diagnosis of distant visceral metastasis. Progression-free survival was defined as the period between the date of the primary melanoma diagnosis (with or without lymph node sentinel biopsy procedure) to the date of the first regional (node or cutaneous) recurrence (stage IIIB minimum). Progression-free survival, distant metastasis-free survival and overall survival curves were estimated using the Kaplan-Meier method, and differences between PFS, DMFS, and OS curves were assessed using the log-rank test.

Survival and histoprognostic markers (age, gender, Breslow index, ulceration and mitotic activity) of *NRAS* Q61 mutated primary melanomas were compared between two groups: one group of 48 melanomas with <60% of M%*NRAS* and another group of 24 tumors with ≥60% of M%*NRAS*.

Student tests were performed for quantitative values, and Chi^2 tests for qualitative values. The results were considered significant when $P < 0.05$.

Results

NRAS mutation frequency and allele quantification

The frequencies of *BRAF* V600 and *NRAS* Q61 mutations were evaluated in 267 FFPE melanoma patients of the series (flow chart in Additional file 2: Figure S2) diagnosed between March 2013 and May 2015. *NRAS*

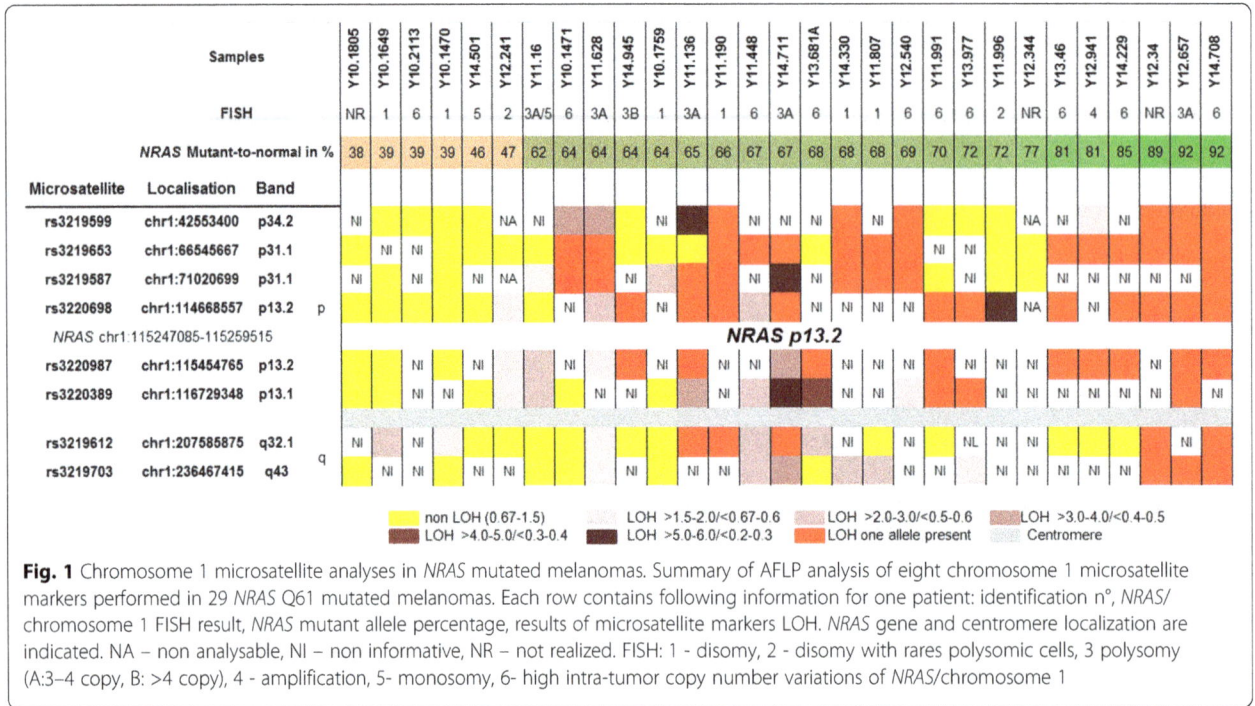

Fig. 1 Chromosome 1 microsatellite analyses in *NRAS* mutated melanomas. Summary of AFLP analysis of eight chromosome 1 microsatellite markers performed in 29 *NRAS* Q61 mutated melanomas. Each row contains following information for one patient: identification n°, *NRAS*/chromosome 1 FISH result, *NRAS* mutant allele percentage, results of microsatellite markers LOH. *NRAS* gene and centromere localization are indicated. NA – non analysable, NI – non informative, NR – not realized. FISH: 1 - disomy, 2 - disomy with rares polysomic cells, 3 polysomy (A:3–4 copy, B: >4 copy), 4 - amplification, 5- monosomy, 6- high intra-tumor copy number variations of *NRAS*/chromosome 1

mutation was detected in 48 melanomas, corresponding to 18% (48/267) of all melanomas and 33.8% (48/142) of *BRAF* V600 wild type cases. Additionally, 63 *NRAS* Q61 mutated melanomas, diagnosed before this period, were included into the molecular analyses. In total, 111 *NRAS* Q61 mutated tumors were collected with 60–95% tumor cells.

Characterization of M%*NRAS* were performed in a larger group of 104 *NRAS* Q61 mutated melanomas containing ≥80% tumor cells. The corresponding mutations were c.182A > G p.Q61R in 58.6% (61/104), c.181C > A p.Q61K in 23.1% (24/104), c.182A > T p.Q61L in 13.5% (14/104), c.183A > T p.Q61H in 2.9% (3/104) and c.183A > C p.Q61H in 1.9% (2/104) of samples. M%*NRAS* was highly heterogeneous, ranging from 15.5 to 94% (Fig. 2). The majority of cases (60.6%, 63/104) had ≥30 to 60% M%*NRAS* and was thus considered as heterozygous (HET). The remaining 41 cases were considered as having non-heterozygous M%*NRAS*: 11.5% (12/104) had <30% of M%*NRAS* (Low non-HET) and 27.9% (29/104) had ≥60% of M%*NRAS* (High non-HET).

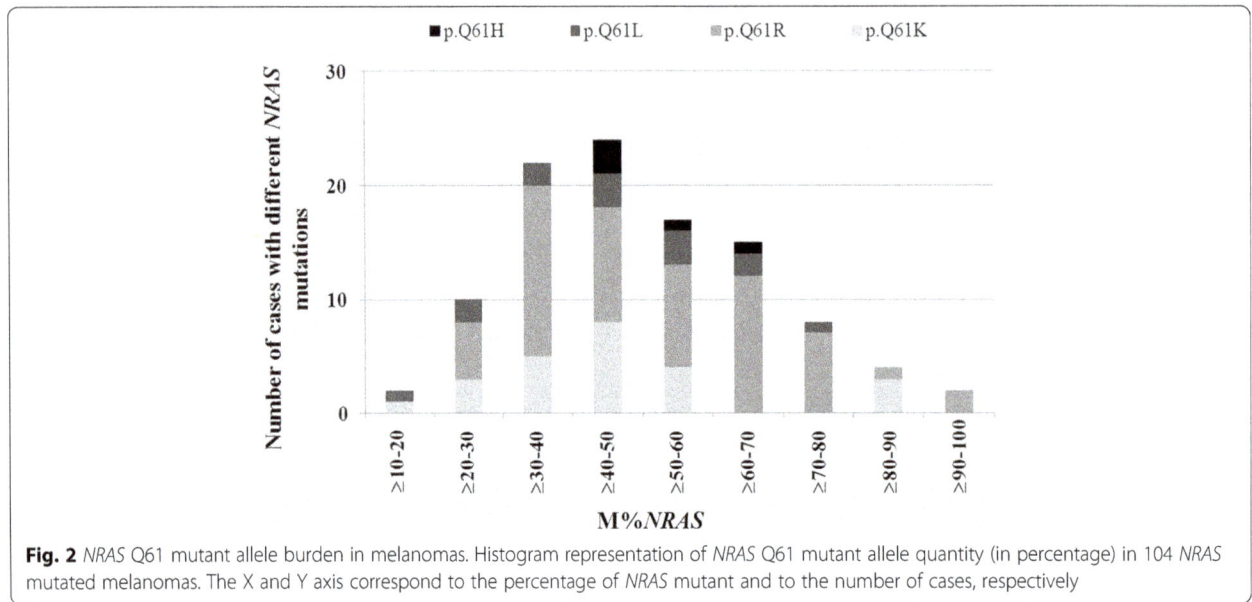

Fig. 2 *NRAS* Q61 mutant allele burden in melanomas. Histogram representation of *NRAS* Q61 mutant allele quantity (in percentage) in 104 *NRAS* mutated melanomas. The X and Y axis correspond to the percentage of *NRAS* mutant and to the number of cases, respectively

We then compared our results with database of the Cancer Genome Atlas (TCGA) analyzed on the CBioPortal platform. Among the 85 *NRAS* mutated cases that were available only 50.6% (43/85) had a heterozygous status of *NRAS* mutation, while 34.1% (29/85) was High non-HET and 15.3% (13/85) was Low non-HET (Additional file 3: Figure S3).

FISH analysis

Among 101 samples (41 *NRAS* WT and 60 *NRAS* Q61) analyzed by FISH with *NRAS* locus and chromosome 1 specific fluorescent probes, different types of alternations were observed: no alteration of *NRAS*/chromosome 1 (disomy), disomy but rare cells with polysomy, polysomy and monosomy, which were detected in 23.1% (24/101), 19.2% (20/101), 9.6% (10/101) and 3.8% (4/101) of cases, respectively. *NRAS* amplification was a rare alteration and observed in 6.7% of melanoma samples (7/101). In 23.1% of samples (24/101), we observed intra-tumor cellular heterogeneity in *NRAS*/chromosome 1 copy numbers. Finally, FISH analysis of *NRAS* gene was non informative in 14.4% of cases (15/101).

To better understand the chromosomal mechanisms leading to M%*NRAS* increase, we compared M%*NRAS* and *NRAS*/chromosome 1 copy number status between 32 *BRAF*/*NRAS* WT and 57 *NRAS* Q61 mutated melanomas (Fig. 3). Disomy of *NRAS*/chromosome 1 (with or without polysomy in few cells) were detected in 59.4% (19/32) of *BRAF*/*NRAS* WT, 50% (15/30) of HET, but in only 28.6% (6/21) of High non-HET melanomas (*P* = 0.08). Polysomy of *NRAS*/chromosome 1 was detected in 13.3% (4/30) of HET, and 28.6% (6/21) of High non-HET

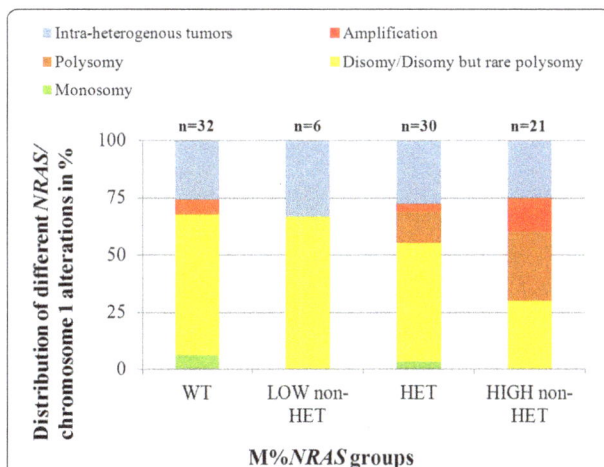

Fig. 3 *NRAS*/chromosome 1 aberrations in *NRAS* mutated (*n* = 57) and *NRAS* WT (*n* = 32) melanomas. Histogram representation of prevalence of *NRAS*/chromosome 1 abnormalities evaluated by FISH in 104 *NRAS* mutated melanomas depending on the amounts of *NRAS* Q61 mutations. WT – wild-type, HET – heterozygous

samples, but was absent in *BRAF*/*NRAS* WT melanomas (*P* < 0.05). Amplification of *NRAS* was detected in 6.3% (2/32) and 9.5% (2/21) of *BRAF*/*NRAS* WT and High non-HET melanomas, respectively. Additionally, in 3.3% (1/30) of HET and 9.5% (2/21) of High non-HET cases, a gain of *NRAS* gene was observed. Deletion of *NRAS* was also a rare event and was observed in 9.4% (3/32) of *BRAF*/*NRAS* WT and 3.3% (1/30) of HET melanomas. A high intra-tumor copy number variation of *NRAS*/chromosome 1 was observed in 25% (8/32) of *BRAF*/*NRAS* WT, 30% (9/30) of HET and 23.8% (5/21) of High non-HET. FISH results of Low non-HET group were excluded from the comparative analysis because of insufficient numbers of samples (only 6 samples).

Chromosome 1 microsatellite analysis

Eight polymorphic microsatellite markers were analyzed in 6 HET and 23 High non-HET tumors melanoma samples. In all HET melanomas, non LOH of *NRAS* locus surrounding microsatellites was detected but one for which microsatellites presented a low LOH, near the upper LOH detection threshold. In the majority of samples of High non-HET group, the microsatellite analysis revealed the presence of only one marker in the regions surrounding *NRAS* gene (Fig. 1). The probability of one *NRAS* allele loss was evaluated as very high in 30% (7/23) and mean in 26.1% (6/23) of tumors. In 26.1% (6/23) of tumors, the LOH results were non informative. In 17.4% (4/23), LOH with the presence of two alleles rather than one allele loss was detected.

Correlation of M%*NRAS* and clinical data

Information on primary tumor was available for 72 patients. The main histological subtypes were SSM and nodular melanomas, in 44.4% (32/72) and 38.9% (28/72) of cases, respectively. Median Breslow was 2.84 mm [0.4–10]. An ulceration was present in 47.2% (34/72) of melanomas, and 58.3% (42/72) had a mitotic activity (> 1 mitosis / mm^2). Among these cases, we found *NRAS* Q61R mutation in 63.9% (46/72) of melanomas, *NRAS* Q61K in 25% (18/72), *NRAS* Q61L in 6.9% (5/72) and *NRAS* Q61H in 4.2% (3/72). M%*NRAS* was quantified by analysis of primary melanoma in 18.1% (13/72) of cases and of metastasis (lymph node, cutaneous or visceral) in 81.9% (59/72). Patients were divided into two groups depending on % of *NRAS* mutant allele. M%*NRAS* was ≥60% in the first group (*n* = 24, 33.3%) and <60% in the second cohort (*n* = 48, 66.7%). The second group contained 41 HET M%*NRAS* and 7 low not-HET M%*NRAS* cases. Clinical and pathological features of primary *NRAS* mutated melanomas were compared between these two groups and they are summarized in Table 2. No statistically significant differences were observed between these two groups with baseline criteria ($P > 0.05$). The median follow-up of the patients was 40 months (range [1–445]). PFS, DMFS and OS in both groups were not different (Fig. 4).

Discussion

In this study, we reported the prevalence of *NRAS* Q61 mutation and, for the first time, the variations of *NRAS* mutant alleles (M%*NRAS*), in a large series of human melanoma samples. We have demonstrated that M%*NRAS*

Table 2 Clinicopathologic characteristics of studied subjects. Comparison of clinical and pathological features of *NRAS* mutated primary melanomas according to the *NRAS* mutant allelic burden (<60% or ≥60%)

	≥60% of M% NRAS n = 24/72 (33.3%)	<60% of M% NRAS n = 48/72 (66.7%)	P-value (statistic test)
Origin of pyrosequencing sample			
From primary melanoma	5	8	0.91 (Chi2with Yates' correction)
From metastasis	19	40	
Age			
Mean, years (SD)	63.1 ± 17.4	65.2 ± 14.7	0.61 (Student)
Median, year [range]	60 [37–93]	66 [32–97]	
Gender			
Ratio M/F	13/11	30/18	0.49 (Chi2)
Breslow index			
Mean, mm (SD)	3.0 ± 2.1	3.3 ± 2.2	0.57 (Student)
Median, mm [range]	3.00 [0.40–10.00]	2.61 [0.50–9.00]	
Ulceration	14	20	0.14 (Chi2)
Mitotic activity	11	31	0.45 (Chi2)
Initial AJCC stage			
I	5	10	0.7 (Chi2)
IA	4	2	
IB	1	8	
II	11	26	
IIA	4	10	
IIB	6	5	
IIC	1	11	
III	7	9	
IIIA	0	2	
IIIB	4	2	
IIIC	3	6	
IV	1	0	
NA	0	2	
Histologic subtype			
Nodular melanoma	9	19	0.63 (Chi2)
SSM	10	22	
Acral melanoma	1	0	
Lentigo maligna melanoma	0	1	
Mucosal melanoma	0	1	
On congenital naevus	0	1	
Inclassable	1	2	
NA	3	2	

SMM superficial spreading melanoma
NA data not available
SD standard deviation
M/F male/female

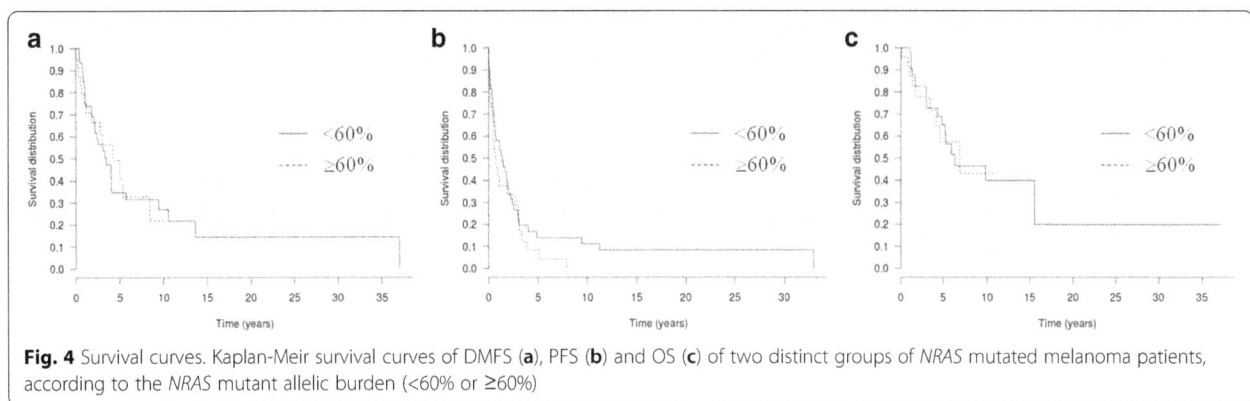

Fig. 4 Survival curves. Kaplan-Meir survival curves of DMFS (**a**), PFS (**b**) and OS (**c**) of two distinct groups of *NRAS* mutated melanoma patients, according to the *NRAS* mutant allelic burden (<60% or ≥60%)

was highly heterogeneous; indeed, only 61% of *NRAS* mutated melanomas were heterozygous, while 30% of cases had a significantly increased M%*NRAS* (≥60%). Our results were confirmed by analysis of the cases of the TCGA database.

NRAS pyrosequencing assays used in this study were developed to identify all hot-spot mutations in the codon 61 of *NRAS* gene. The specificity of these assays for different mutations was confirmed by Sanger sequencing. Additionally, the genotyping accuracy of 40 *NRAS* mutated melanomas, 27 of which were p.Q61R was confirmed by immunohistochemistry with an antibody against Q61R [27]. In a recent study, we have demonstrated that pyrosequencing was a robust molecular technique for oncogenic mutant allele quantification, by comparing it with quantitative real time PCR and picodroplet digital PCR [20]. This previous study was focused on *BRAF* mutations, and similar M%*BRAF* heterogeneity was demonstrated in melanomas, with 19% of cases having an increased M%*BRAF*. Altogether, we estimate from both series that 36.2% of melanomas with *BRAF/NRAS* mutations have a non-heterozygous oncogenic allele.

Few studies have investigated M%*NRAS* in melanomas. Recently, we reported two cases with an increase of M%*NRAS* during metastatic melanoma progression; suggesting that M%*NRAS* may enhance metastatic capacities of melanomas [28]. Additionally, a large screening study of 833 cells lines from the database of Cancer Genome Project, Sanger Institute, focused on frequently mutated genes (six suppressor gene and five oncogenes), has identified *NRAS* homozygous mutation in 10% of cell lines [29]. However, the zygosity status was only determinate by manual examination of sequencing electropherograms.

Interestingly, in vitro studies of mutant RAS family members had demonstrated a high oncogenic potential of increased mutant allele frequency. The oncogenic potential of $NRAS^{G12D/G12D}$ was highly increased as compared

to heterozygous or hemizygous *NRAS* cells in *NRAS*-driven hematopoietic transformation [30]. Additionally, progenitors of hematopoietic cells expressing the highest levels of $NRAS^{G12D}$ demonstrated cytokine-independent CFU-GM colony growth and exhibited an increased level of pAkt, pErk and pS6 proteins. Endogenous expression of $HRAS^{G12V}$ promotes papilloma and angiosarcoma development and these neoplasm initiations have been strongly associated with $HRAS^{G12V}$ allelic and gene copy number imbalances [31, 32].

Mutation in one allele of an oncogene is sufficient for activation of its targets and M%*NRAS* is expected to be around 50% in diploid cells. However, in tumours with high chromosome instability, chromosome number is rarely disomic and M%*NRAS* could widely exceeded 50%. To better understand the chromosome mechanisms leading to *NRAS* mutant allele increase in the proportion of *NRAS* mutated melanoma, we firstly performed FISH analyses with 2 BAC probes covering *NRAS* region and another region of chromosome 1, telomeric to this gene, in a large series of 104 melanomas. Different types of *NRAS*/chromosome 1 status were observed. Polysomy was mainly observed in *NRAS* mutated tumours and disomic and/or disomic but rare polysomic cells were less frequent in High non-HET M%*NRAS* than in M%*NRAS* WT tumours. Amplification and deletion of *NRAS* gene were rarely observed and were seen in both *NRAS* WT and *NRAS* mutated melanomas. Genomic analysis of human cutaneous melanoma genomes have been described in several studies. However, in most of them, only melanoma cell lines were studied. The analysis of 60 melanoma cell lines by Gast [33] have revealed targeted focal amplifications of *NRAS* genes in 11% of them ($n = 7/60$) and amplification were detected in both *NRAS* mutated and *NRAS* WT melanomas. This frequency is higher that the frequency of *NRAS* amplification detected in the present series and in other reports. In a subset of cutaneous melanocytic lesions,

NRAS amplification was found to be restricted to a few cases with *NRAS* mutations [34]. Additionally, Stark and colleagues reported rare instances of focal amplification including *NRAS* gene in two cell lines with *NRAS* mutation; however, a poor correlation between copy number increase and concomitant mutation in this oncogene was described [35]. Polysomy of chromosome 1 and intra-tumour *NRAS*/chromosome 1 heterozygosity were frequently found in our series and was preferentially observed in *NRAS* mutated cancers. Correlation between mutant burden and gene copy gains have already been described for *KRAS* [36] and *BRAF* gene [20]. To our knowledge, *NRAS*/chromosome 1 copy number variations have never been described in melanomas with regard to the *NRAS* mutant allele burden.

Secondly, we analyzed chromosome 1 microsatellite polymorphism in normal and tumor DNA in a group of 29 *NRAS* mutated cancers by ALFP method. As expected, LOH with WT allele loss was mostly restricted to the High non-HET M%*NRAS* group. However, unlike in haematological malignancy [37, 38], acquired copy-neutral LOH was not a predominant mechanism of mutant allele imbalance in *NRAS* Q61 mutated melanomas; indeed this aberration was detected in only 23% of our samples. Other mechanisms of High non-HET M%*NRAS* were amplification and gain of *NRAS* gene (14%) and polysomy of chromosome 1 (23.8%). In 9 melanomas (38.1%), an intra-tumor copy number variation of *NRAS*/chromosome 1 was detected. As most melanomas have copy number variations of whole chromosomes and of chromosome segment, *NRAS* mutant allele increase could be a consequence of chromosome instability and clonality in these tumors.

Correlation of M%*NRAS* with clinical data revealed no association with age, sex, histological melanoma subtypes, nor with histoprognostic markers of the patients with *NRAS* Q61 mutated melanomas. Moreover, no differences in patient survival outcomes were observed between patients with <60% and ≥60% of M%*NRAS*. However, this cohort is a retrospective monocentric study, and the analyses were limited by small number of patients. Furthermore, the value of M%*NRAS* has to be investigated for prediction of response to targeted therapy, as done for M%*NRAS* with promising results. We hypothesize that High non-HET M%*NRAS* could have an oncogenic addiction effect, which could improve the sensitivity of targeted therapy in this subgroup of *NRAS* Q61 mutated melanoma.

Conclusion

We report herein for the first time that 30% of cutaneous *NRAS* mutant melanomas have a high M%*NRAS*.

Chromosome instability, (chromosome 1 polysomy, intra-tumor copy number variation of chromosome1/*NRAS*) rather than the acquired copy neutral LOH seems to be responsible for most of the cases with high M%*NRAS*. Histoprognostic markers and survivals were not different when comparing patients with <60% and ≥60% of M%*NRAS*; however this should be checked in a larger and multicentric series.

Additional files

> **Additional file 1: Figure S1.** Identification of *NRAS* WT and different *NRAS* mutations. Sequence of *NRAS* wild type allele (A) and of different *NRAS* mutant alleles and the corresponding pyrosequencing profiles. Pyrosequencing profiles by assays 1 (A, B, D, E) and by assay 2 (C and F) are present
>
> **Additional file 2: Figure S2.** Flow chart. Flow chart for melanoma samples regarding the *NRAS* gene status and the type of molecular analysis carried out
>
> **Additional file 3: Figure S3.** *NRAS* Q61 mutant allele burden in ATGC melanomas. Histogram representation of *NRAS* Q61 mutant allele quantity (in percentage) in 85 ATGC *NRAS* mutated melanomas. The X and Y axis correspond to the percentage of *NRAS* mutant and to the number of cases, respectively

Abbreviations

ALFP: Amplified fragment length polymorphism; DMFS: Distant metastasis free survival; FISH: Fluorescence in situ hybridization; HET: Heterozygous; LOH: Loss of heterozygosity; M%*NRAS*: *NRAS* mutant allele frequency; OS: Overall survival; PFS: Progression-free survival

Acknowledgements

The authors thank Mariama Bakari, Dominique Pechaud, Yolaine Pothin and Catherine Le Gall for technique contribution and/or data collection.

Funding

This work was supported partly by grants from the Association Vaincre le Mélanome, Ligue Contre le Cancer (Comité 92 WB2013–232), and Association pour la Recherche et l'Enseignement en Pathologie (AREP).

Authors' contributions

Conception and design: ZHR, EFB, JFE; Development of the methodology, Acquisition of data: ZHR, EFB; NT, CM, UZ; Analysis and interpretation of data: ZHR, EFB, AB, NT, UZ, CM, PS, JFE; Writing and revision of the manuscript: ZHR, EFB, JFE; Study supervision: JEF, PS. All authors have read and approved the final manuscript.

Competing interests

JF.E. received honoraria from Roche and Glaxo Smith Kline for counseling on patients with melanomas on the diagnosis and/or treatment with BRAF inhibitors. P.S. received honoraria for counseling on diagnosis and/or treatment of patients with melanomas from Roche and Glaxo Smith Kline.

Author details

[1]Research Unit EA4340 Biomarkers in Cancerology and Hemato Oncology, Versailles SQY University, Paris-Saclay University, 9, Avenue Charles de Gaulle, 92104 Boulogne-Billancourt, France. [2]Department of Pathology, Ambroise Paré Hospital, AP-HP, Boulogne-Billancourt, France. [3]Department of Dermatology, Ambroise Paré Hospital, AP-HP, Boulogne-Billancourt, France. [4]Department of Public Health, Ambroise Paré Hospital Ap-HP, Boulogne-Billancourt, France.

References

1. Albino AP, Nanus DM, Mentle IR, Cordon-Cardo C, McNutt NS, Bressler J, et al. Analysis of ras oncogenes in malignant melanoma and precursor lesions: correlation of point mutations with differentiation phenotype. Oncogene. 1989;4:1363–74.

2. Davies H, Bignell GR, Cox C, Stephens P, Edkins S, Clegg S, et al. Mutations of the BRAF gene in human cancer. Nature. 2002;417:949–54.

3. Curtin JA, Fridlyand J, Kageshita T, Patel HN, Busam KJ, Kutzner H, et al. Distinct sets of genetic alterations in melanoma. N Engl J Med. 2005;353:2135–47.

4. Tsao H, Chin L, Garraway LA, Fisher DE. Melanoma: from mutations to medicine. Genes Dev. 2012;26:1131–55.

5. Cancer Genome Atlas Network. Genomic Classification of Cutaneous Melanoma. 2015. Cell 2015, 161:1681–1696.

6. Long GV, Menzies AM, Nagrial AM, Haydu LE, Hamilton AL, Mann GJ, et al. Prognostic and clinicopathologic associations of oncogenic BRAF in metastatic melanoma. J Clin Oncol. 2011;29:1239–46.

7. Greaves WO, Verma S, Patel KP, Davies MA, Barkoh BA, Galbincea JM, et al. Frequency and spectrum of BRAF mutations in a retrospective, single-institution study of 1112 cases of melanoma. J Mol Diagn. 2013;15:220–6.

8. Omholt K, Platz A, Kanter L, Ringborg U, Hansson J. NRAS and BRAF mutations arise early during melanoma pathogenesis and are preserved throughout tumor progression. Clin Cancer Res. 2003;9:6483–8.

9. Akslen LA, Angelini S, Straume O, Bachmann IM, Molven A, Hemminki K, et al. BRAF and NRAS mutations are frequent in nodular melanoma but are not associated with tumor cell proliferation or patient survival. J Invest Dermatol. 2005;125:312–7.

10. Thumar J, Shahbazian D, Aziz SA, Jilaveanu LB, Kluger HM. MEK targeting in N-RAS mutated metastatic melanoma. Mol Cancer. 2014;13:45.

11. Devitt B, Liu W, Salemi R, Wolfe R, Kelly J, Tzen CY, et al. Clinical outcome and pathological features associated with NRAS mutation in cutaneous melanoma. Pigment Cell Melanoma Res. 2011;24:666–72.

12. Ellerhorst JA, Greene VR, Ekmekcioglu S, Warneke CL, Johnson MM, Cooke CP, et al. Clinical correlates of NRAS and BRAF mutations in primary human melanoma. Clin Cancer Res. 2011;17:229–35.

13. Jakob JA, Bassett RL Jr, Ng CS, Curry JL, Joseph RW, Alvarado GC, et al. NRAS mutation status is an independent prognostic factor in metastatic melanoma. Cancer. 2012;118:4014–23.

14. Chapman PB, Hauschild A, Robert C, Haanen JB, Ascierto P, Larkin J, et al. BRIM-3 study group. Improved survival with vemurafenib in melanoma with BRAF V600E mutation. N Engl J Med. 2011;364:2507–16.

15. Hauschild A, Grob JJ, Demidov LV, Jouary T, Gutzmer R, Millward M, et al. Dabrafenib in BRAF-mutated metastatic melanoma: a multicentre, open-label, phase 3 randomised controlled trial. Lancet. 2012;380:358–65.

16. Long GV, Stroyakovskiy D, Gogas H, Levchenko E, de Braud F, Larkin J, et al. Combined BRAF and MEK inhibition versus BRAF inhibition alone in melanoma. N Engl J Med. 2014;371:1877–88.

17. Long GV, Stroyakovskiy D, Gogas H, Levchenko E, de Braud F, Larkin J, et al. Dabrafenib and trametinib versus dabrafenib and placebo for Val600 BRAF-mutant melanoma: a multicentre, double-blind, phase 3 randomised controlled trial. Lancet. 2015;386:444–51.

18. Robert C, Karaszewska B, Schachter J, Rutkowski P, Mackiewicz A, Stroiakovski D, et al. Improved overall survival in melanoma with combined dabrafenib and trametinib. N Engl J Med. 2015;372:30–9.

19. Dummer R, Schadendorf D, Ascierto PA, Arance Fernández AM, Dutriaux C, Maio M,et al. Results of NEMO: A phase III trial of binimetinib (BINI) vs dacarbazine (DTIC) in NRAS-mutant cutaneous melanoma. J Clin Oncol 2016, ASCO Meeting Abstracts 34:9500.

20. Hélias-Rodzewicz Z, Funck-Brentano E, Baudoux L, Jung CK, Zimmermann U, Marin C, et al. Variations of BRAF mutant allele percentage in melanomas. BMC Cancer. 2015;15:497.

21. Lebbé C, How-Kit A, Battistella M, Sadoux A, Podgorniak MP, Sidina I, et al. BRAF(V600) mutation levels predict response to vemurafenib in metastatic melanoma. Melanoma Res. 2014;24:415–8.

22. Colomba E, Hélias-Rodzewicz Z, Von Deimling A, Marin C, Terrones N, Pechaud D, et al. Detection of BRAF p.V600E mutations in melanomas: comparison of four methods argues for sequential use of immunohistochemistry and pyrosequencing. J Mol Diagn. 2013;15:94–100.

23. Moreau S, Saiag P, Aegerter P, Bosset D, Longvert C, Hélias-Rodzewicz Z, et al. Prognostic value of BRAFV600 mutations inmelanoma patients after resection of metastatic lymph nodes. Ann SurgOncol. 2012;2012(19):4314–21.

24. Balschun K, Haag J, Wenke AK, von Schönfels W, Schwarz NT, Röcken C. KRAS, NRAS, PIK3CA exon 20, and BRAF genotypes in synchronous and metachronous primary colorectal cancers diagnostic and therapeutic implications. J Mol Diagn. 2011;2011(13):436–45.

25. Lourenço N, Hélias-Rodzewicz Z, Bachet JB, Brahimi-Adouane S, Jardin F. Tran van Nhieu J, Peschaud F, Martin E, Beauchet A, Chibon F. Emile JF Copy-neutral loss of heterozygosity and chromosome gains and losses are frequent in gastrointestinal stromal tumors Mol Cancer. 2014;13:246.

26. Gao J, Aksoy BA, Dogrusoz U, Dresdner G, Gross B, Sumer SO,et al Integrative analysis of complex cancer genomics and clinical profiles using the cBioPortal. Sci Signal 2013, 6:pl1.

27. Ilie M, Long-Mira E, Funck-Brentano E, Lassalle S, Butori C, Lespinet-Fabre V, et al. Immunohistochemistry as a potential tool for routine detection of the NRAS Q61R mutation in patients with metastatic melanoma. J Am Acad Dermatol. 2015 May;72:786–93.

28. Funck-Brentano E, Hélias-Rodzewicz Z, Longvert C, Mokhtari K, Saiag P, Emile JF. Increase in NRAS mutant allele percentage during metastatic melanoma progression. Exp Dermatol. 2016;25:472–4.

29. Soh J, Okumura N, Lockwood WW, Yamamoto H, Shigematsu H, Zhang W, et al. Oncogene mutations, copy number gains and mutant allele specific imbalance (MASI) frequently occur together in tumor cells. PLoS One. 2009;4:e7464.

30. Xu J, Haigis KM, Firestone AJ, McNerney ME, Li Q, Davis E, et al. Dominant role of oncogene dosage and absence of tumor suppressor activity in Nras-driven hematopoietic transformation. Cancer Discov. 2013;3:993–1001.

31. Chen X, Mitsutake N, LaPerle K, Akeno N, Zanzonico P, Longo VA, et al. Endogenous expression of Hras(G12V) induces developmental defects and neoplasms with copy number imbalances of the oncogene. Proc Natl Acad Sci U S A. 2009;106:7979–84.

32. Chen X, Makarewicz JM, Knauf JA, Johnson LK, Fagin JA. Transformation by Hras(G12V) is consistently associated with mutant allele copy gains and is reversed by farnesyl transferase inhibition. Oncogene. 2014;33:5442–9.

33. Gast A, Scherer D, Chen B, Bloethner S, Melchert S, Sucker A, et al. Somatic alterations in the melanoma genome: a high-resolution array-based comparative genomic hybridization study. Genes Chromosomes Cancer. 2010;49:733–45.

34. Dubruc E, Balme B, Dijoud F, Disant F, Thomas L, Wang Q, et al. Mutated and amplified NRAS in a subset of cutaneous melanocytic lesions with dermal spitzoid morphology: report of two pediatric cases located on the ear. J Cutan Pathol. 2014;2014(41):866–72.

35. Stark M, Hayward N. Genome-wide loss of heterozygosity and copy number analysis in melanoma using high-density single-nucleotide polymorphism arrays. Cancer Res. 2007;67:2632–42.

36. Modrek B, Ge L, Pandita A, Lin E, Mohan S, Yue P, et al. Oncogenic activating mutations are associated with local copy gain. Mol Cancer Res. 2009;2009(7):1244–52.

37. Rumi E, Pietra D, Guglielmelli P, Bordoni R, Casetti I, Milanesi C, et al. Associazione Italiana per la Ricerca sul Cancro Gruppo Italiano Malattie Mieloproliferative. Acquired copy-neutral loss of heterozygosity of chromosome 1p as a molecular event associated with marrow fibrosis in MPL-mutated myeloproliferative neoplasms. Blood. 2013;121:4388–95.

38. Dunbar AJ, Gondek LP, O'Keefe CL, Makishima H, Rataul MS, Szpurka H, et al. 250K single nucleotide polymorphism array karyotyping identifies acquired uniparental disomy and homozygous mutations, including novel missense substitutions of c-Cbl, in myeloid malignancies. Cancer Res. 2008;2008(68): 10349–57.

Permissions

The contributors of this book come from diverse backgrounds, making this book a truly international effort. This book will bring forth new frontiers with its revolutionizing research information and detailed analysis of the nascent developments around the world.

We would like to thank all the contributing authors for lending their expertise to make the book truly unique. They have played a crucial role in the development of this book. Without their invaluable contributions this book wouldn't have been possible. They have made vital efforts to compile up to date information on the varied aspects of this subject to make this book a valuable addition to the collection of many professionals and students.

This book was conceptualized with the vision of imparting up-to-date information and advanced data in this field. To ensure the same, a matchless editorial board was set up. Every individual on the board went through rigorous rounds of assessment to prove their worth. After which they invested a large part of their time researching and compiling the most relevant data for our readers.

The editorial board has been involved in producing this book since its inception. They have spent rigorous hours researching and exploring the diverse topics which have resulted in the successful publishing of this book. They have passed on their knowledge of decades through this book. To expedite this challenging task, the publisher supported the team at every step. A small team of assistant editors was also appointed to further simplify the editing procedure and attain best results for the readers.

Apart from the editorial board, the designing team has also invested a significant amount of their time in understanding the subject and creating the most relevant covers. They scrutinized every image to scout for the most suitable representation of the subject and create an appropriate cover for the book.

The publishing team has been an ardent support to the editorial, designing and production team. Their endless efforts to recruit the best for this project, has resulted in the accomplishment of this book. They are a veteran in the field of academics and their pool of knowledge is as vast as their experience in printing. Their expertise and guidance has proved useful at every step. Their uncompromising quality standards have made this book an exceptional effort. Their encouragement from time to time has been an inspiration for everyone.

The publisher and the editorial board hope that this book will prove to be a valuable piece of knowledge for researchers, students, practitioners and scholars across the globe.

Contributors

Ioannis Bassukas and Athanasios Petridis
Department of Skin and Venereal Diseases, University of Ioannina, Ioannina, Greece

Georgios Chaidemenos
Department of Dermatology, Hospital for Skin and Venereal Diseases, Thessaloniki, Greece

Andreas Katsampas, Marita Kosmadaki, Georgia Avgerinou and Panagiotis Stavropoulos
Department of Dermatology, University of Athens, Hospital "A. Syggros", Athens, Greece

Dimitrios Sotiriadis
Department of Dermatology, Medical School, Aristotle University of Thessaloniki, Thessaloniki, Greece

Theofanis Spiliopoulos
Department of Dermatology, University of Patras, Patras, Greece

Evgenia Toumpi
Department of Dermatology and Venereology, "Attikon" General University Hospital, Athens, Greece

Loukas Xaplanteris
Janssen Cilag Pharmaceutical SACI, Athens, Greece

Hara Kousoulakou
PRMA Consulting Ltd, Hampshire, UK

Brad Schenkel
Janssen Scientific Affairs, LLC, Horsham, PA, USA

Maryam Salimi and Graham Ogg
Department of Medicine, MRC Human Immunology Unit, NIHR Biomedical Research Centre, Radcliffe University of Oxford, Oxford, UK

Fiona Bath-Hextall, Arun Kumar and Karen Cox
School of Health Sciences, Faculty of Medicine and Health Sciences, University of Nottingham, Queen's Medical Centre, Nottingham NG7 2UH, UK

Cris Glazebrook
Division of Psychiatry, School of Community Health Sciences, Queen's Medical Centre, Nottingham NG7 2UH, UK

Jo Leonardi-Bee
Division of Epidemiology and Public Health, Clinical Sciences Building, City Hospital, Nottingham NG5 1PB, UK

William Perkins
Department of Dermatology, Queen's Medical Centre, University Hospital, Nottingham NG7 2UH, UK

Claire Jenkinson
Nottingham Clinical Trials Unit, University of Nottingham, Queen's Medical Centre, Nottingham NG7 2UH, UK

Anne Marie Nyholm, Catharina M Lerche, Valentina Manfé, Edyta Biskup, Martin Glud and Robert Gniadecki
Department of Dermatology, Faculty of Health and Medical Sciences, University of Copenhagen, Bispebjerg Hospital, Copenhagen, Denmark

Peter Johansen and Niels Morling
Department of Forensic Medicine, Section of Forensic Genetics, Faculty of Health and Medical Sciences, University of Copenhagen, Copenhagen, Denmark

Birthe Mørk Thomsen
Department of Pathology, University of Copenhagen, Faculty of Health and Medical Sciences, Bispebjerg Hospital, Copenhagen, Denmark

Selina K Tour, Kim S Thomas and Jonathan M Batchelor
Centre of Evidence Based Dermatology, The University of Nottingham, Nottingham, UK

Dawn-Marie Walker and Paul Leighton
Faculty of Medicine and Health Sciences, University of Nottingham, Nottingham, UK

Adrian SW Yong
Norfolk and Norwich University Hospitals NHS Foundation Trust, Norwich, UK

Michela Tinelli
Centre of Academic Primary Care and Health Economics Research Unit, University of Aberdeen, Aberdeen, UK

Mara Ozolins, Fiona Bath-Hextall and Hywel C Williams
Centre of Evidence Based Dermatology, University of Nottingham, A103, King's Meadow Campus, Lenton Lane, Nottingham NG7 2NR, UK

Fernando Valenzuela
Department of Dermatology, Faculty of Medicine, University of Chile and Probity Medical Research, Santiago, Chile

Kim A Papp
Clinical Research and Probity Medical Research, Waterloo, ON, Canada

David Pariser
Department of Dermatology, Eastern Virginia Medical School and Virginia Clinical Research Inc., Norfolk, VA, USA

Stephen K Tyring
Department of Dermatology, University of Texas Medical School, Houston, TX, USA

Robert Wolk, Marjorie Buonanno and Huaming Tan
Pfizer Inc, Groton, CT, USA

Jeff Wang
Quintiles, Cambridge, MA, USA Present address: Statistical Consulting and Solutions, LLC, Brookline, MA, USA

Hernan Valdez
Pfizer Inc, New York, NY, USA Specialty Care Medicines Development Group, Pfizer Inc, 219 E 42nd Street, 7th Floor Room 50, NYO 219/07/01, New York, NY 10017, USA

Xiang Gao
The First Department of Health Care, Weifang People's Hospital, Shandong, China
Departments of Rheumatology and Occupational Medicine, Huashan Hospital of Fudan University, Shanghai, China

Lei Han and Ling Lu
Departments of Rheumatology and Occupational Medicine, Huashan Hospital of Fudan University, Shanghai, China

Lan Yuan
Center for Clinical Molecular Medicine; Ministry of Education Key Laboratory of Child Development and Disorders, Key Laboratory of Pediatrics in Chongqing, Chongqing, China Chongqing International Science and Technology Cooperation Center for Child Development and Disorders, Children's Hospital of Chongqing Medical University, Chongqing, China

Yongchen Yang, Guimei Gou and Hengjuan Sun
Shanghai Children's Hospital, Shanghai Children's Hospital Affiliated to Shanghai Jiao Tong University School of Medicine, Shanghai, China

Liming Bao
Center for Clinical Molecular Medicine; Ministry of Education Key Laboratory of Child Development and Disorders, Key Laboratory of Pediatrics in Chongqing, Chongqing, China Chongqing International Science and Technology Cooperation Center for Child Development and Disorders, Children's Hospital of Chongqing Medical University, Chongqing, China Department of Pathology, Geisel School of Medicine at Dartmouth College, Lebanon, New Hampshire, USA

Charlotta Remröd and Åke Svensson
Department of Dermatology and Venereology, University of Lund, Hudkliniken, Skåne University Hospital, Jan Waldenströmsg. 16, Malmö 205 02, Sweden

Karin Sjöström
Psychiatric consultant at the Department of Dermatology and Venereology, Hudkliniken, Skåne University Hospital, Jan Waldenströmsg. 16, Malmö 205 02, Sweden

Arne Johannisson
Department of Health Sciences, Lund University, Box 157, 221 00 Lund, Sweden

Ann Pontén
Department of Occupational and Environmental Dermatology, Lund University, Malmö, Sweden
Department of Occupational and Environmental Dermatology, Malmö University Hospital, Malmö, Sweden

Åke Svensson
Department of Dermatology, Lund University, Malmö, Sweden
Department of Dermatology, Malmö University Hospital, Malmö, Sweden

Noor Hasnani Ismail and Zahara Abdul Manaf
Dietetic Program, School of Healthcare Sciences, Faculty of Health Sciences, Universiti Kebangsaan Malaysia, Jalan Raja Muda Abdul Aziz, 50300 Kuala Lumpur, Malaysia

Noor Zalmy Azizan
Department of Dermatology, Hospital Kuala Lumpur, 50300 Kuala Lumpur, Malaysia

Teresa Løvold Berents and Jørgen Rønnevig
Institute of Clinical Medicine, University of Oslo, Oslo, Norway
Department of Dermatology, Oslo University Hospital, Oslo, Norway

Elisabeth Søyland
Department of Research, Education and Innovation, Oslo University Hospital, Oslo, Norway

Peter Gaustad
Institute of Clinical Medicine, University of Oslo, Oslo, Norway Department of Microbiology, Oslo University Hospital, Oslo, Norway

Gro Nylander and Beate Fossum Løland
Norwegian National Advisory Unit on Breastfeeding, Womens and Children´s Division, Oslo University Hospital, Oslo, Norway

Huibin Man and Weiping Bi
Wendeng Central Hospital, Shandong, P.R. China

Shujun Xin and Chengzhi Lv
The Center for Skin Physiology Research, Dalian Skin Disease Hospital, Liaoning 116021, P.R. China

Theodora M Mauro and Peter M Elias
Dermatology Service, Veterans Affairs Medical Center, San Francisco, CA, USA
Department of Dermatology, University of California, 4150 Clement Street, San Francisco, CA 94121, USA

Mao-Qiang Man
The Center for Skin Physiology Research, Dalian Skin Disease Hospital, Liaoning 116021, P.R. China
Dermatology Service, Veterans Affairs Medical Center, San Francisco, CA, USA
Department of Dermatology, University of California, 4150 Clement Street, San Francisco, CA 94121, USA

Ian F Burgess, Elizabeth R Brunton and Nazma A Burgess
Medical Entomology Centre, Insect Research and Development Limited, 6 Quy Court, Colliers Lane, Stow-cum-Quy, Cambridge CB25 9AU, UK

Susanne Stemmler and Sabine Hoffjan
Department of Human Genetics, Ruhr-University, Universitätsstrasse 150, 44801 Bochum, Germany

Qumar Parwez
Private medical practice, Gladbeck, Germany

Elisabeth Petrasch-Parwez
Department of Neuroanatomy and Molecular Brain Research, Ruhr-University Bochum, Bochum, Germany

Joerg T Epplen
Department of Human Genetics, Ruhr-University, Universitätsstrasse 150, 44801 Bochum, Germany
Faculty of Health, Witten/Herdecke University, Witten, Germany

Javaria Mona Khalid and Andrew Maguire
United Biosource Corporation, London, UK

Gary Globe and Dina Chau
Amgen Inc., Thousand Oaks, CA, USA

Kathleen M Fox
Strategic Healthcare Solutions, LLC, Monkton, MD 21111, USA

Chio-Fang Chiou
Janssen Global Services, Companies of Johnson and Johnson, New Jersey, USA

Scott A. Reisman, Angela R. Goldsberry, Chun-Yue I. Lee, Megan L. O'Grady, Joel W. Proksch, Keith W. Ward and Colin J. Meyer
Reata Pharmaceuticals, Inc., 2801 Gateway Dr. Ste 150, Irving, TX 75063, USA

Moussa Soleimani-Ahmadi
Social Determinants in Health Promotion Research Center, Hormozgan University of Medical Sciences, Bandar Abbas, Iran Department of Medical Entomology and Vector Control, Faculty of Health, Hormozgan University of Medical Sciences, Bandar Abbas, Iran

Alireza Sanei-Dehkordi
Department of Medical Entomology and Vector Control, Faculty of Health, Hormozgan University of Medical Sciences, Bandar Abbas, Iran

Seyed Aghil Jaberhashemi
Bashagard Health Center, Hormozgan University of Medical Sciences, Bashagard, Iran

Mehdi Zare
Department of Occupational Health Engineering, Faculty of Health, Hormozgan University of Medical Sciences, Bandar Abbas, Iran

Tomke Cordts, Johannes Horter, Julian Vogelpohl, Thomas Kremer, Ulrich Kneser and Jochen-Frederick Hernekamp
Department of Hand, Plastic and Reconstructive Surgery – Burn Center, BG Trauma Center Ludwigshafen, Ludwig-Guttmann-Strasse 13, 67071 Ludwigshafen, Germany

Abeer Shaheen and Jamal Khaddam
Department of dermatology, Tishreen University, Lattakia, Syria

Fadi Kesh
Department of Plastic and Reconstructive Surgery, Tishreen University, Lattakia, Syria

Awatef kelati, Hanane Baybay, Salim Gallouj, Mariame Meziane and Fatima Zahra Mernissi
Department of dermatology, University Hospital Hassan II, 202 Hay Mohamadi, Fez, Morocco

Mariam Atassi and Samira Elfakir
Department of clinical epidemiology and scientific research, University Hospital Hassan II, Fez, Morocco

Abraham Getachew Kelbore
Mekelle University, Tropical Dermatology, Mekelle, North Ethiopia

Workalemahu Alemu
Dermatovenereology Department, Mekelle University, Mekelle, North Ethiopia

Ashenafi Shumye
Public Health Department, Mekelle University, Mekelle, North Ethiopia

Sefonias Getachew
Addis Ababa University, School of Public Health, Addis Ababa, Ethiopia

Murlidhar Rajagopalan
Department of Dermatology, Apollo Hospital, Chennai, India Department of Dermatology, Apollo Hospital, Greams Road No: 21, Greams Lane, Off Greams Road, Chennai, India

Arun Inamadar
Department of Dermatology, SBMP Medical College, BLDE Deemed University, Bijapur, India

Asit Mittal
Department of Dermatology, R.N.T. Medical College and Hospital, Udaipur, India

Autar K. Miskeen
Dr Miskeen's Central Clinical Microbiology Lab, Thane, India

C. R. Srinivas
Department of Dermatology, PSG Hospitals, Peelamedu, Coimbatore, India

Kabir Sardana
Department of Dermatology, Venereology and Leprosy Dr. Ram Manohar Lohia Hospital and Post Graduate Institute of Medical Education and Research, New Delhi, India

Kiran Godse
Department of Dermatology, Padmashree Dr D Y Patil University, Navi Mumbai, India

Krina Patel
Department Of Dermatology, GMERS Medical College and Hospital, Sola, Ahmedabad, India

Madhu Rengasamy
Department of Dermatology (Mycology), Madras Medical College, Chennai, India

Shivaprakash Rudramurthy
Mycology Division, Department of Medical Microbiology, Postgraduate Institute of Medical Education and Research (PGIMER), Chandigarh, India

Sunil Dogra
Department of Dermatology, Postgraduate Institute of Medical Education and Research (PGIMER), Chandigarh, India

Kim A. Papp
K Papp Clinical Research and Probity Medical Research Inc, Waterloo, ON, Canada

Robert Bissonnette
Innovaderm Research, Montreal, QC, Canada

Melinda Gooderham
SKiN Centre for Dermatology and Probity Medical Research Inc, Peterborough, and Queens University, Kingston, ON, Canada

Steven R. Feldman
Wake Forest Baptist Health, Winston-Salem, NC, USA

Lars Iversen
Aarhus University Hospital, Aarhus, Denmark

Jennifer Soung
Southern California Dermatology, Santa Ana, CA, USA

Zoe Draelos
Dermatology Consulting Services, High Point, NC, USA

Carla Mamolo, Vivek Purohit, Cunshan Wang and William C. Ports
Pfizer Worldwide Biopharmaceuticals, Global Innovative Pharma Business, Groton, CT, USA

Rosarin Sruamsiri
Health Economics, Janssen Pharmaceutical KK, 5-2, Nishikanda 3-chome Chiyoda-ku, Tokyo 101-0065, Japan Center of Pharmaceutical Outcomes Research, Naresuan University, Phitsanulok, Thailand

Kosuke Iwasaki and Wentao Tang
Milliman, Tokyo, Japan

Jörg Mahlich
Health Economics and Outcomes Research, Janssen-Cilag GmbH, Johnson and Johnson Platz 1, Neuss 41470, Germany Düsseldorf Institute for Competition Economics (DICE), University of Düsseldorf, Düsseldorf, Germany

Joo-Heung Lee
Department of Dermatology, Samsung Medical Center, Sungkyunkwan University School of Medicine, 50 Irwon-dong, Gangnam-gu, Seoul, Korea

Jai-Il Youn
Department of Dermatology, National Medical Center, Seoul, Korea

Tae-Yoon Kim and Chul-Jong Park
Department of Dermatology, College of Medicine, The Catholic University of Korea, Seoul, Korea

Jee-Ho Choi
Department of Dermatology, Asian Medical Center, University of Ulsan College of Medicine, Seoul, Korea

Yong-Beom Choe
Department of Dermatology, Konkuk University School of Medicine, Seoul, Korea

Hae-Jun Song
Department of Dermatology, College of Medicine, Korea University, Seoul, Korea

Nack-In Kim
Department of Dermatology, College of Medicine, Kyung Hee University, Seoul, Korea

Kwang-Joong Kim
Department of Dermatology, Hallym University Sacred Heart Hospital, Seoul, Korea

Jeung-Hoon Lee
Department of Dermatology, School of Medicine, Chungnam National University, Daejeon, Korea

Hyun-Jeong Yoo
Pfizer Pharmaceuticals Korea Limited, Seoul, Korea

Emmanuel Armand Kouotou
Biyem-Assi District Hospital, Yaoundé, Cameroon
Department of Medicine and Medical Specialties, Faculty of Medicine and Biomedical Sciences, University of Yaoundé I, Yaoundé, Cameroon
Yaoundé General Hospital, Yaoundé, Cameroon

Anne-Cécile Zoung-Kanyi Bissek, Elie Claude Ndjitoyap Ndam and Defo Defo
Department of Medicine and Medical Specialties, Faculty of Medicine and Biomedical Sciences, University of Yaoundé I, Yaoundé, Cameroon
Yaoundé General Hospital, Yaoundé, Cameroon

Jobert Richie N Nansseu
Sickle Cell Disease Unit, Mother and Child Centre, Chantal Biya Foundation, Yaoundé, Cameroon
Department of Public Health, Faculty of Medicine and Biomedical Sciences, University of Yaoundé I, Yaoundé, Cameroon

Isidore Sieleunou
School of Public Health, University of Montréal, Montréal, Canada

George Moncrieff
Mayfield Clinic Summertown, Oxford OX2 7DE, UK

Annie Lied-Lied, Gill Nelson
Johnson and Johnson Ltd (UK), Maidenhead, Berkshire, UK

Chantal E Holy and David Wei
Johnson and Johnson, Inc, New Brunswick, NJ, USA

Rachel Weinstein
Janssen Research and Development, LLC, Titusville, NJ, USA

Simon Rowe
NHS Wakefield Clinical Commissioning Group, West Yorkshire, UK

Surjit Singh
Department of Pharmacology, All India Institute of Medical Sciences (AIIMS), Jodhpur 342005, India

Anil Bhansali
Department of Endocrinology, Post Graduate Institute of Medical Education and Research (PGIMER), Chandigarh 160012, India

Raúl de Lucas
Hospital Universitario La Paz, Madrid, Spain

Gerardo Moreno-Arias
Hospital Quirón Teknon, Barcelona, Spain

Montserrat Perez-López
Clínica Dermatológica de Moragas, Barcelona, Spain

Ángel Vera-Casaño
Hospital Carlos Haya,, Málaga, Spain

Sonia Aladren and Massimo Milani
Isdin S.A. Medical Department, Provençals 33, Barcelona, Spain

Nathalie Terrones
Research Unit EA4340 Biomarkers in Cancerology and Hemato Oncology, Versailles SQY University, Paris-Saclay University, 9, Avenue Charles de Gaulle, 92104 Boulogne-Billancourt, France

Zofia Hélias-Rodzewicz, Ute Zimmermann, Cristi Marin and Jean-François Emile
Research Unit EA4340 Biomarkers in Cancerology and Hemato Oncology, Versailles SQY University, Paris-Saclay University, 9, Avenue Charles de Gaulle, 92104 Boulogne-Billancourt, France
Department of Pathology, Ambroise Paré Hospital, AP-HP, Boulogne-Billancourt, France

Elisa Funck-Brentano and Philippe Saiag
Research Unit EA4340 Biomarkers in Cancerology and Hemato Oncology, Versailles SQY University, Paris-Saclay University, 9, Avenue Charles de Gaulle, 92104 Boulogne-Billancourt, France
Department of Dermatology, Ambroise Paré Hospital, AP-HP, Boulogne-Billancou

Alain Beauchet
Department of Public Health, Ambroise Paré Hospital Ap-HP, Boulogne-Billancourt, France

Index

A

Acitretin, 133, 226-234, 255, 261

Acne Vulgaris, 99-106, 173-174, 263-264, 268

Adalimumab, 1-2, 4-5, 7, 15, 72, 133, 215-216, 219, 221-225

Atopic Dermatitis, 10, 13-15, 17, 98, 112-113, 127, 132, 182, 186-191, 214, 242, 245, 250-251

Atopic Eczema, 14, 87, 98, 107, 109-111, 191, 241-242, 247, 250-251

B

Basal Cell Carcinomas, 18

Beck Depression Inventory, 80, 82, 84, 87

Biological Therapies (BTS), 215-216

Bromelain, 157-158

Burn Intensive Care Unit, 158, 163

C

Chi-square Test, 74, 101, 104, 165, 168-172, 227, 254, 257-258

Childhood Eczema, 88-89, 91-92, 95-96, 98

Chronic Inflammatory Skin Disorder, 127

Chronic Obstructive Pulmonary Disease, 10, 15, 134

Chronic Viral Infection, 71

Colloidal Oatmeal, 241-242, 244, 251

Combination Therapy, 192, 197-199, 226-227, 233, 255

Cytomegalovirus, 62, 64-65, 67-72

D

Delphi Method, 193-194

Dermatophytosis, 192-202

Dimeticone, 120-126

Discrete Choice Experiment (DCE), 52, 56

E

Electrocardiogram, 146, 149

Emollient, 107, 109-112, 241-246, 248-251, 263-264

Enzymatic Debridement, 157-158, 163

Epidemiology, 3, 26, 71, 98, 112, 138, 151, 156, 174-176, 180-181, 190, 193, 225, 233, 251, 268

Epidermal Differentiation Complex, 131-132

Epstein-barr Virus, 62, 64-65, 67-68, 70-72

Erythema, 109, 146-147, 195, 205, 252-254, 256-258

Etanercept, 1-2, 5, 7, 9, 63, 70-72, 133, 204, 213, 225-234

F

Flow Cytometry, 28-29, 31

G

Glycemic Index, 99-100

Gross Domestic Product, 114-115

H

Hand Eczema, 88-98, 245

Hardy-weinberg Equilibrium, 132

Head Louse Infestation, 120, 126, 156

Human Leukocyte Antigen, 73, 78

Human Scabies, 235-239

I

Immunohistochemistry, 142, 149, 275, 277

In Situ Hybridization, 30, 269-270, 276

Inflammatory Skin Disease, 133

Infliximab, 1-2, 5, 7, 70, 72, 133, 215-216, 219, 221-224

Innate Lymphoid Cell, 17

J

Janus Kinase Inhibition, 62

K

Keloid, 164-165, 167, 169-174

L

Laminin 5, 127-130, 132

Logistic Regression Model, 59-60, 82, 104, 182, 205, 244

M

Mesenteric Lymph Nodes, 11, 15

Metabolic Syndrome, 135, 252-253, 257-258, 261

Metformin, 252-262

Mixed Logit Model, 51, 54, 59, 61

N

Non Melanoma Skin Cancer, 18-19, 23, 25-26

O

Oncogene-induced-senescence, 28, 36

P

Patient-reported Outcome, 39-40

Pediculosis, 120, 156

Pharmacokinetic, 212

Pioglitazone, 252-262

Plexus Catheter, 157, 160-161, 163

Polymyositis, 73, 78-79

Post-scabies Pruritus, 235, 237, 239

Primary Human Keratinocytes, 140-141, 143-144

Pruritus, 81-82, 108-109, 146-147, 178, 185, 199, 203, 206, 209, 211, 213-214, 231-232, 235-239, 245

Psoriasis, 1-10, 15, 17, 62-64, 69-72, 80-87, 133-139, 203-218, 221, 223-234, 252-258, 260-261

Psychic Trait Anxiety, 80, 82-85

Psychological Morbidity, 18-19, 85-86

R
Radiation Dermatitis, 140, 149

Randomised Controlled Trial, 39, 51, 56, 71, 121, 125, 156, 251, 277

Recalcitrant Tinea Infection, 195

Rhino-conjunctivitis, 89-92, 96-97

S
Secukinumab, 215, 219, 221, 224

Skin Grafting, 157-158, 160-163

Somatic Trait Anxiety, 80, 83-84

Squamous Cell Carcinomas, 26

Ssp-stress Susceptibility, 80, 83-85

Steroid Phobia, 107-108, 112

T
Tofacitinib, 62-65, 67-72, 203-214

U
Ustekinumab, 1-9, 204, 215-216, 219, 221-225

V
Vitiligo, 39-50, 243

W
Western Blotting, 28